Published by Andrew Newman.
Illustrations by Marcelle Marais.

First Printing, 2014
ISBN 978-0-9567645-3-9

P O Box 485
Constantia 7848
Western Cape
South Africa

to all who seek

Once upon a time
There was a little fish

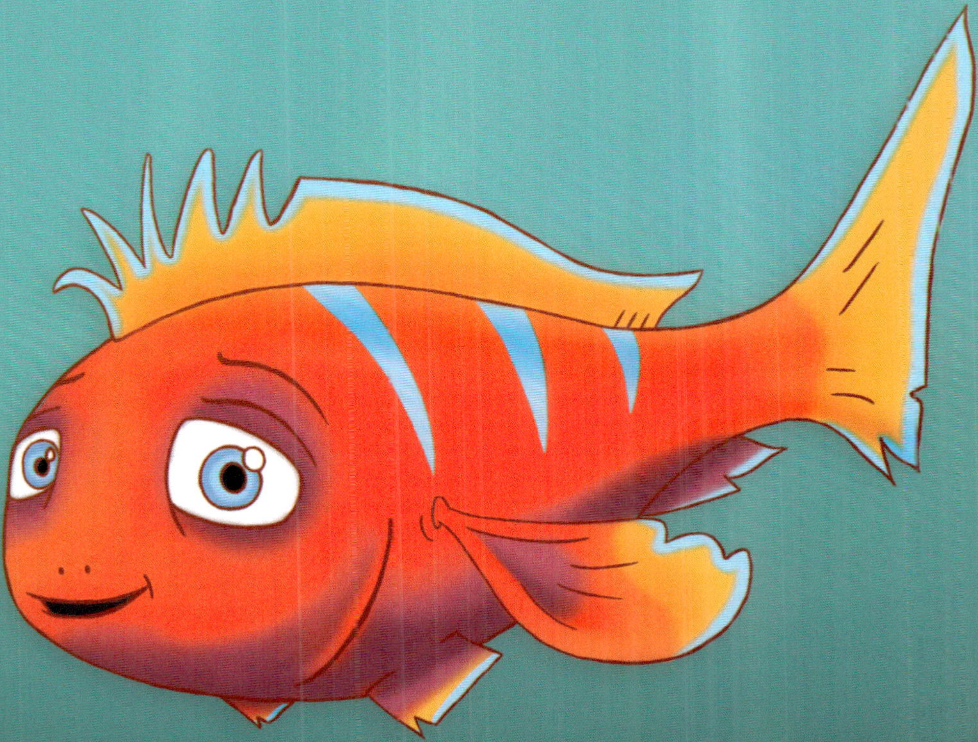

Who never felt at home.
He had a special wish

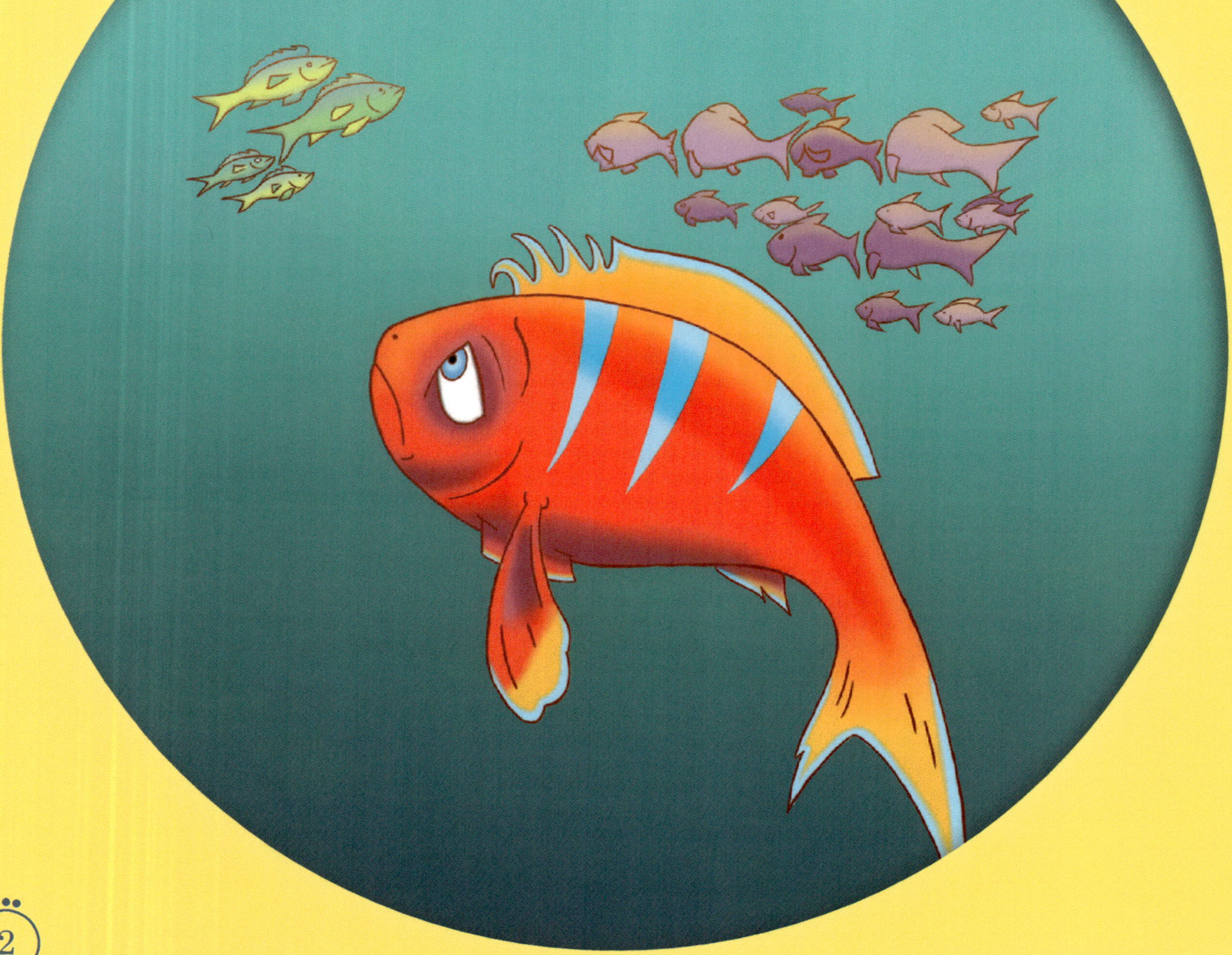

He dreamt of finding water
Enough to quench his soul

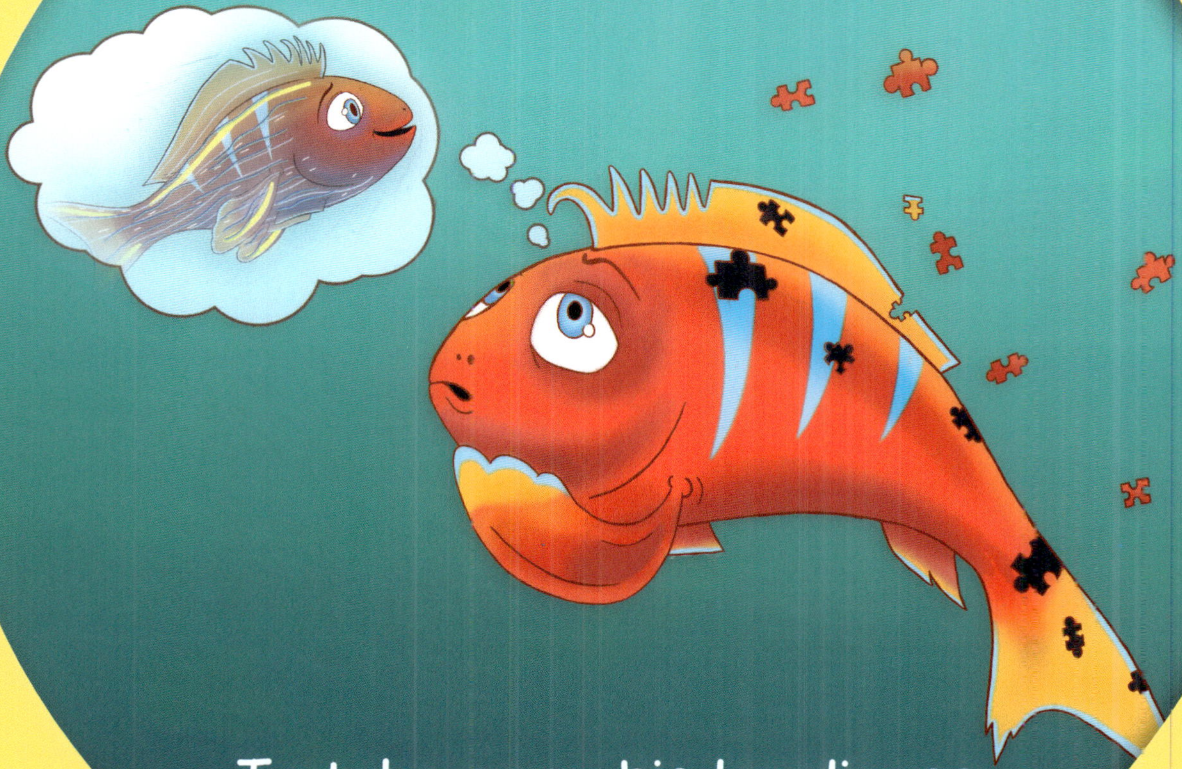

To take away his loneliness
And make his pieces whole

"Where O Where is water?"
Sought the little fish
"I will shrivel up if I can't fulfill this wish."

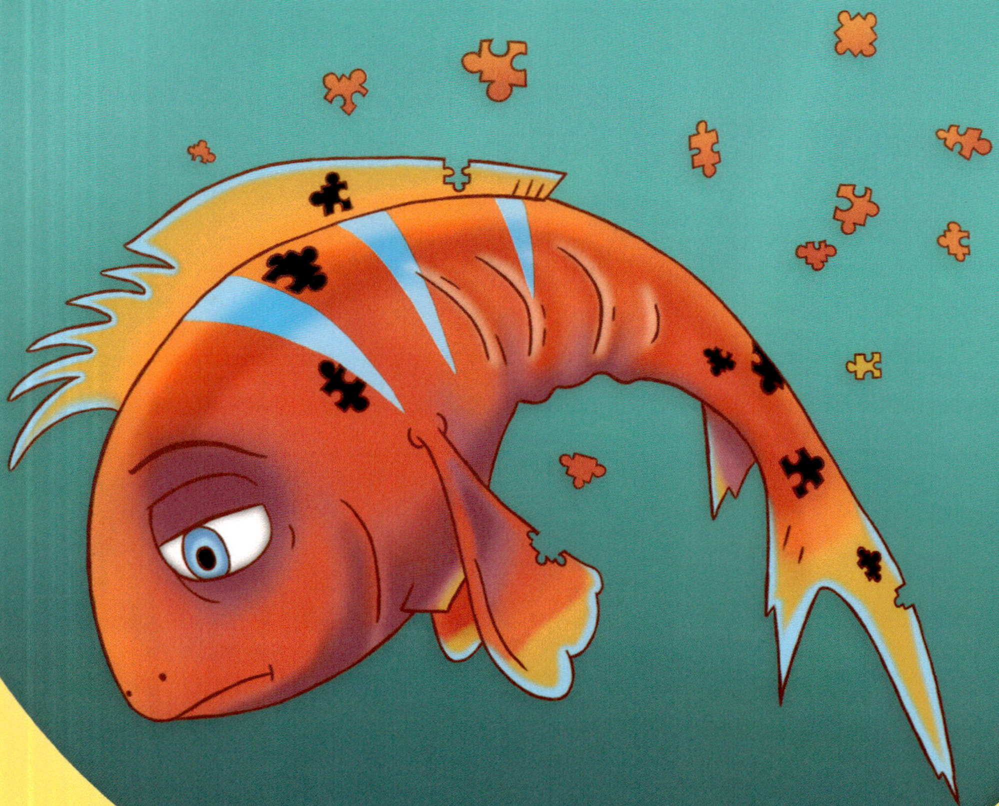

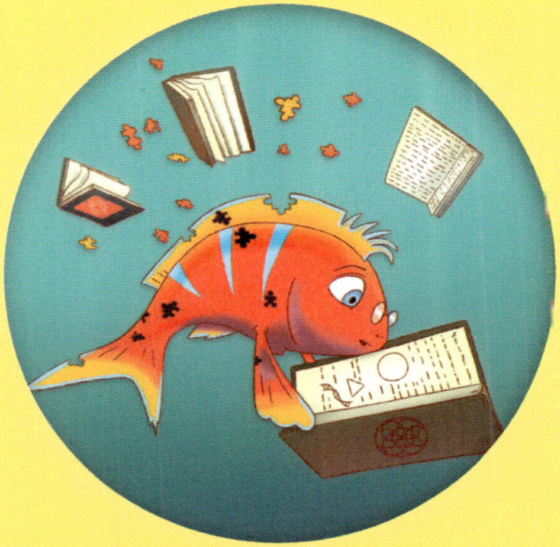

Is it here?

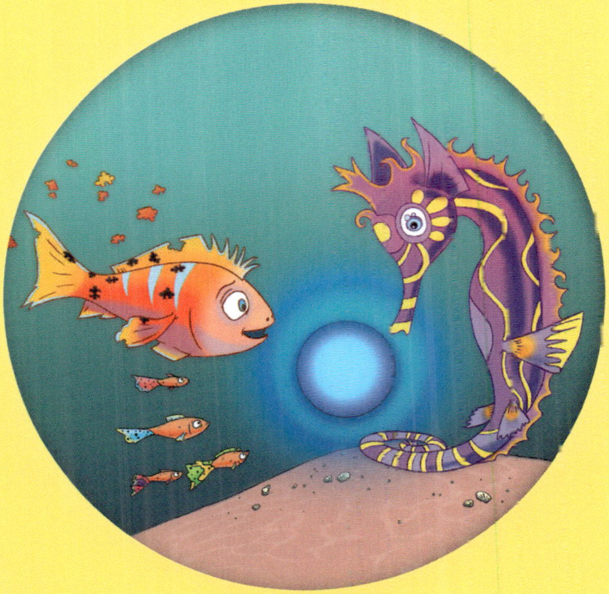

Or here?

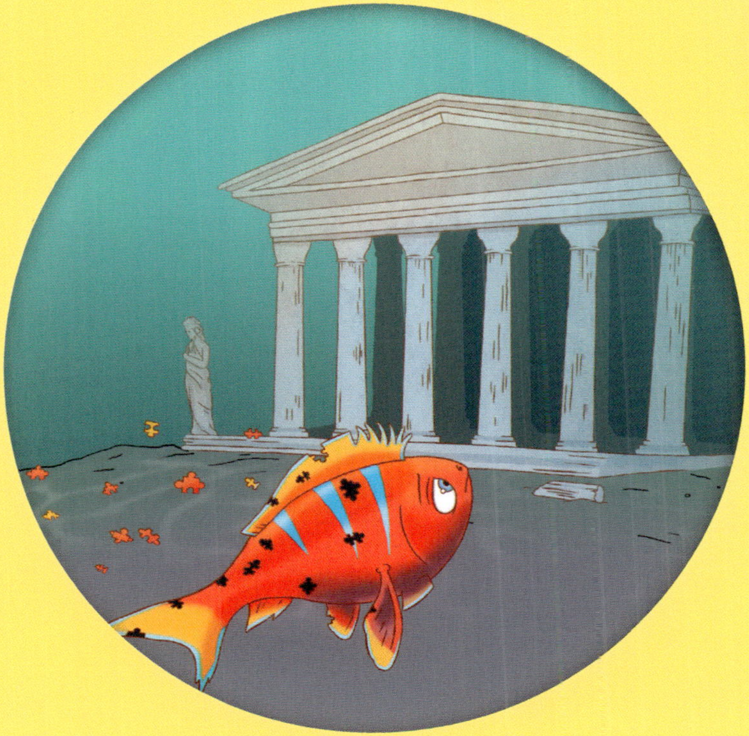

Maybe here?

No one had the answers
That he'd believe or trust

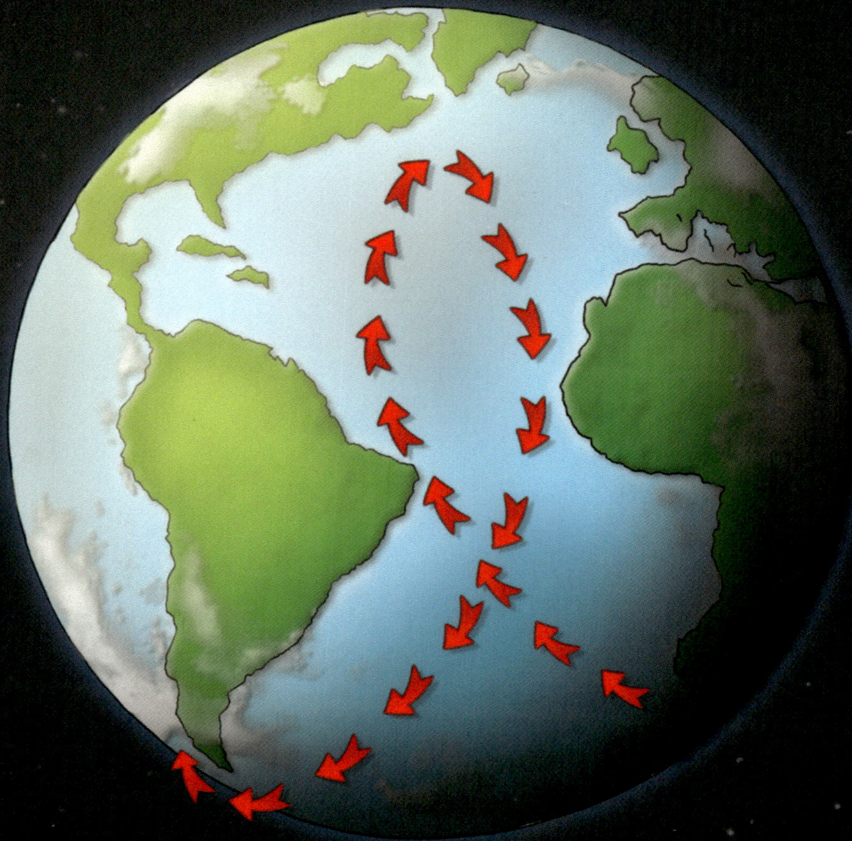

So onward he went swimming
Thinking that he must

He swam

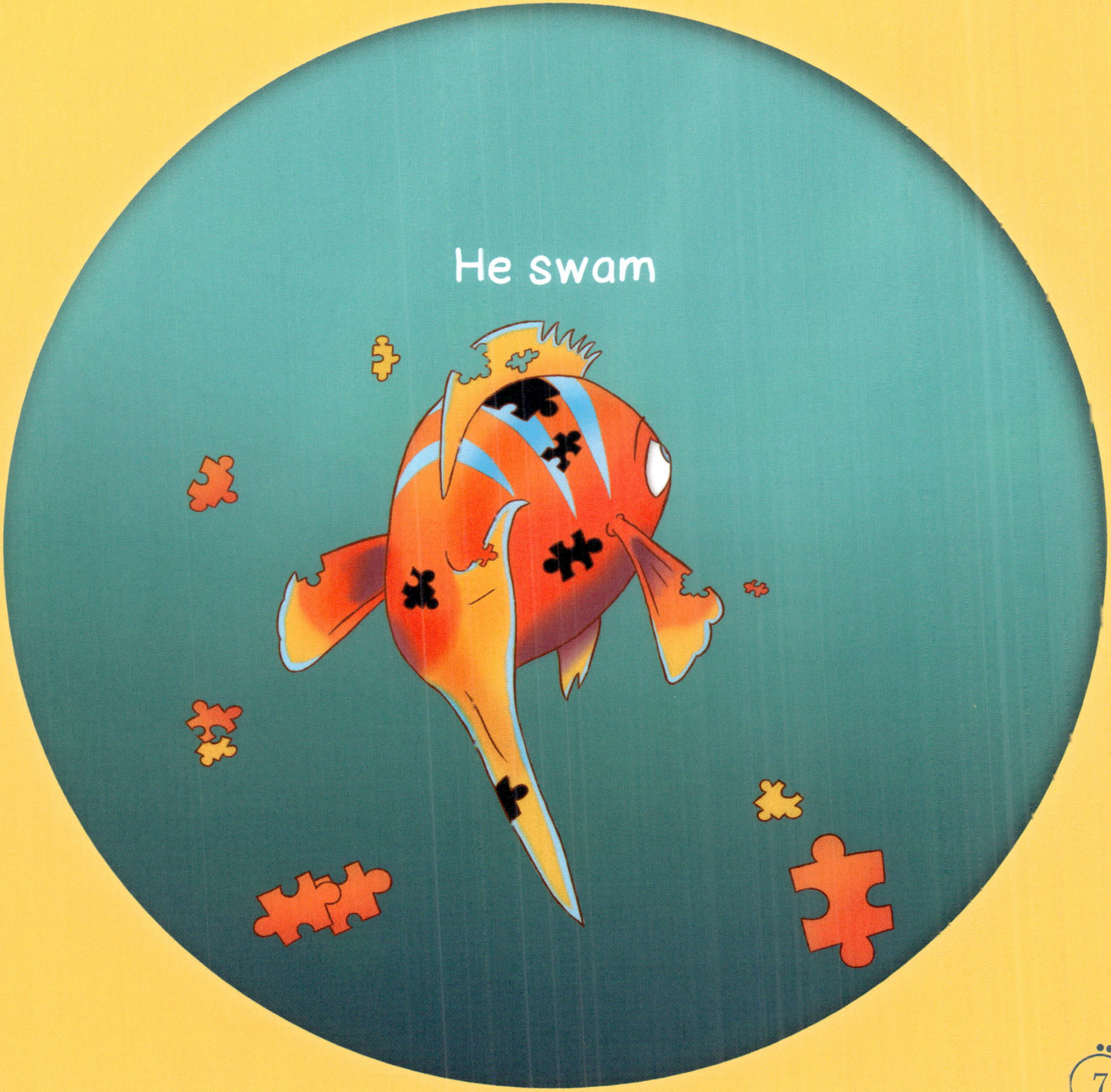

And swam

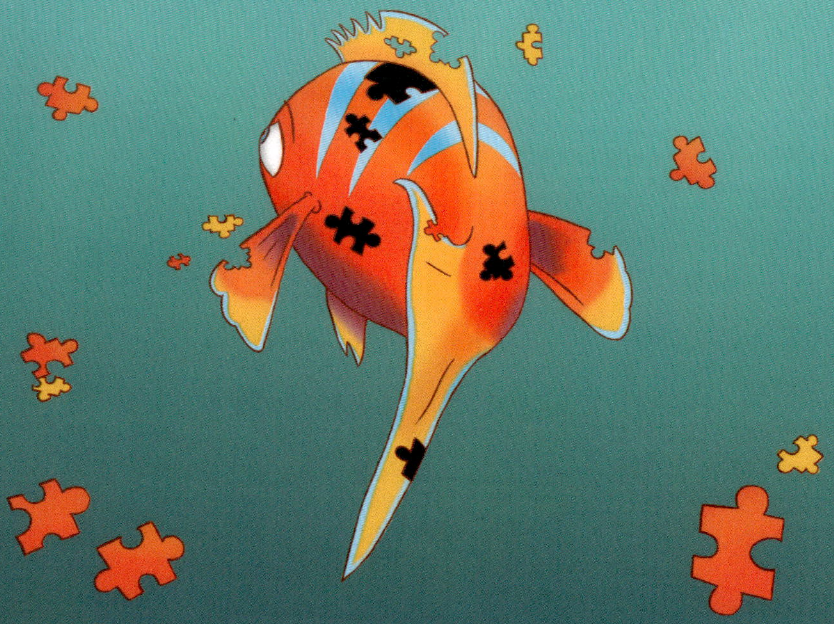

And swam

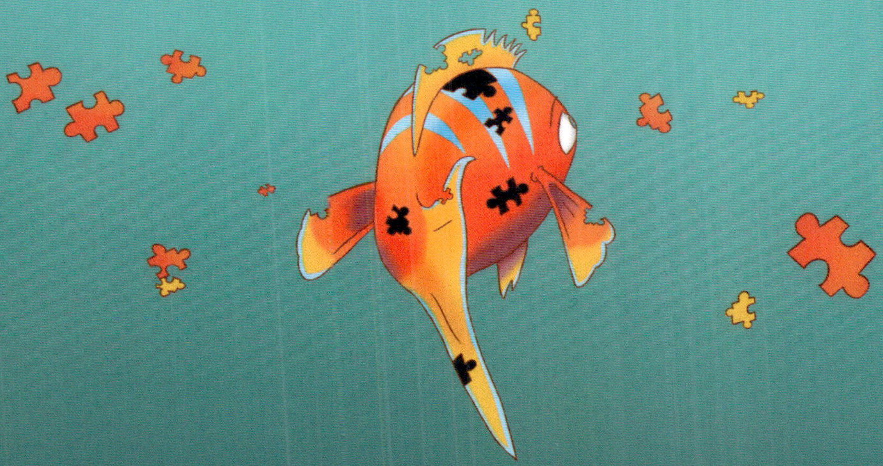

He paused at a few places
to have a little sip

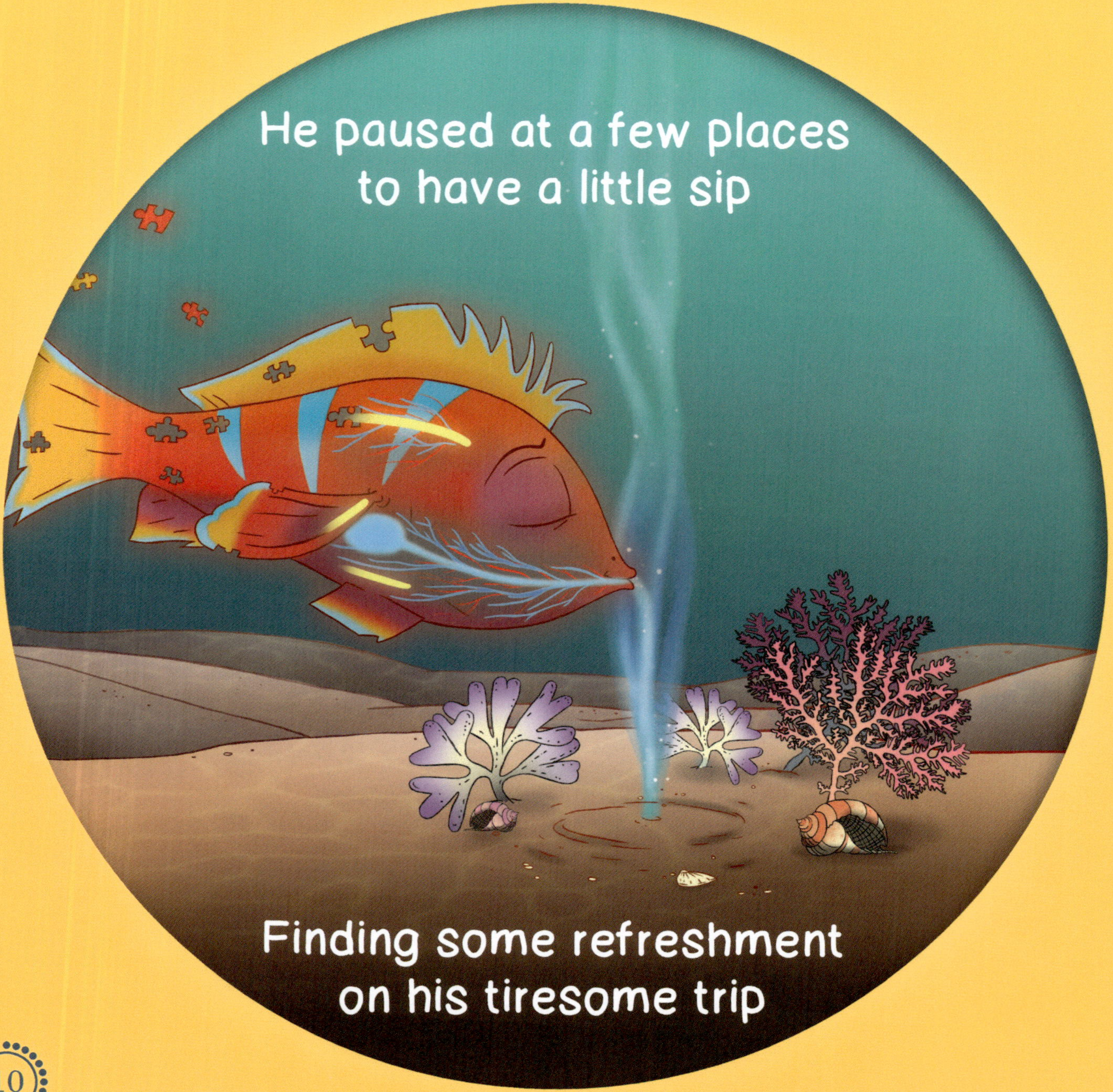

Finding some refreshment
on his tiresome trip

On he swam
Thirsty for more
What he had found
Couldn't be all

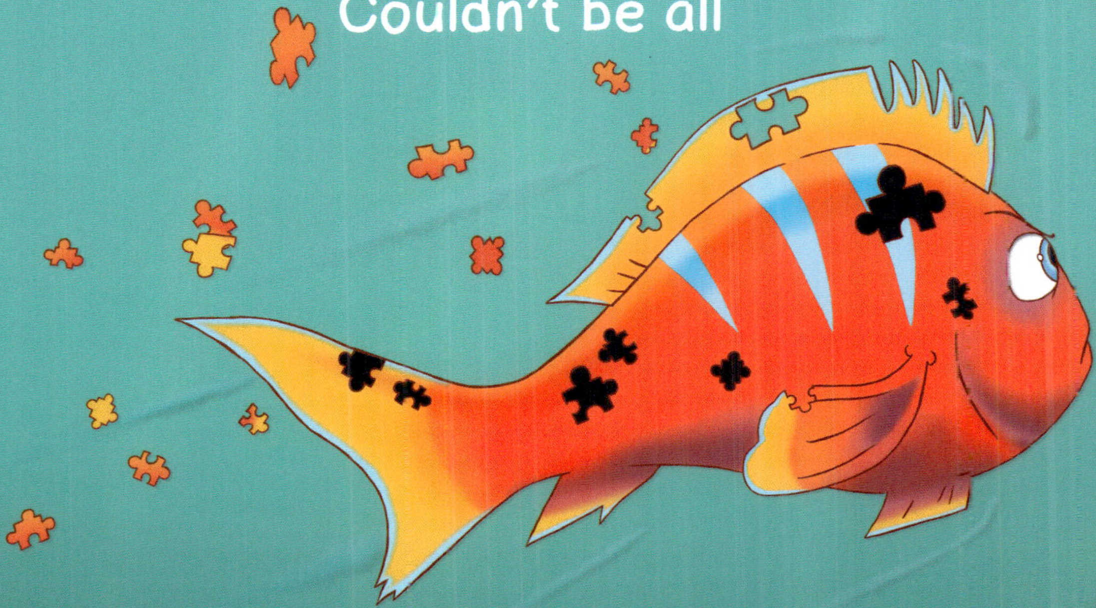

One day he leapt up in the air

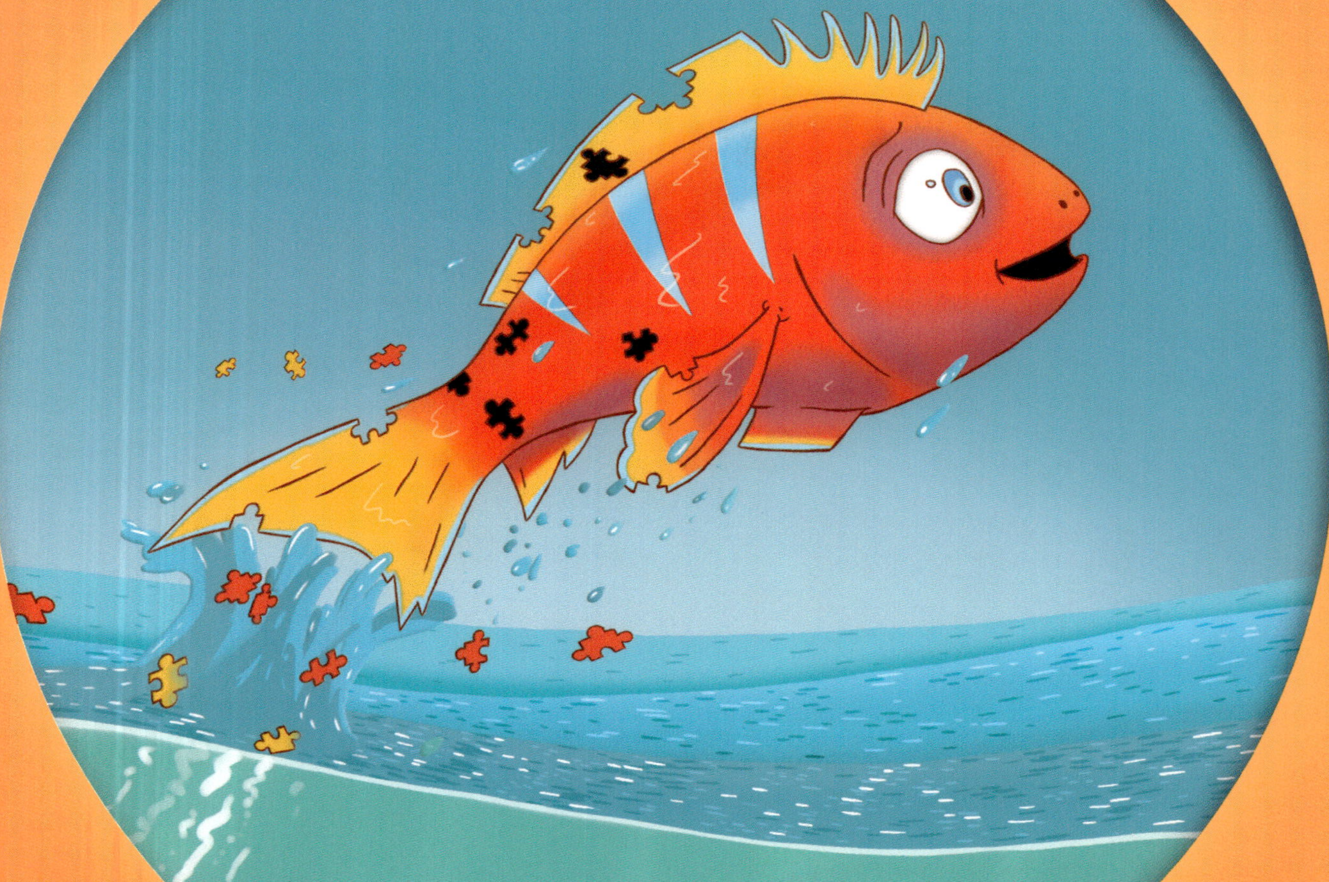

It was brave and bold
and done on a dare

He thought,
“If I could get the view of a bird..”

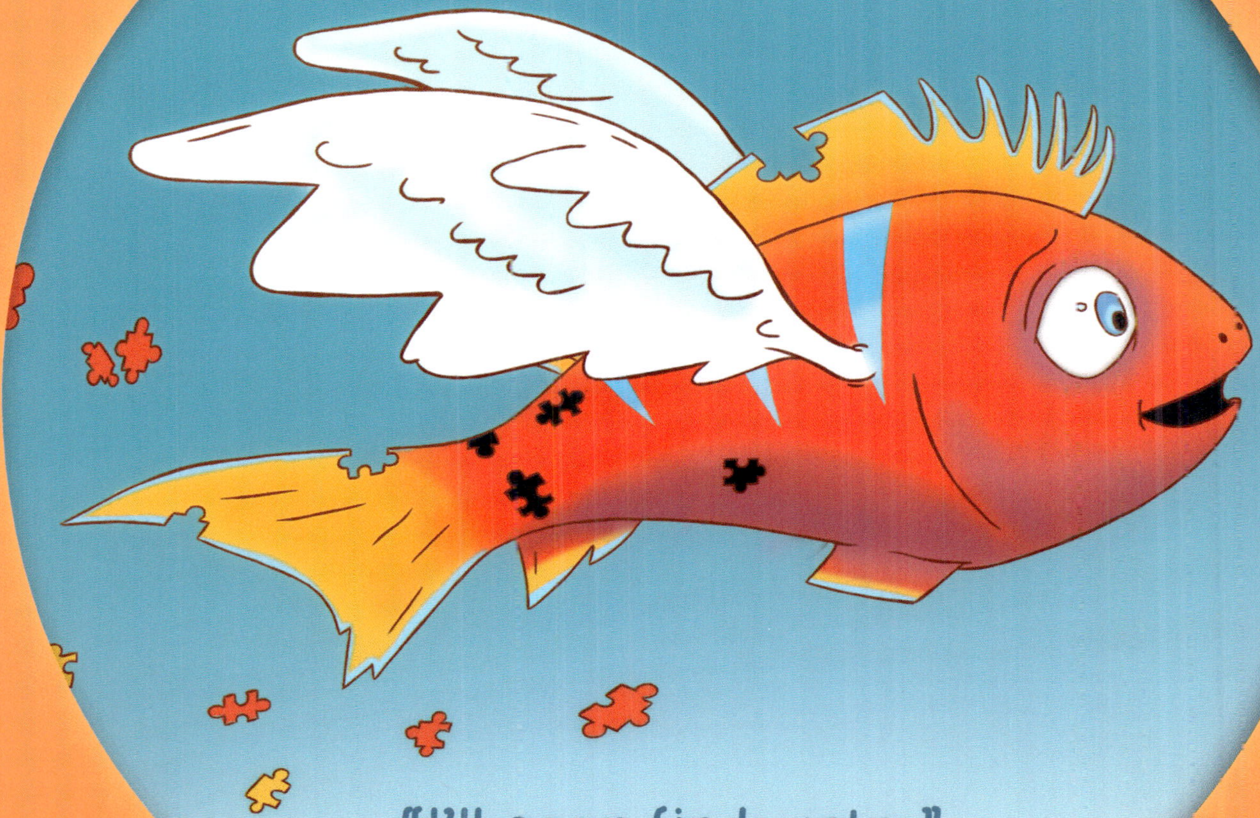

“I’ll soon find water”
So he had heard

He leapt in the air
Took a huge big gasp

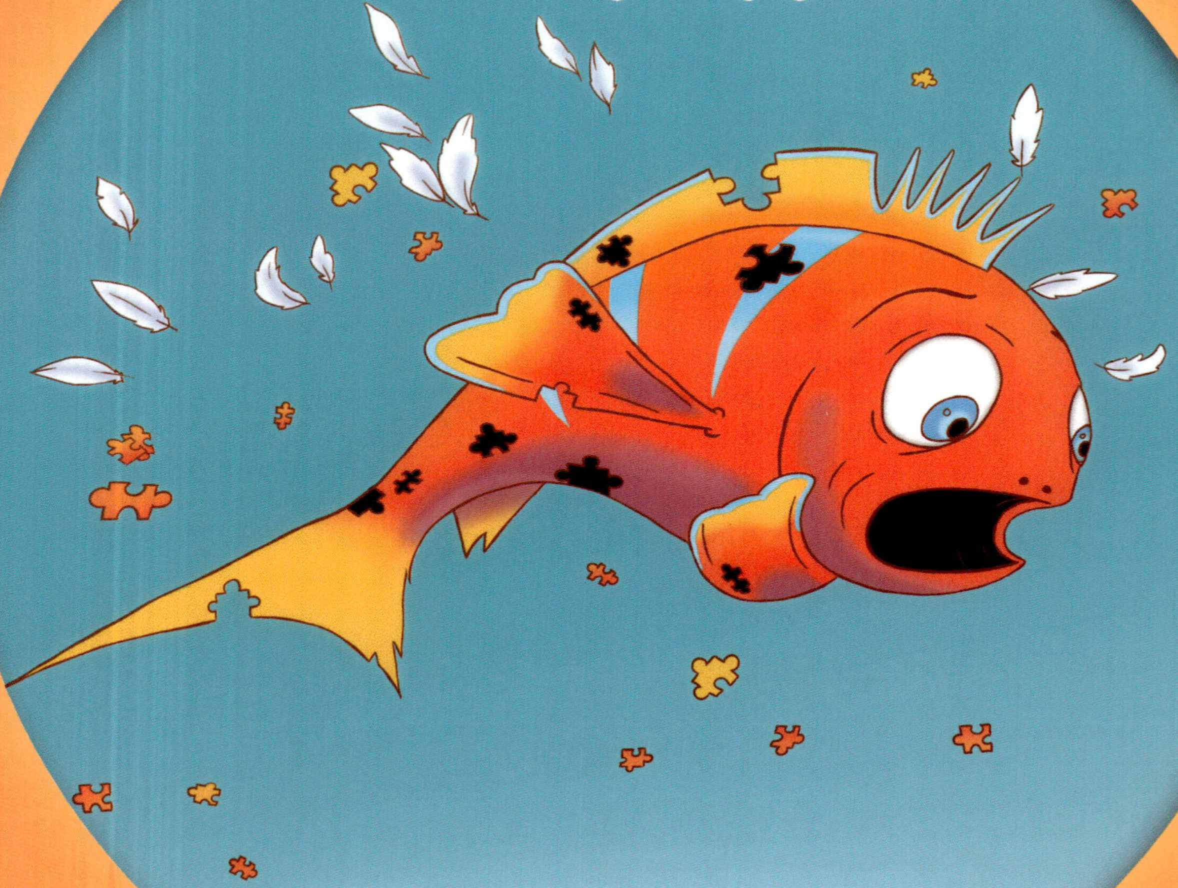

BUT his gills shut down
Drowned with the blast

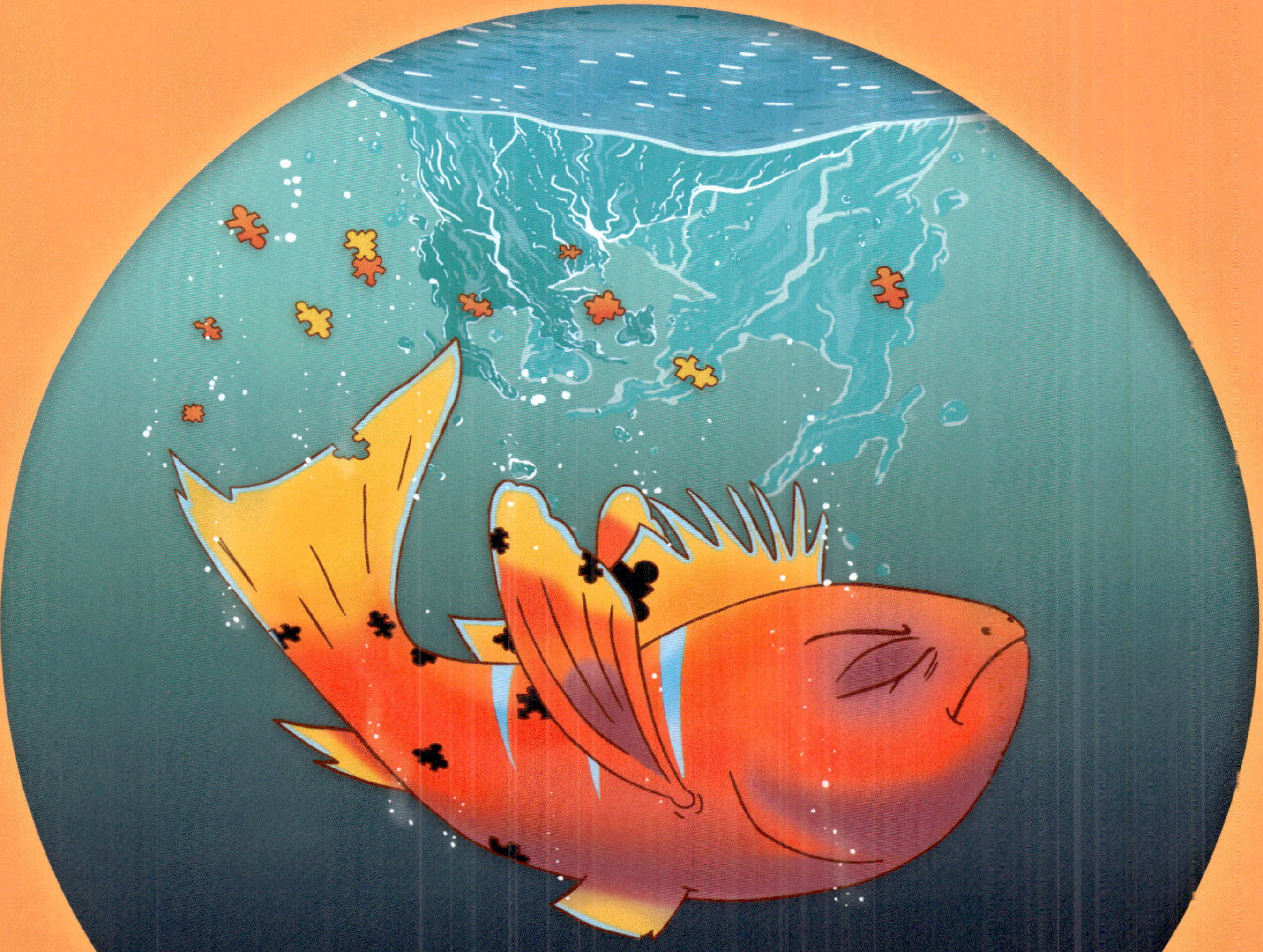

Thankfully gravity pulled him back in.
To where he could breathe
And where he could swim

He nearly drowned
with all that fresh air

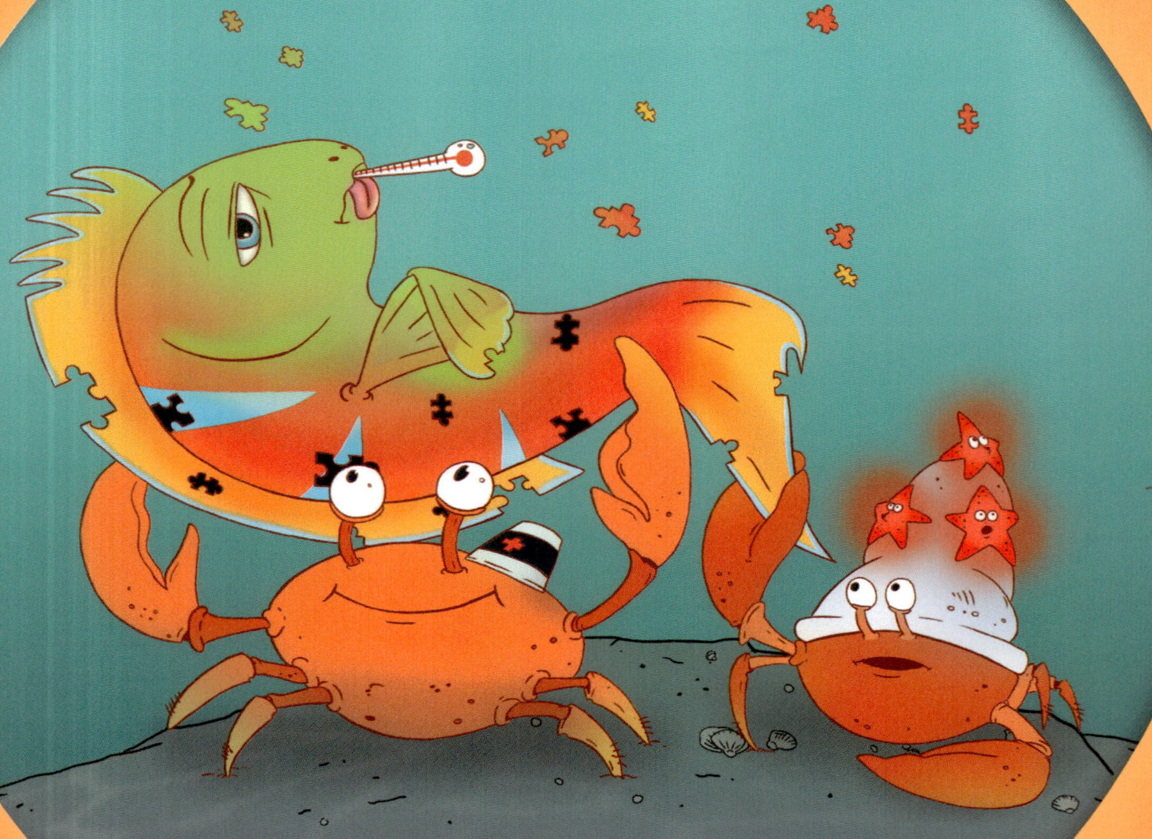

It was empty of something
that offered fish care

It was empty of fluid
And flow and delight.

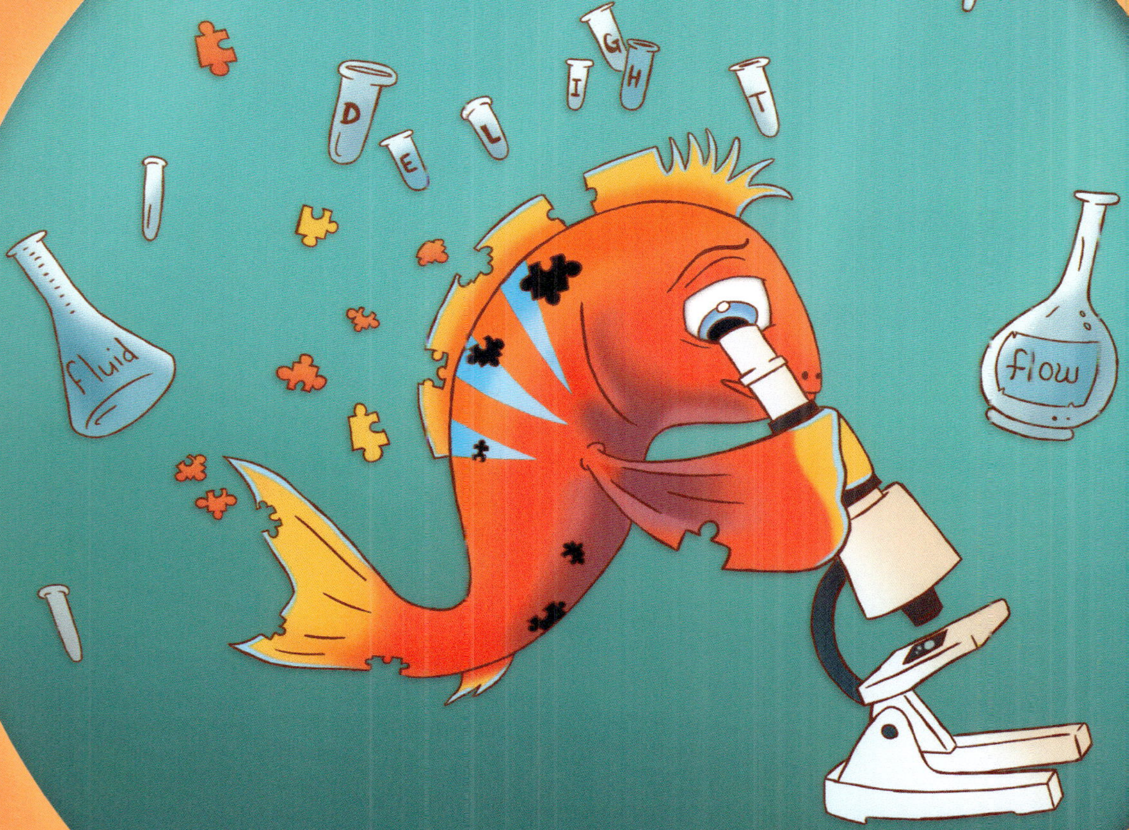

It was empty of water!!
That shook the fish right

"I see" said the fish in an
ungraspable way.

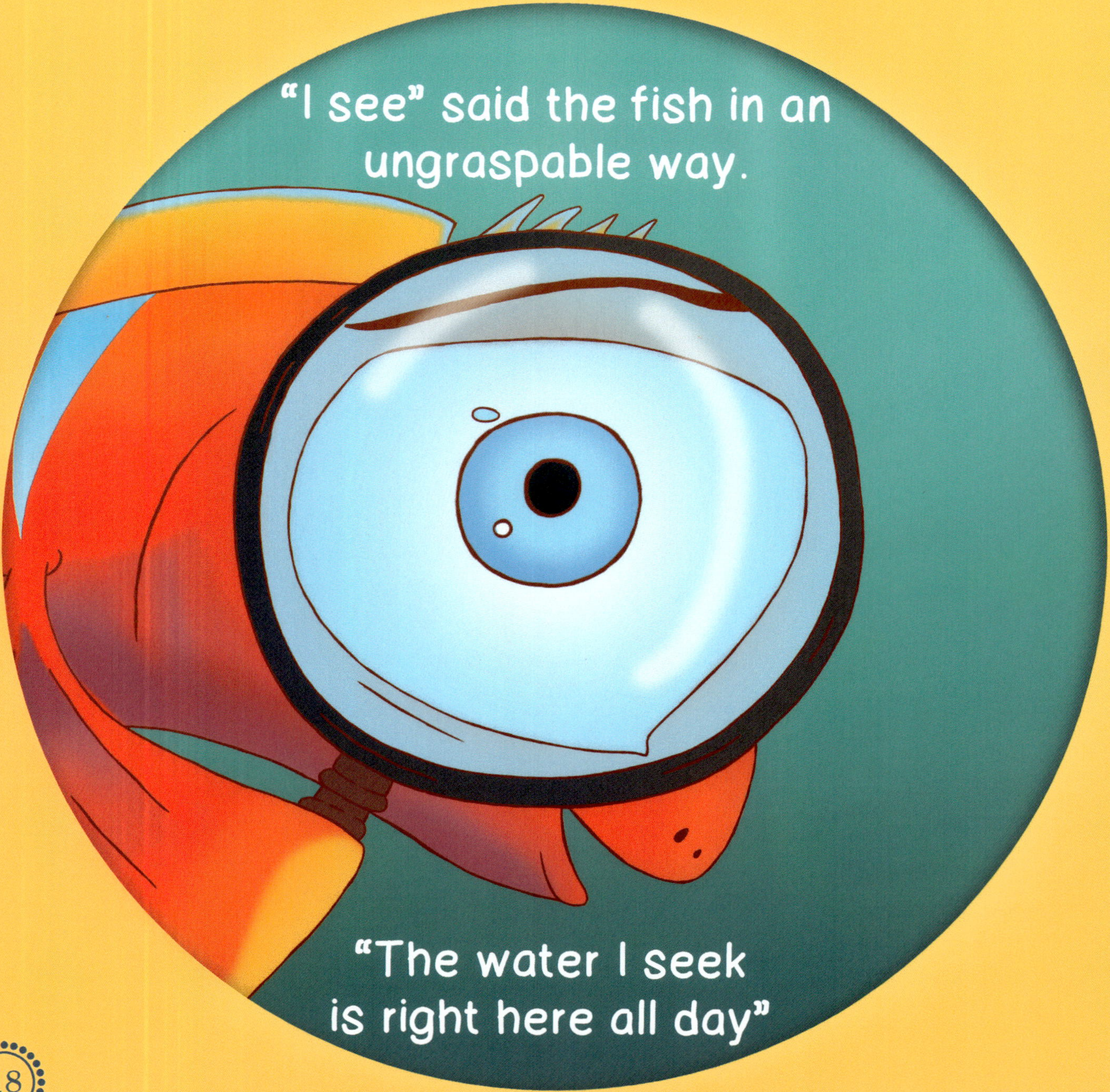

"The water I seek
is right here all day"

The water I seek
surrounds me right now.
Somehow it seems it's inside me

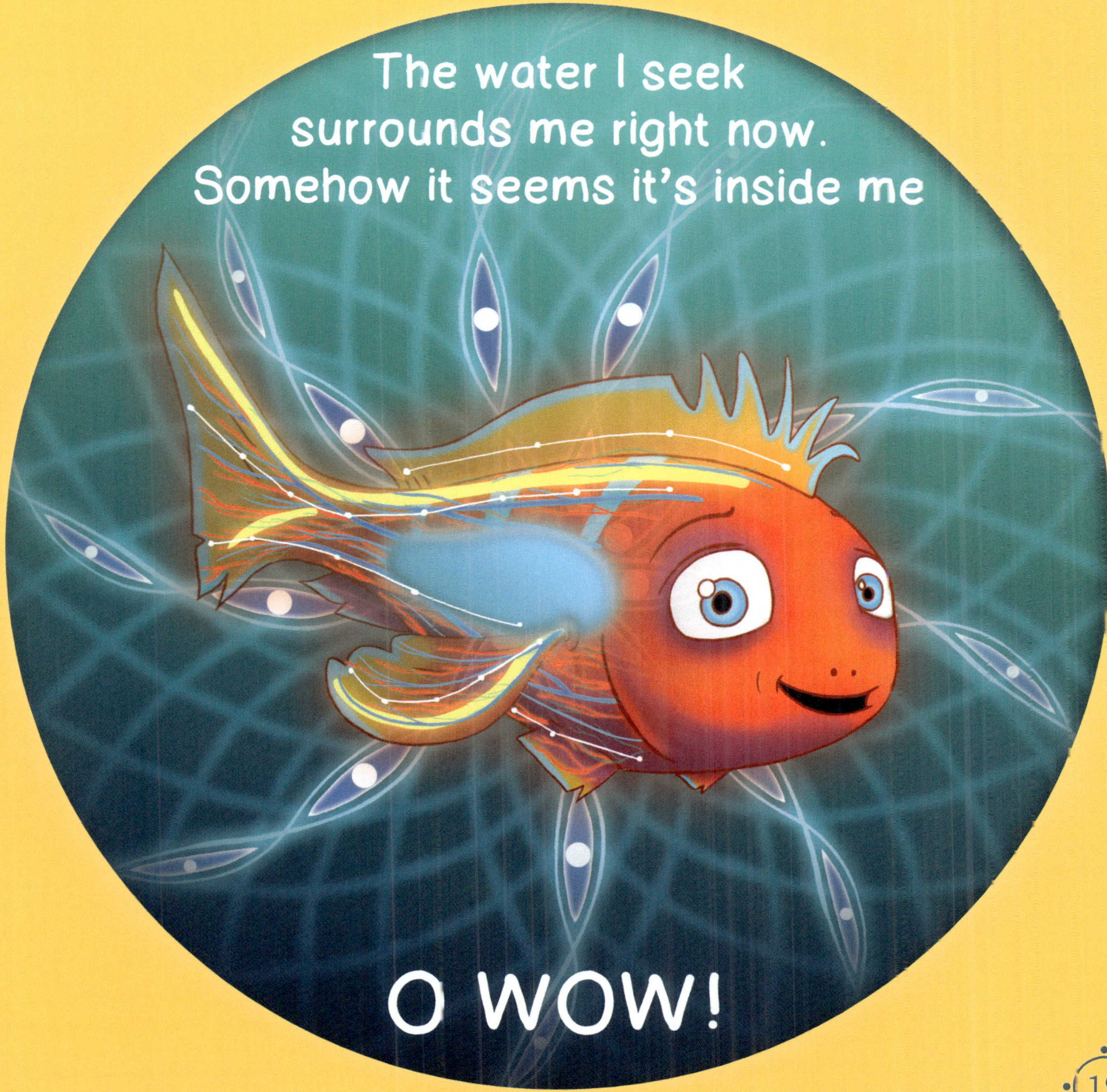

O WOW!

I don't need to swim
Or to seek or to look

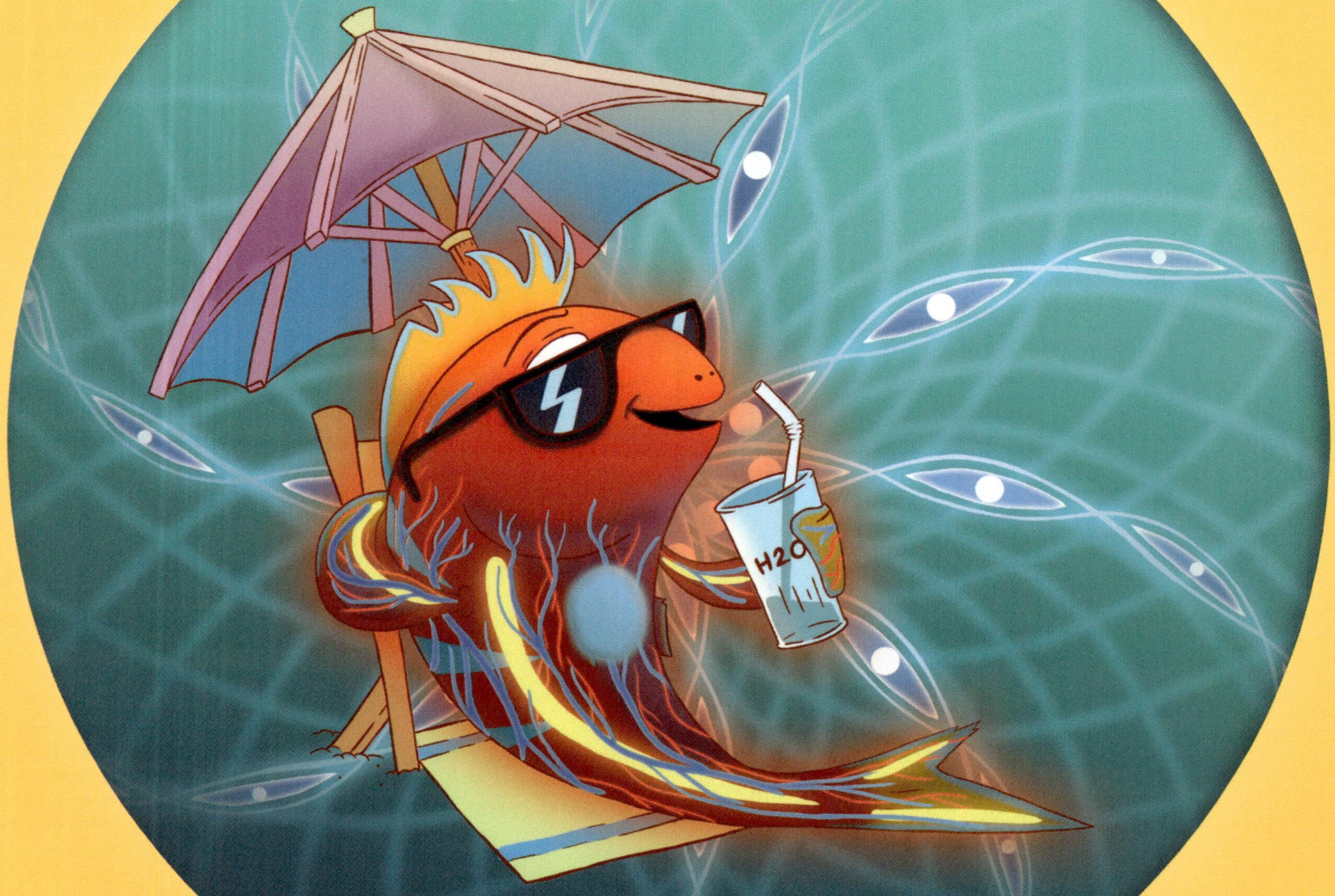

To discover the water
I simply mistook

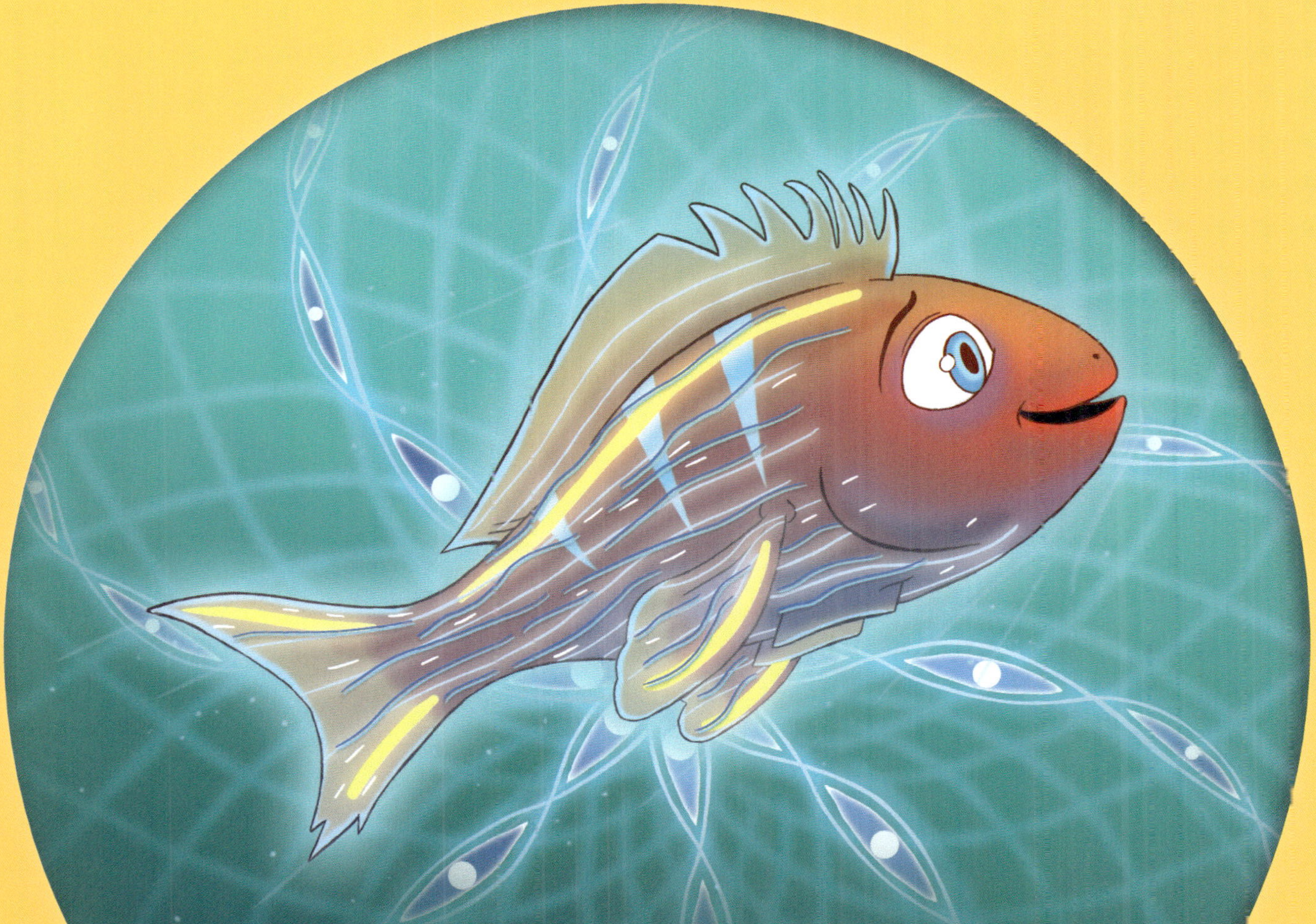

I don't need to effort
Or quest or breathe air
To experience water
IT'S ALREADY THERE!

THE END

Note to self:

When the shrivelling restarts
And I think I oughta
Go out and seek.....

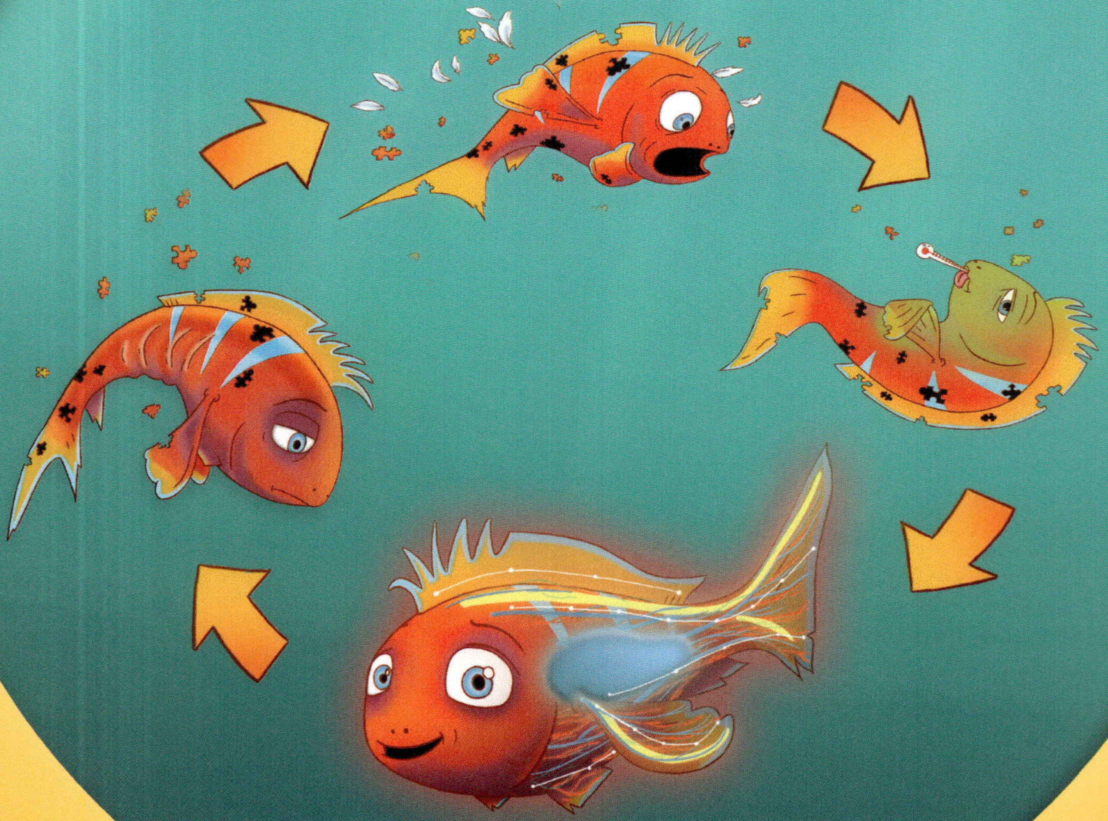

I REMEMBER THE WATER

REMEMBER THE WATER

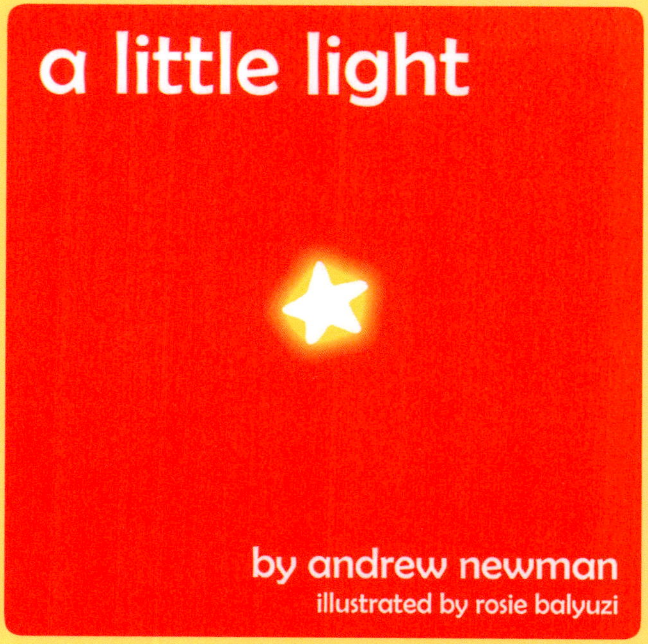
a little light
by andrew newman
illustrated by rosie balyuzi

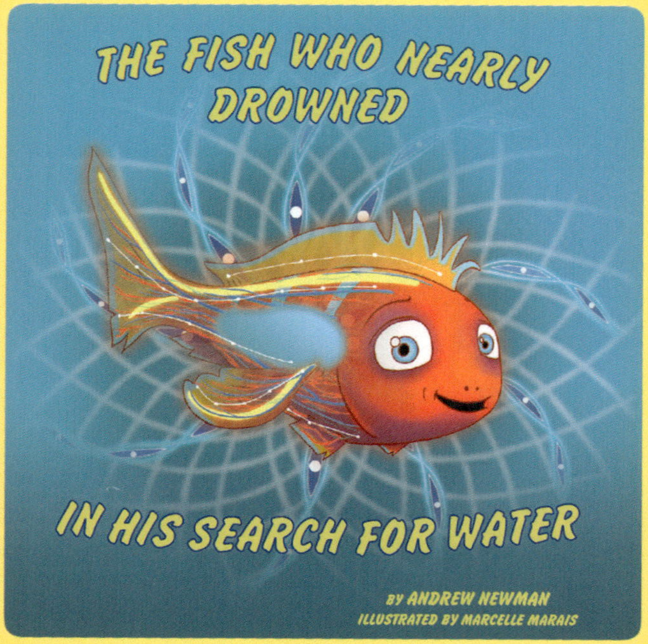
THE FISH WHO NEARLY DROWNED
IN HIS SEARCH FOR WATER
BY ANDREW NEWMAN
ILLUSTRATED BY MARCELLE MARAIS

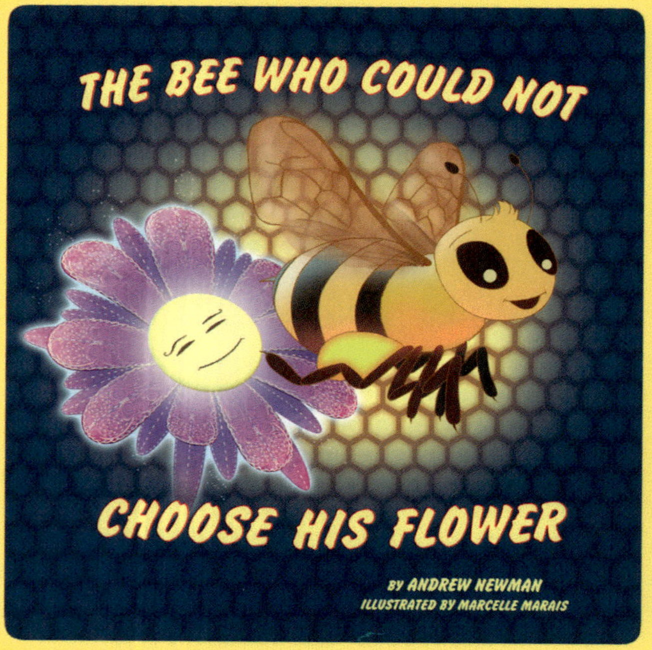
THE BEE WHO COULD NOT
CHOOSE HIS FLOWER
BY ANDREW NEWMAN
ILLUSTRATED BY MARCELLE MARAIS

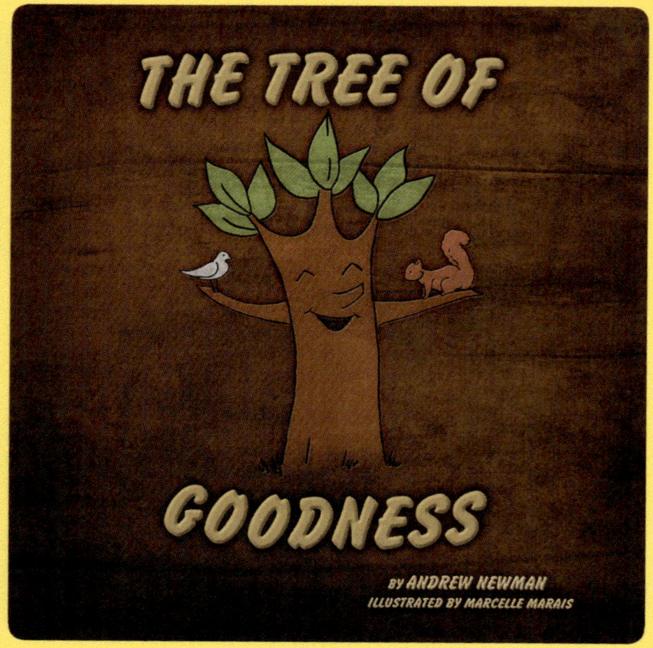
THE TREE OF
GOODNESS
BY ANDREW NEWMAN
ILLUSTRATED BY MARCELLE MARAIS

Andrew Newman

One day I sat down and wrote a poem.
Another day, I sat down and begged strangers to write me poems for Haiti.

It seems that I like poems.

Once-in-a-while a very special poem comes to me and says "Please will you make me into book". Then it usually dances around my head when I am trying to sleep. This keeps me awake until I say "YES, I will make you into a book."

These special poems have simple, easy to read messages that seem to be deeply familiar for everyone who reads them. I like that. They make life a little brighter, happier, easier, simpler and enjoyable. "That's a good thing", I think.

Please smile as you read them. That will make me happy.

www.andrewnewman.co.za

Marcelle Marais - illustrator

Marcelle Marais is an illustrator and animator born in South Africa, with 10 years experience working on a variety of projects from music videos and illustrating books to supplying the local and international advertising industry. He resides near the ocean and has a love for nature, art, literature and anything aquatic.

www.barnaclescreative.com

Tony Grogan's

EASTERN CAPE

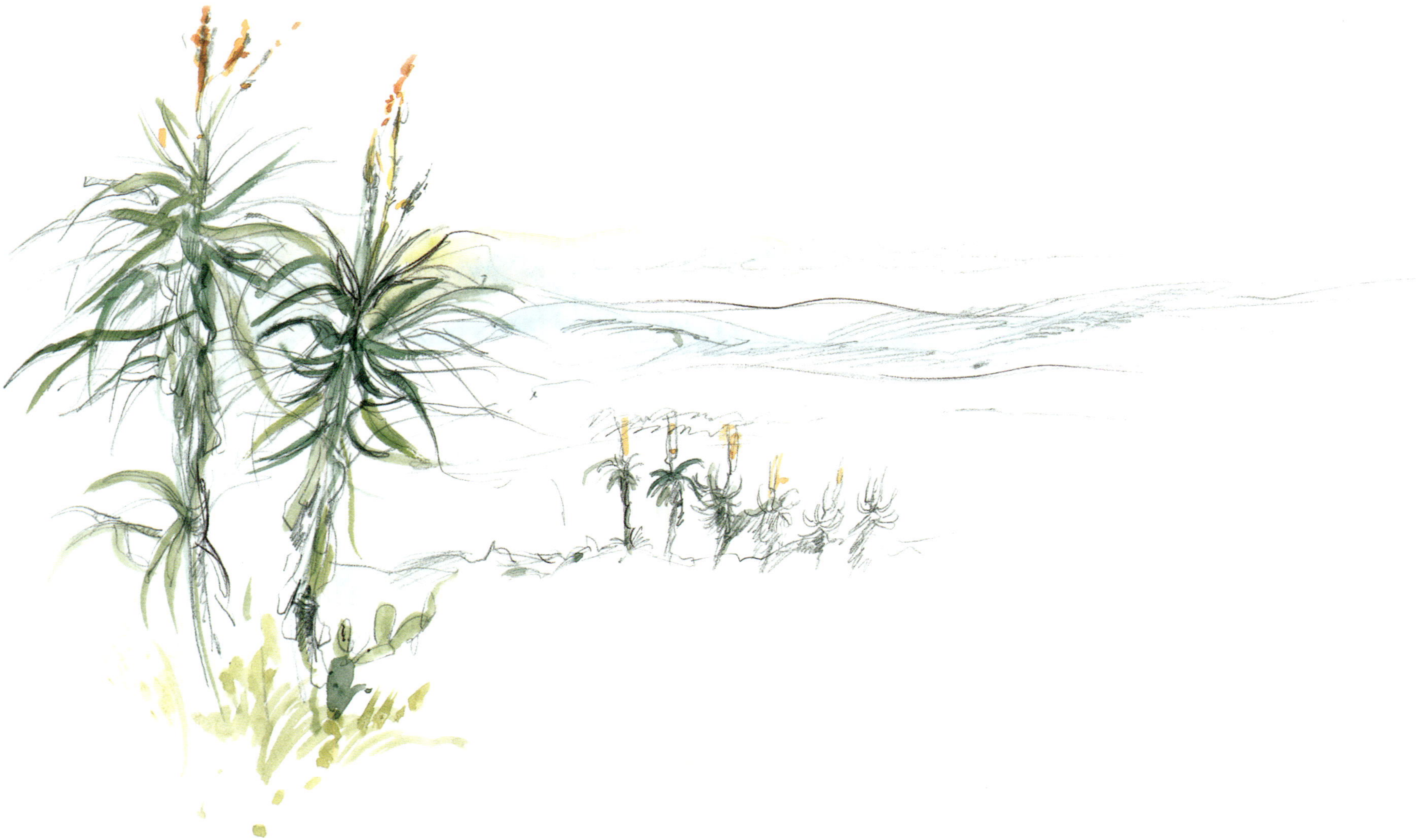

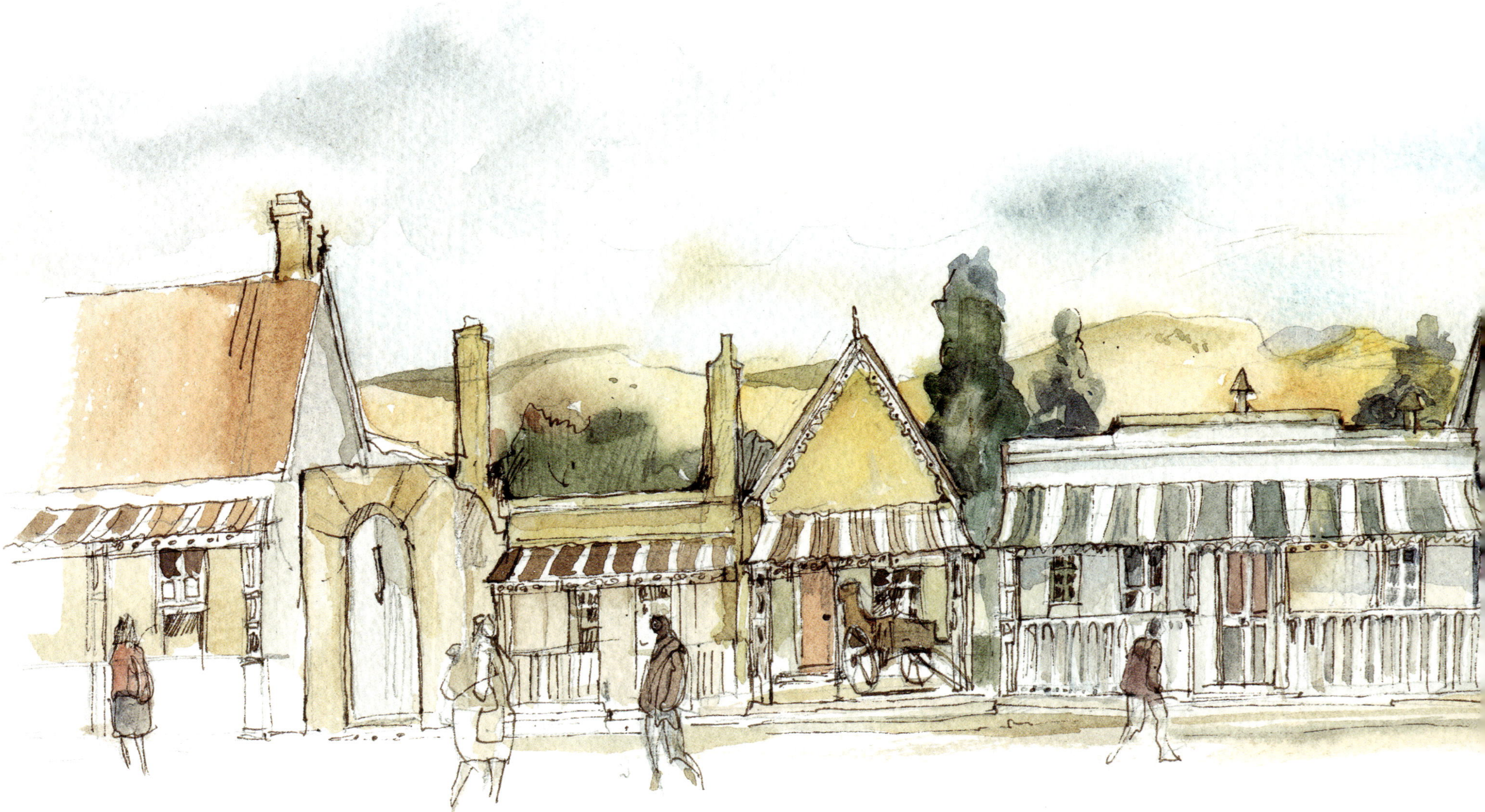

Tony GROGAN'S

EASTERN CAPE

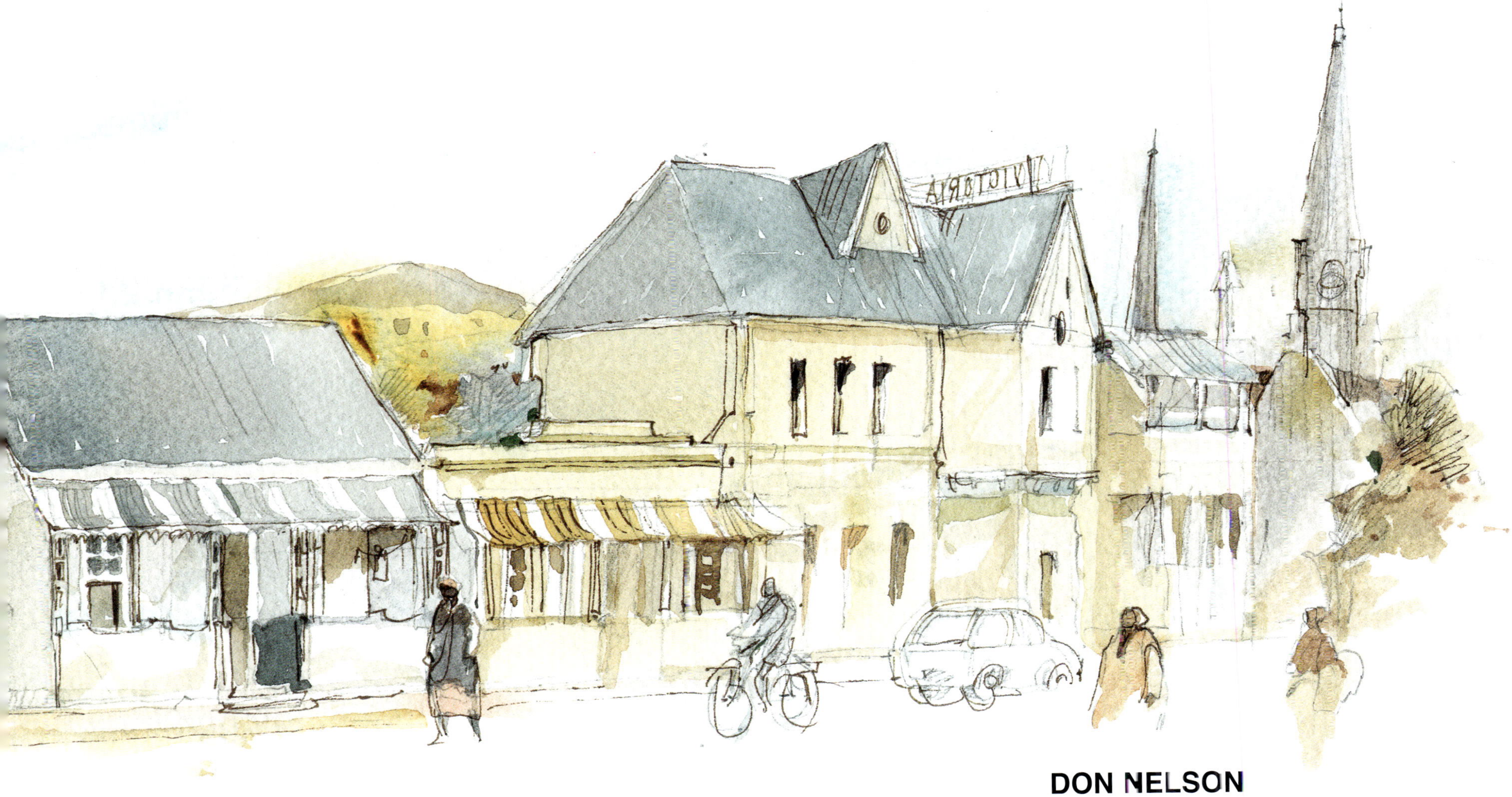

DON NELSON
Cape Town

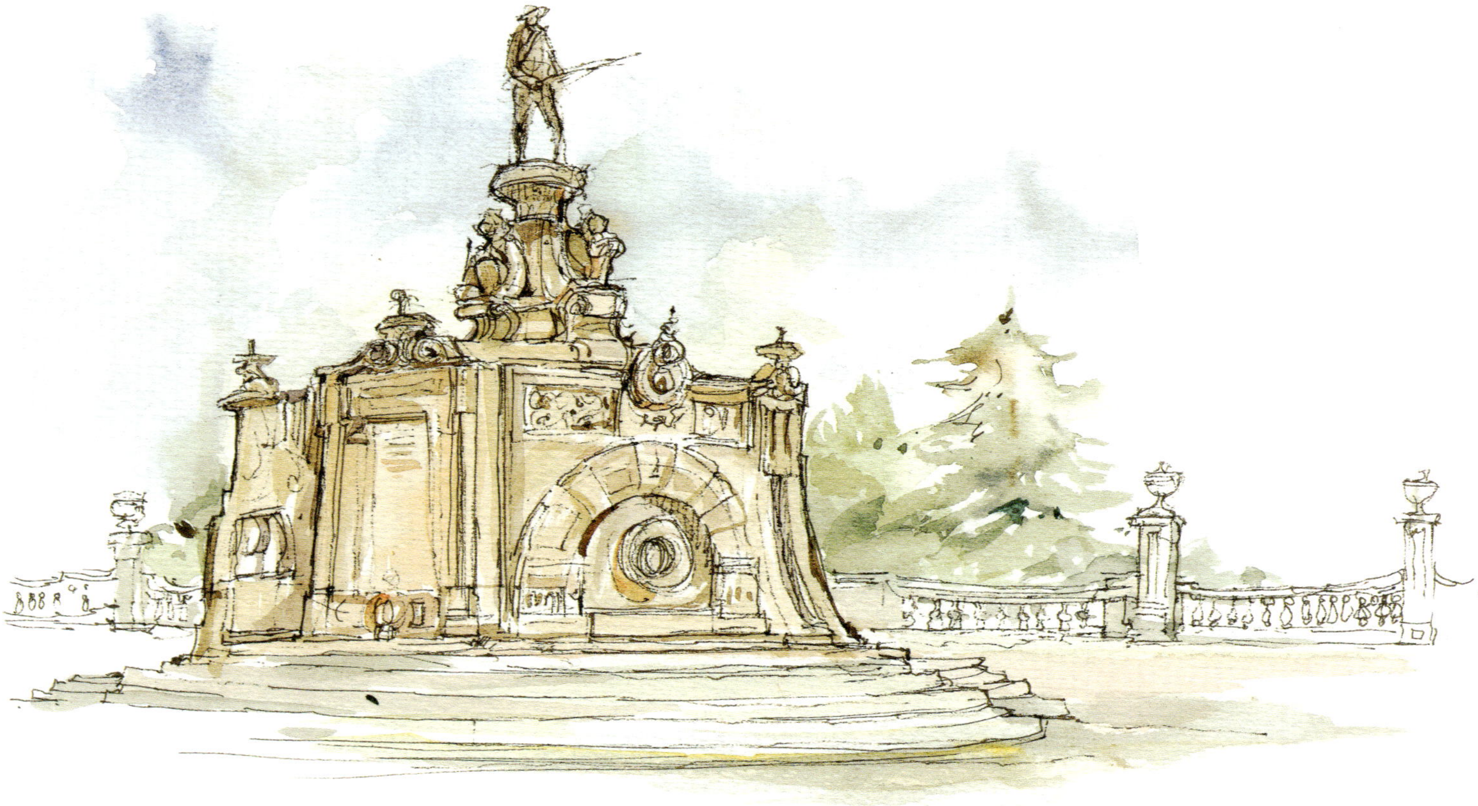

ISBN 1 86806 223 6

First edition 2005

Publisher: Don Nelson Publishers,
PO Box 18600, Wynberg 7824

Design and layout: Sarah-Anne Raynham

Reproduction by Virtual Colour, Cape Town

Printed and bound by Tien Wah Press
Pte Limited, Singapore

Thanks and acknowledgements

I want to thank all the kind and friendly people of the Eastern Cape for the advice, information, assistance and generous hospitality, without which this book would not have been possible, and in particular: Ivor Markman, Eira Maasdorp, Chris and Tamsin Bush, Kim and Ian van Niekerk, Erica McNalty, Dave and Verity Hobson Rosemary and Bill Fowldes, Mike and Sandra Antrobus, Ernest Pringle, Nomitsi Mhana, Cynthia Stali, Steve and Rita Bax, Dave and Jen Henderson, Adrian Gardiner, Dave Cox, the James family, Richard, Rob and Marian Rubidge, Paul and Jannis Sephton, Alex and Marianne Palmer, Bill, Alison and Doreen Brown, Jen and Jonny Louw, Lyndon and Hanrie Snelling, Graeme Resell, Trevor Wigley, Dorothea and Tony Moores, and my beloved wife, Jen, for her patience, encouragement and her invaluable help in putting this book together.

Bibliography

TV Bulpin: *Discovering South Africa*
(TV Bulpin Publications)

Jeanette Eve: *Eastern Cape Literature*
(Double Storey Books)

Nelson Mandela: *Long walk to Freedom*
(McDonald Purnell)

NC Mapham: *The War of Mlangeni in the Waterkloof*
(The Prophet)

Noel Mostert: *Frontiers*
(Jonathan Cape)

Eve Palmer: *The Plains of Camdeboo*
(Lowrie Publishers)

Thomas Pringle: *Narrative of a residence in South Africa*
(Struik Publishers)

Joan Southey: *Footprints in the Karoo*
(Jonathan Ball)

Edited by Guy Butler: *The 1820 Settlers*
(Human and Rousseau)

For my grandchildren:

Keenan, Cassandra, Derrin and Hannah

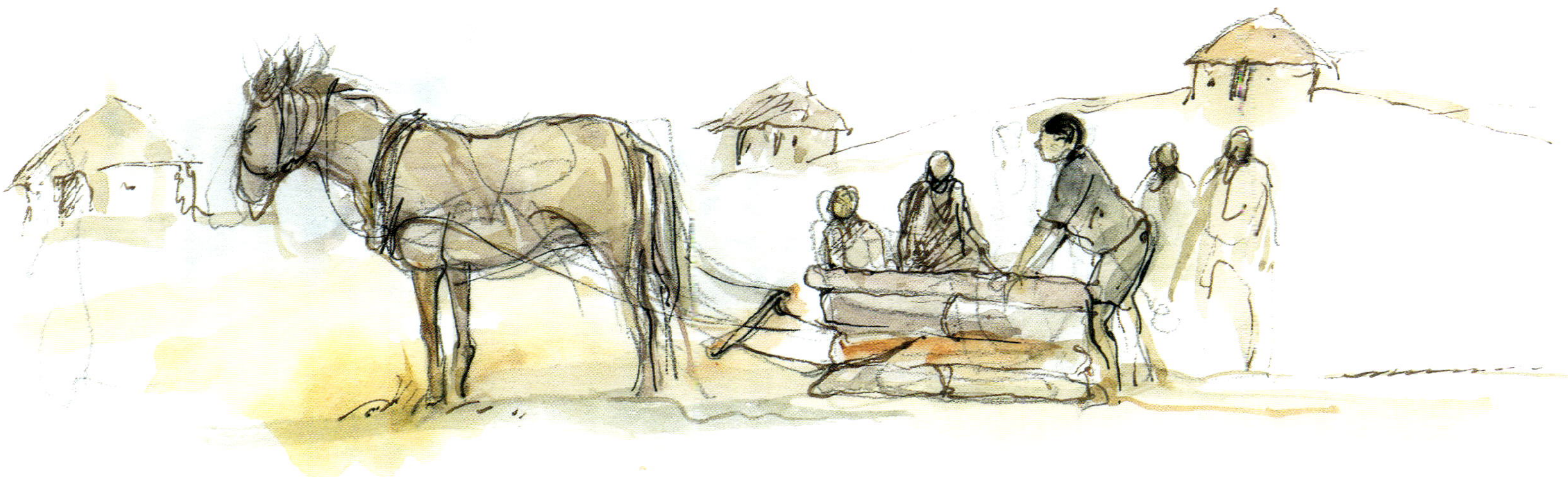

Introduction

This is my second book of drawings of the Eastern Cape; the other was published 25 years ago under the title *Settler Country*. As that book concentrated mainly on the Albany area and the old frontier regions of the Cape Colony, the reach of the present volume has been extended to include a wider area of this large province of South Africa. The province is too vast to represent the entire extent of the Eastern Cape, but I have tried within the limits of space to give a personal diary with sketches and notes of my experiences and observations, which I hope will reflect the general ambience of the province and its history, beauty and character. I had a general plan of the places I wanted to visit and the subject matter I needed, but always remained open to chance encounters upon my travels.

I have lived in Cape Town for the past 30 years, but I was born and grew up in the Eastern Cape and it was where my three children were born, so my roots are still very much there. Early in the century, my grandfather was port captain at various harbours on the east coast. Starting at Port St Johns – a relaxed posting I am told, as only two or three boats entered the harbour during the year at that time – he graduated to harbour master of Mossel Bay, East London and finally Port Elizabeth. I was born in Port Elizabeth at the beginning of the Second World War and when my father returned from active service, we moved to East London, a small town then with beautiful rivers and beaches, and a very pleasant place to spend your childhood. It still is.

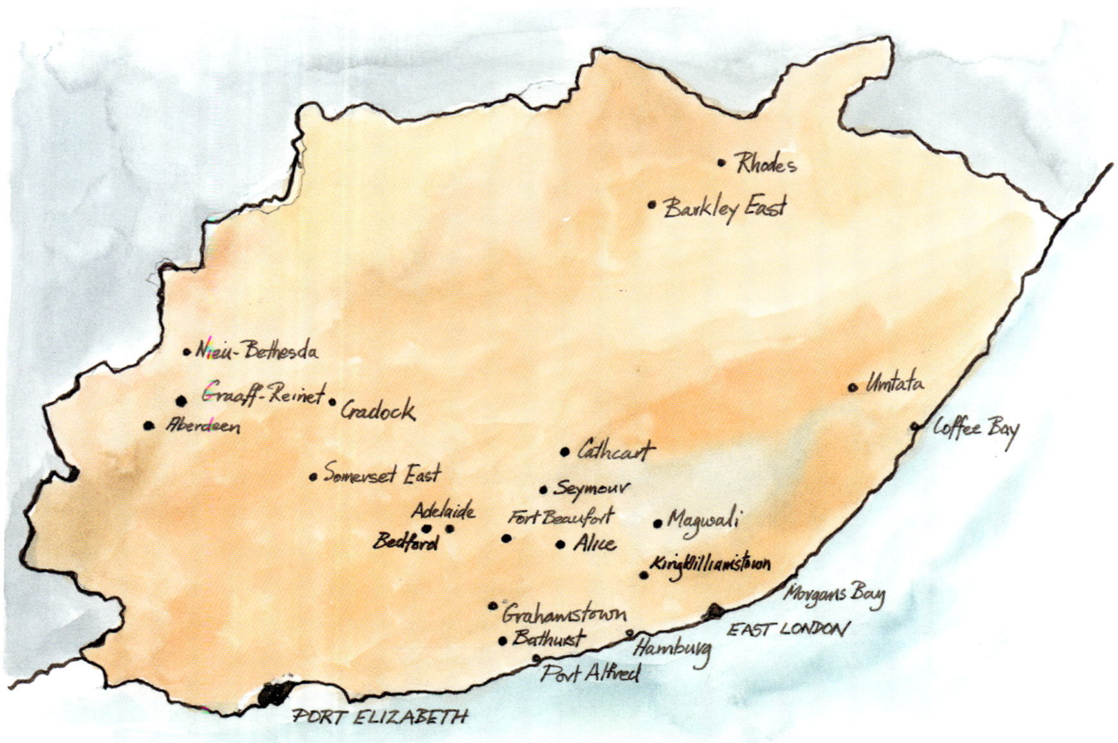

Happily my link with the Eastern Cape has been re-established by my son-in-law and daughter Chris and Tamsin Bush moving to Adelaide where they own a private game reserve, Molweni, in the heart of the old frontier area.

This book has been in preparation for several years. I have travelled extensively, meeting and talking to people, painting and jotting down impressions, and have found that wherever you travel in the Eastern Cape, you can be assured of helpfulness and a warm welcome. Of course, it's useful if you've grown up in the Eastern Cape because you are part of a network and inevitably you will have some link with whoever you meet, either through school, sport, university or the person you meet has a relative or a friend who knows your father, aunt or cousin. It's a close-knit network which also survives among those who move away from the province. Go to the Western Province Cricket Club on a Friday evening and you'll find a cluster of these exiles who have been gathering at the pub for the last 30 years to share a beer and the bonhomie so dear to the heart of the Eastern Capers.

The Eastern Cape was the original interface between so many elements of South African people which affected our subsequent history. It was the anvil on which were forged our later attitudes and prejudices. It is a theme explored exhaustively by Noel Mostert in his excellent book, *Frontiers*, a history of the Eastern Cape. It was here that the Xhosa, the early trekboers, the Khoisan people, the British settlers, the military, the missionaries and all those strands that formed the web of South Africa's social and political history came into contact. Exploring the old battle sites, and visiting the

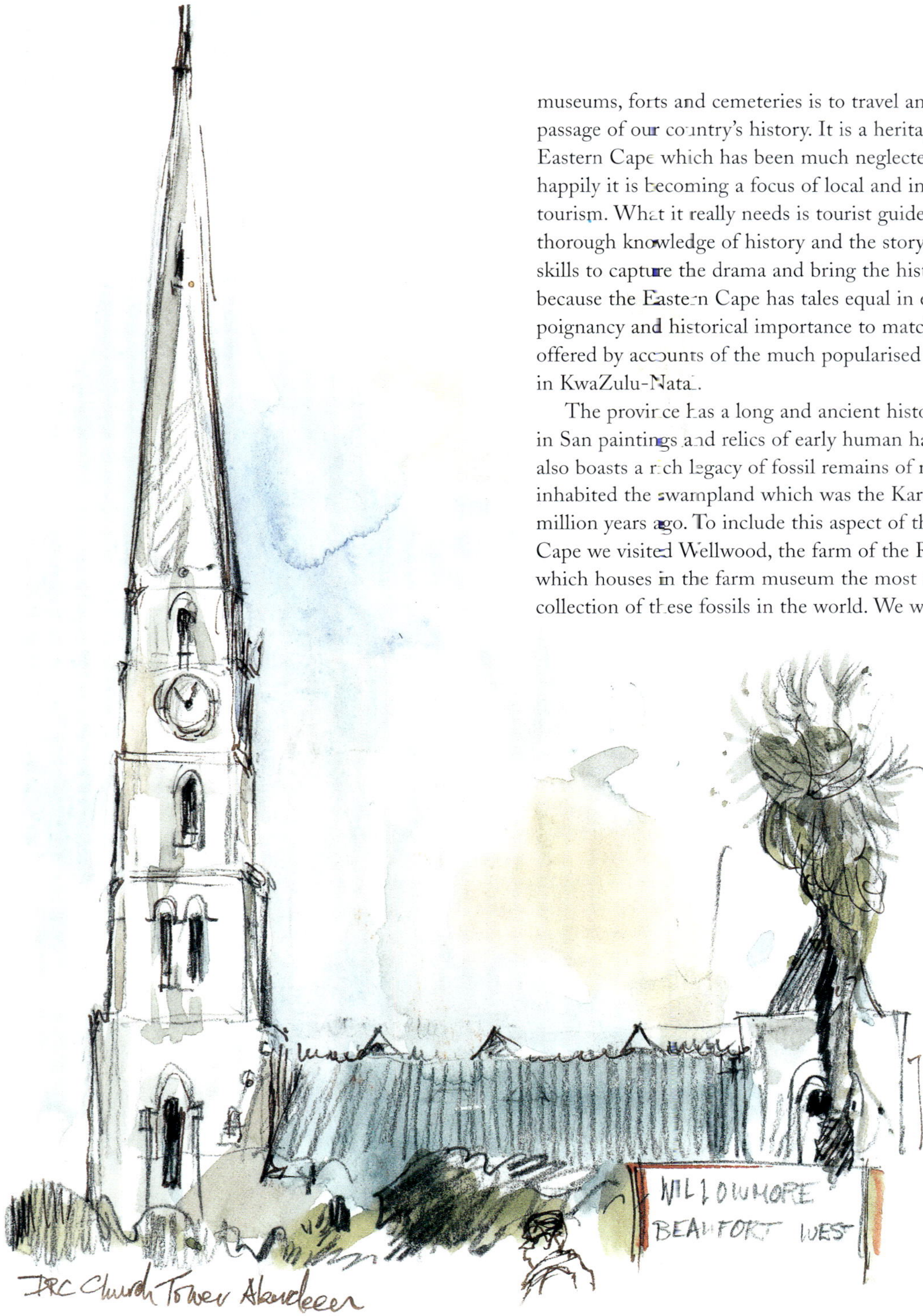

museums, forts and cemeteries is to travel an important passage of our country's history. It is a heritage of the Eastern Cape which has been much neglected but happily it is becoming a focus of local and international tourism. What it really needs is tourist guides with a thorough knowledge of history and the story-telling skills to capture the drama and bring the history alive, because the Eastern Cape has tales equal in excitement, poignancy and historical importance to match anything offered by accounts of the much popularised Zulu wars in KwaZulu-Natal.

The province has a long and ancient history reflected in San paintings and relics of early human habitation. It also boasts a rich legacy of fossil remains of reptiles that inhabited the swampland which was the Karoo 200 million years ago. To include this aspect of the Eastern Cape we visited Wellwood, the farm of the Rubidges, which houses in the farm museum the most complete collection of these fossils in the world. We were invited to lunch by Alex and Marianne Palmer of the farm Cranemere, immortalised in Eve Palmer's classic book of the Karoo, The Plains of Camdeboo. Here, too, the family has a museum displaying fossils, artefacts and remains of early human habitation discovered on the farm over the years.

I was enchanted with the variety and contrast of the Eastern Cape landscape, particularly its remote and wild places – the harsh, barren spaces of the Karoo and its shimmering distances; the thickly forested mountains with foothills sprinkled with thorn trees; remote and uninterrupted stretches of sandy coastline; lovely inlets and lagoons of placid dark water separated by barriers of sand from a wild and tumultuous ocean; undulating grassy hills ending abruptly in black cliffs which plunge precipitously into the sea – all stimulating challenges to an artist's brush.

I have also tried to represent the traditional life of the Xhosa people, and my approaches and requests to be allowed to make drawings was met with touching eagerness to share and explain their traditions and ceremonies. We came across a group of women beautifully attired in traditional dress at a bus stop, and were invited to follow them and join the celebrations at the coming out party of one of their sons. I arranged a portrait session with a sangoma in Adelaide and when I arrived at her hut, anxious that she might regard my visit as an intrusion, was surprised to find not one but two sangomas and three novices all dressed up in their finery for the occasion and only too willing to explain the details of their profession and share their rituals with refreshing openness and enthusiasm.

We travelled from Cape Town along the N1, then turned off at Beaufort West on the road to Aberdeen, at which point you can put your car into autodrive because the road ahead is as straight as an arrow with scarcely a turn for the next 150km. Your first landmark to indicate you are approaching the Eastern Cape is the spire of the church in Aberdeen which can be seen in the distance like a shining white needle in the arid landscape. The townsfolk of Aberdeen claim that it is the highest church spire in the country.

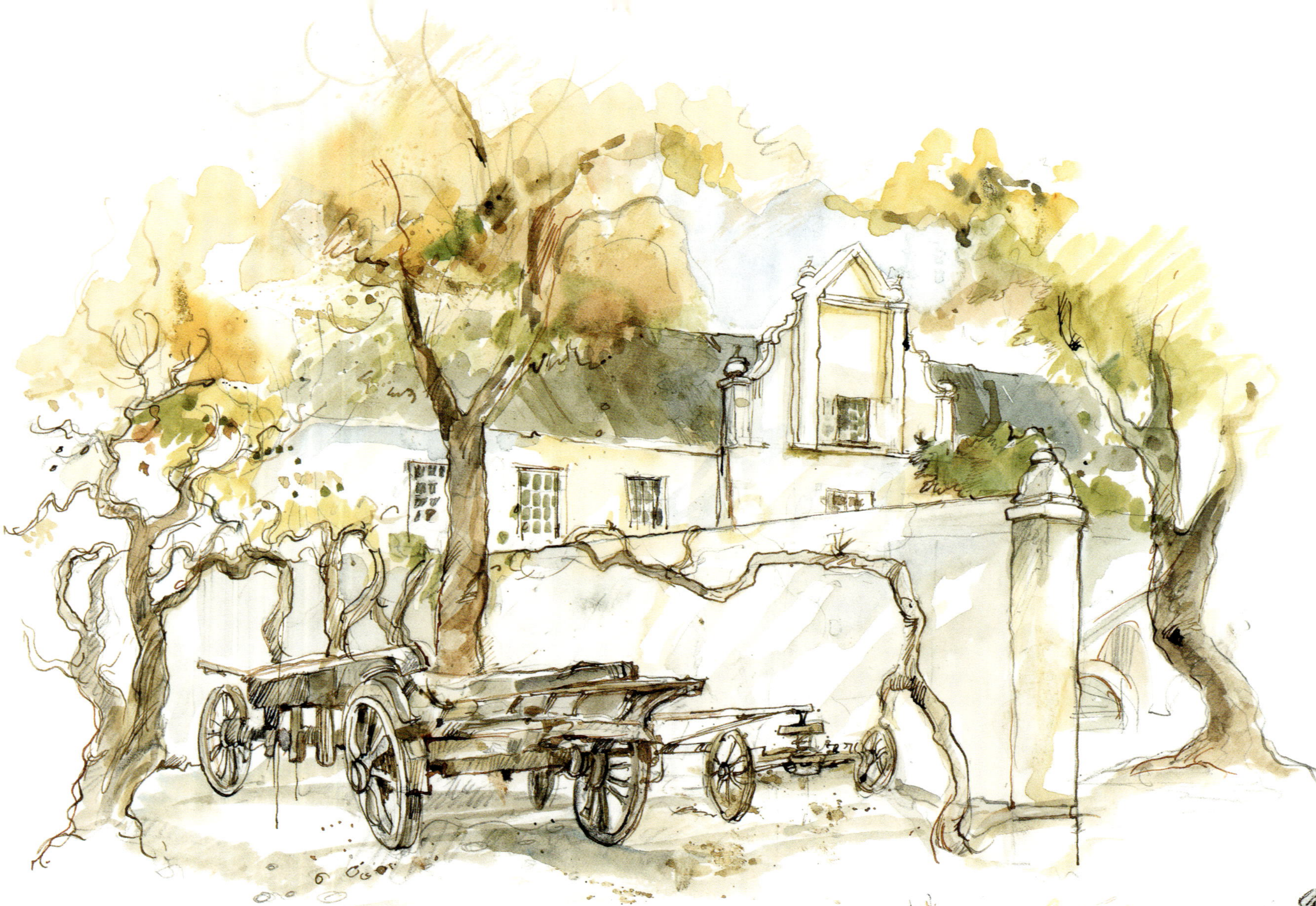

Graaff-Reinet: Reinet House

Reinet House, built in 1805, was the first parsonage of the Dutch Reformed Church, and is a superb example of Cape Dutch architecture. The grape vine at the back of the house is the oldest in the country. A *brandewyn* (brandy) festival is taking place in the garden behind the house, where experts who have retained the art of distilling are supervising logs of wood being fed into the oven of the still. They are watched by interested onlookers.

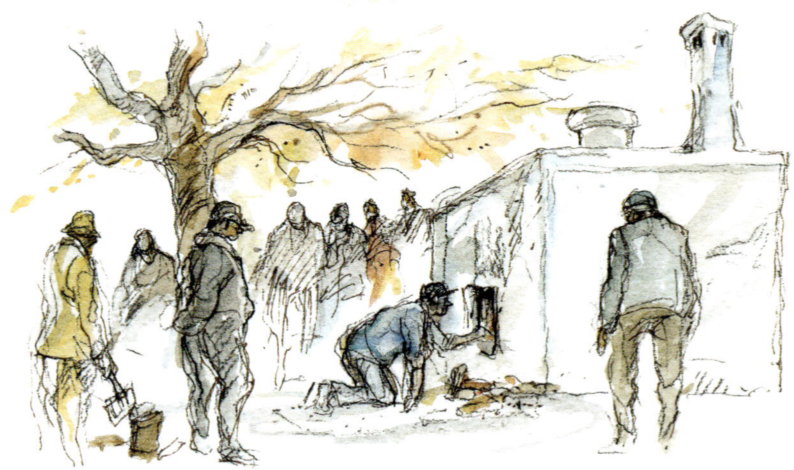

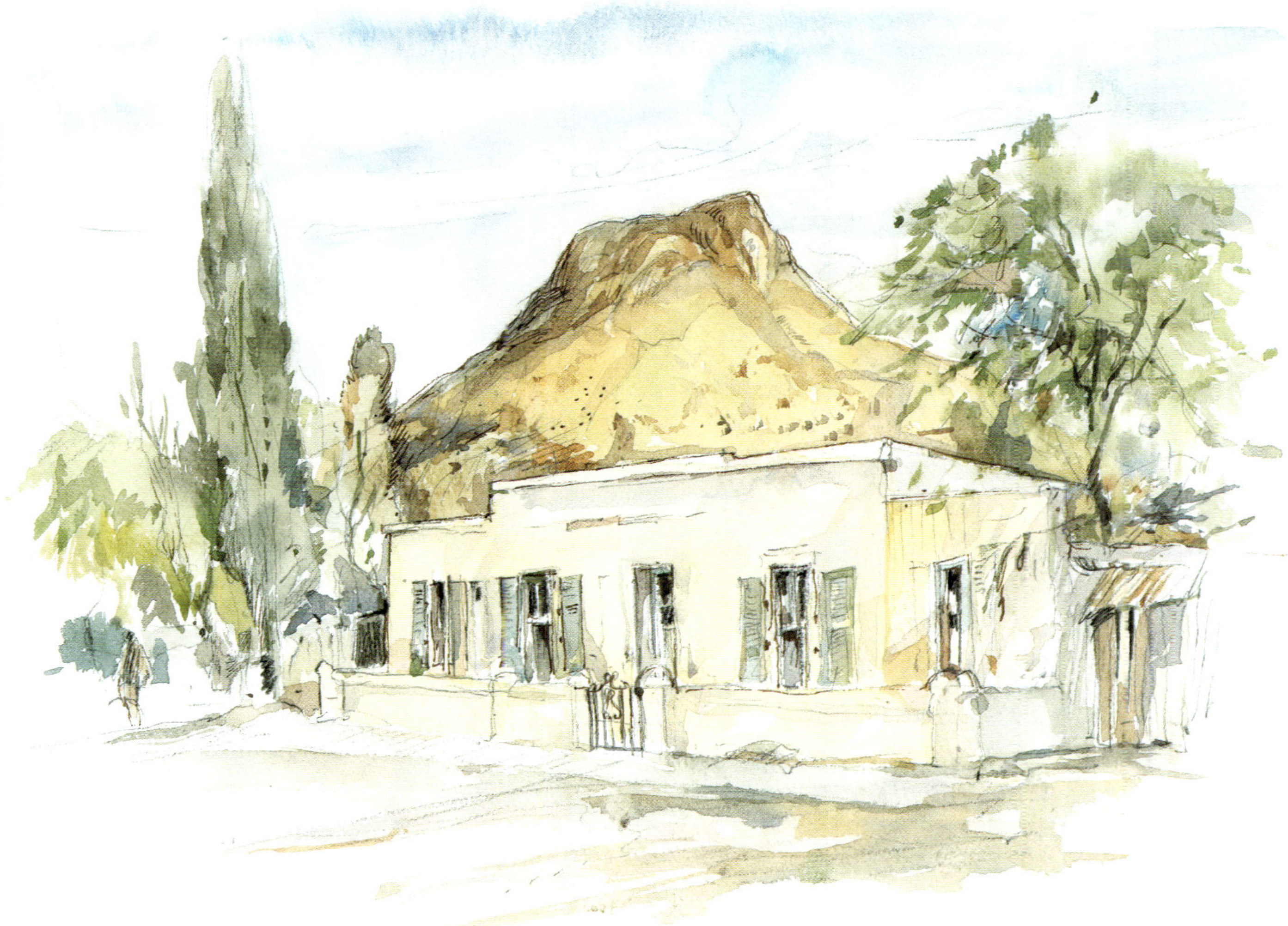

Donkin Street

One of the old houses in Donkin Street, now beautifully renovated belongs to Hillary Palmé. She invites me to look inside. The garden behind the house is a peaceful, rural idyll with a large swathe of immaculate lawn running down to the river. A horse grazes peacefully under the trees. Spioenkop, the battlefield where British and Boer forces met in 1900, forms a stunning backdrop.

She tells me the large erven in Donkin and Plasket streets were once vegetable gardens whose owners sold their produce to the local market until the system of agricultural boards (official committees under the old government that dictated the marketing of agricultural produce) put a stop to this. Some then turned to distilling illegal brandy and used to sell it from convenient backstreet windows with the shutters open for the purpose. The smell of the fermenting grapes was disguised with evil-smelling fires to avoid the local policeman being guided to the scene of the crimes by his nose.

One of the charms of living in Graaff-Reinet in years gone by were the water furrows which supplied water to gardens in the town. Each resident had a designated time to tap into the water supply and irrigate his or her garden. The temptation to cheat and take more than their share of this precious commodity by putting a pebble under the sluice gate revealed flaws in the most upright of characters. Junius in *Stoep Stories*, a journal of Graaff-Reinet's heritage, expresses his shock and disillusion in the conduct of one gentleman 'in every respect of the highest quality, a gentleman, quiet and dignified who presented a picture of respectable old age, a man of moderation, kind to children and animals, who gave generously to the church, but he stole water! I came to see him as he really was.' Nobody's perfect, I guess.

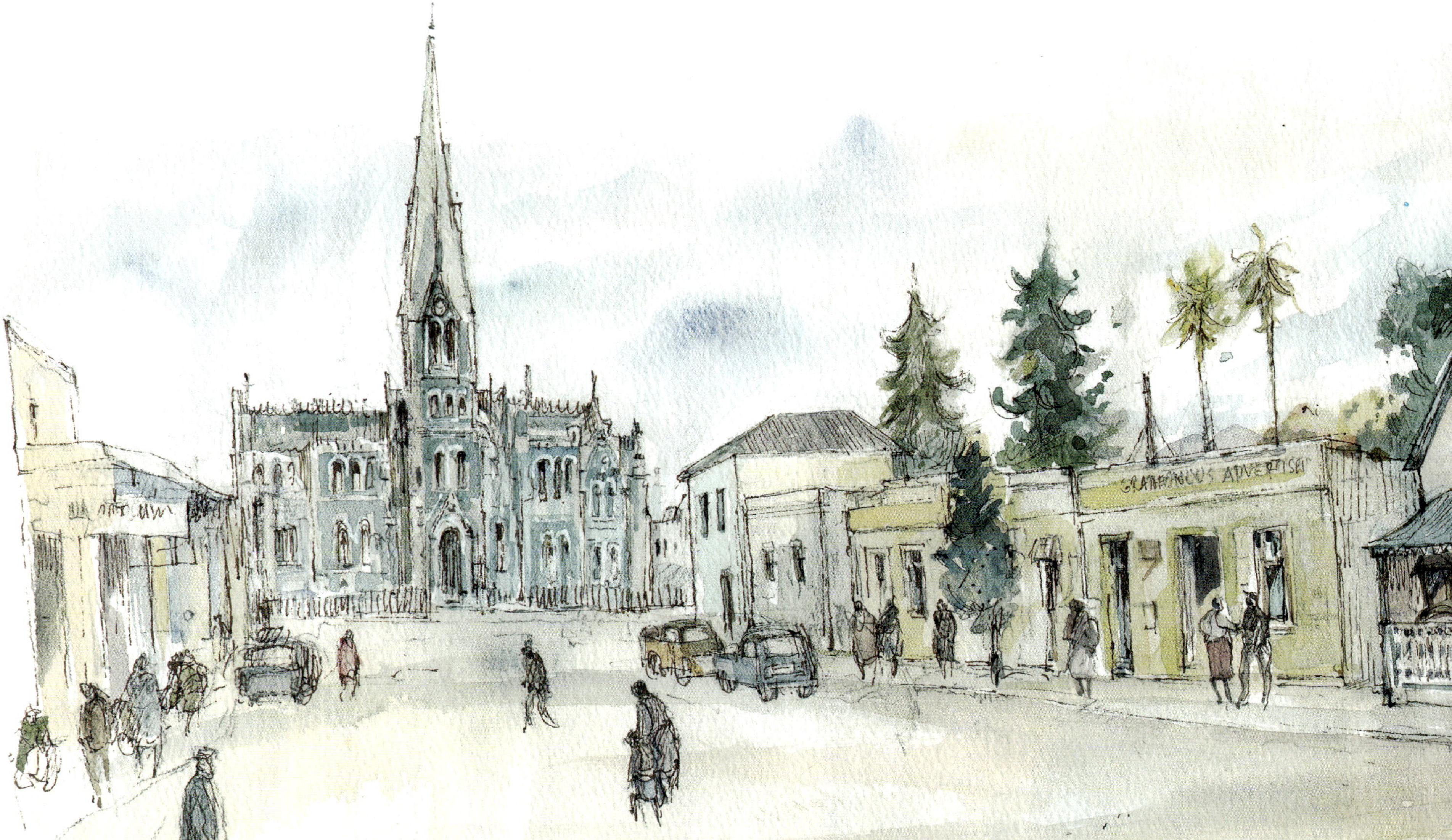

Graaff-Reinet

Graaff-Reinet was established in 1786 as the seat of a magistracy required to maintain order on a troubled frontier. An admirable programme of preservation and restoration of its unique architecture over the years has retained the town's charming 19th-century atmosphere and character. The main street, Church Street, is lined with historic buildings and leads the eye to its main focus, the impressive Dutch Reformed Church, modelled on Salisbury Cathedral in England.

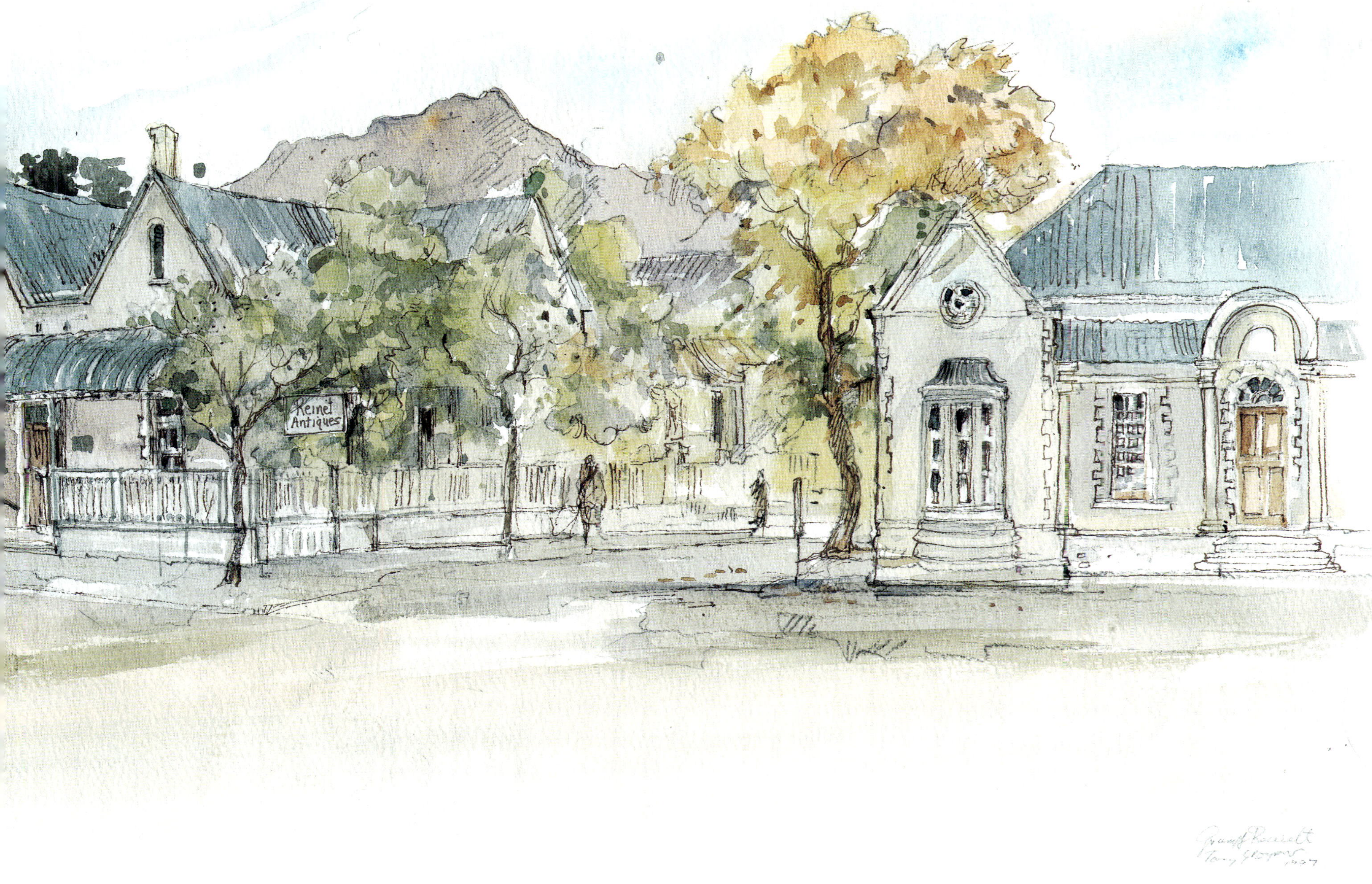
Reinet
Antiques

Nooitgedacht

Eira Maasdorp took us to the historic farm, Nooitgedacht in the Graaff-Reinet district, on which she grew up. The old ox wagon at the gate was the one on which her father brought his young bride to the farm. On the way they passed a small hovel on the side of the road and he stopped the wagon and jokingly announced to his bride that this was their new home. Such was her mother's happiness and contentment with her new husband, Eira said, that she expressed no disappointment at the meanness of the abode and immediately started unpacking.

The rambling Cape Dutch homestead, Nooitgedacht, with its fine proportions and pleasing lines, must have come as a very pleasant surprise when the couple arrived there. The house was built in 1836 and has been beautifully restored by the new owners.

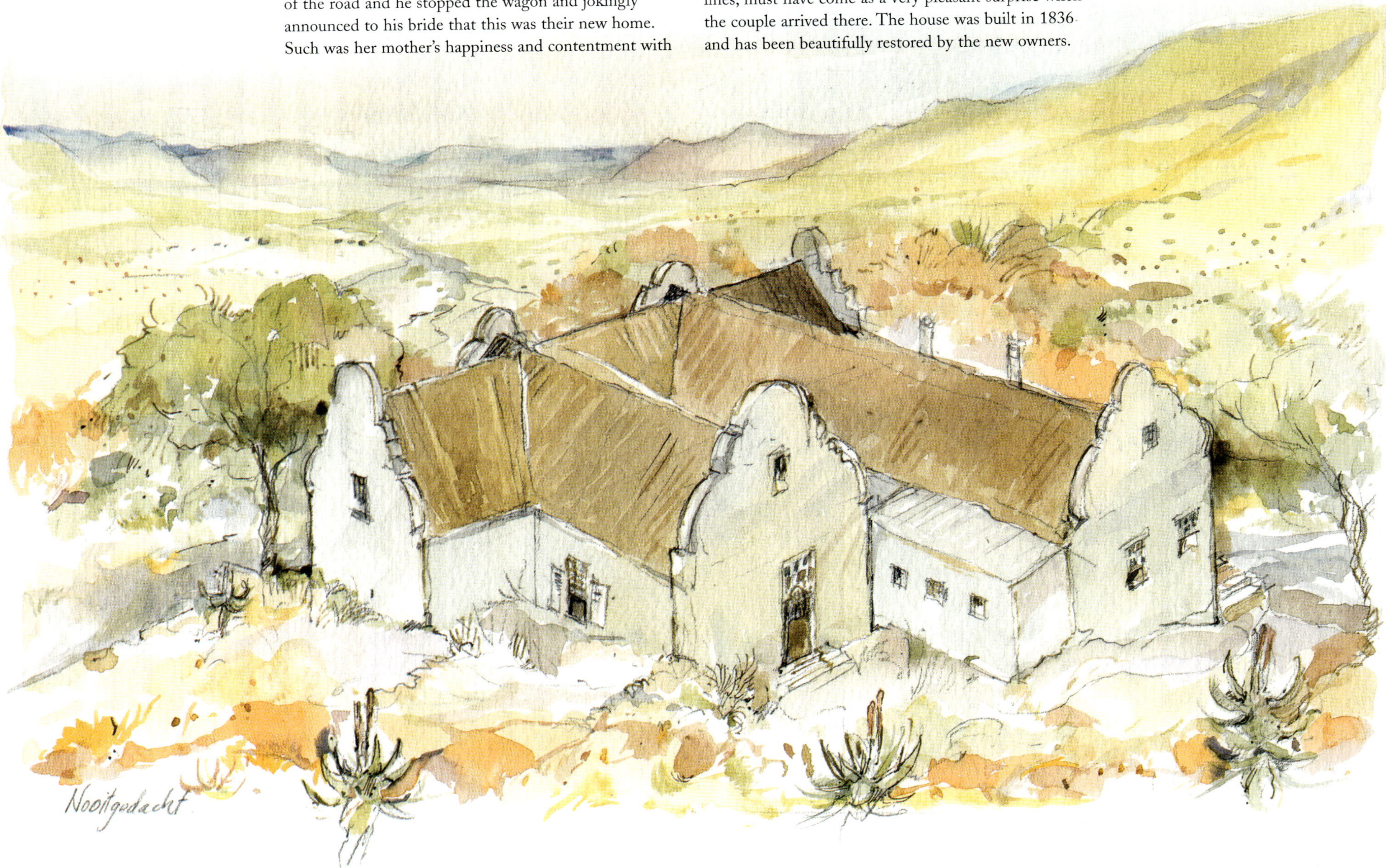

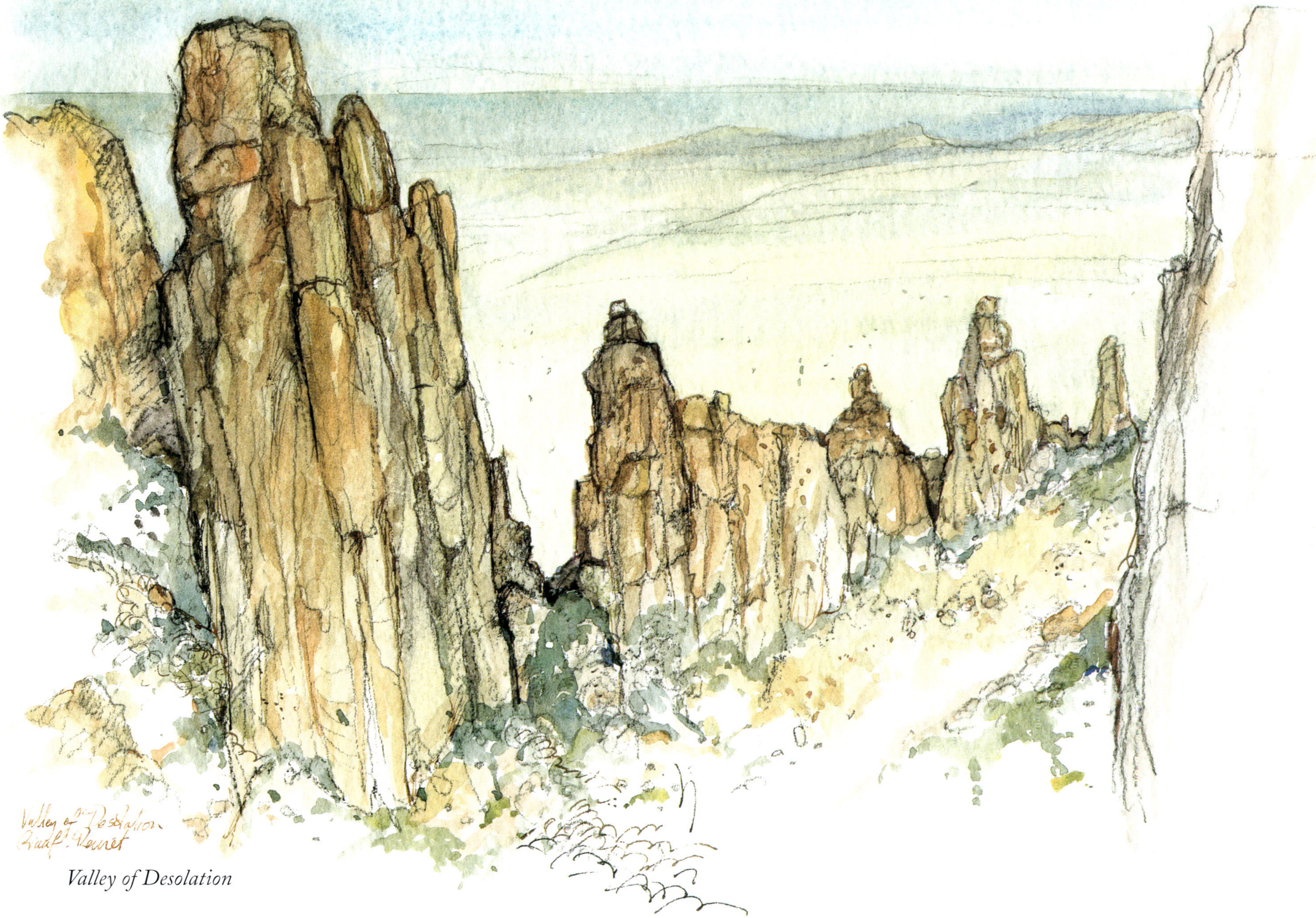

Valley of Desolation

Nature has carved a chasm into the plateau on the summit of the mountain massif behind Graaff-Reinet. The Valley of Desolation is a place of weathered turrets and towers of stone with rocks and boulders tumbled down to the valley floor in wild confusion. The view from the top is a breathtaking scene of the desolate, dry plains of the Karoo. An immense stillness pervades, and we drink in the great panorama which stretches away in all its exquisite beauty and grandeur to the end of the world.

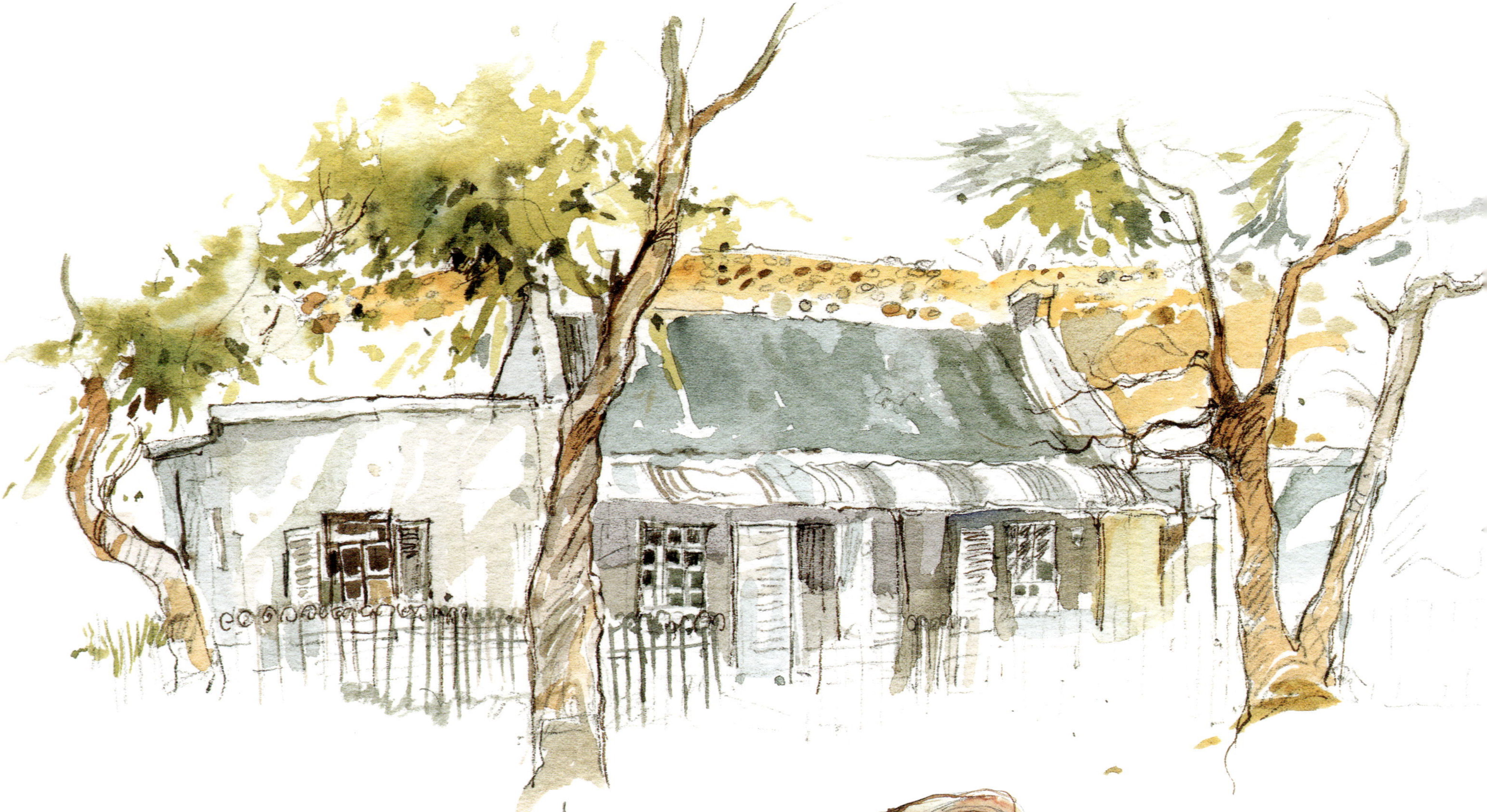

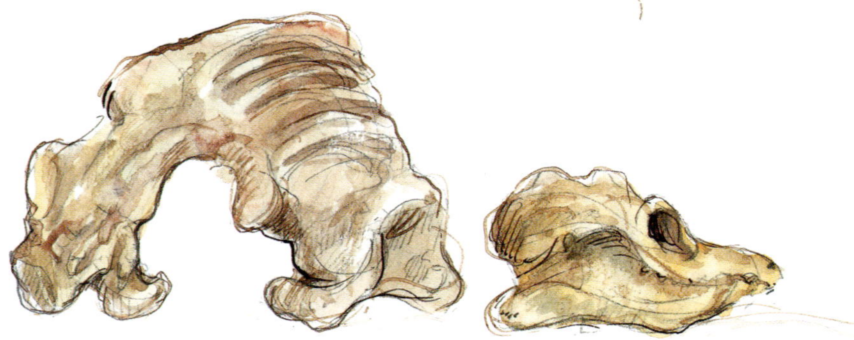

Wellwood

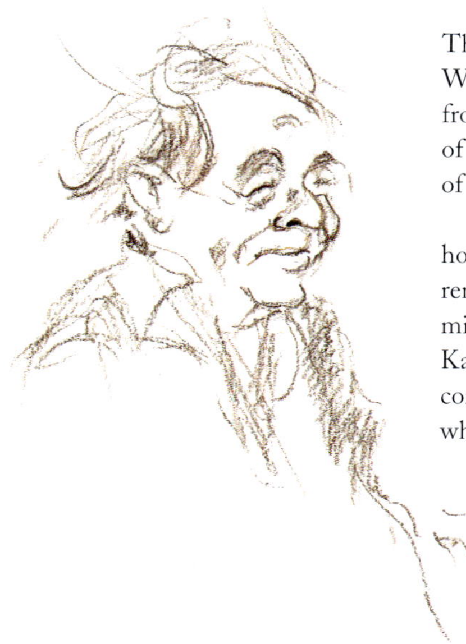

The first house built by Charles Rubidge on the farm, Wellwood, was set in the lee of a ridge that protected it from the prevailing wind. Robert is the fifth generation of Rubidges farming this beautiful, productive farm, one of the best known in the Karoo for its merino stud.

The farm is also famous for its museum which houses a unique and extensive collection of fossil remains of reptiles which inhabited the Karoo 200 million years ago. It is hard to imagine that the arid Karoo was then a damp, tepid swampland, ideal conditions for the formation and preservation of fossils which are richly embedded in the rock strata. The great palaeontologist, Robert Broom, estimated that here were preserved in the Karoo formations about 800,000 million specimens, of which at any one time at least a million specimens are lying on the surface waiting to be picked up.

Robert's father, Richard, whom I have drawn here, told me that his father Sydney used to range the stock camps on horseback and became an expert at spotting fossils embedded in the rock strata on the farm. His interest was quickened when he read a newspaper article on the antiquity of fossils. Richard told us that his sister Peggy had a school assignment to write on fossils. On 10 July 1934 her father took her and some friends into the veld to see what they could find. They found a number of 'boney-stones' as he called them. Included was the snout of a large carnivorous reptile. In the ensuing months, when his farming duties allowed, he patiently carved out the entire skull using a hammer and chisel. From this moment Sydney's interest became a consuming passion. Robert Broom, with whom he was to have a friendship of 17 years, heard of his extraordinary discovery and named the fossil *Dinogorgon rubidgei*. He told Sydney that that name would survive as long as human culture remained.

Richard conducted us on a tour of the exhibition, which is indeed remarkable. The skulls range from monstrous Jurassic creatures to tiny mouse like reptiles. The Eastern Cape is full of unexpected discoveries but to find a fossil collection of such value and significance housed on a farm on the Karroo was extraordinary.

A world renowned paleantologist, who visited the farm in 1949, wrote in Syndney's diary: "Mr Sydney Rubidge's collection of Karoo reptiles is the most interesting and important in the world. There is no parallel to the building up in ten years of so magnificent a series of fossils reptiles, essentially from one set of rocks, by one man actively engaged in the management of a difficult farm."

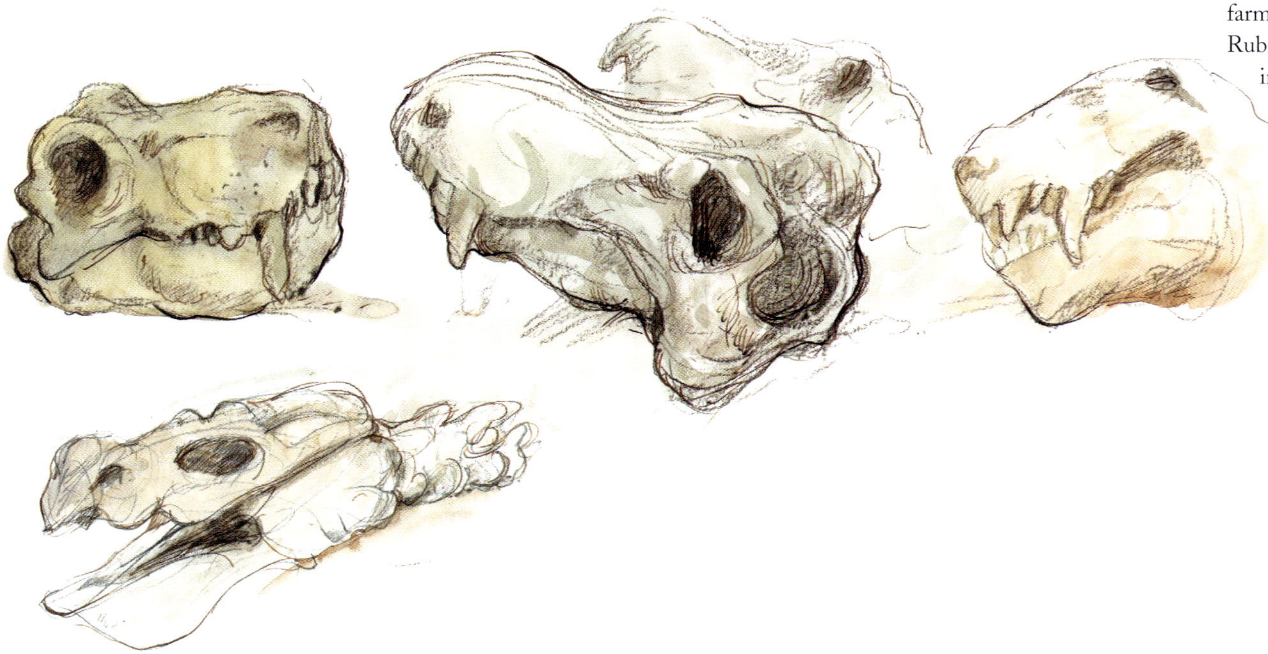

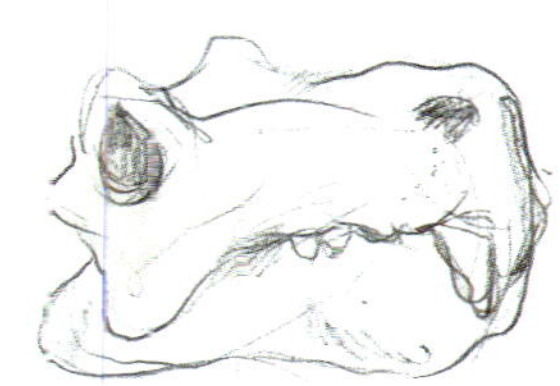

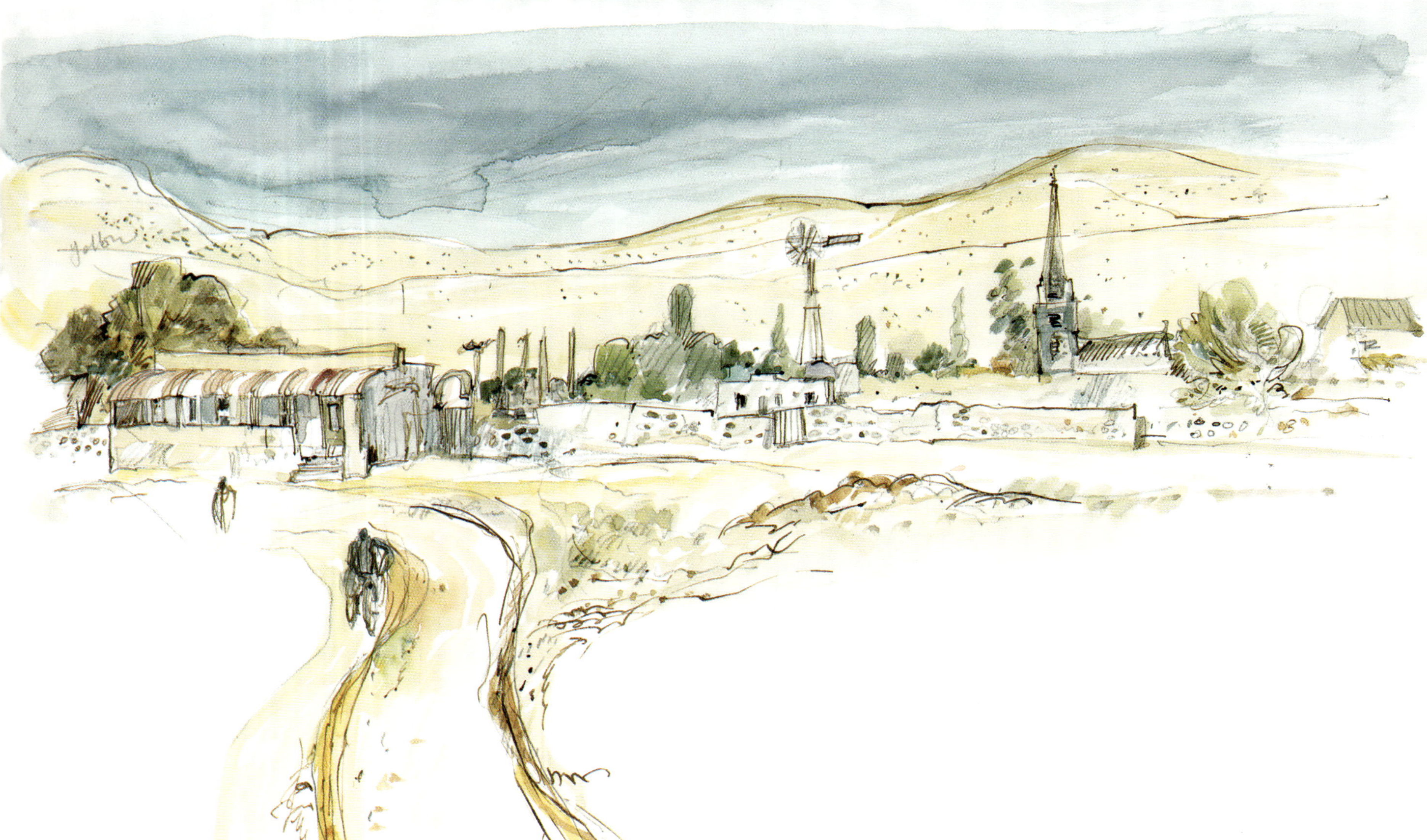

Nieu-Bethesda

Nieu-Bethesda is a remote, tiny village virtually unheard of until the recluse artist Helen Maarten's extraordinary Owl House was discovered. With the help of two men, first Piet van der Merwe and then Koos Malgas, residents of the local township, she created in her garden a strange, crowded fantasy of dream-like figures, birds and animals made of wire and cement and decorated with pieces of coloured glass.

Learned theses have been written about the artistic merit of these sculptures. I find them strangely affecting and disturbing, and walking through her house, which is open to the public, embarrassingly intrusive. It is an intensely private space with its strange shrines, personal paraphernalia and treasures displayed for all to see as it was when Helen lived here. She had a preoccupation with light, which shines through coloured glass and is reflected in mirrors and sparkles on the walls plastered with ground glass. The strange light creates a haunted and unearthly atmosphere.

We visit Koos Malgas in the bleak little township on the hill above the village. He and his family have set up a small business manufacturing owls and Koos is scrap-

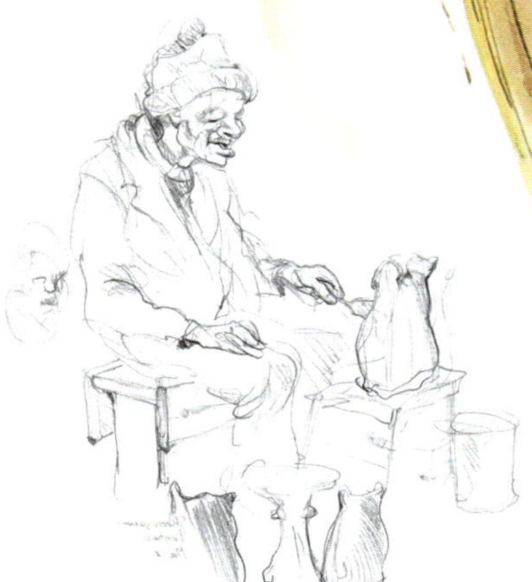

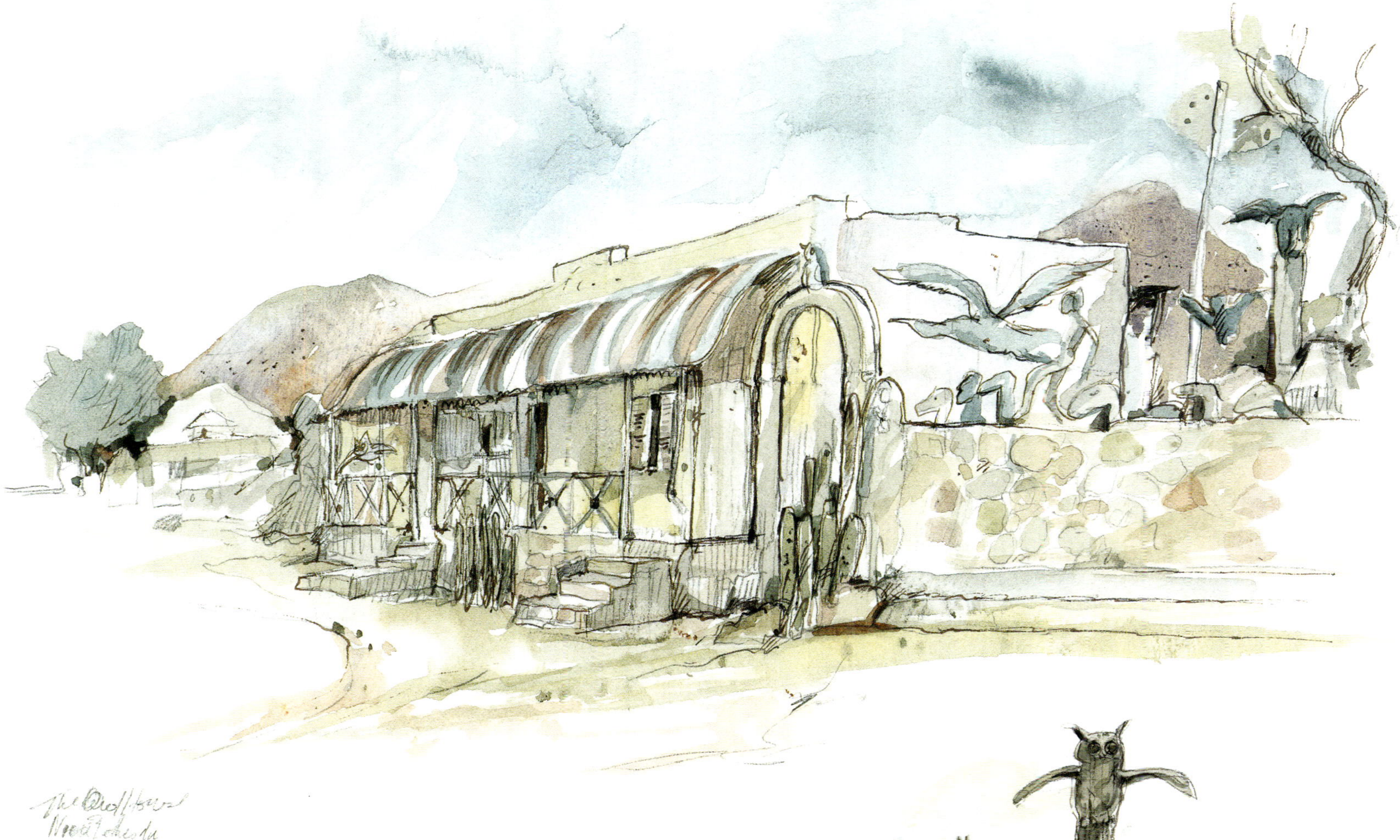

ing away listlessly at his newest creation. He is old, bent and embittered. I sense that he feels exploited by the media and has not been given enough credit, or for that matter reward, for the part he played in creating Helen Maarten's world. Artist Peggy Delport said he did much more than carry out Helen's instructions. "The interpretive process and the forms with their particular elegance were his."

I can barely make out what he is saying as his voice is ruined, either by smoking or inhalation of ground glass, or both, and he pipes and wheezes his way with difficulty through our conversation.

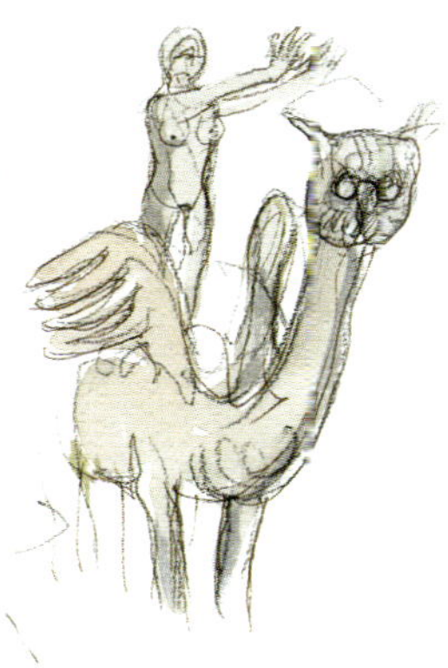

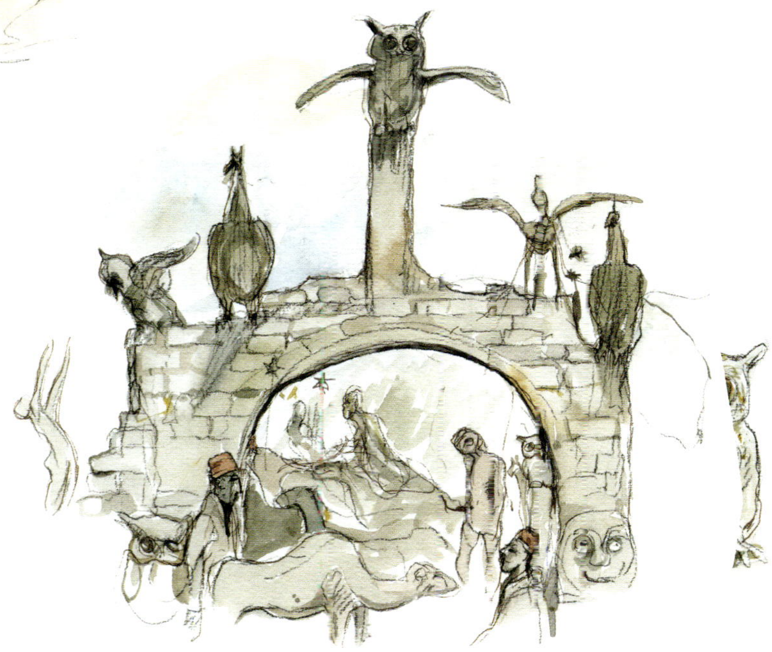

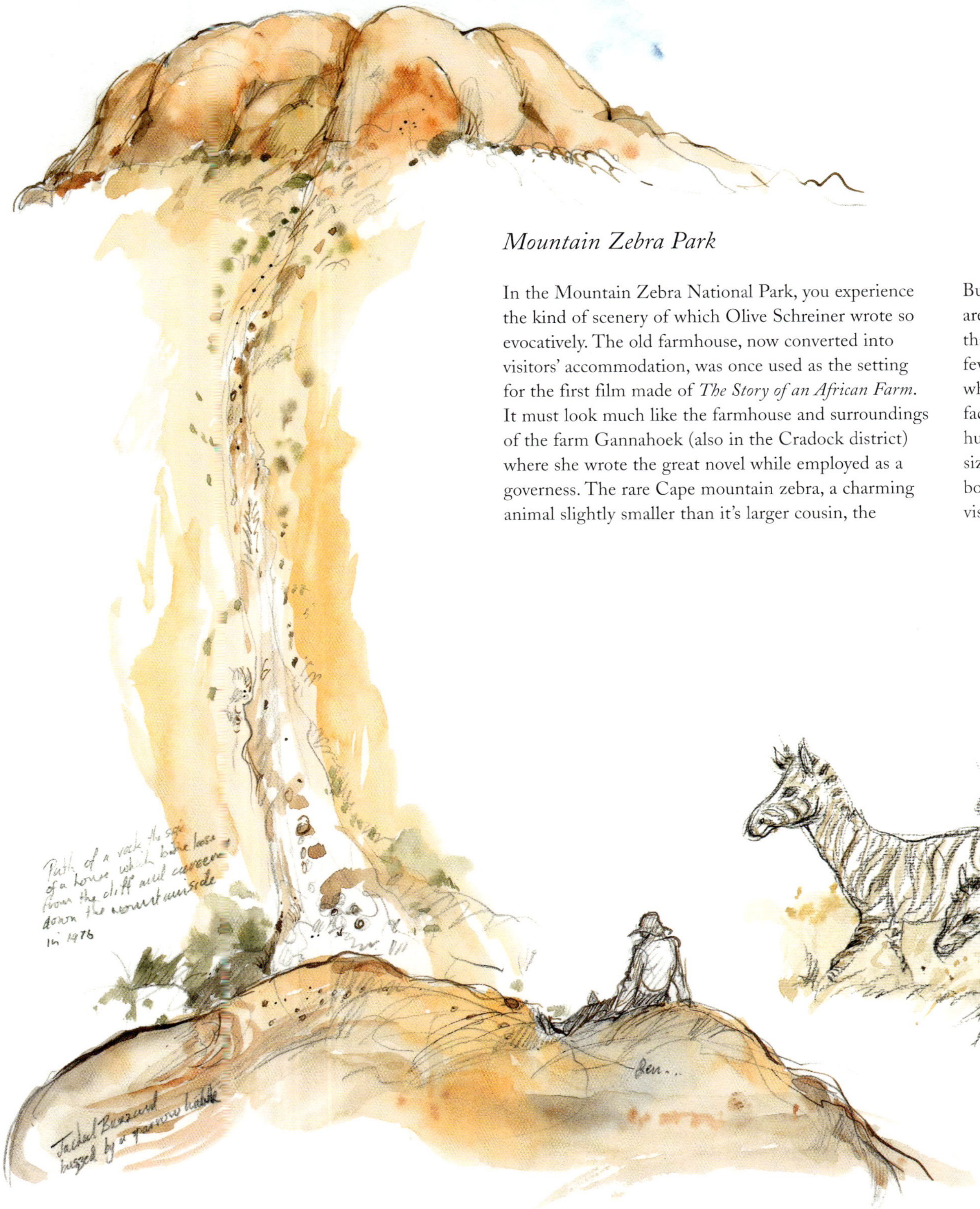

Mountain Zebra Park

In the Mountain Zebra National Park, you experience the kind of scenery of which Olive Schreiner wrote so evocatively. The old farmhouse, now converted into visitors' accommodation, was once used as the setting for the first film made of *The Story of an African Farm*. It must look much like the farmhouse and surroundings of the farm Gannahoek (also in the Cradock district) where she wrote the great novel while employed as a governess. The rare Cape mountain zebra, a charming animal slightly smaller than it's larger cousin, the Burchell's zebra, has a home in the park and its numbers are growing. It is a very pleasant place to walk on tracks that wend their way around the mountain foothills. A few years ago, rangers were startled by a thunderous roar which echoed through the valley when a piece of cliff face from one of the surrounding koppies broke off and hurtled down the mountainside. The huge boulder, the size of a small house, eventually came to rest at the bottom, its destructive path down the mountain still visible today.

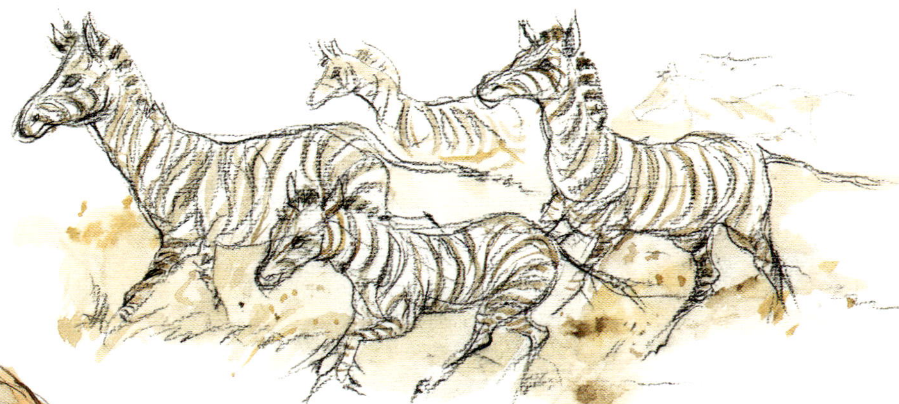

Cradock

Cradock is one of the oldest towns in the Eastern Cape. It takes its name from Governor John Cradock who, in 1814, visited the area and chose the site of a new town on the farm Buffelskloof owned by one of the early trekboers, Pieter van Heerden. Situated on a bend of the Great Fish River, Cradock is a town of considerable charm. Like the Graaff-Reinet Dutch Reformed Church, the town's elegant DRC Church is also based on the design of an English church: St Martin-in-the-Fields in Trafalgar Square, London.

Olive Schreiner is closely associated with the town. She lived here from 1868 to 1870 and later on farms in the district. The Karoo landscape and its people profoundly influenced her and became the context of much of her fiction. We spend time in Schreiner House, a small flat-roofed house in Cross Street, in which there is an exhibition telling the story of her remarkable life.

We overnight in one of Sandra Antrobus' beautifully restored bed-and-breakfast houses in Market Street, where the saddle makers, wagon makers and other craftsmen in the transport industry used to live. With the advent of the car they fell on hard times and couldn't afford to alter their homes, so these houses are the same as they were at the turn of the century. Sandra has collected furniture that dates from that time and the rooms are filled with authentic items, including little improving tomes placed on bedside tables. I was intrigued to hear an elderly Dutch couple enthusing about the furnishings and I asked them why they were so fascinated, coming from a country with a history dating back hundreds of years. "That's just it," they said. "We have retained much from centuries back, but these are things that we can remember from our own lives, and most of that we have thrown away."

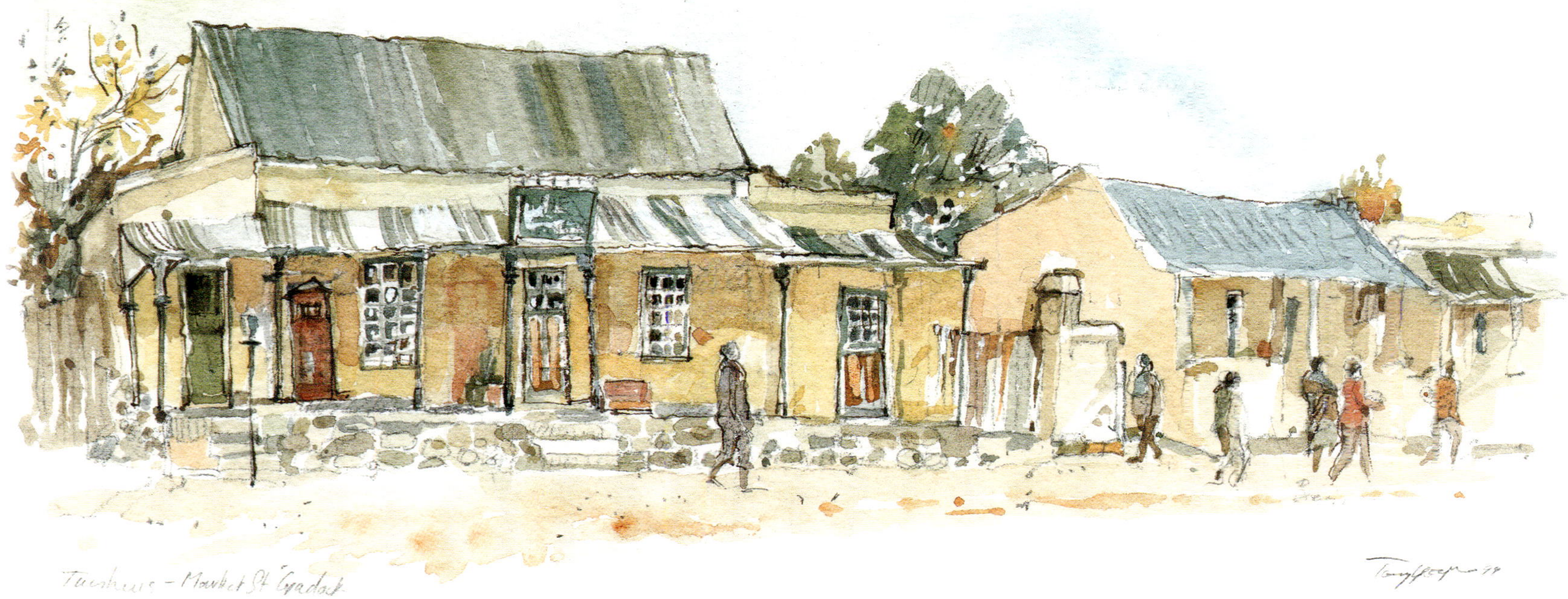

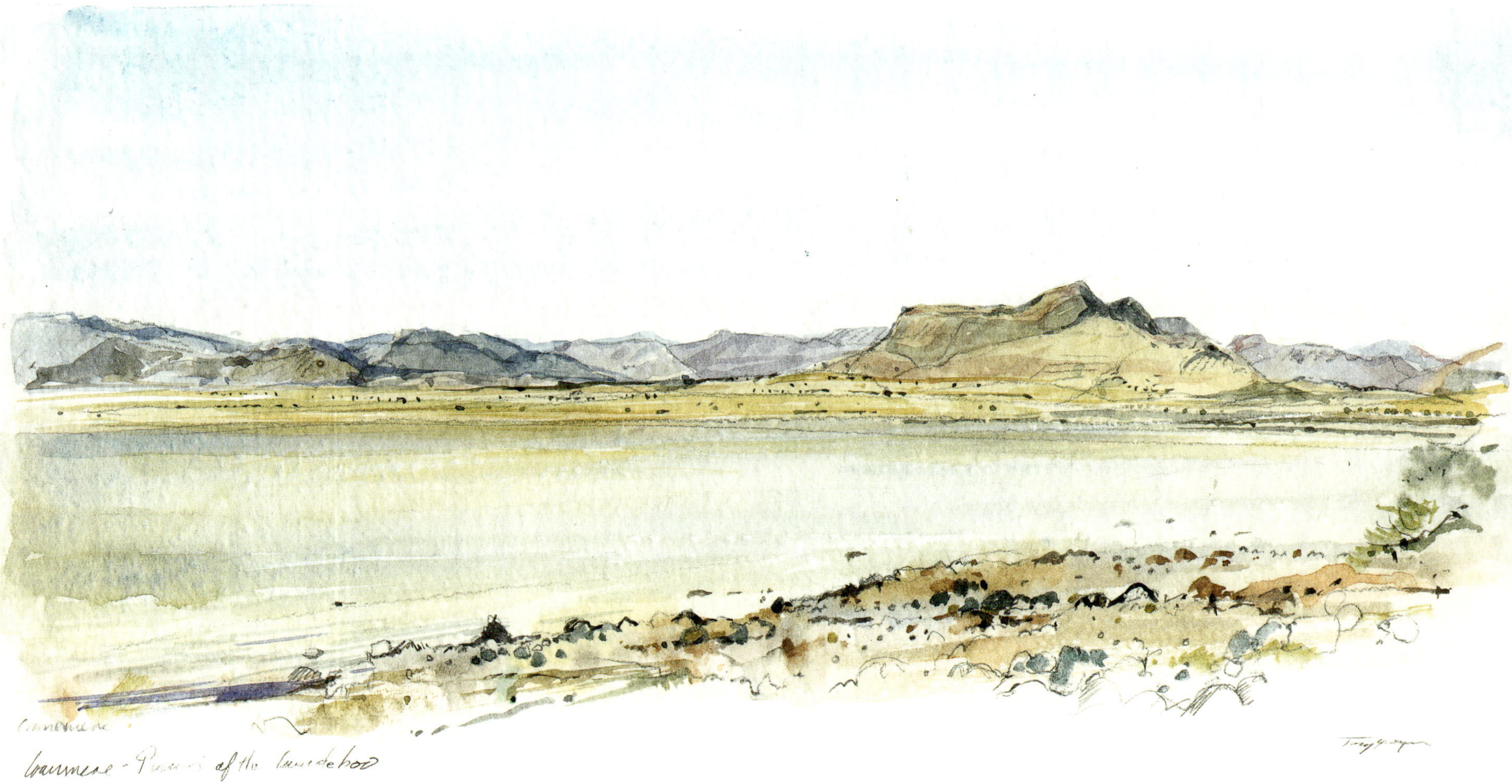

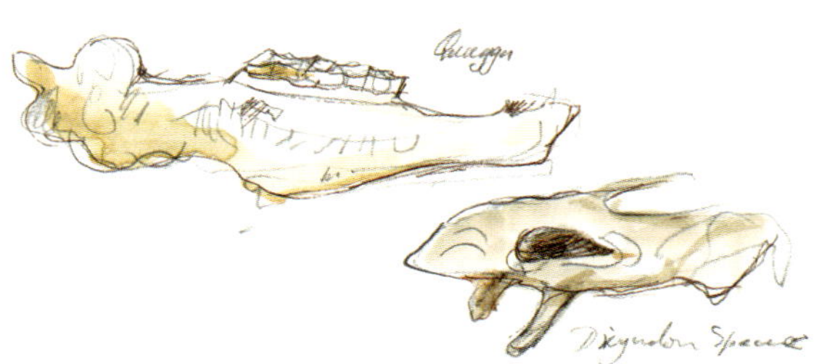

Cranemere

We visit Cranemere, the farm featured in Eve Palmer's classic book of the Karoo, *The Plains of Camdeboo*. It is a windless day and the large dam from which it derives its name shines like glass in the bright morning sun. Eve Palmer has written an engaging and absorbing story of the farm, its natural environment, its prehistory, the family and the fascinating people who have passed this way.

We are met by Eve Palmer's nephew, Alex, who extends a warm Eastern Cape welcome. He invites us to see the farm museum which has a fascinating display of fossils and artefacts collected on Cranemere. One family dig revealed the bones of buffalo, quagga and lions at what must have been a Stone Age slaughtering site. There is the tibia of a wildebeest splintered to serve as a cutting tool. The skull of a young San has a hole in the temple area and scratches in the bone around the wound as evidence of some primitive surgery.

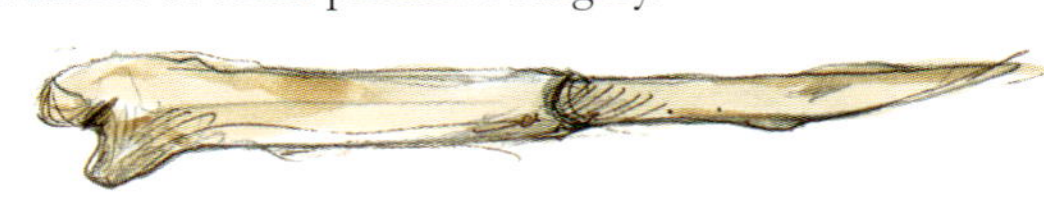

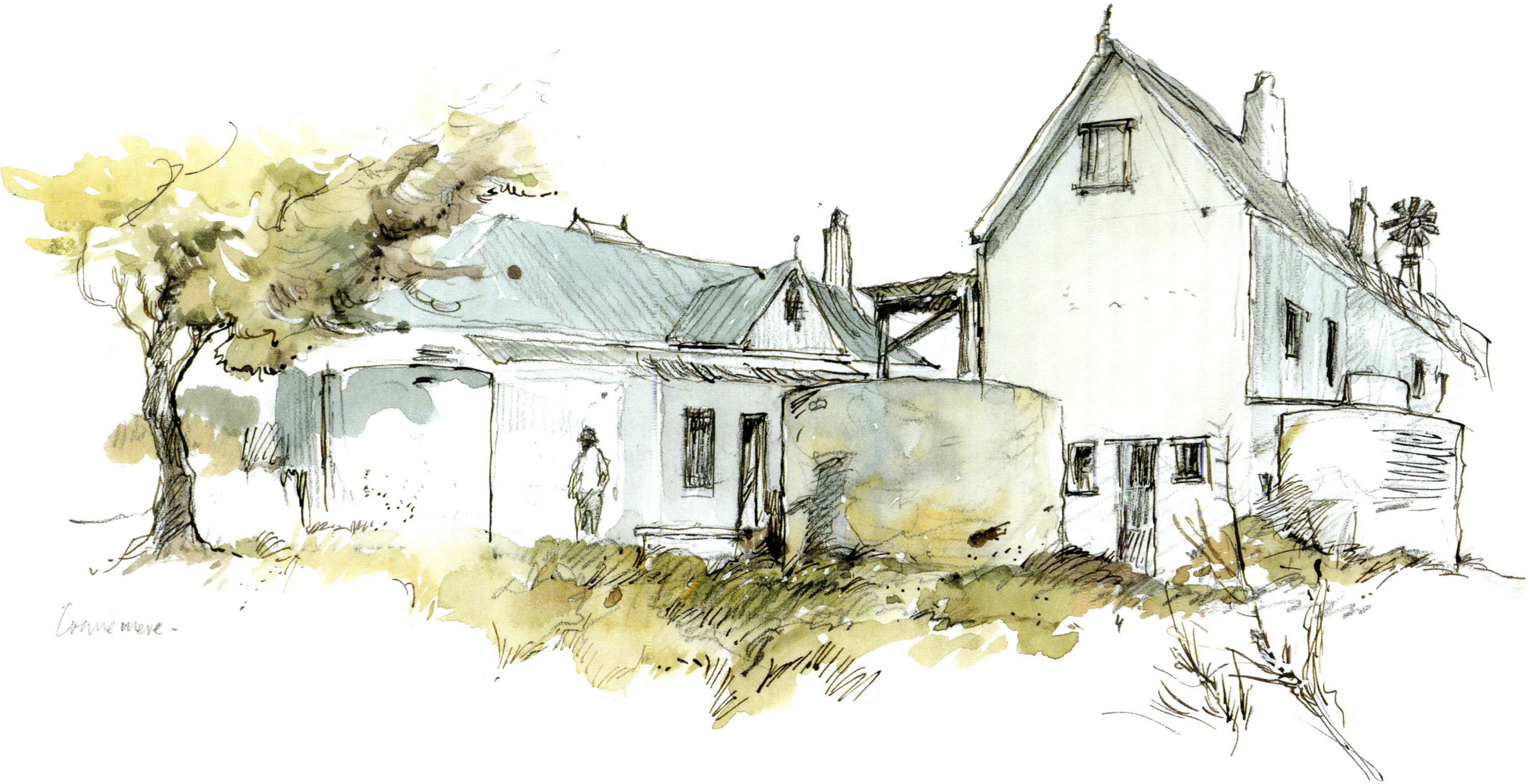

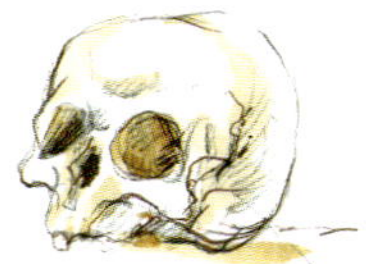

Photographs, drawings and memorabilia of great interest include the old-fashioned typewriter on which Eve Palmer typed the manuscript of *The Plains of Camdeboo* and the original manuscript itself.

Marianne, Alex's wife, has invited us to lunch, which on a Karoo farm is a delicious repast with Karoo lamb, which has its own unique flavour, and a full range of vegetables. Alex's mother, Sita, visiting for the day from Graaff-Reinet, is at 92 a picture of grace and elegance, her ensemble set off by a silk scarf and broad-brimmed straw hat. She is wonderfully animated and keeps us entertained with amusing stories of her experiences when she was a young woman and mistress of the farm. It seems we are lucky to have Alex with us, as Sita once discovered him sleeping peacefully with a Cape cobra coiled up in the shade of his pram. She is not aware that I am making a drawing of her as she relates the story.

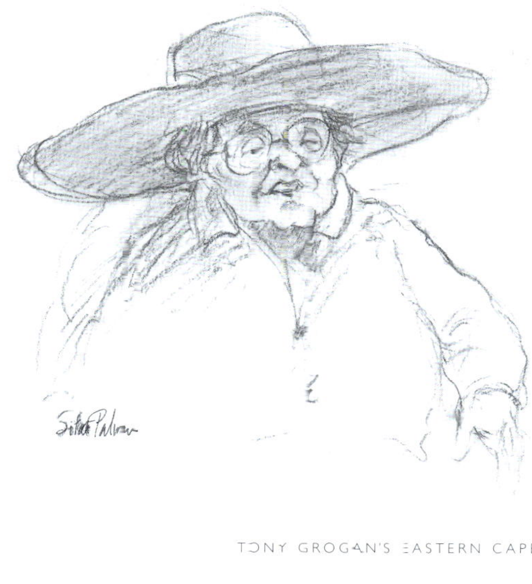

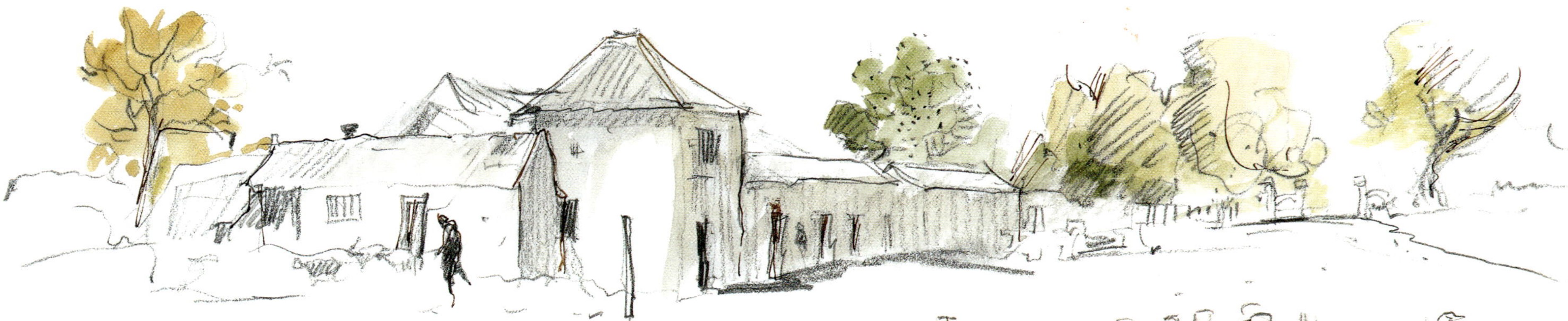

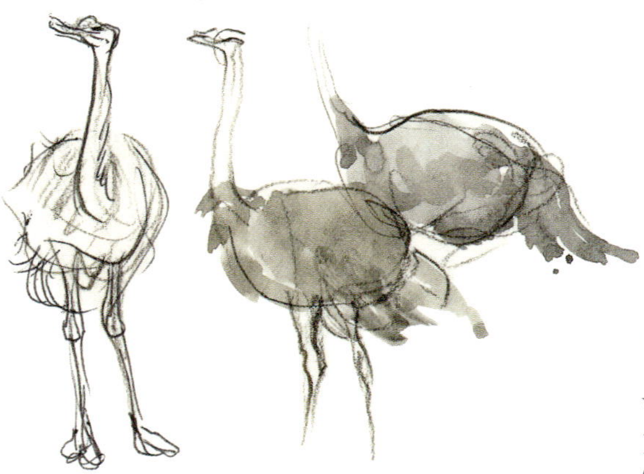

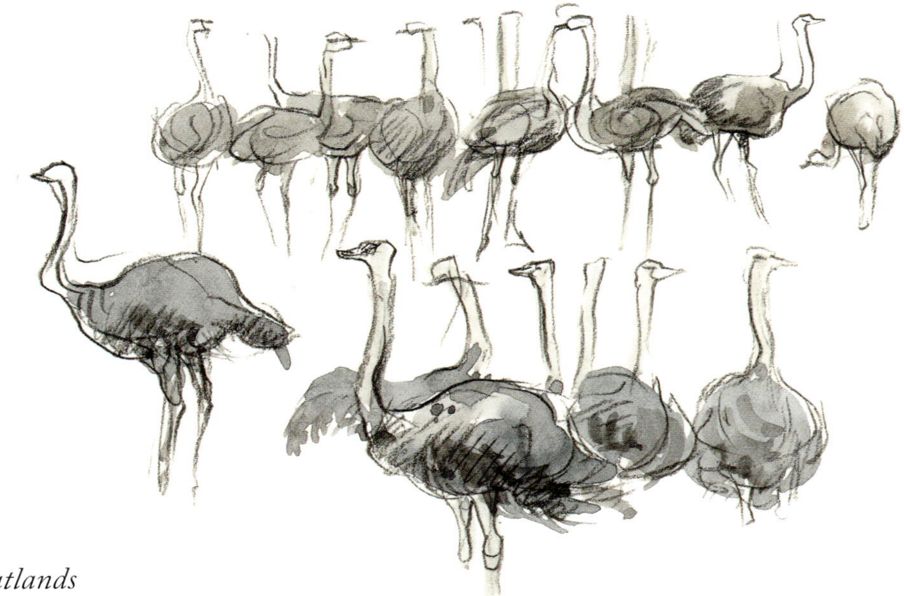

Wheatlands

Wheatlands is a beautiful farm in the Karoo, near Pearston. It was bought in 1849 by an Irishman, Thomas Parks, who first immigrated to Argentina but then decided to leave because of political uncertainties in that country and came to South Africa instead. How times have changed.

The farm first became renowned for its production of brandy – Parks Brandy at 10 shillings a gallon in 1874 became known throughout the country. Arthur Parks, the grandnephew of Thomas, discontinued th distilling, no doubt encouraged by his wife Lily, the daughter of a missionary. Keeping the fires alive was also a problem with labourers tending the furnace fir ing it difficult to refrain from taking the odd *dop* to warm themselves in the freezing Karoo nights. Arth found a more profitable enterprise in ostrich feathers

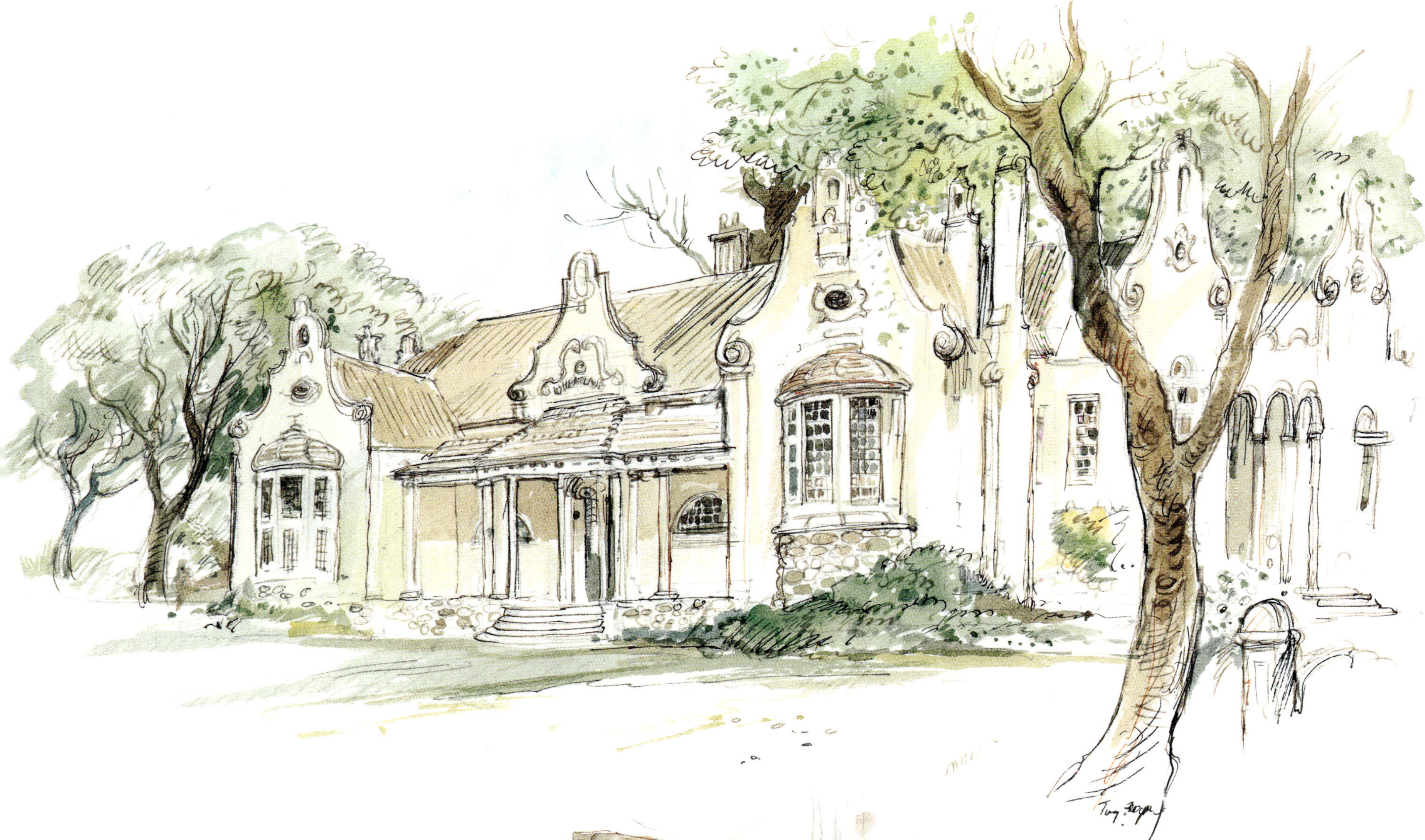

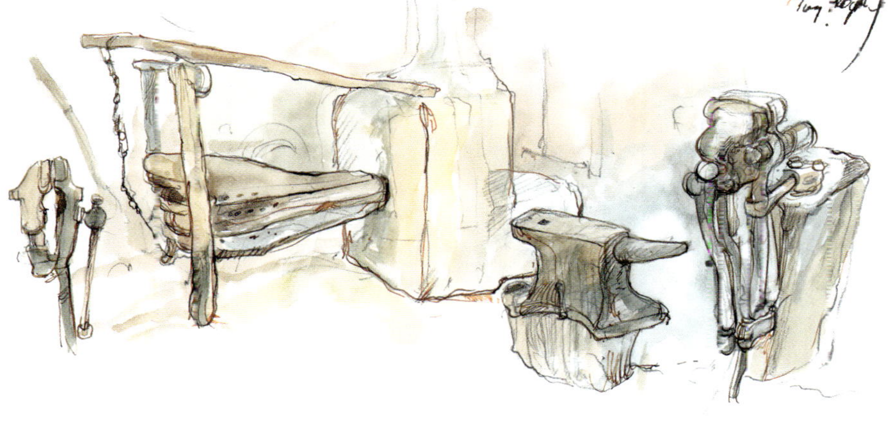

He did extremely well, enabling him to build a beautiful, spacious and sumptuously furnished manor house on Wheatlands. Arthur Short, who represents the fifth generation on the farm, and his wife Di run an elegant bed-and-breakfast establishment in the old house. Jen and I were the only guests and felt most esteemed, as the two of us were attended, at a table laid with fine silverware, which could have seated 20.

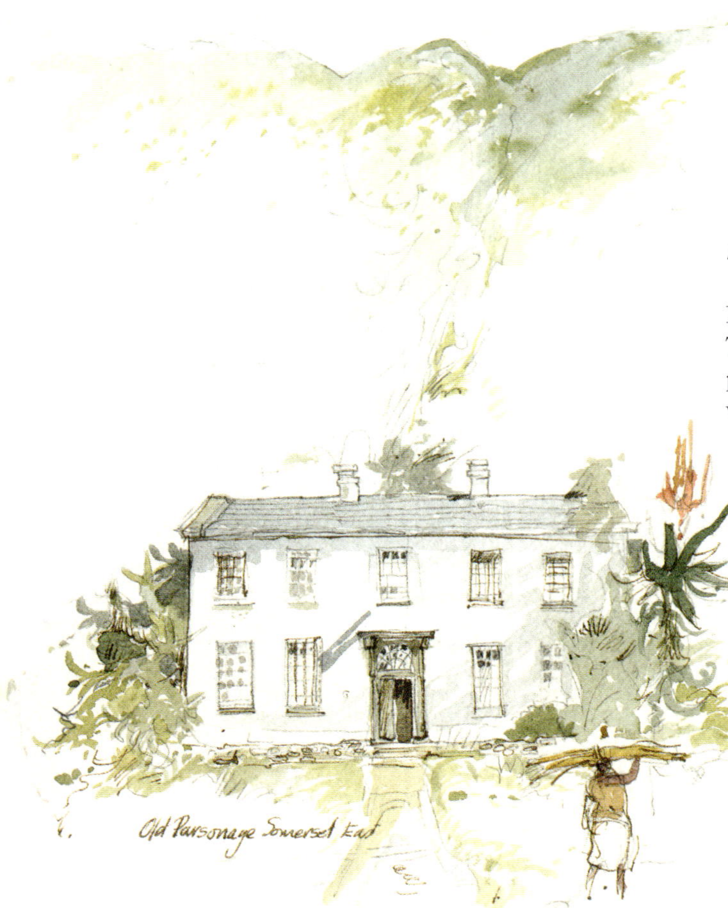
Old Parsonage Somerset East

Somerset East

It is Sunday in Somerset East and the streets are quiet. The only sound is the clinking of bottles carried in a plastic bag by a one-legged man on crutches making his way to the shop at this early hour.

Somerset East was originally established as a farm in 1815 to supply food to the frontier garrisons. The village later laid out on its precincts was named after the then governor, Lord Charles Somerset.

An oak-lined street leads directly to the old Dutch Reformed Church parsonage, now the stately Somerset East Museum. Behind it the densely forested Bosberg mountain provides a lovely backdrop to the town. Across the road from the parsonage is the Walter Battiss Museum which is the house in which the artist grew up. He was not only a great artist but also a great character. I remember meeting Walter Battiss once in the East London Museum. A bohemian figure in an unravelling Aran sweater, faded jeans and a different coloured sandshoe on each foot, he was studying a map of the Eastern Cape coast, looking for an island on which to start an art colony. The only possibility seemed to be a bare rock off Coega and that was already occupied by seabirds, so nothing came of it. The idea later blossomed as an imaginary island called Fook, for which the artist designed a series of stamps.

The farm was originally given to Robert Hart in recognition of the work he did in laying out and administering Somerset Farm for the governor.

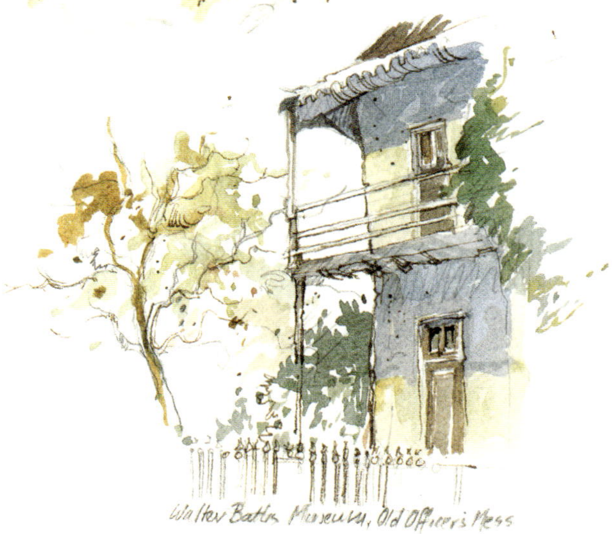
Walter Battis Museum, Old Officer's Mess

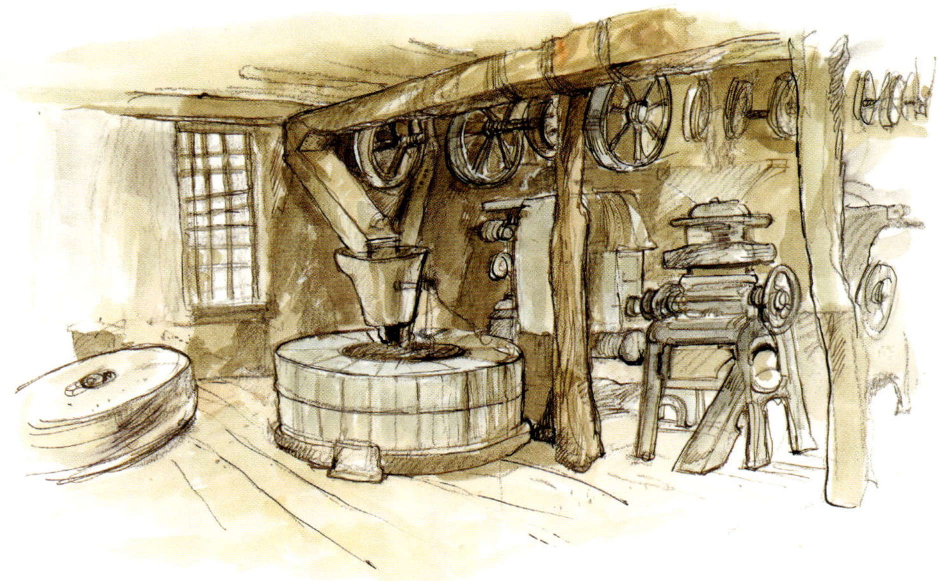

Glen Avon Mill

The old mill on Glen Avon farm, owned by Bill and Alison Brown. The mill, built in 1823, has one of the largest wheels in South Africa and is unusual as it top-driven. The mill was working until 20 years ago. The mill house is three stories high and when we visited, the machinery was intact and the mill wheels still in place. Early transactions written on the beams are still visible and a notice reads 'No spitting or smoking'.

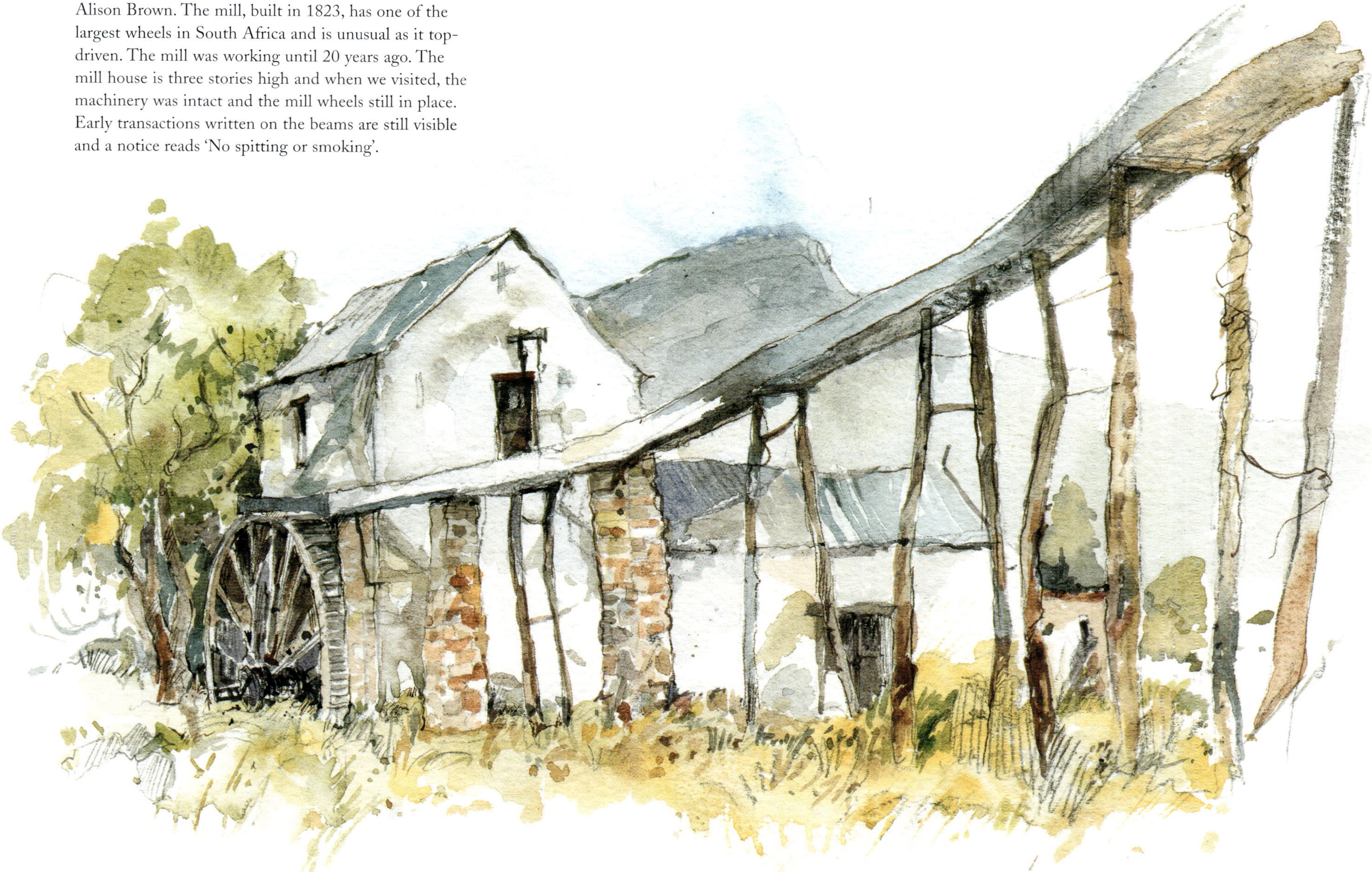

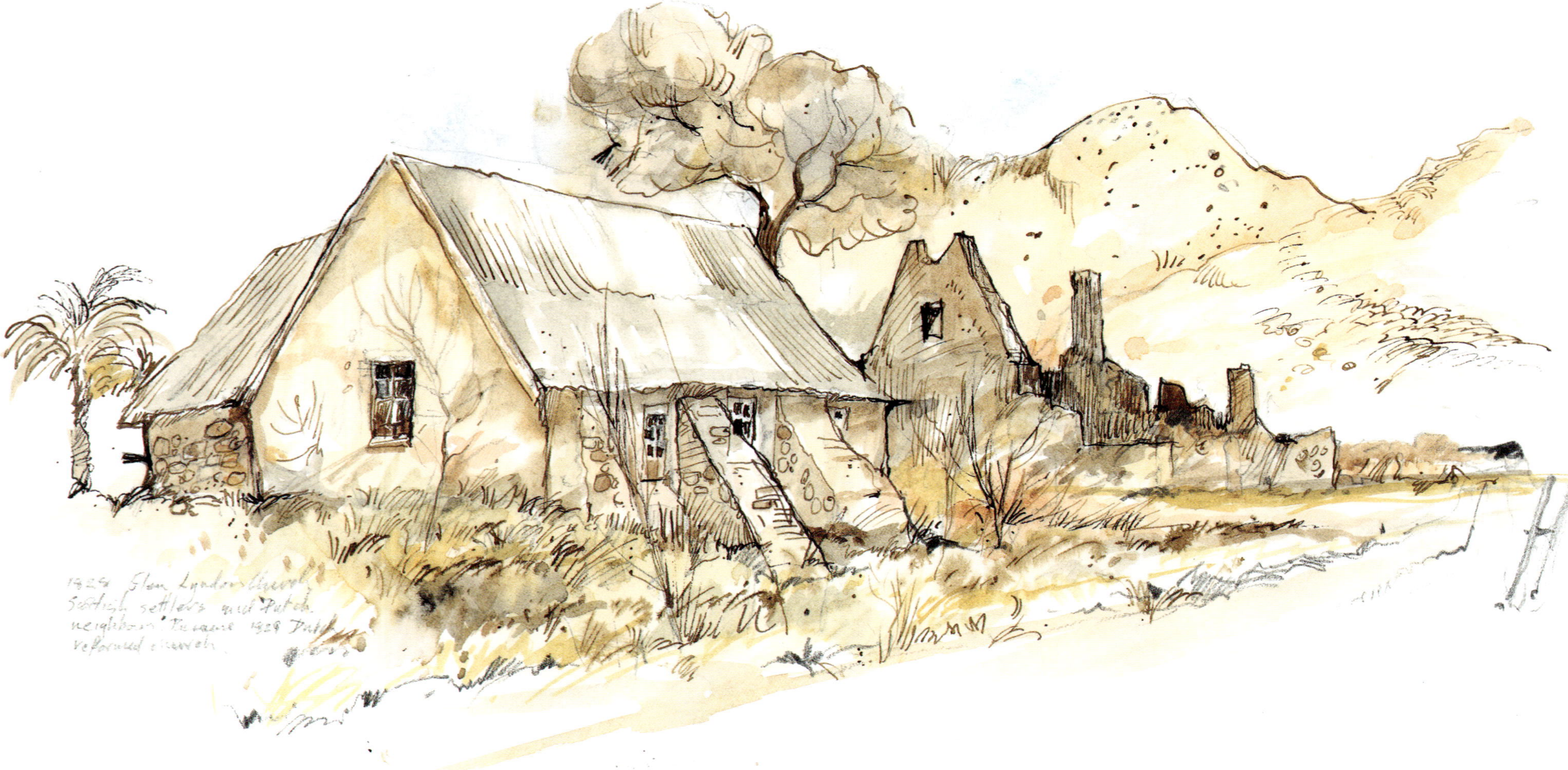
Glen Lynden Church
Scottish settlers and Dutch
neighbours
reformed church

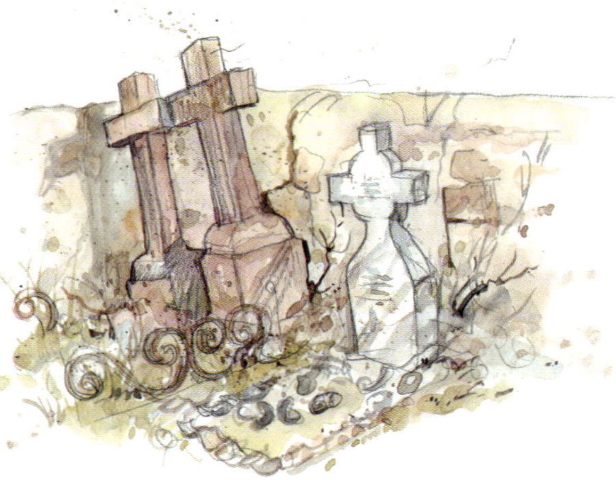

Baviaans Valley

The Baviaans Valley is Pringle country. Thomas Pringle's party of Scottish settlers was given land in this secluded valley in 1820, far from the main body of settlers in the Albany area south of Grahamstown. The witgat tree under which Thomas Pringle built his beehive hut can still be seen on the farm Glen Eildon, owned by Alex and Barrie Pringle.

Pringle describes his location in approving and elegant prose in his *Narrative of a Residence in South Africa*: "The bottom of the valley, through which the

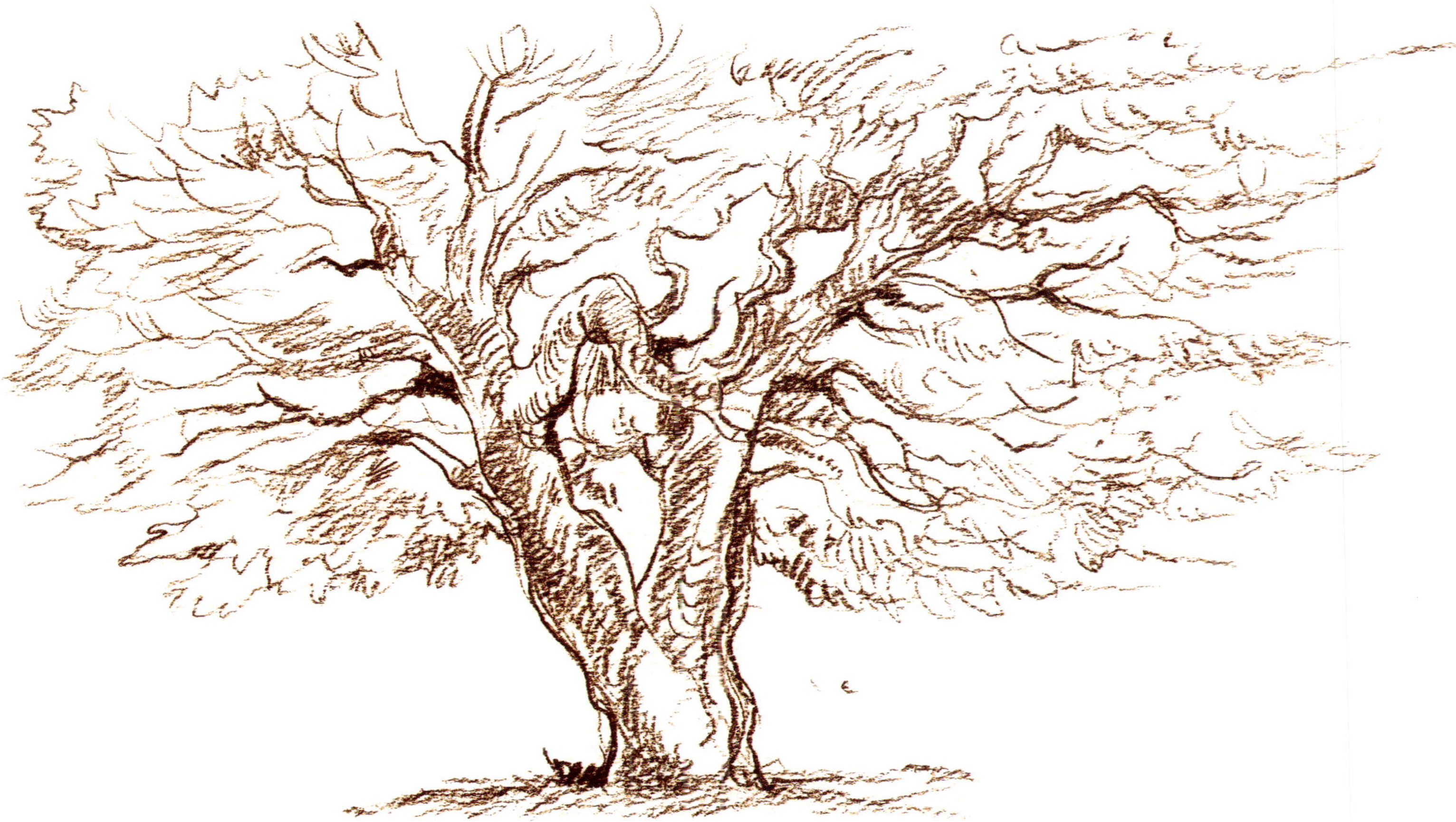

infant river meandered, presented a warm, pleasant, and secluded aspect; spreading itself into the verdant meadows, sheltered and embellished, without being encumbered, with the groves of mimosa trees among which we observed in the distance herds of wild animals – antelopes and quaggas – pasturing in undisturbed quietude."

The first church built in 1828 by the settlers is the Glen Lyndon church, which can be seen on the side of the tortuous road winding its way through the Baviaans River Valley. From the church, a straggling footpath through dry, thorny scrub leads to an overgrown, neglected graveyard. The heat at this time of the year is ferocious. There is no water in the river, and flanks of smooth black ironstone in the river bed lie exposed and shining in the blazing sun. Ironically, a marble stone in the unkempt graveyard has a poignant inscription: 'In loving memory of William Nash, son of BM and MA Webber, who drowned while bathing at Glen Lyndon 20.1.1880.'

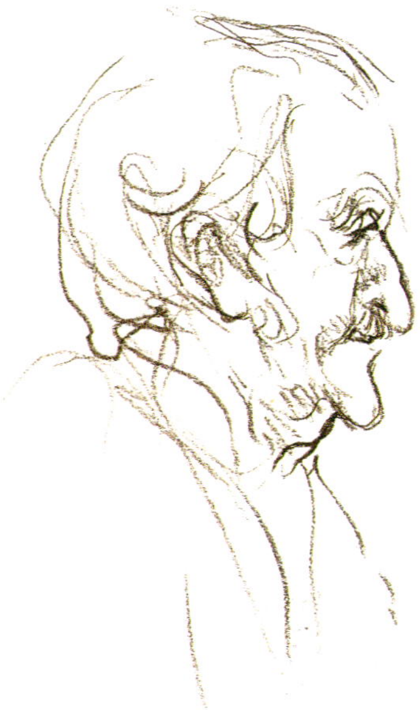

Victor Pringle

On an earlier visit, Kim van Niekerk took us up the Baviaans River Valley in driving rain to meet Ernest Pringle, lawyer, farmer and lepidopterist. On his remote farm, Huntly Glen, he showed us his incredible collection of butterflies which includes every species and variant known in South Africa, several named after him. We met his father, Victor, who has since died. In the same room, presented just as immaculately and annotated with a complete record of how and where each specimen was found, is Victor's egg collection, begun when he was a boy. Victor was also renowned as the best rooikat (caracal) hunter in the district. A stuffed specimen peered over his shoulder as I drew him. He told the story of how he was called by a farmer to get rid of one of the cats that was decimating his sheep. Arriving at the farmhouse door at six in the morning, Victor was offered a cup of coffee by the farmer before he got on with the job of tracking down the rooikat. "Actually, I've already done it," he said pointing at the dead cat lying near the front door.

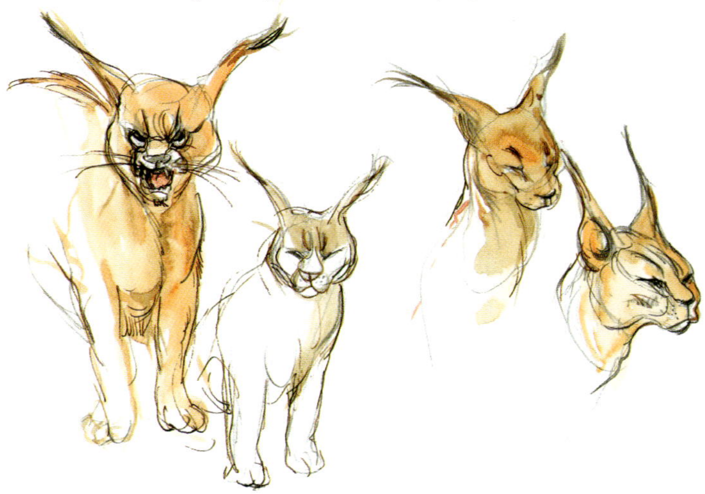

Ernest Pringle

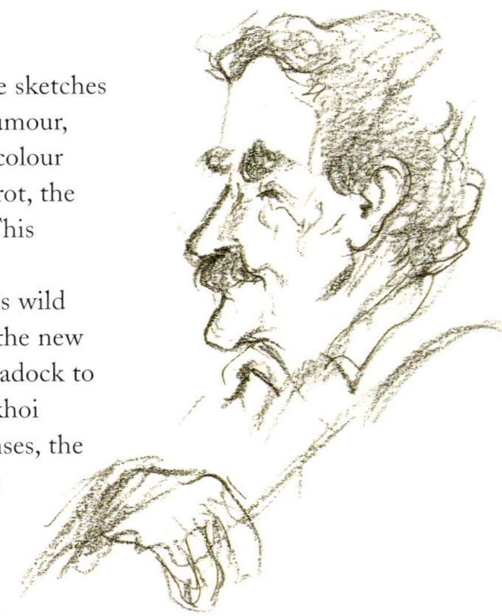

Ernest Pringle is also a keen local historian. He sketches the history of the valley with animation and humour, padding it out with a few ghost stories to add colour and mystery. He takes us to Bezuidenhout's Grot, the scene of Frederick Bezuidenhout's last stand. This gentleman, one of the trekboers, a people of independent and unruly spirit who lived on this wild frontier in the early 1800s, was summoned by the new British administration to appear in court in Cradock to answer charges of mistreating one of his Khoikhoi servants. After he had ignored several summonses, the authorities sent a military detachment to bring him in. These troops consisted mainly of pandoors (Khoikhoi levies), which further inflamed him. Bezuidenhout, defiant to the last, hid himself and an unwilling and terrified farmhand believed to have been his half-breed son, in a cleft in a rocky outcrop overlooking the river from which vantage point he opened fire on the approaching party. In the ensuing standoff, after a brisk exchange of fire, Bezuidenhout was shot and killed.

This resulted in the so-called Slagter's Nek rebellion, a half-baked effort easily and ruthlessly put down by the British. After a lengthy trial, the ringleaders were sentenced to death and subjected to an appallingly blundered and callous execution. In the early part of the 20th century, the incident was frequently seized upon and used for propaganda purposes by the National party to stir up anti-English sentiment.

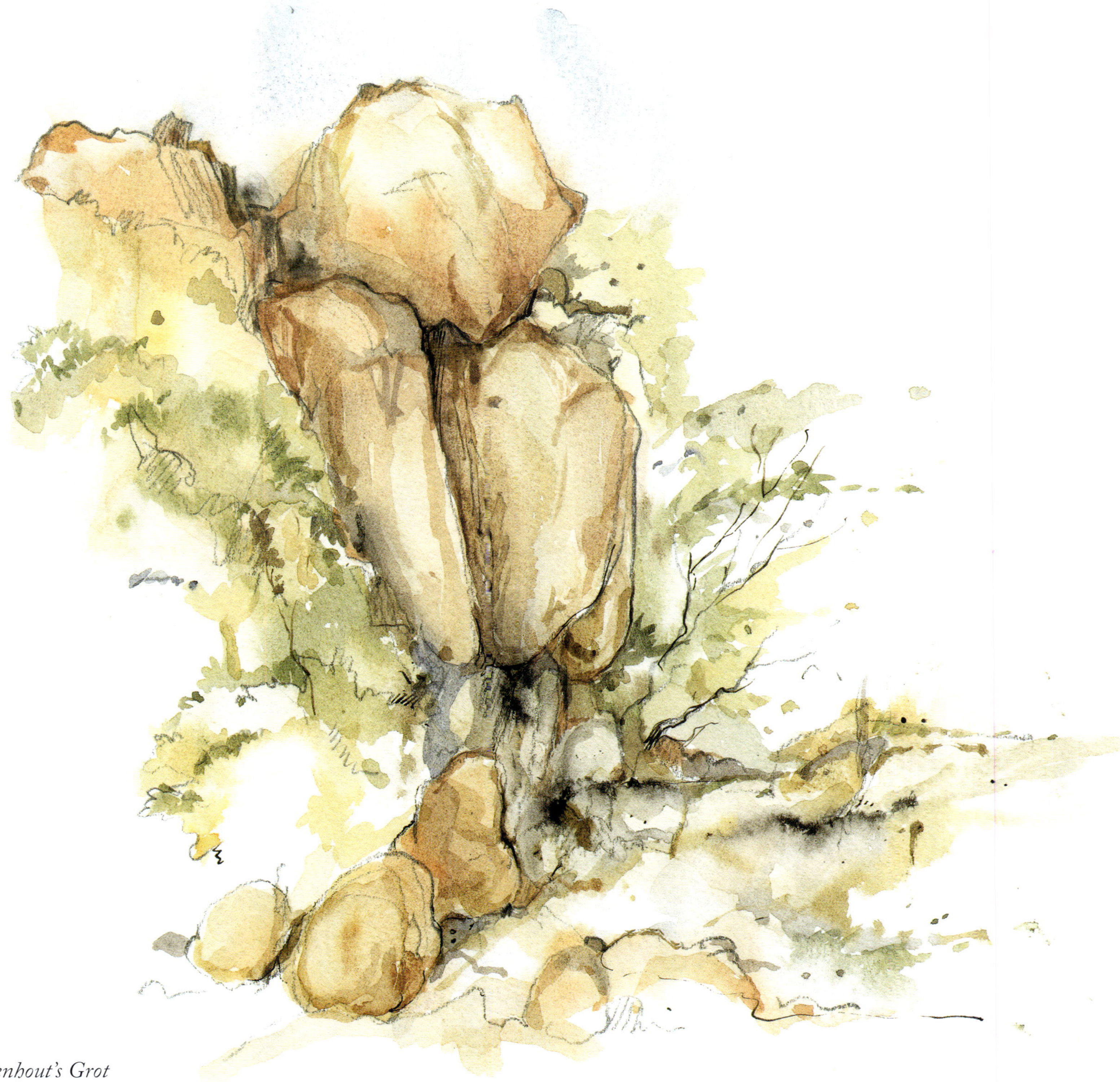

Bezuidenhout's Grot

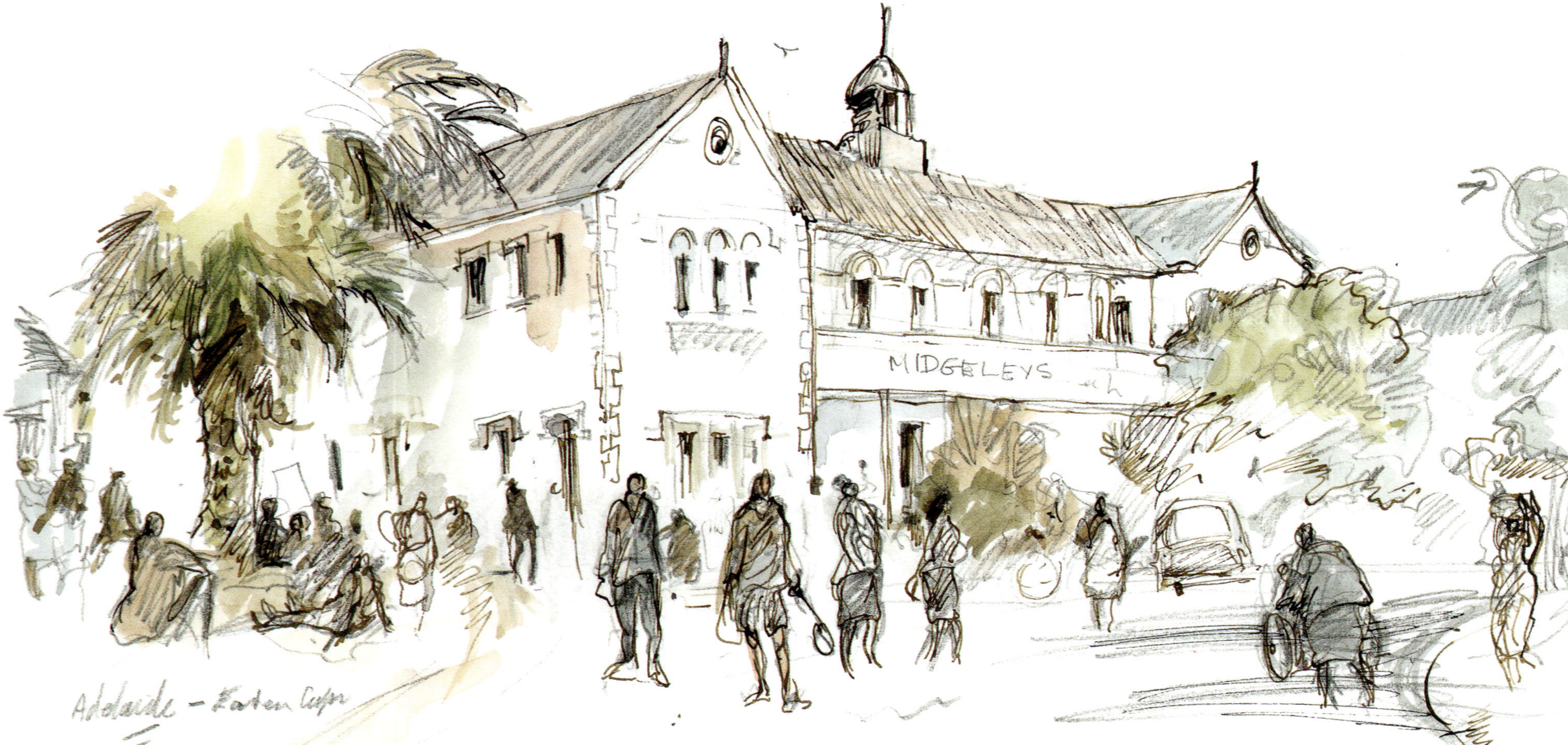

Adelaide voting day

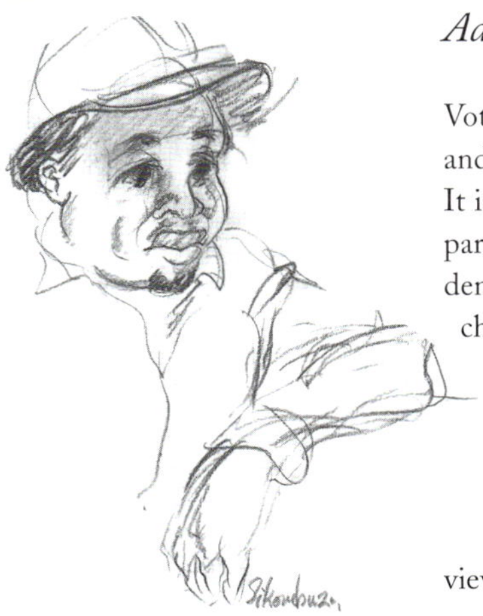

Voting day in Adelaide. It is five o'clock in the evening and some farmers have brought their workers in to vote. It is a languid, desultory affair. No one seems particularly excited about exercising his or her democratic rights, and a few voters idle away their time chatting. A large overweight policeman lolls in a canvas chair at the door of the voting hall. He is a token security provision, like the razor wire draped at various points around the hall and the ribbons of no-entry tape, which most voters casually ignore.

Sikumbuza, leaning on a bakkie, takes a jaundiced view of proceedings. "There you are," he says, gesturing to a large black limousine bearing an official presence. "They drive around in big cars, make promises and give you a T-shirt, and that's the last you see of them."

The election in the little Eastern Cape dorp has been a quiet affair. This morning there was a demonstration and placards waved in the township, which was quelled by the police. The protesters were expressing their disappointment at non-delivery.

Weary cynicism seems to be the prevailing attitude of the farmers.

"Who are you going to vote for?" a farmer asked his guys. "Promises, promises are that all you'll get. Who

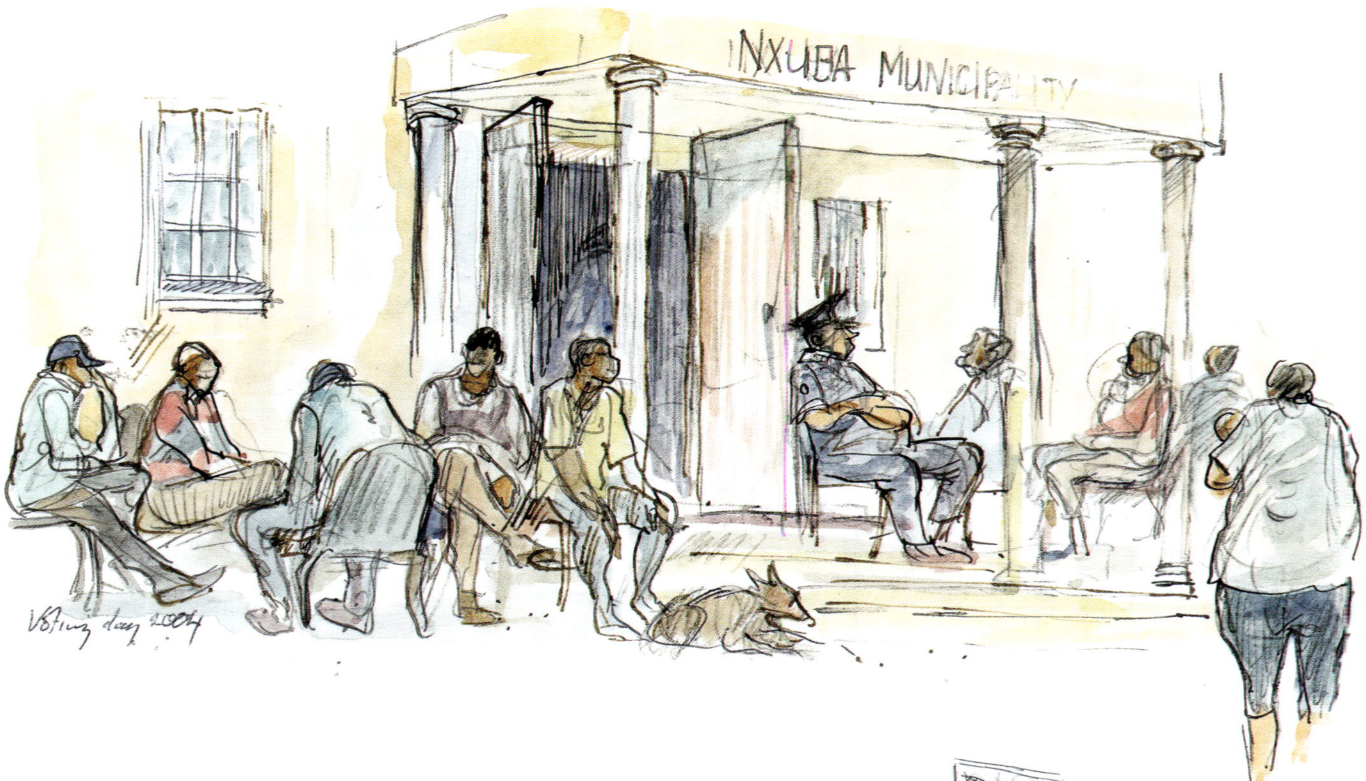

am I going to vote for? A heifer, that's who I'm going to vote for. If a heifer promises me milk, I'll get milk!"

Three hefty farmers are discussing the affairs of the day. "What you need to bring on to your land are camels," says one authoritively. "They'll eat up all those mimosas and their droppings will nutrify the soil."

"What am I going to tell an American hunter who is looking for kudu and comes across a camel in the bush?" asks Chris, who has a game farm.

"Anyway, if you want to sort out the problem, get camels. The problem is goats." He refers to another farmer who has allowed goats to run riot on his land. "If you want to see a f.....ed up farm, go and see ... 's." He mentions the name of a farmer in the district.

We repair to the local pub. Somebody observes that voting isn't over yet so the pub shouldn't be open. But it's late in the day, it's been hot all day, voting is nearly over; it's only a small town in the Eastern Cape and who cares anyway?

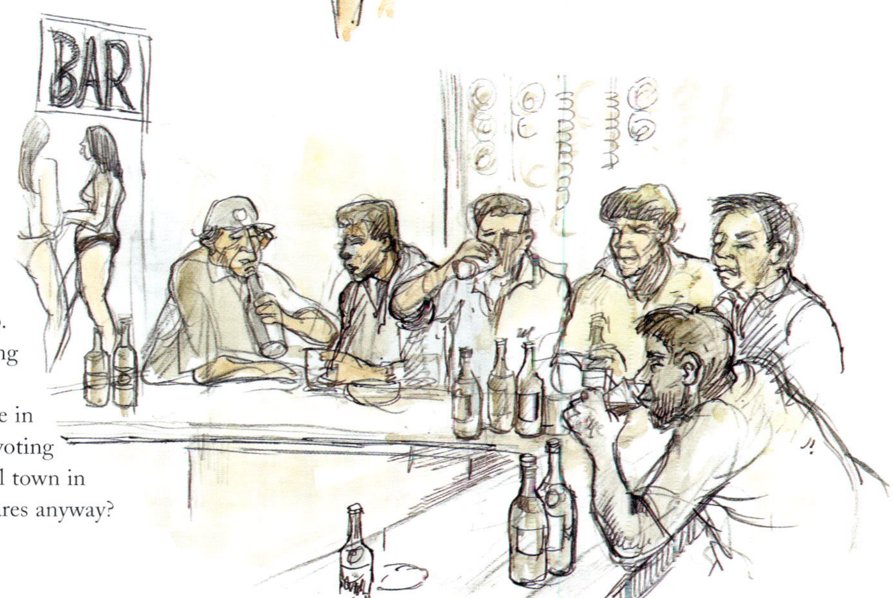

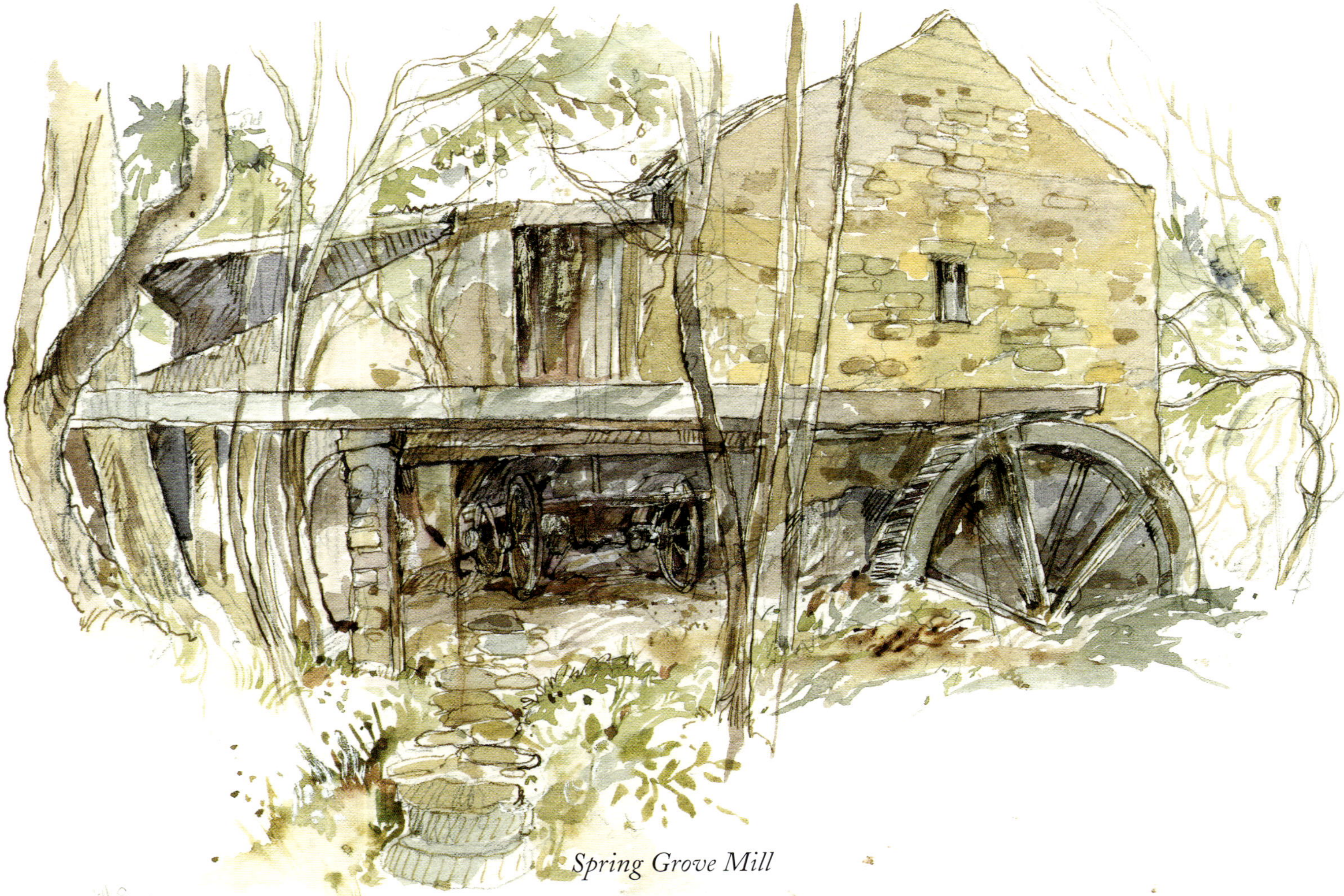

Spring Grove Mill

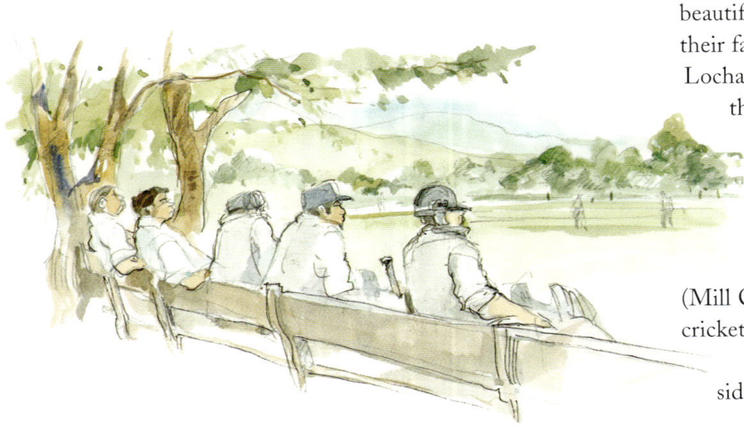

The Anslie family have owned their farm in the beautiful Cowie Valley for six generations. The mill on their farm Spring Grove was in use until fairly recently. Lochart Ainslie tells me of the terrible accident when the miller was entangled in the machinery and killed. His father never used the mill again after the tragedy.

I made this drawing before Lochart had converted the mill into a characterful pub, the Mill, which serves as the clubhouse for the MCC (Mill Cricket Club). Matches are played on the Mill cricket field, ringed by ancient oaks with a beautiful mountain backdrop. There is a match against a side from Port Elizabeth today. It is a picture of serene gentility, the click of ball on bat, the occasional shouts and appeals from the players, and wives and children picnicking in the shade of the oaks. In the farmhouse, some of the ladies are settling down to a game of bridge.

This drawing now doesn't show the huge stone slabs now used as outside tables for the pub. Lochart explains that they are completely weather resistant so there's no need for treatment with Woodoc.

Farms in the Cowie Valley are renowned for their beautiful gardens and are visited by garden lovers from all over the country. Cavers is a fine example.

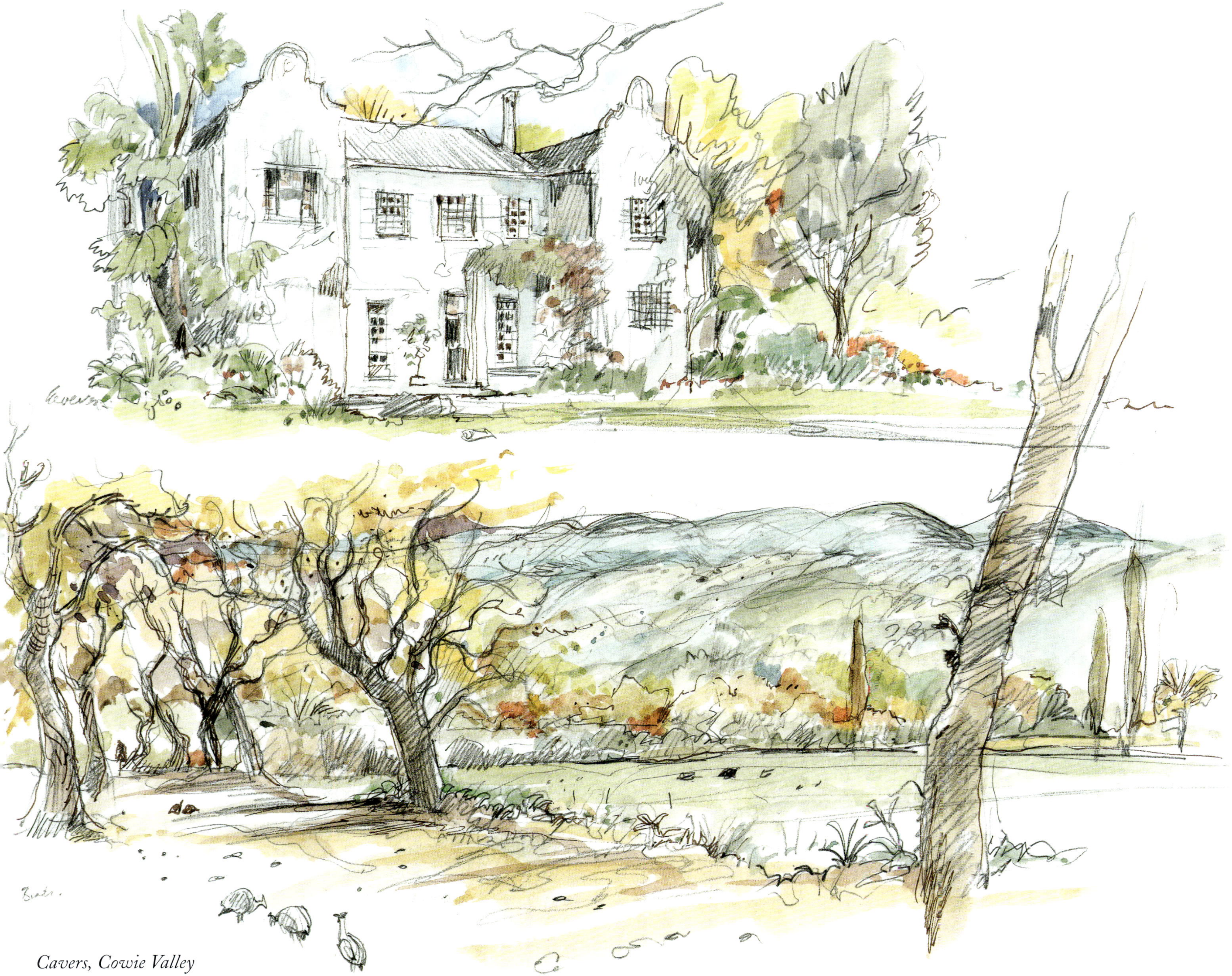

Cavers, Cowie Valley

Stock sale

Stock sales are important events on the Eastern Cape farming and social calendar. Watch these tough, sun-browned farmers leaning on the pens earnestly discussing sheep dip, cattle-sickness, the weather or sneering at the latest disastrous performance of the Springbok rugby side, and you sense their camaraderie and realise that events like these are what makes farming still a worthwhile occupation. I took my sketchbook along to a couple of these sales and sketched the scene – the confused animals milling about and some of the rough-hewn countenances of the farmers scrutinising them. Someone leaned over my shoulder and made the unkind remark that the goats were better looking. Some of them were perfect prototypes of the characters affectionately and hilariously parodied in David Mullins and Alan Weyer *Boet and Swaer* sketches which capture to perfection the perplexed, slow-talking, rural types baffled and buffeted by fate and the weather, and trying to make sense of an unkind and increasingly complex world.

The auctioneer is a star performer, whipping up flagging interest when a group of sleek heifers is driven into the paddock.

"My goodness, what have we here?" he announces in awe and wonder. "I have never seen such beautiful beasts! Where have they come from?!" His tone suggests they are divine beasts herded in from a celestial pasture.

It's a smooth and uninterrupted flow of wisecracks and exaggerated claims. "Come on now," he says, "You'll

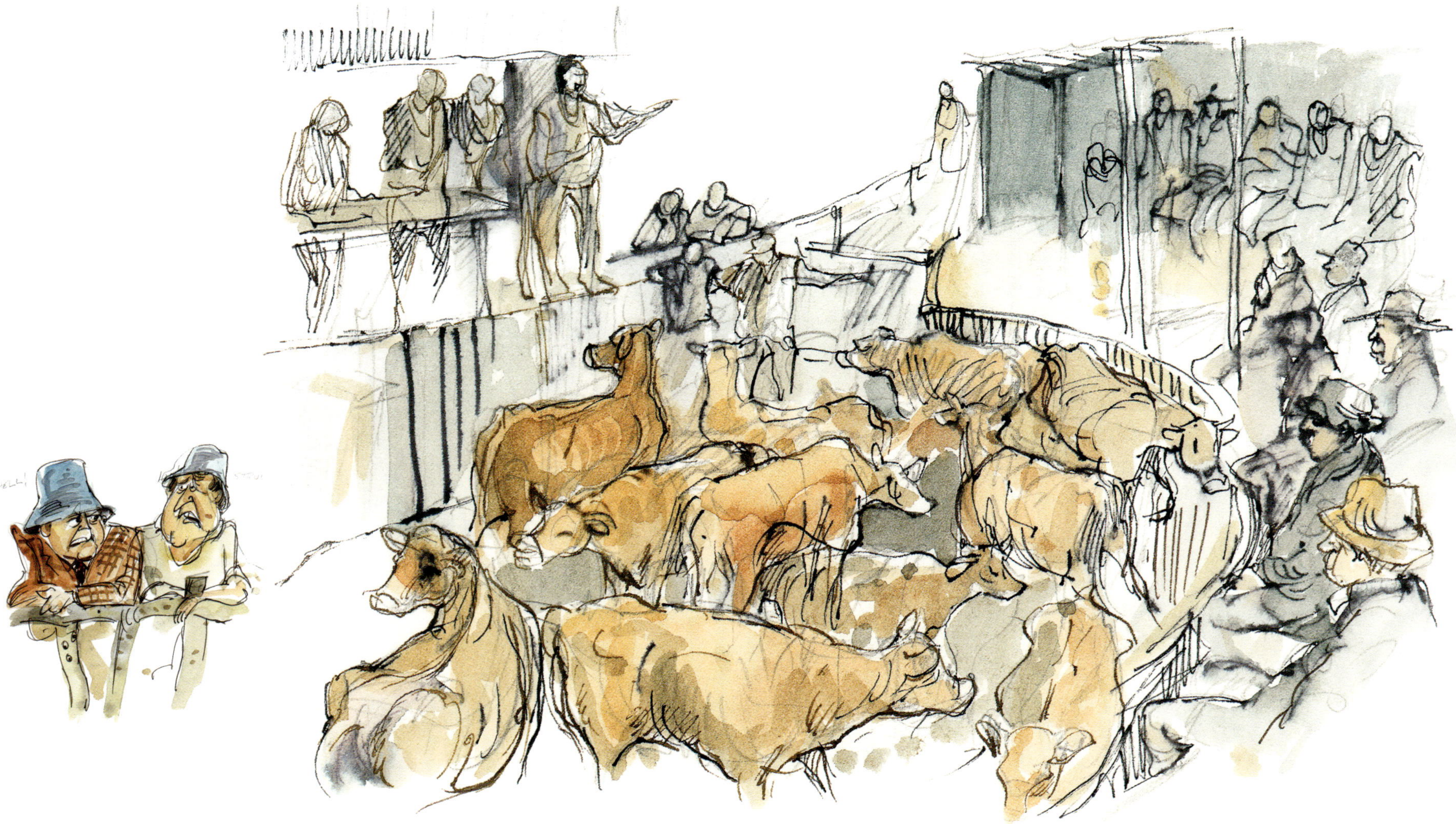

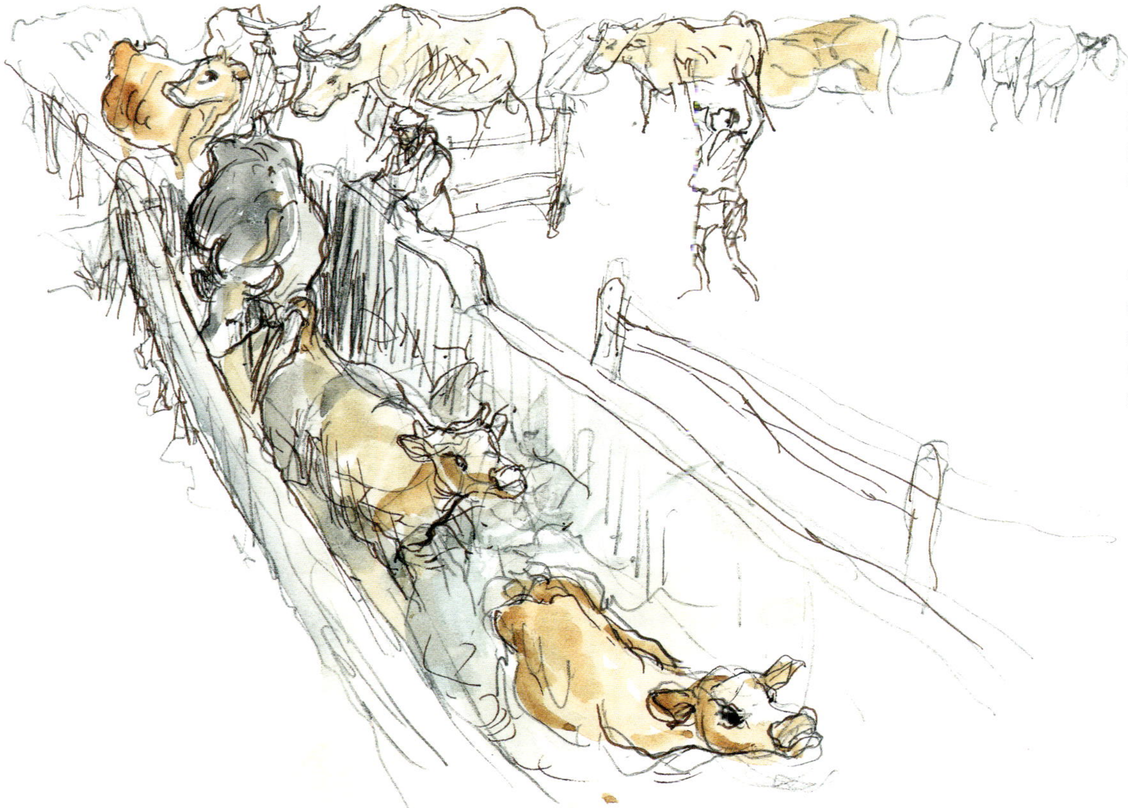

never get a bargain like this again. There's Bob...". He points to one of the farmers placidly watching proceedings. 'He's so rich, if he stood on his wallet and stepped off, he'd sprain his ankle."

I position myself at the far side of the tank to draw cattle being dipped. There is a lot of whistling and shouting by the herders but the cattle seem quite accepting of the process, each one teetering on the edge of the tank before launching itself into the water with a thunderous splash.

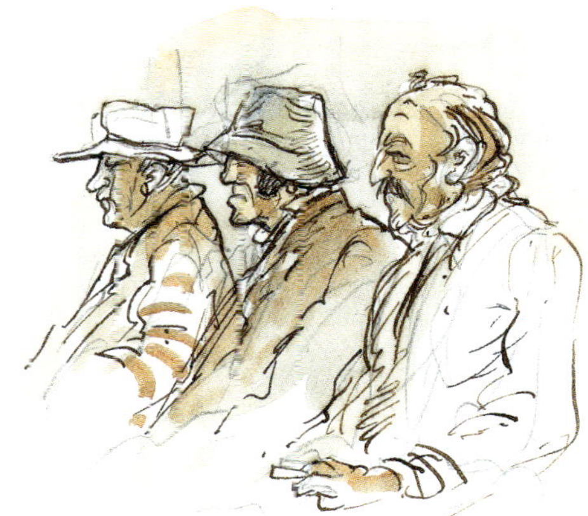

Farmers at Bedford Stock auction.

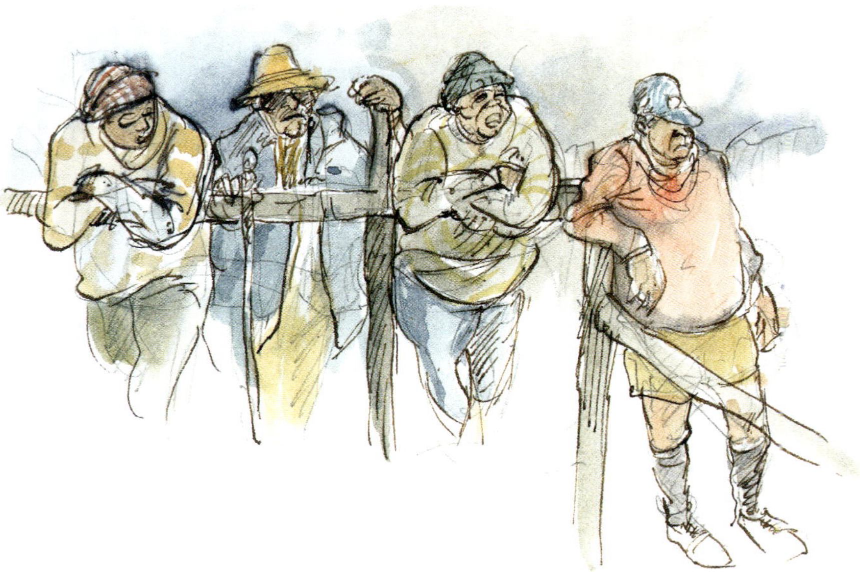

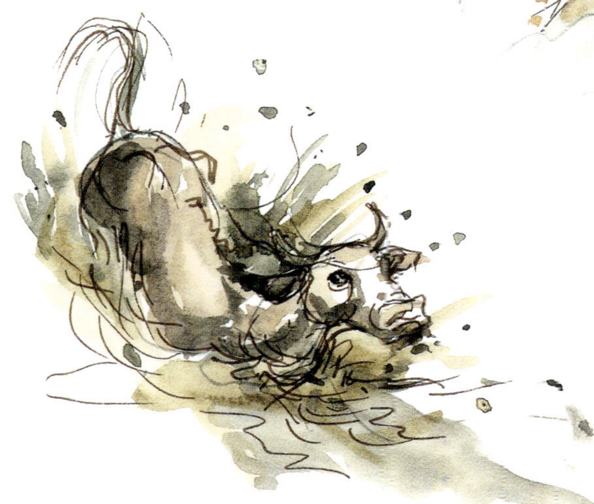

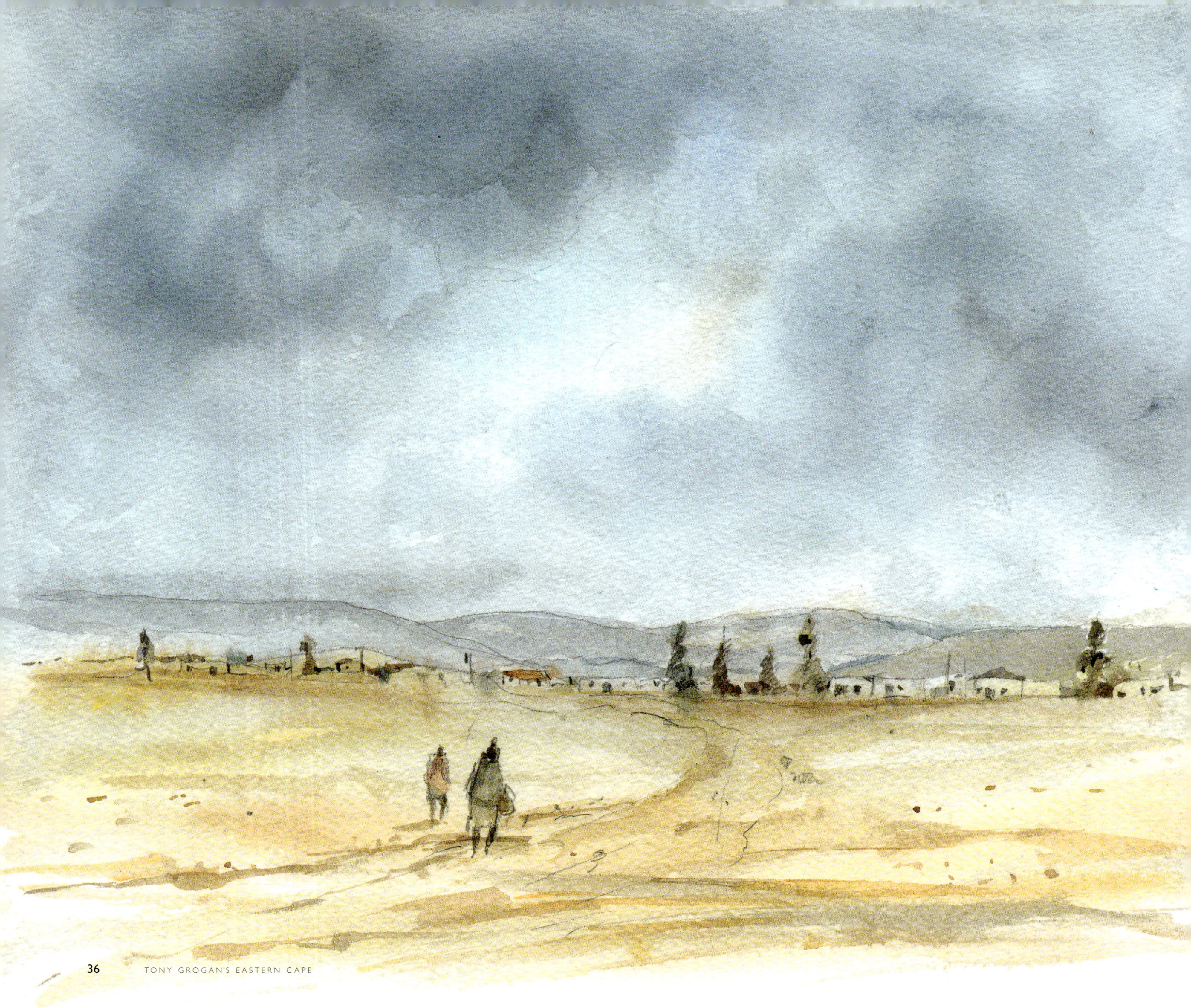

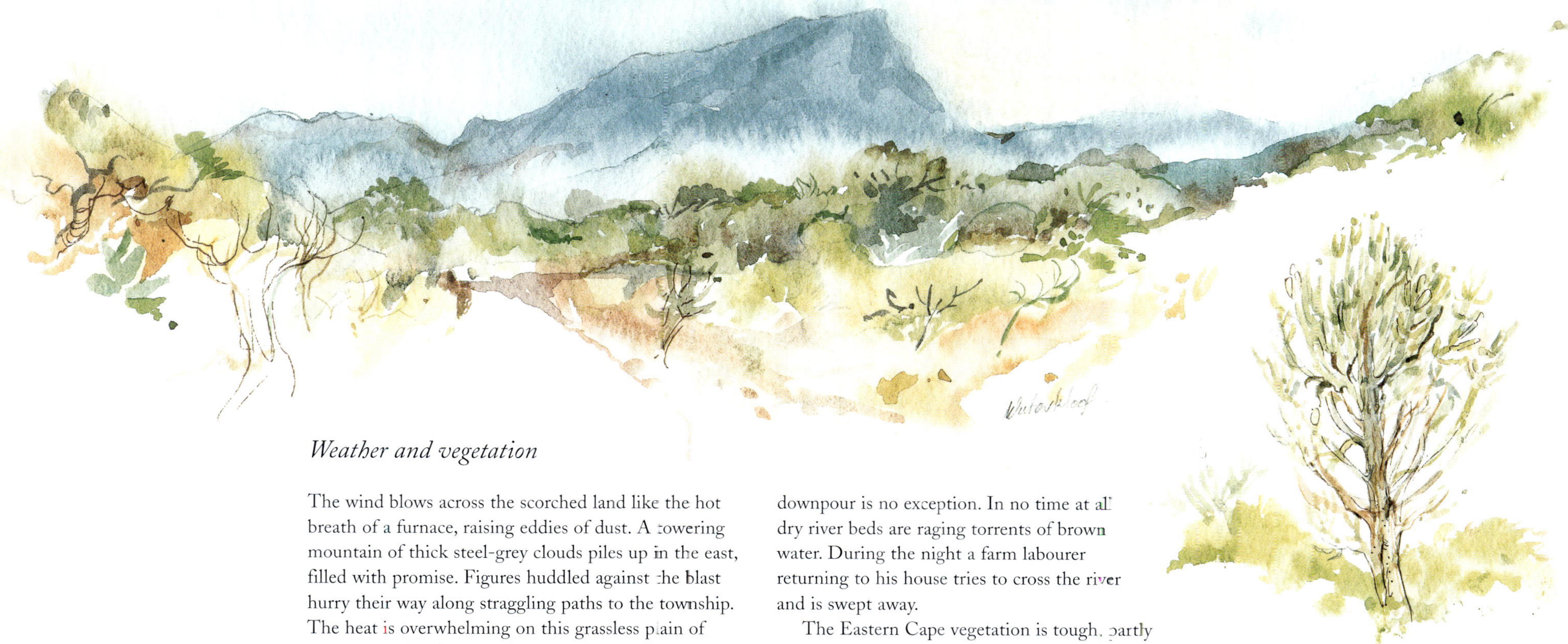

Weather and vegetation

The wind blows across the scorched land like the hot breath of a furnace, raising eddies of dust. A towering mountain of thick steel-grey clouds piles up in the east, filled with promise. Figures huddled against the blast hurry their way along straggling paths to the township. The heat is overwhelming on this grassless plain of gravel and stones, but soon the sun disappears behind the clouds, the land darkens, lightning flashes and thunder rolls across the hills. When the rain comes, it pours down in torrents – too much in too short a time. This seems to be the lot of the Eastern Cape. In accounts of the experiences of the early settlers, you will read time and again of their suffering either through flood or drought. This downpour is no exception. In no time at all dry river beds are raging torrents of brown water. During the night a farm labourer returning to his house tries to cross the river and is swept away.

The Eastern Cape vegetation is tough, partly because the country was originally inhabited by large animals and the plants had to adapt to being heavily grazed and trampled. Plants like the spekboom could be broken into pieces and the broken branches would take root where they fell. Two of the most typical of Eastern Cape plants are the aloe and the euphorbia. The cactus is an import and although useful for fodder during drought, has become an invasive pest.

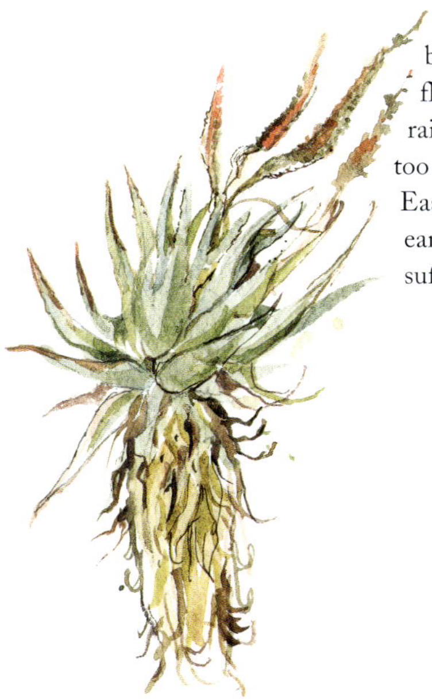

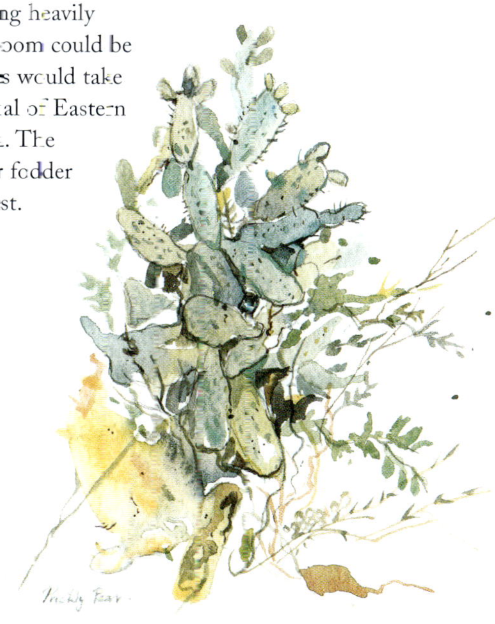

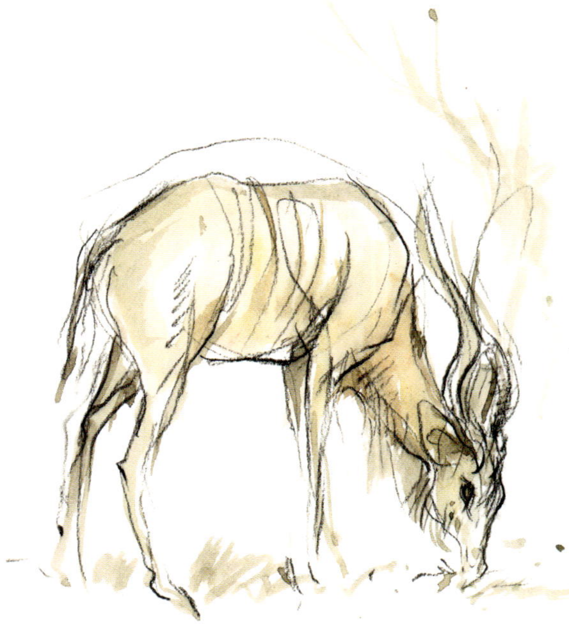

Game farming

Because of recurring stock theft, many of the farms in the Eastern Cape have converted to game, and with the removal of sheep and goats, overgrazed veld is recovering and many of the animals which thrived in these parts in earlier years are once again found here in large numbers.

Thomas Pringle in the poem *The Desolate Valley*, quoted in *Literary Guide to the Eastern Cape* by Jeanette Eve, evocatively captures the profusion of game in the 1800s before it was shot out in this area in the foothills of the Winterberg:

"Round this secluded region circling rise
A billowy waste of mountains, wild and wide;
Upon whose grassy slopes the pilgrim spies
The gnu and quagga, by the greenwood side,
Tossing their shaggy manes in tameless pride;
Or troop of elands near some sedgy fount;
Or kudu fawns, that from the thicket glide
To seek their dam upon the misty mount
With harts, gazelles, and roes more than the eye can count."

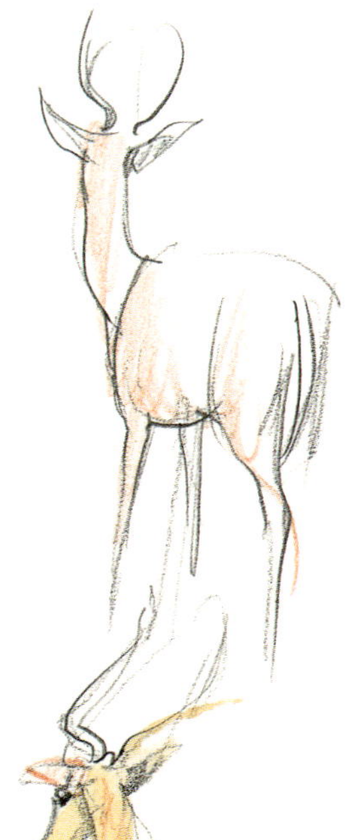

Many of these animals now thrive on the Molweni Private Game Reserve where these sketches were done.

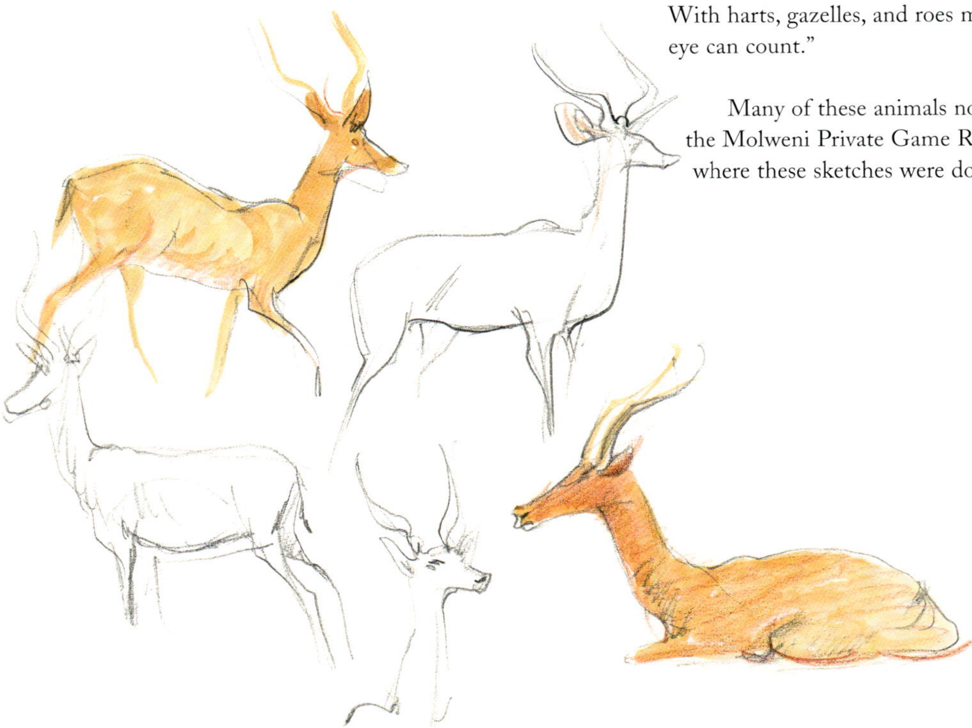

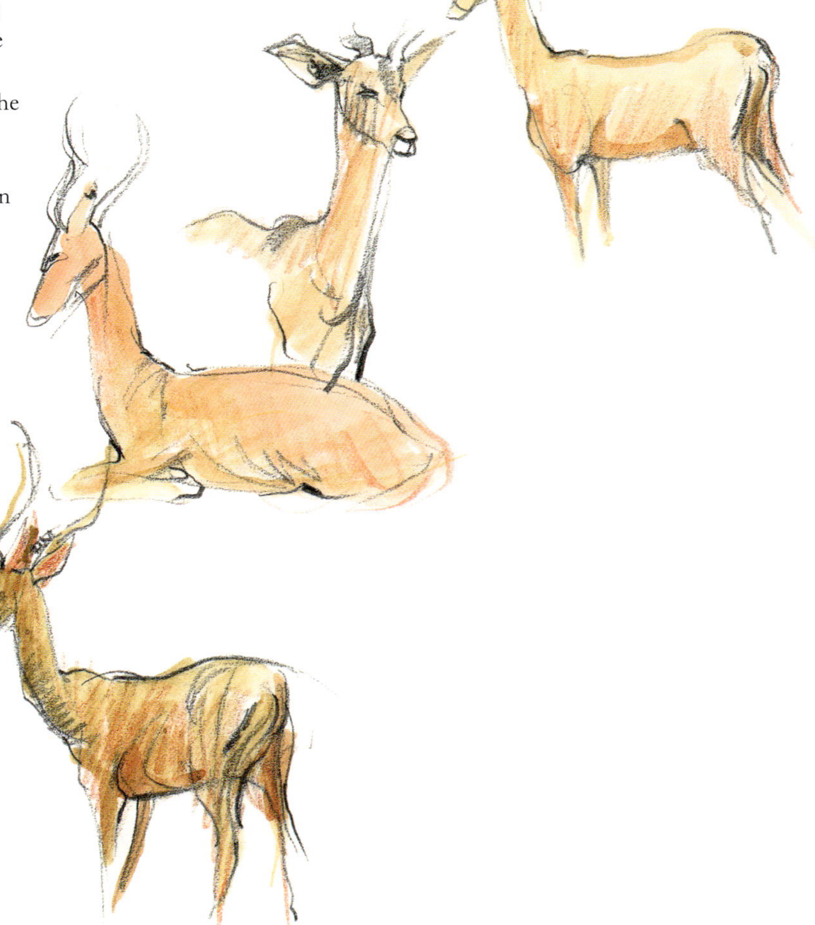

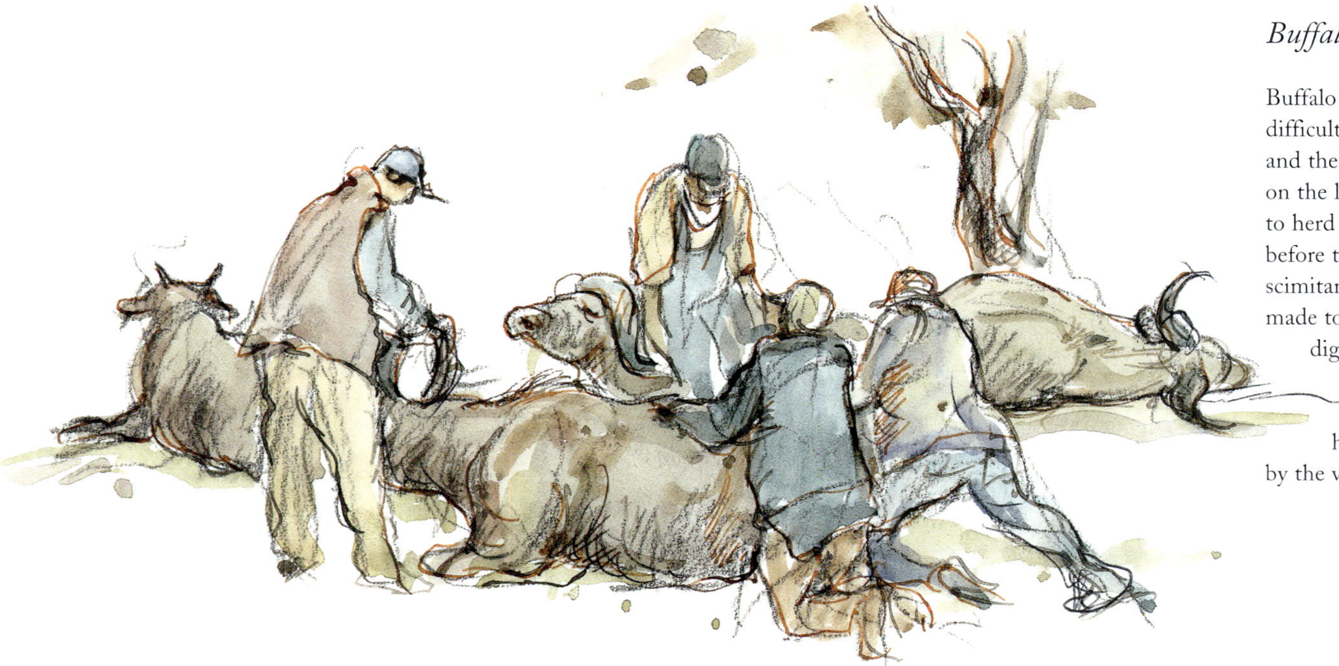

Buffalo

Buffalo usually confine themselves to thick bush and are difficult to see in the undergrowth. The herd has grown and the owner Chris Bush want to sells some of them on the local game auction, so a helicopter is brought in to herd the animals into a boma where they are darted before transporting them. A large bull with impressive, scimitar horns refuses to leave his harem and an effort is made to drive him out of the boma with a mechanical digger. But he is determined to stay, and with his blood up, is not prepared to be pushed around by any machine. Before he does damage to himself – and the digger loader – he is darted by the vet.

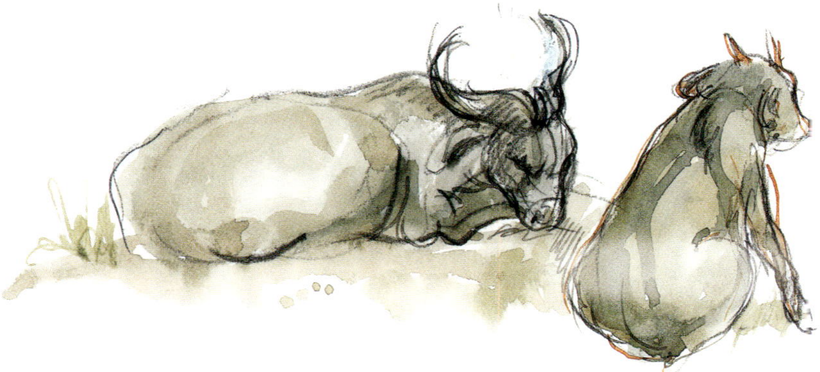

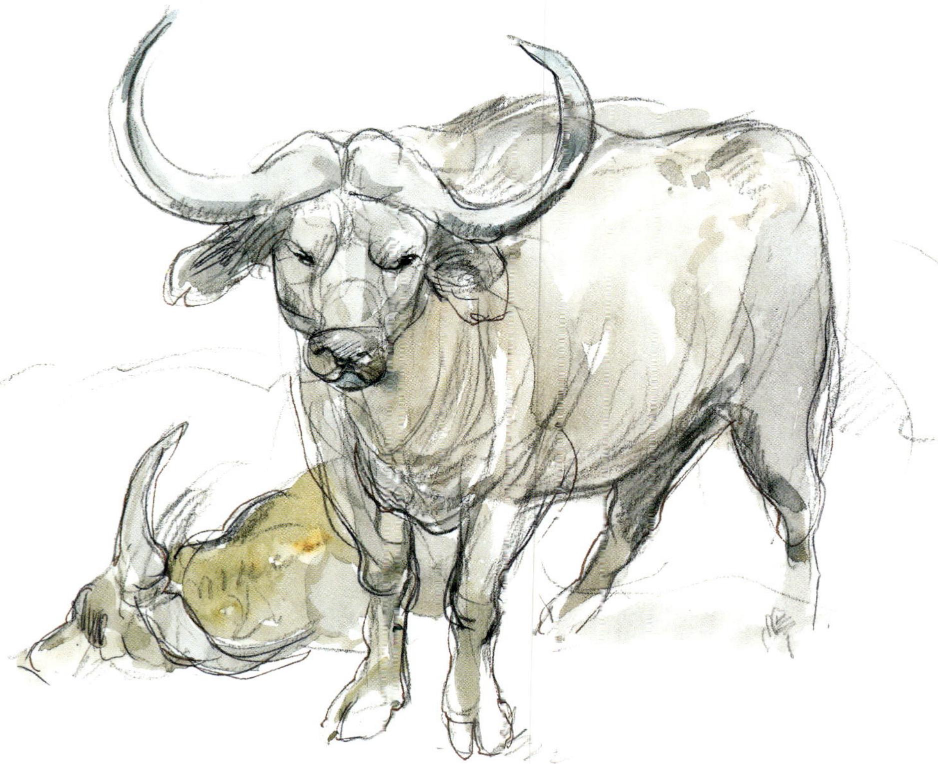

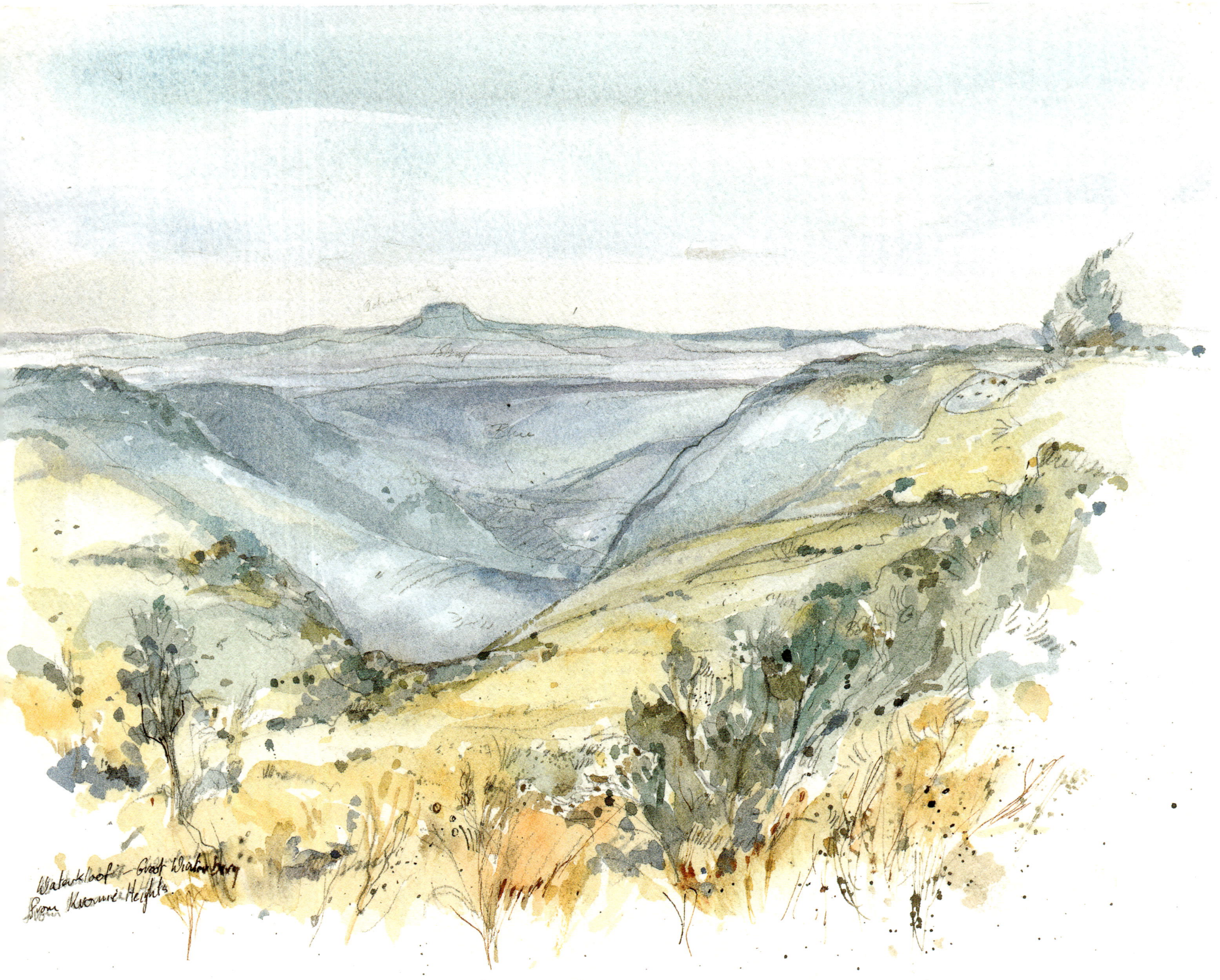
Waterkloof – Groot Winterberg

Waterkloof

The Waterkloof, a general title given to a configuration of valleys, deep kloofs and crags, densely wooded ravines and steep mountainsides, rising to sunlit and grass-covered plateaux, presents a breathtaking panorama looking north towards the Winterberg. In this beautiful place, one of the cruellest and nastiest of the frontier wars was fought from 1851-1852. The Waterkloof was lovely to the eye but an awful place for raw, young British troopers, ill-trained for bush warfare, unaccustomed to the climate and led by incompetent officers. Suffocating in hot tunics and lumbered with kitbags containing 25kg of equipment, fighting an enemy familiar with the terrain and flitting like shadows through the forest, they blundered through the bush led by the chief blunderer, Colonel Henry Somerset, who was in overall command of operations. This genial buffoon, not renowned for courage, efficiency or military brilliance, eased the rigours of war by being accompanied on the campaign trail by several 'comely wenches'. With this kind of leadership it was not surprising that the toll in men and officers was high, a fact bemoaned by Queen Victoria – particularly the loss of officers.

The Eastern Cape bush is thick and impenetrable, full of snagging thorns and obstructive branches and foliage. I have gone off the beaten track on more than one occasion – once carrying a bicycle – to experience what it must have been like for those soldiers.

For two years the great Xhosa chief, Maqoma, a brilliant military strategist, defied the British in this mountain stronghold. The cost of the campaign and the inefficiency with which it was fought strained the patience of the British government and eventually led to the dismissal of the governor, Sir Harry Smith. Like so many of the frontier wars, this one did not end with a conclusive victory. The Xhosa and their allies were worn down by a process of attrition – they were unable to sow their crops and eventually bombarded out of the Waterkloof by artillery barrages.

It is a place haunted by the echoes of those distant battles. We sat under the stars around a fire one night in the company of Jock and Piet, two ex-army generals who were making a study of the battle sites. While they related stories of the battles, suddenly out of the darkness issued the stirring skirl of bagpipes. With them had come Hammie, a piper from a Port Elizabeth regiment. As the strains echoed through the valley in the darkness, one of the generals observed that no doubt the souls of many young soldiers of the 74th Infantry who had lost their lives in those kloofs would stir in their lonely graves at that yearning, hauntingly lovely sound from the land of their birth.

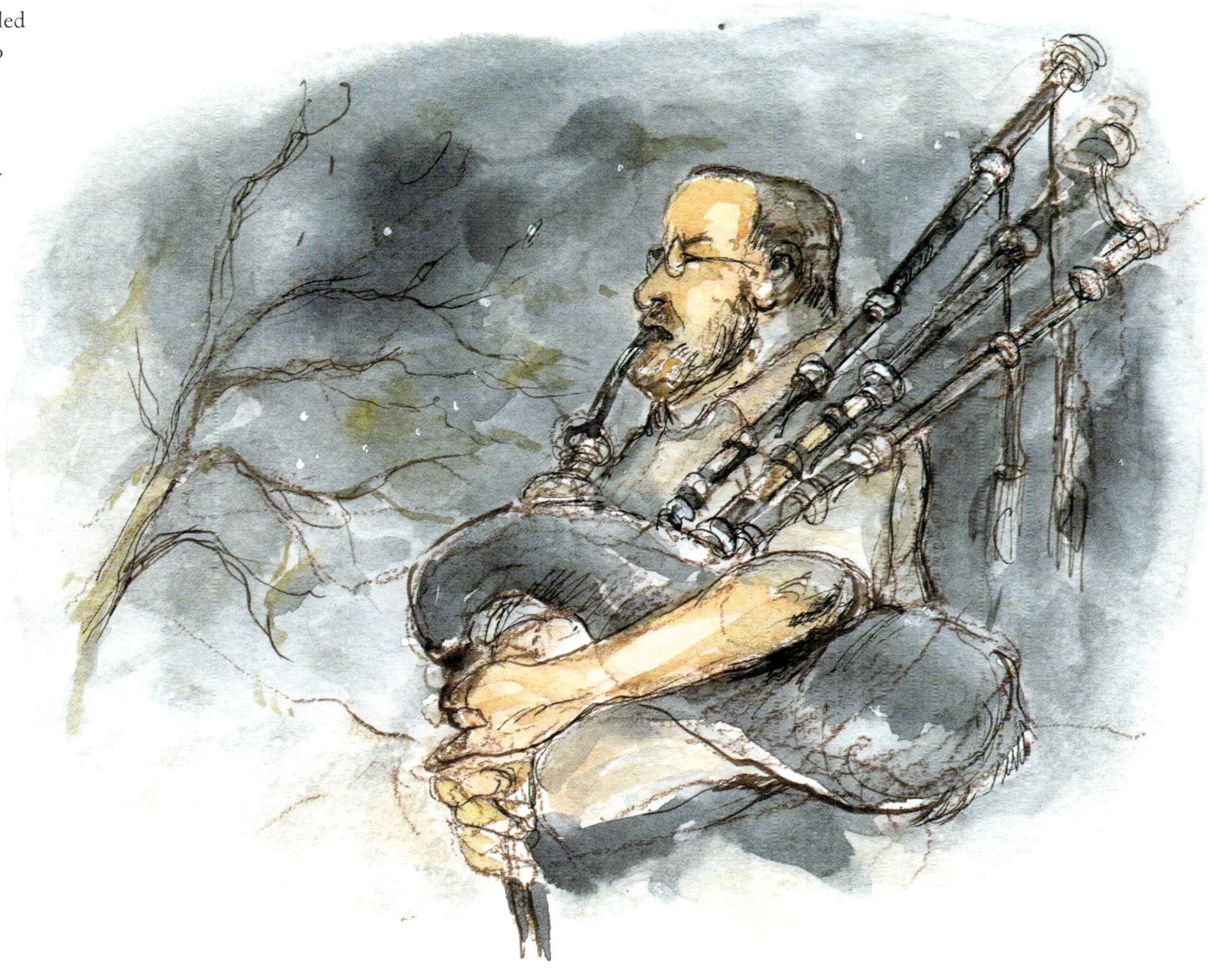

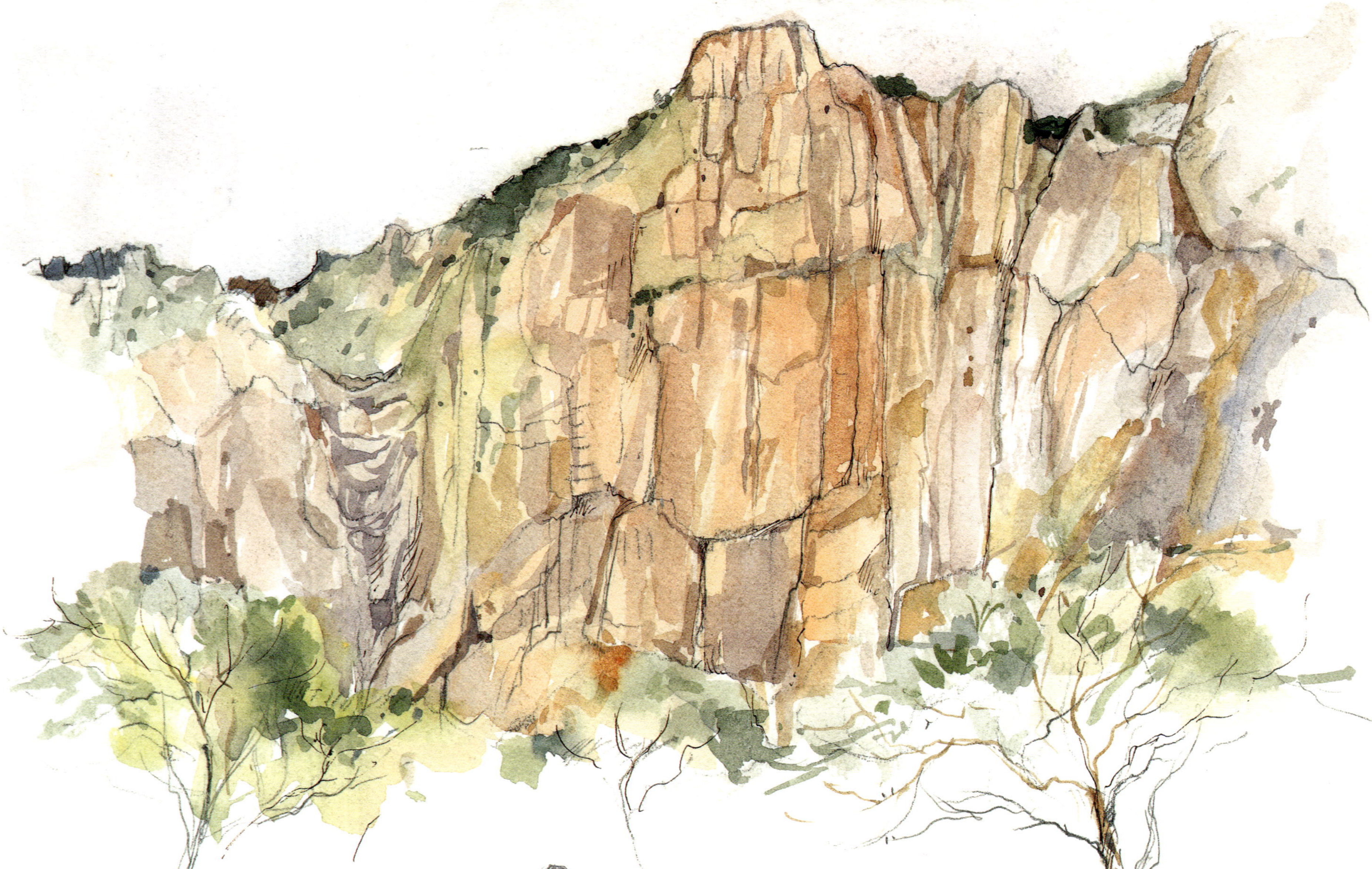

Waterkloof: Mundell's Krantz

The farmer has recovered an old road leading to the top of the plateau in the Waterkloof. From the valley below, it twists and zigzags its way tortuously through thick bush up the steep incline. He has used a bulldozer to open it, but we marvel at the doggedness and skill of the original road maker who toiled without modern machinery to follow the contours of the precipitous slope and lay out the road in its steady incline. At the top we discover the remains of a simple fort. Overgrown by grass and weeds are the foundation stones and slabs of stone which paved the floor. This must have been one of Governor Cathcart's 'castles' built at the end of the 1851-52 war to establish military points from which to harass and finally drive out Chief Maqoma's Xhosa from this mountain fastness.

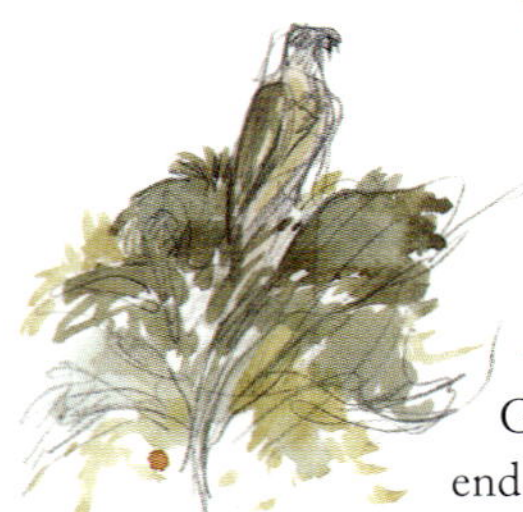

From the top there is a view over Mundell's Krantz to the valley below, where a Xhosa camp was attacked on one of the engagements in the war. John Fisher recalled the encounter many years later: "We reached the brow of Mundell's Krantz, an immense cliff with a chasm in its centre like the portal of some ruined castle and columns on every side, perpendicular and divided by horizontal fractures. We burned the huts and destroyed a great deal of ammunition and firearms in the huts, the artillery playing with them from the top. The Fingoes brought out fifteen or twenty women, loaded with the plunder of their own kraals for the behoof of their captors."

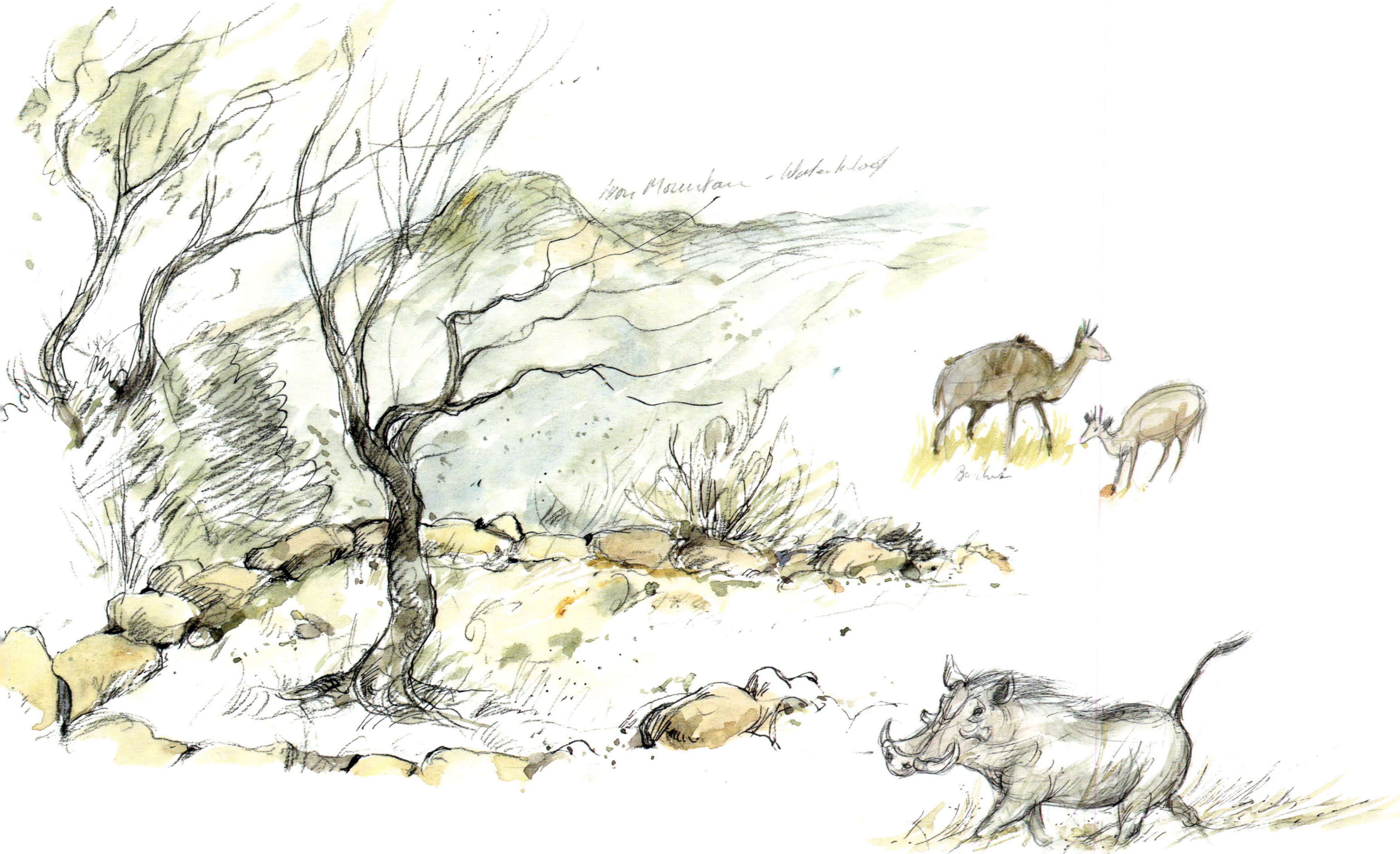

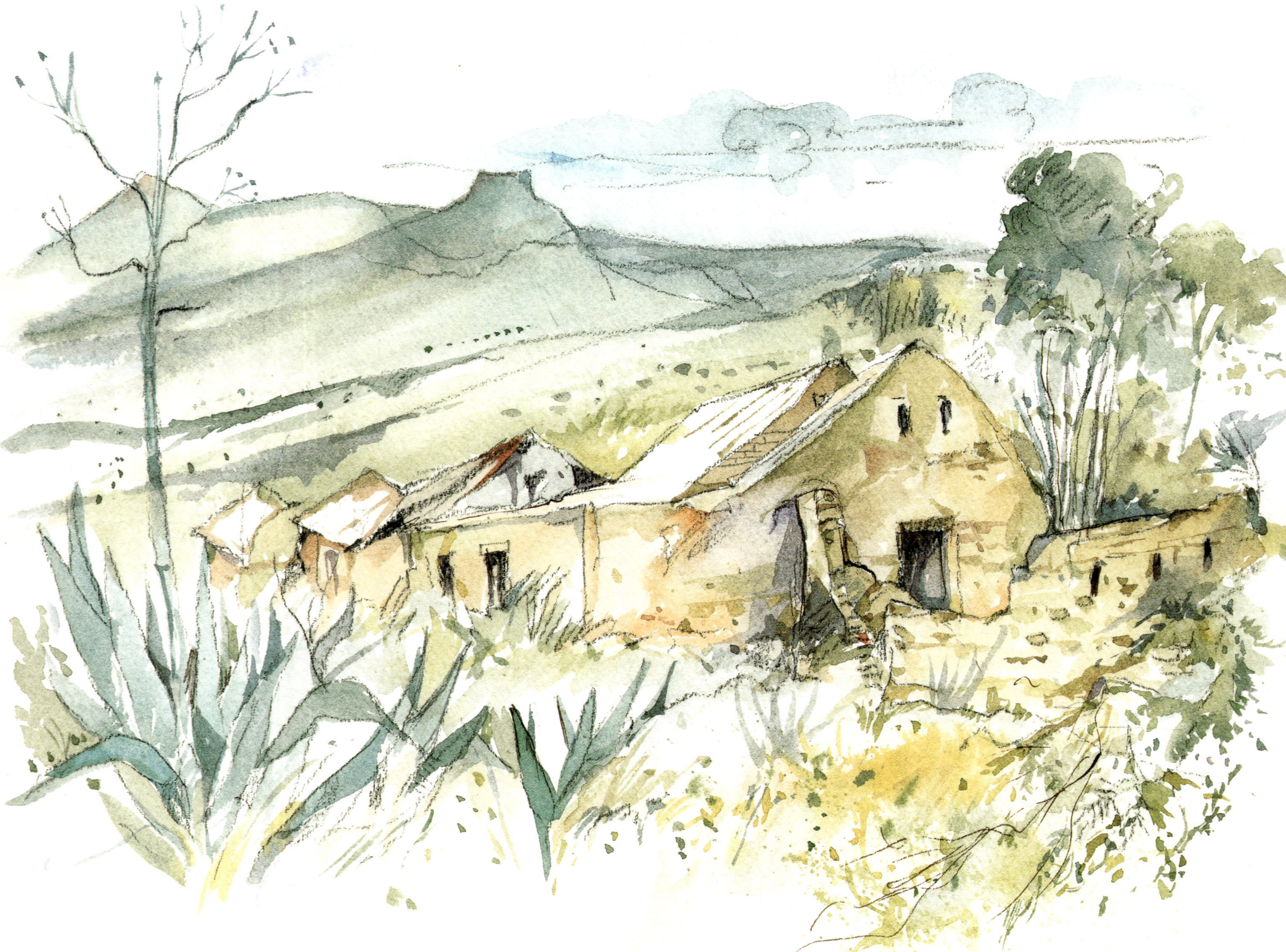

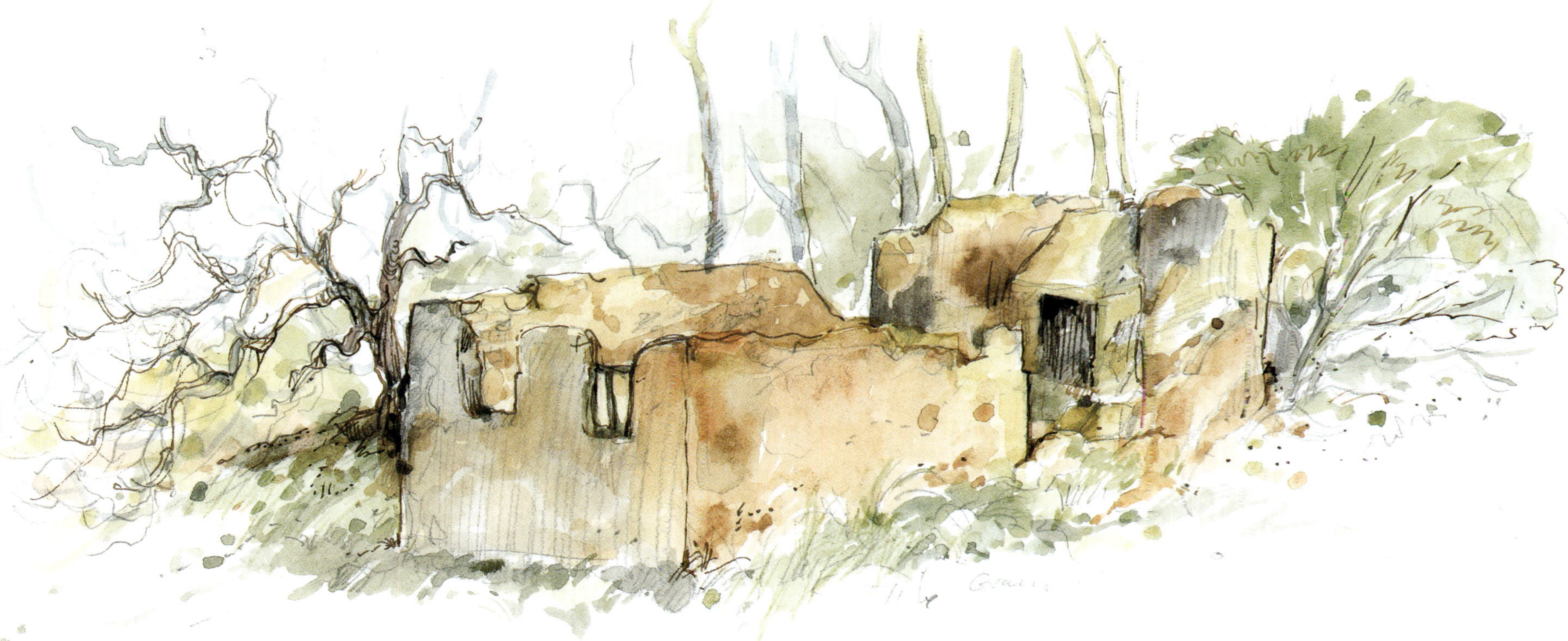

Post Retief and John James

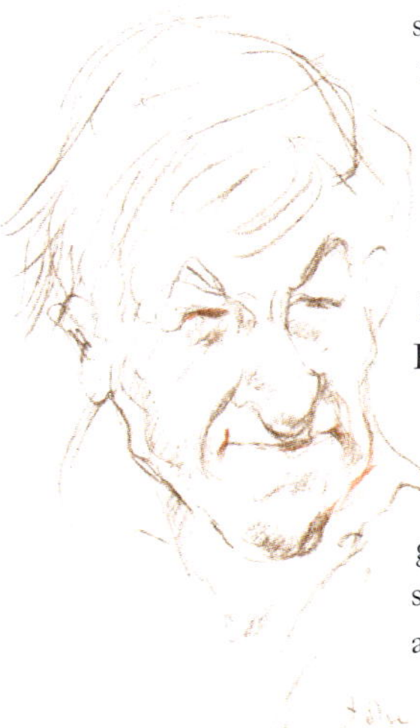

Post Retief, a remote military outpost in the foothills of the Winterberg, served as a hospital and fortified sanctuary for farmers and their families during the 1851–2 War of Mlangeni. It was named after the Voortrekker leader Piet Retief who built it, and was attacked and under siege on several occasions. A farmer who showed me around looked at the crumbling wall, sniffed, and remarked that he couldn't have been much of a builder. There is a sign pointing to Piet Retief's house but there is nothing left of it apart from a few foundation stones

Nearby is the James's farm, Foot's Cray, which has been in the family for five generations. John James is a keen teller of stories. He shows us the ruins of the original farmhouse and describes in graphic detail how, at the end of the war, the family had returned to their home thinking the war was over, when they were surprised by a band of Xhosa and rebel Khoikhoi. The servant who opened the door was shot as they burst into the house and Mr James pursued out of the back door where he too was shot. The fig tree under which he died is still there.

The weather is harsh up here. It's freezing cold in winter and the wind roars down from the mountains with incredible force, which is the reason you don't see any windmills in these parts, John explains.

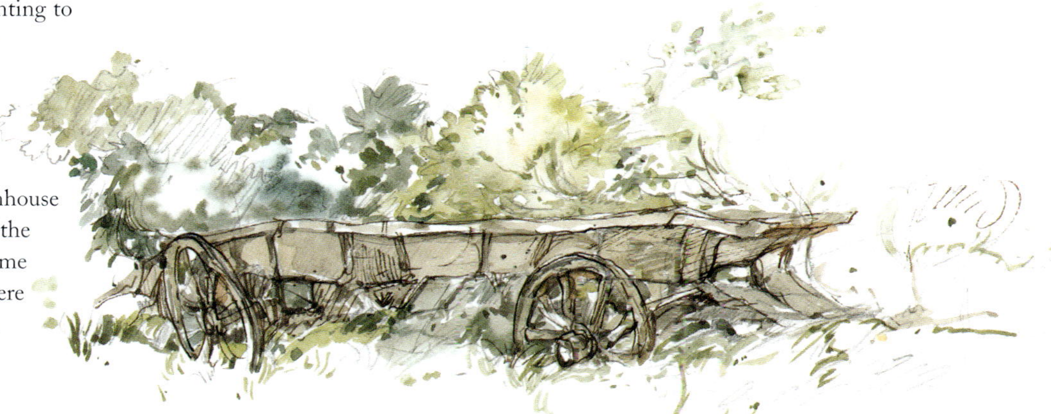

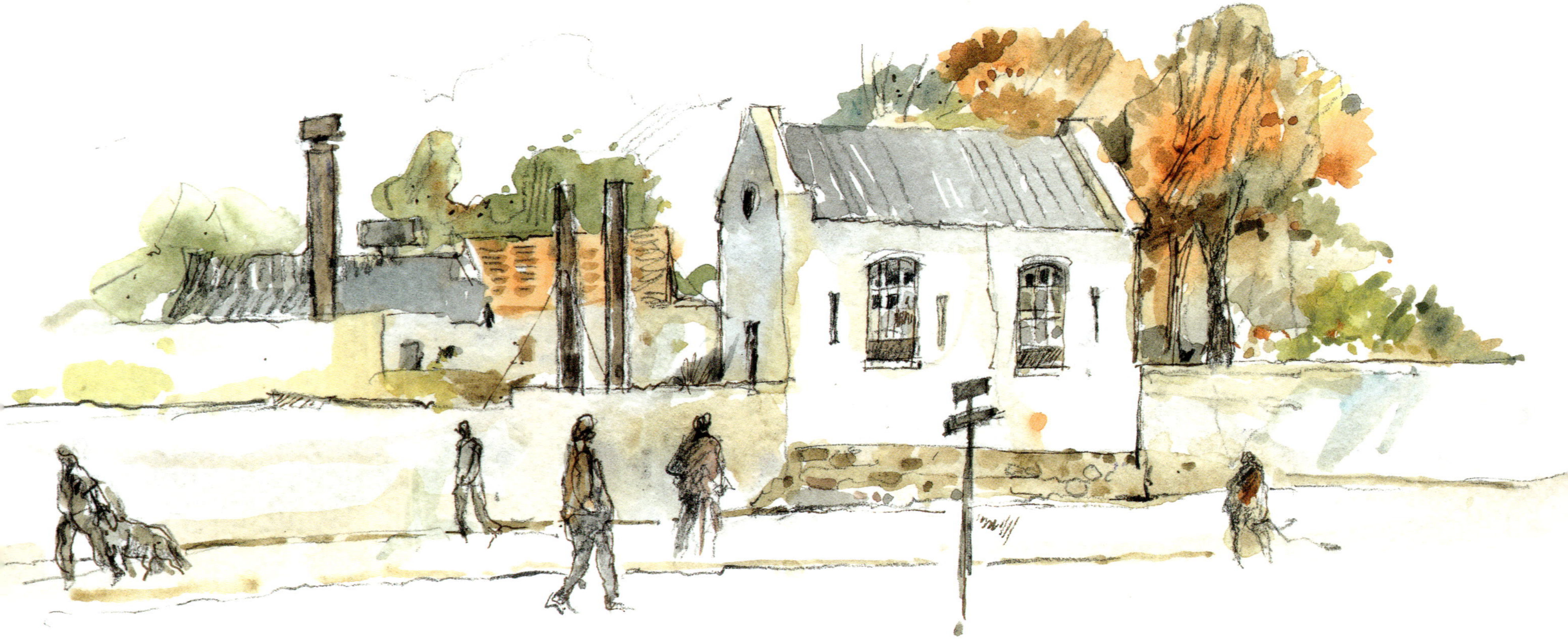

Fort Beaufort

Fort Beaufort began its existence in 1823 as a military outpost with a Martello tower (a round, tower-like fortress with a cannon mounted at the top), which is still in perfect condition. Some of the old military buildings are still to be seen in the streets of the town.

The battle of Fort Beaufort took place in 1852 when the small town was attacked by a combined force of Xhosa and rebel Khoikhoi under the leadership of one Hermanus Matroos, who made a fetching picture as he galloped into town wearing a woman's bonnet and very little else. One of the defenders shot him neatly through the head, which shows it doesn't pay to make yourself conspicuous in battle. A short exchange of fire ensued before the attackers were put to rout.

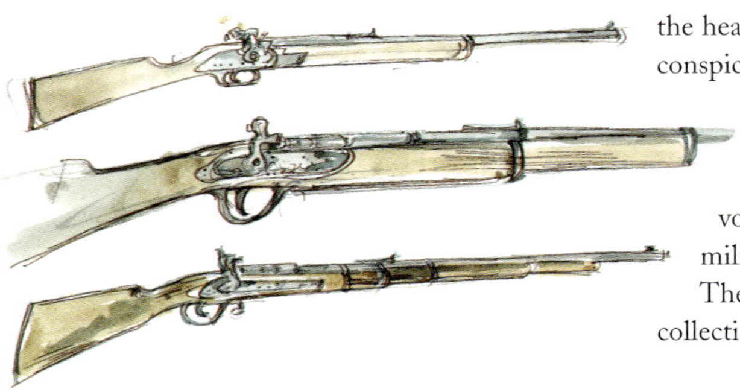

Unaccountably, the local militia didn't stir from their barracks and all the fighting was done by volunteers and Fingo levies. This was not the militia's finest hour.

The Fort Beaufort Museum has an interesting collection of guns and other armaments. An item which catches my attention is a shop dummy wearing a woman's sun bonnet, fragile and faded with age. I am intrigued to read the label which says that the bonnet was worn by Janet Brown. I recall a moving account in Mosterts book, *Frontiers*, of the desperate flight of this missionary's wife, compelled to leave her mission station in a time of war and cross the country in search of her husband. She was in terror of meeting wandering bands of raging Xhosa warriors who had invaded the colony on that dread Christmas day in 1850, one of the hottest days in living memory. It is an epic tale of danger, fortitude and the most amazing humanity shown by Xhosa people who encountered her during her flight and helped and protected her. The bonnet looks oddly incongruous on the dummy with its painted face and pert, beguiling smile.

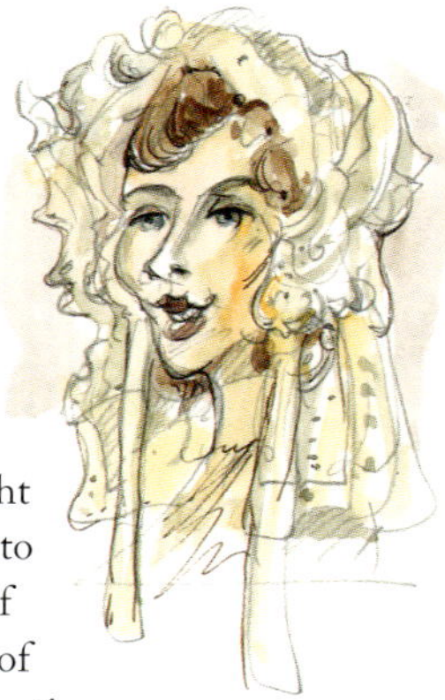

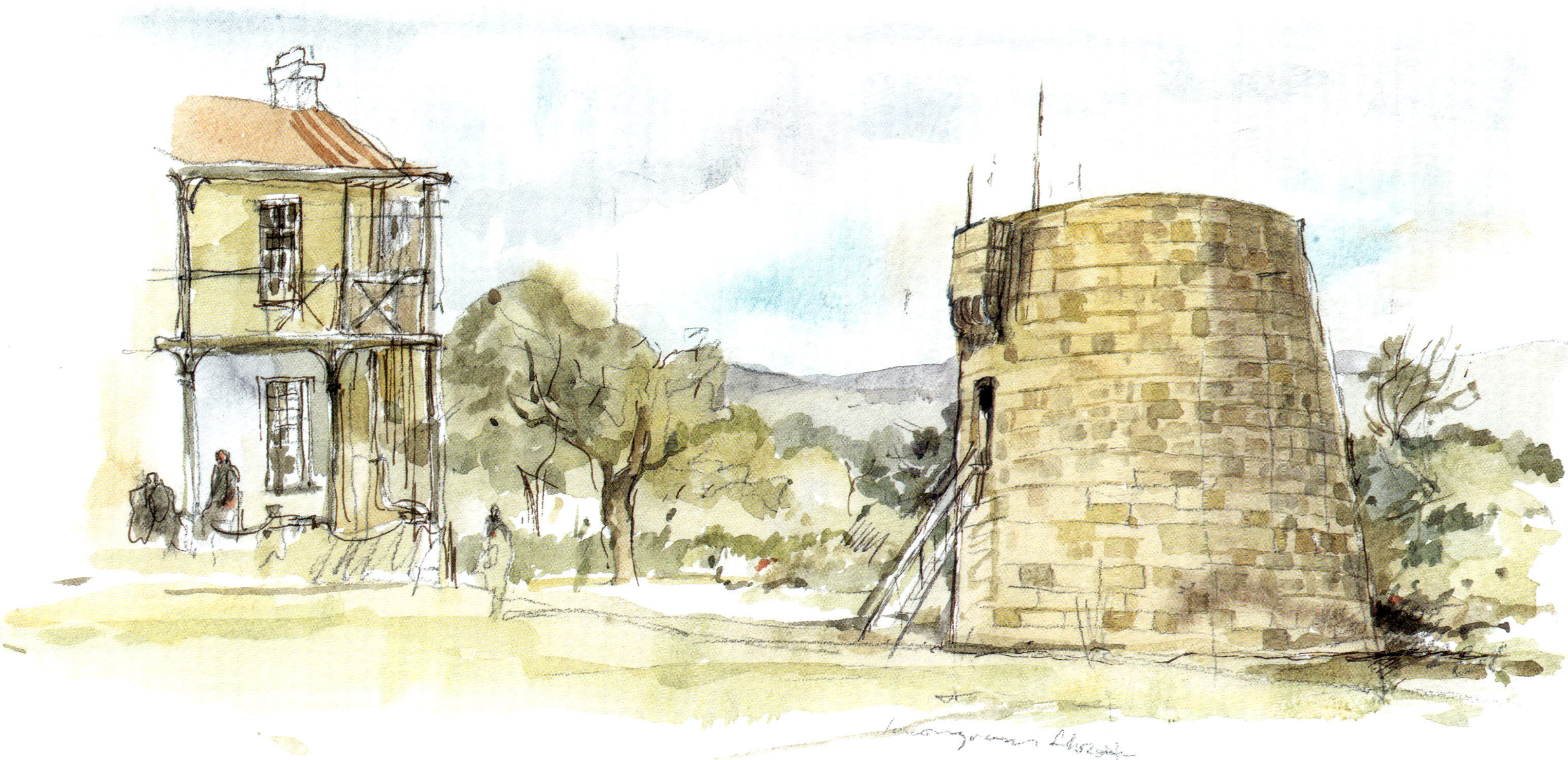

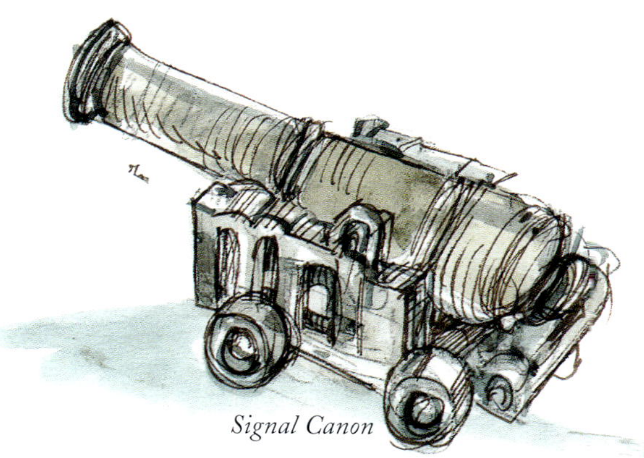

Signal Canon

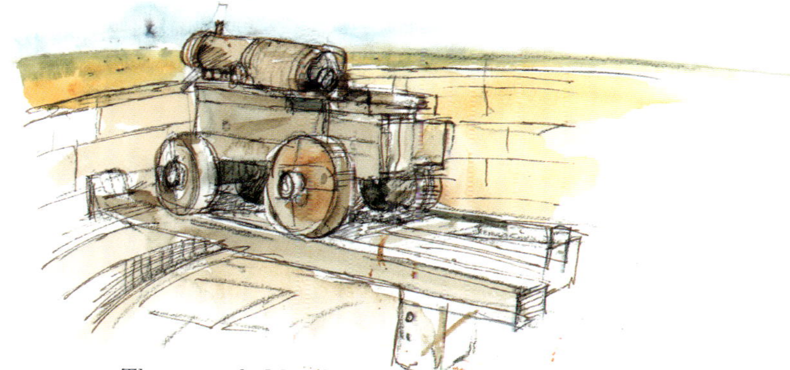

The gun on the Martello tower

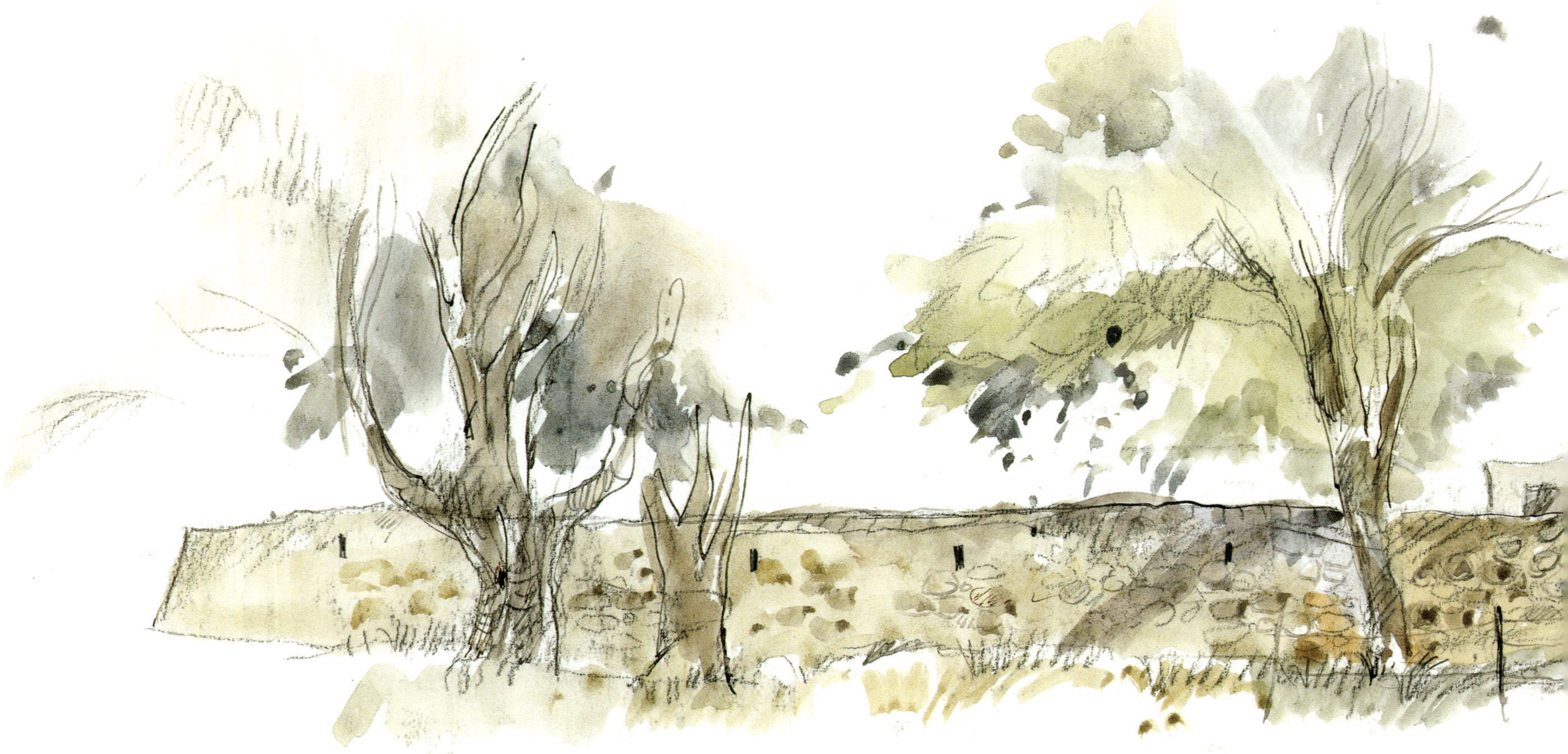

Sipton Manor

I visit Sipton Manor, a short distance from Fort Beaufort. It is a fine example of a fortified farm with a surrounding, protective wall and tower on which a cannon was once mounted. The house was designed and owned by William Gilbert who sent a plan of it to the governor as a suggested prototype for all farm houses built on that troubled frontier. The house is little altered from those times. Gilbert and his family

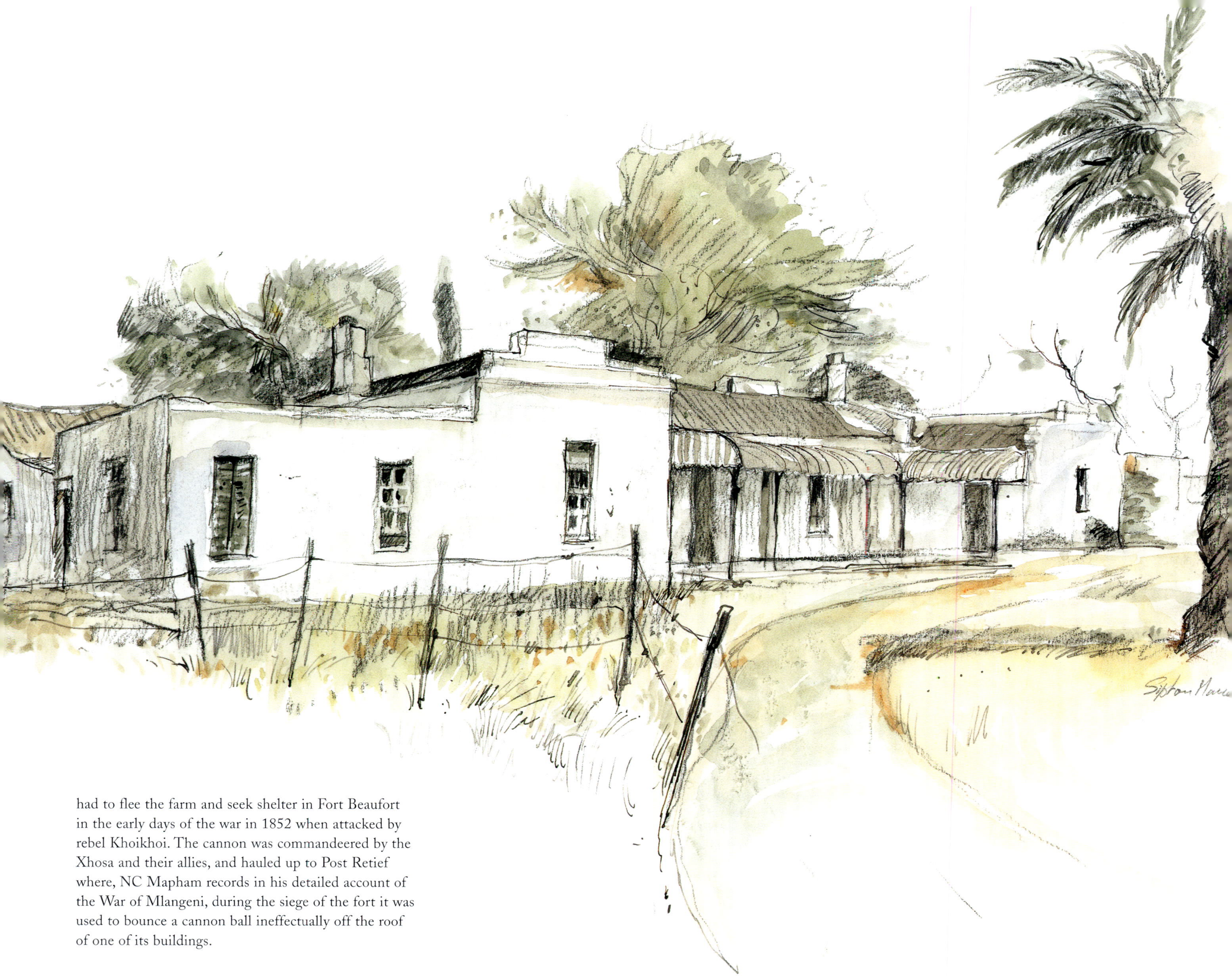

had to flee the farm and seek shelter in Fort Beaufort in the early days of the war in 1852 when attacked by rebel Khoikhoi. The cannon was commandeered by the Xhosa and their allies, and hauled up to Post Retief where, NC Mapham records in his detailed account of the War of Mlangeni, during the siege of the fort it was used to bounce a cannon ball ineffectually off the roof of one of its buildings.

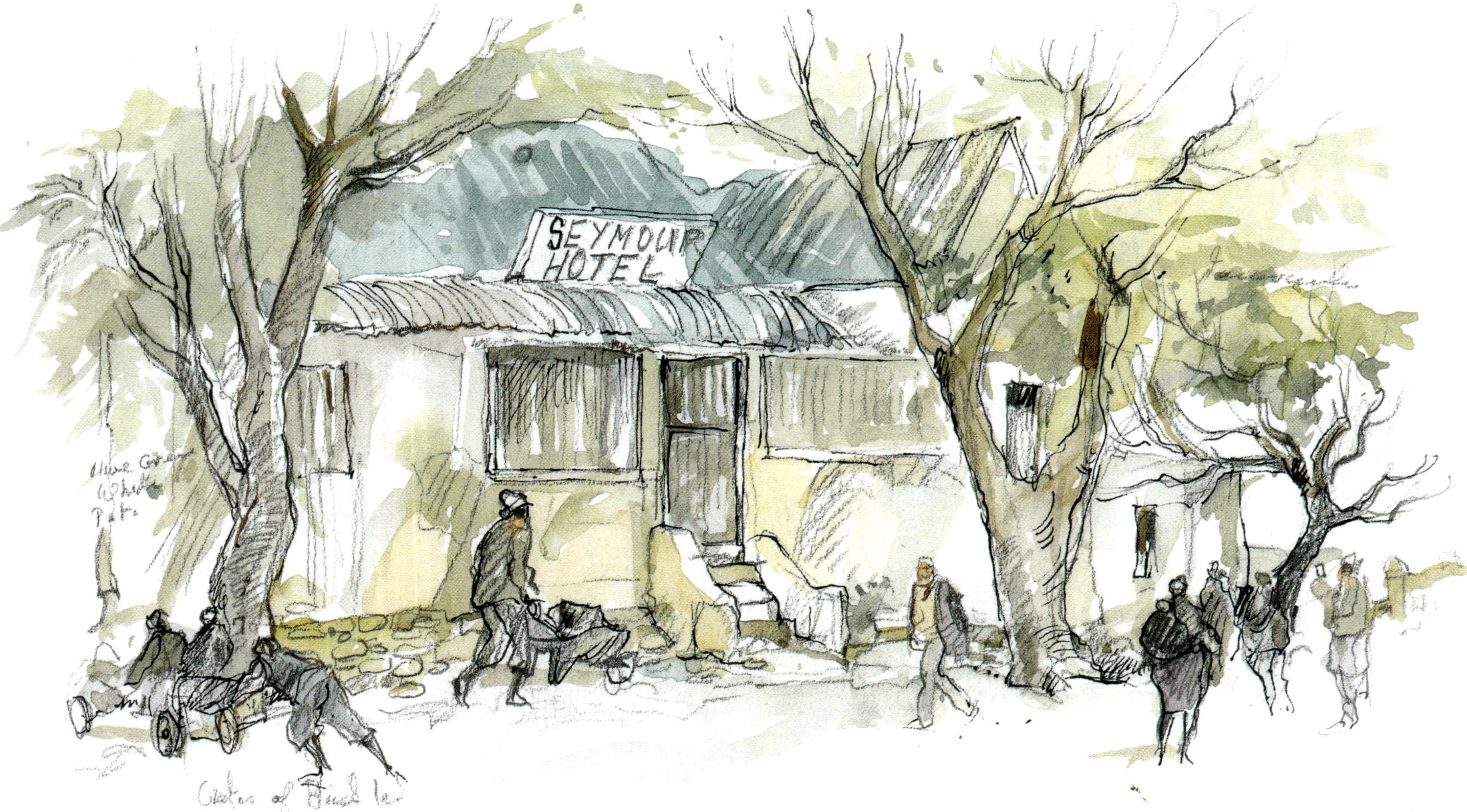

Seymour

I spent the night in the Seymour Hotel many years ago before Seymour become incorporated into that fictional independent national state at the time, Ciskei. It had a very cosy, companionable pub decorated with well-polished copperware, assorted weapons and a few trophy heads. A few of the locals were sitting at the bar staring moodily into their beer, forecasting gloomily that it would all go to the dogs. Alas, their worst fears have been realised. The hotel is shabby and run down, and weeds choke the once well-tended garden. There seems to be an electricity failure because the hotel appears dark inside. Nevertheless, there is a brisk trade going on at the off-sales. A few crates of beer are being loaded on to a donkey cart and someone has arrived with a wheelbarrow to transport his supplies.

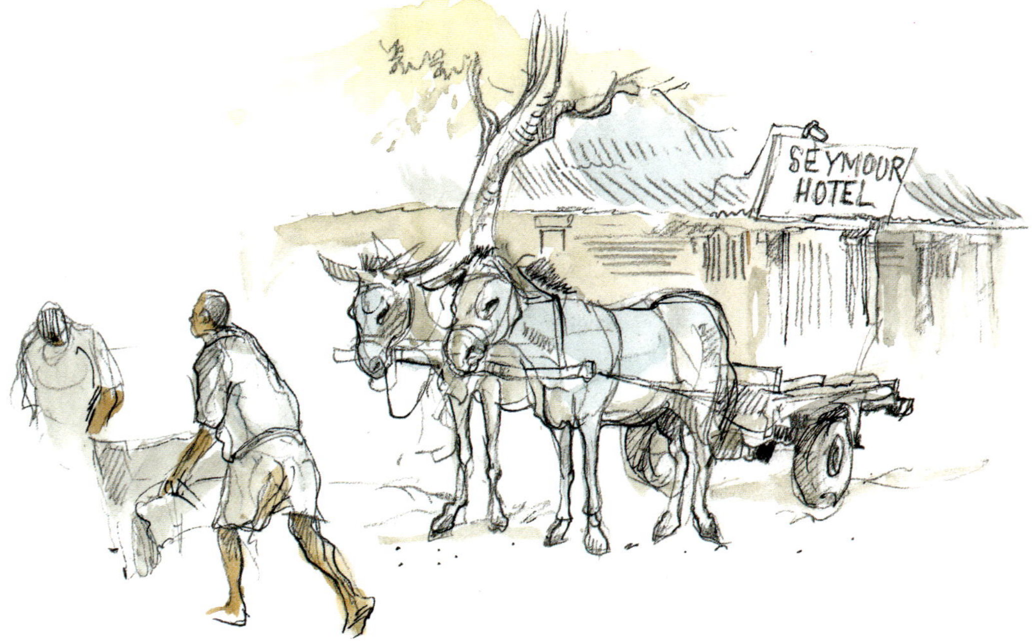

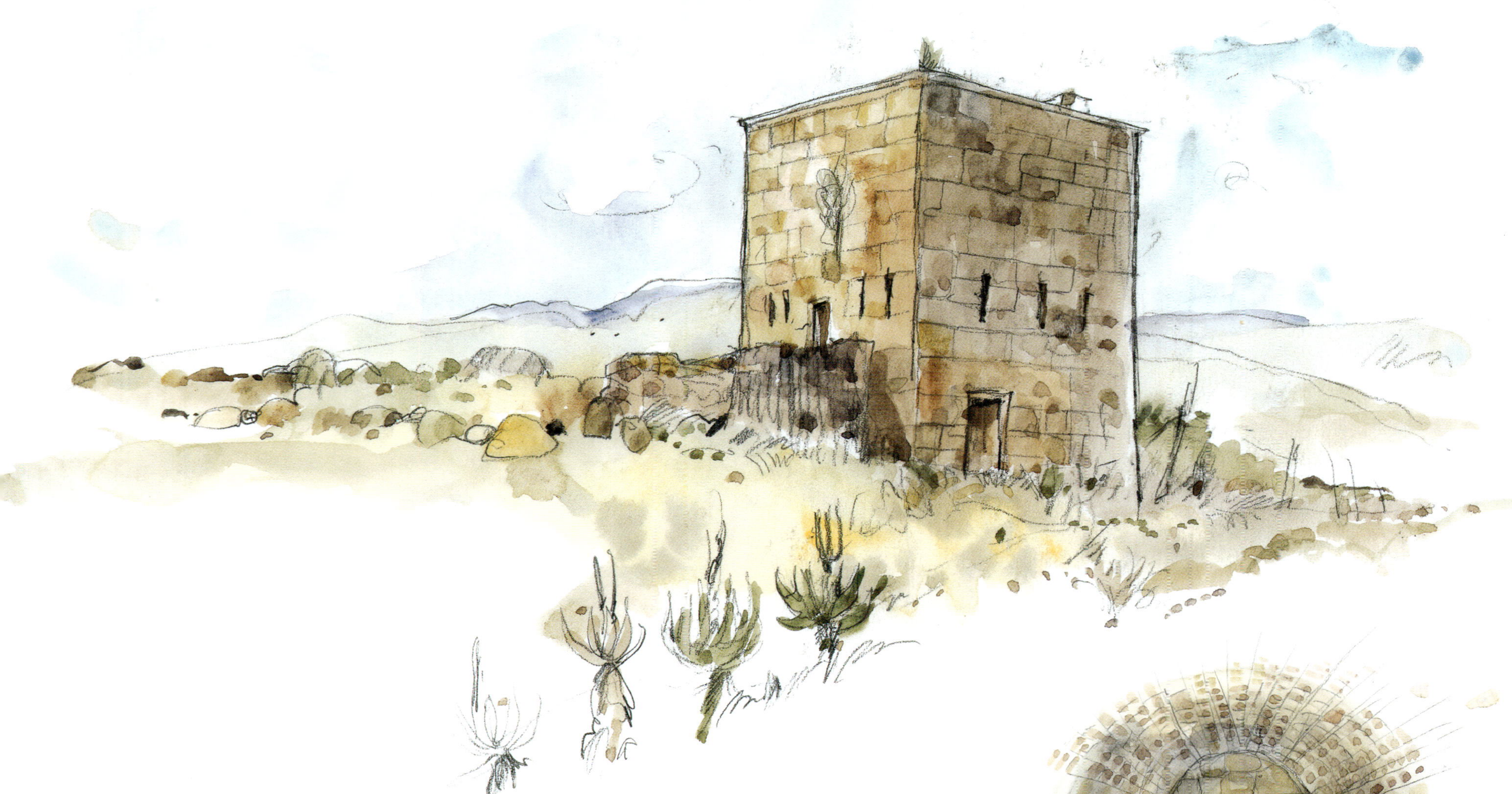

Fort Armstrong

Fort Armstrong near Seymour is one of the forts built during the 1830s as a defensive system to secure the eastern frontier. The site chosen is strategically sound, being on a rise on a tongue of land formed by a tight bend of the Kat River. It was occupied by rebel Khoikhoi troops at the beginning of the Eighth Frontier War, the War of Mlangeni. The fort remained the stronghold of the rebels under their leader, Willem Uithaalder, until it was retaken by a government force armed with artillery.

Today only the main tower of the fort is standing. Scattered stones in the grass are all that remain of the original surrounding walls and buildings. The door is secured only with a piece of wire and I open it to make a drawing of the solid, barrel-vaulted interior. I marvel at the superb masonry skills of the military engineers. The stone is beautifully dressed and laid with absolute precision.

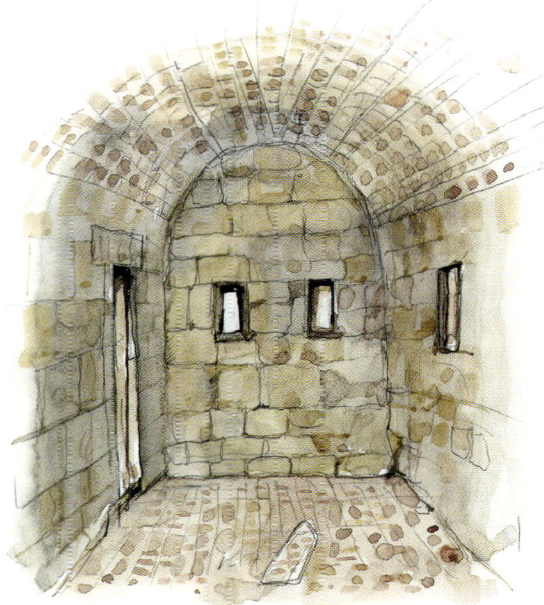

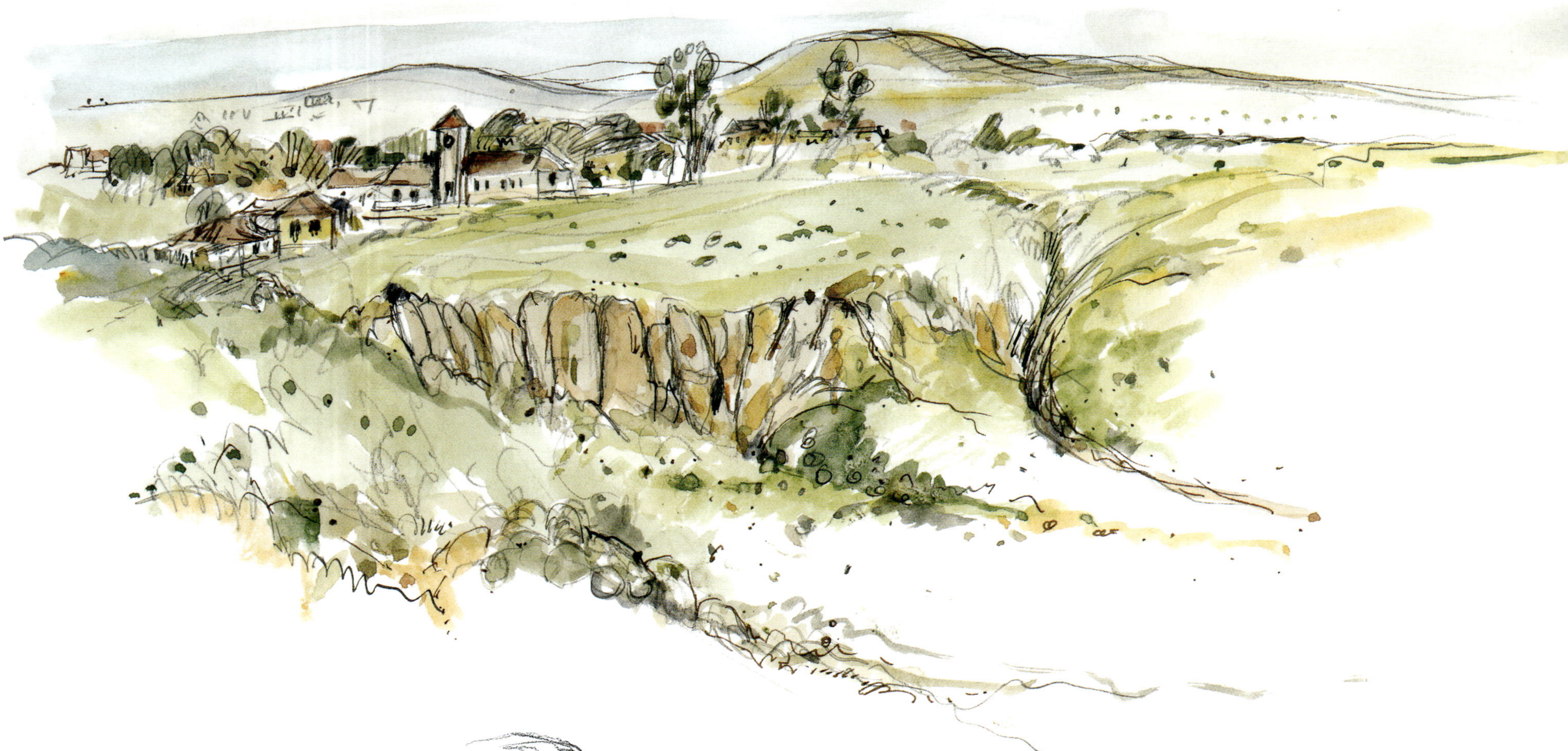

Healdtown

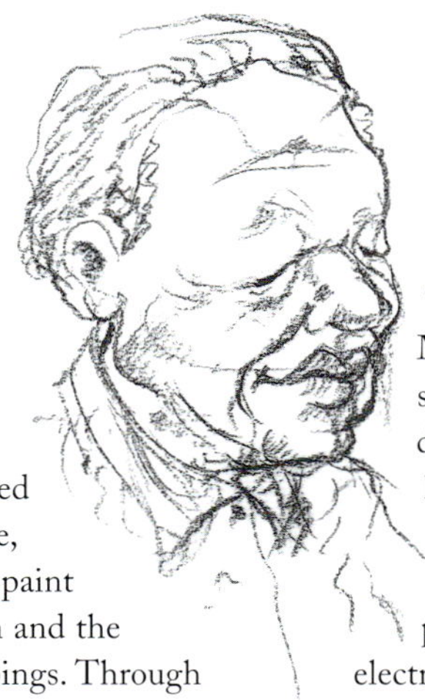

Healdtown is not what it used to be. In his autobiography *A Long Walk to Freedom*, Nelson Mandela describes graceful, ivy-covered colonial buildings and tree-shaded courtyards. What I find is a depressing scene of dereliction and decay. Some of the old classrooms are used as storerooms for surplus school furniture, and others have fallen into disrepair, the paint peeling, timbers rotting, windows broken and the floors covered with pigeon and rat droppings. Through a door hanging on its hinges, I enter the old kitchen where the rusted coal stoves are still in place. In the adjacent dining room, which also served as a school hall, there is a raised platform.

It was here that Mandela recalls experiencing a defining moment in his life. The distinguished Xhosa poet, Krune Mqhayi, had been invited to address the school. Behind the stage was a door, which led directly to the principal's, Dr Wellington's, house through which no one but he entered, so it was a surprise when the headmaster came through the door accompanied by the poet. Mqhayi proceeded to deliver an electrifying oration, urging the pupils to remember their Xhosa culture and to guard it from domination by a foreign European culture. He foresaw the day when they would cast off these foreign notions. That a black man should have the boldness to speak out like this on such a delicate matter in front of whites astounded the young Mandela, and he recalls that it was from that moment he began to alter his perception of men like Dr Wellington, whom he had until then uncritically regarded only as his benefactors.

I think of this as I draw the outside of the dilapidated building with its rusted roof and multiple chimneys. A large sow snuffles around the courtyard, finally lies down ponderously, gives a few snorts of contentment and falls asleep.

Back in Fort Beaufort, the chairman of the Museum Board tells me of ambitious plans to restore the school to its former glory because of its association with past-distinguished pupils like Nelson Mandela and Govan Mbeki.

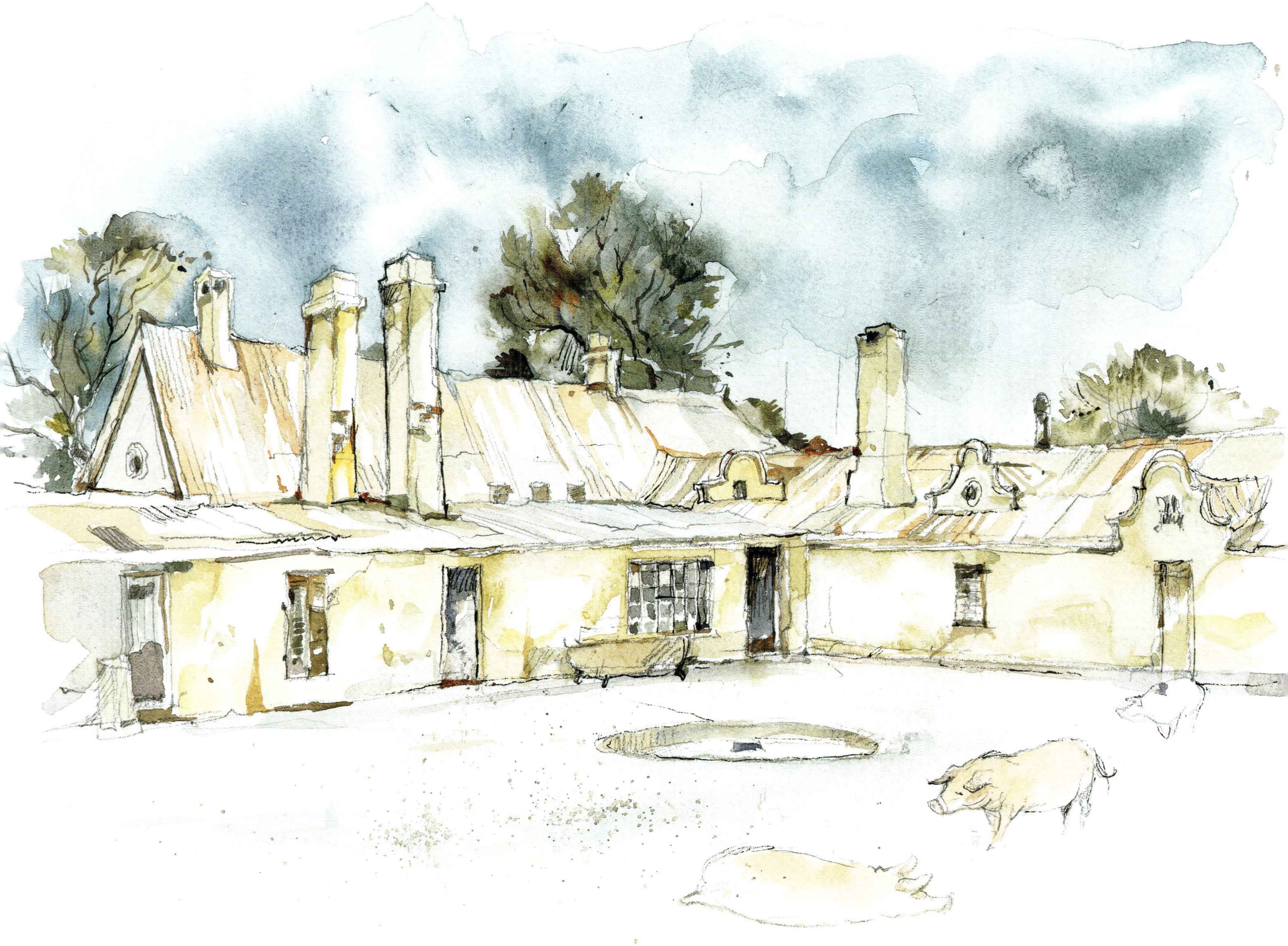

Fort Hare and the Tyume Valley

The clock tower of Fort Hare University in Alice. The university had its roots in a mission station established by John Brownlee in 1820. It produced many distinguished black scholars and intellectuals, such as ZK Mathews, John Tengu Jabavu and JL Dube. Vigorous political debate was encouraged and flourished on the campus, and many political leaders are counted among its alumni, including Nelson Mandela, Oliver Tambo, Govan Mbeki as well several presidents of African countries. During the apartheid years, the university was in frequent ferment as students protested against waves of repressive legislation. Against this background it is

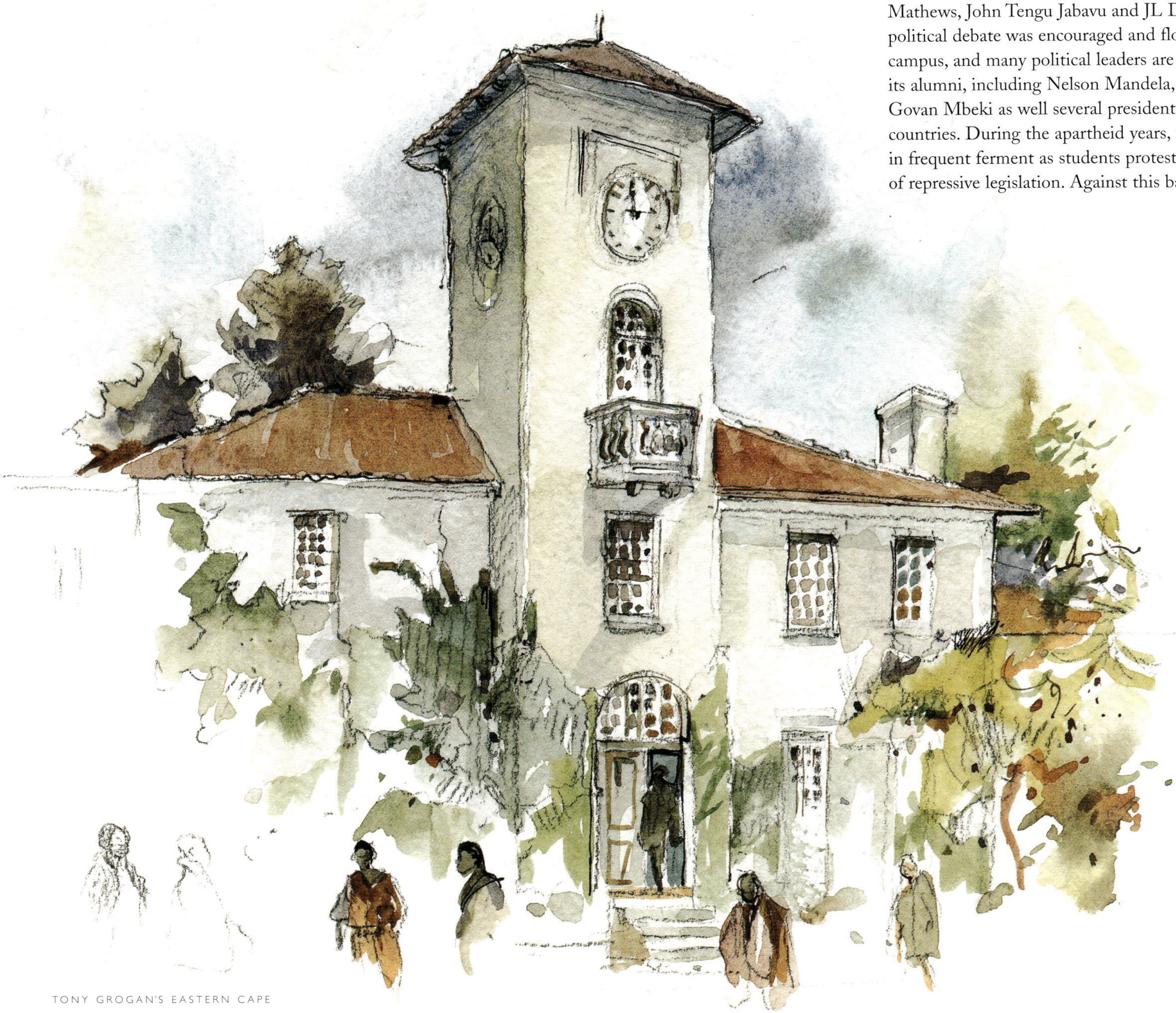

fitting that Fort Hare has been chosen as the repository of the archives of the liberation movement.

We lunch with friends who teach at Fort Hare. They have an interesting collection of clay animals which have become distinctive in the area. The models are much more skilfully made and more varied than the one's I remember being sold at the roadside in the Tyume Valley when I was a child. Then they were almost exclusively, rather crudely modelled red clay oxen.

The Tyume Valley forms a lush green basin in the shadow of the Amatolas below Hogsback. It presents a peaceful rural scene now, but it wasn't always so. Three small villages – Juanesburg, Auckland and Woburn, inhabited mainly by demobilised soldiers who had done serving in the frontier wars – were established here after the War of the Axe in 1846, to prevent the Xhosa reclaiming land from which they had been removed and engaging in sorties across the frontier. On Christmas day of 1850, thousands of warriors swept down from the mountains, drove women and children from the villages, slaughtered their menfolk and burned their houses to the ground. It was the start of the Eighth Frontier War.

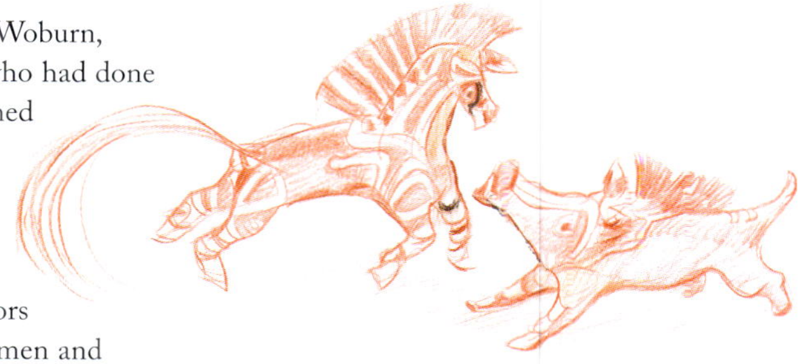

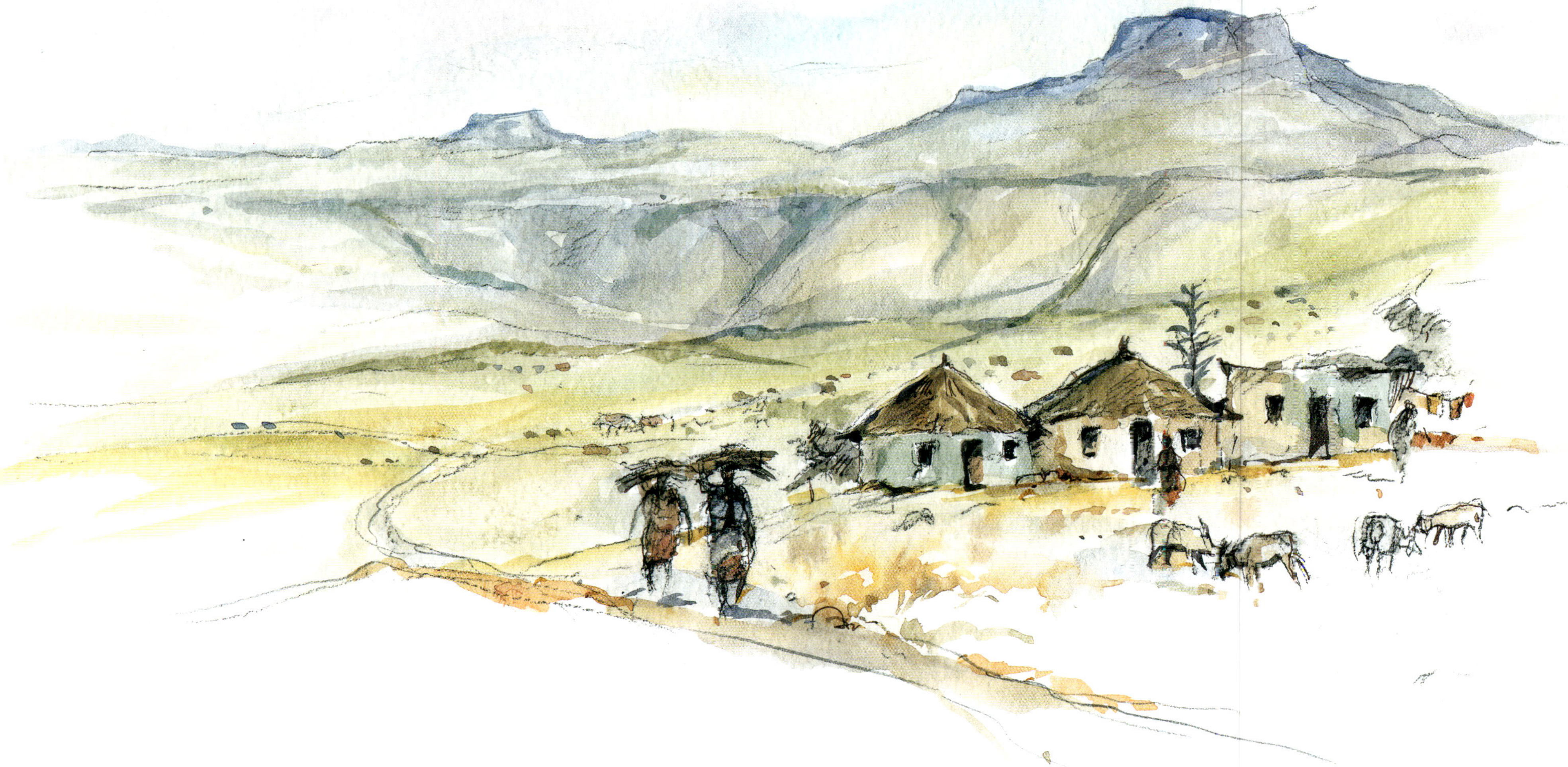

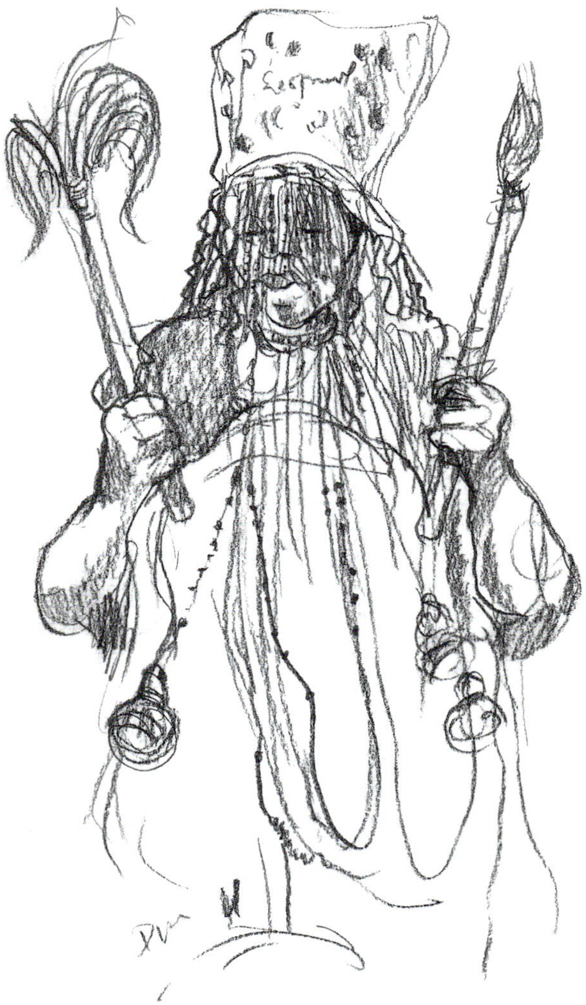

Sangomas

Adelaide is well supplied with traditional healers. Nomitsi Mhana arranges for me to visit a sangoma to do some drawings. I am surprised when I arrive at the sangoma's hut to find not one, but two sangomas and three novices. My anxiety that they might think my visit an intrusion is dispelled by their willingness to answer my questions about their traditions and rituals. Becoming a sangoma is an answer to a call by the ancestors and is not a decision but an obligation. Qualification takes three years under the tutelage of a sangoma.

They demonstrate some of their rituals, including the anointing of one of the novices. Pale liquid in a tin is beaten to a froth with a forked stick turned between the palms of the hands, and the froth is them dabbed on her back and head, all accompanied by an earnest monologue, which sounds like a prayer. It is all very mysterious and I am not sure what this means. Drums are beaten and they sway, clap and stamp their feet, chanting and singing. One of them trills and utters little plaintive cries as she responds to the voices of the ancestors who whisper in her ears.

I am touched by the emotional intensity of the women and the obvious sincerity of their belief.

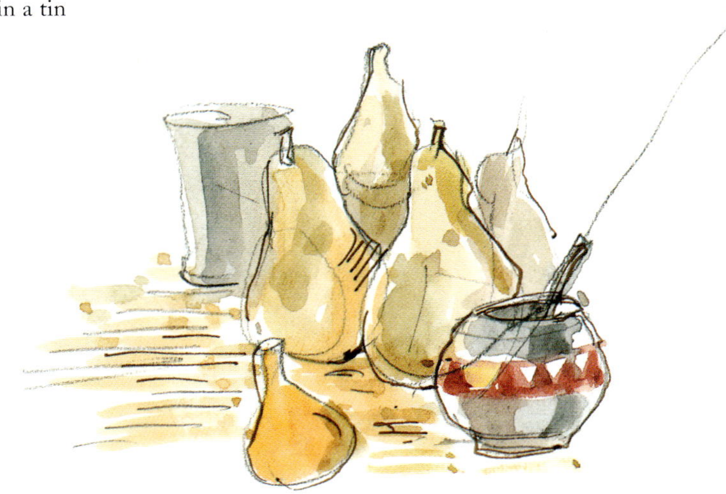

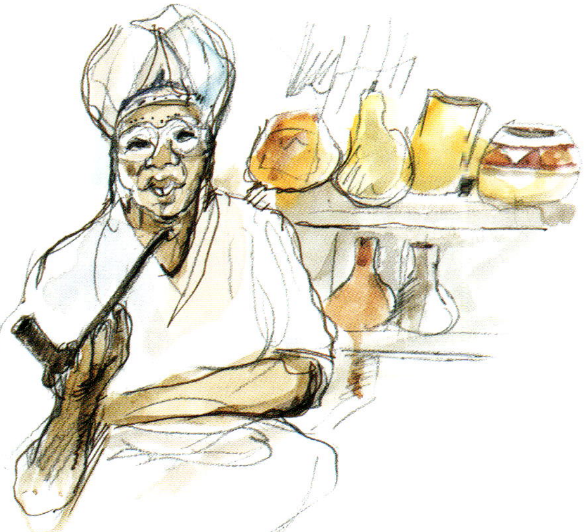

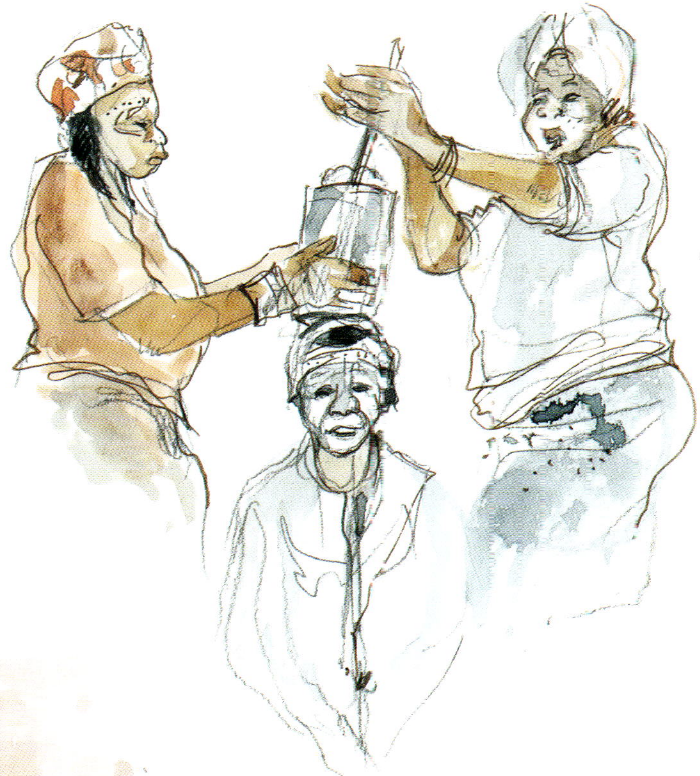

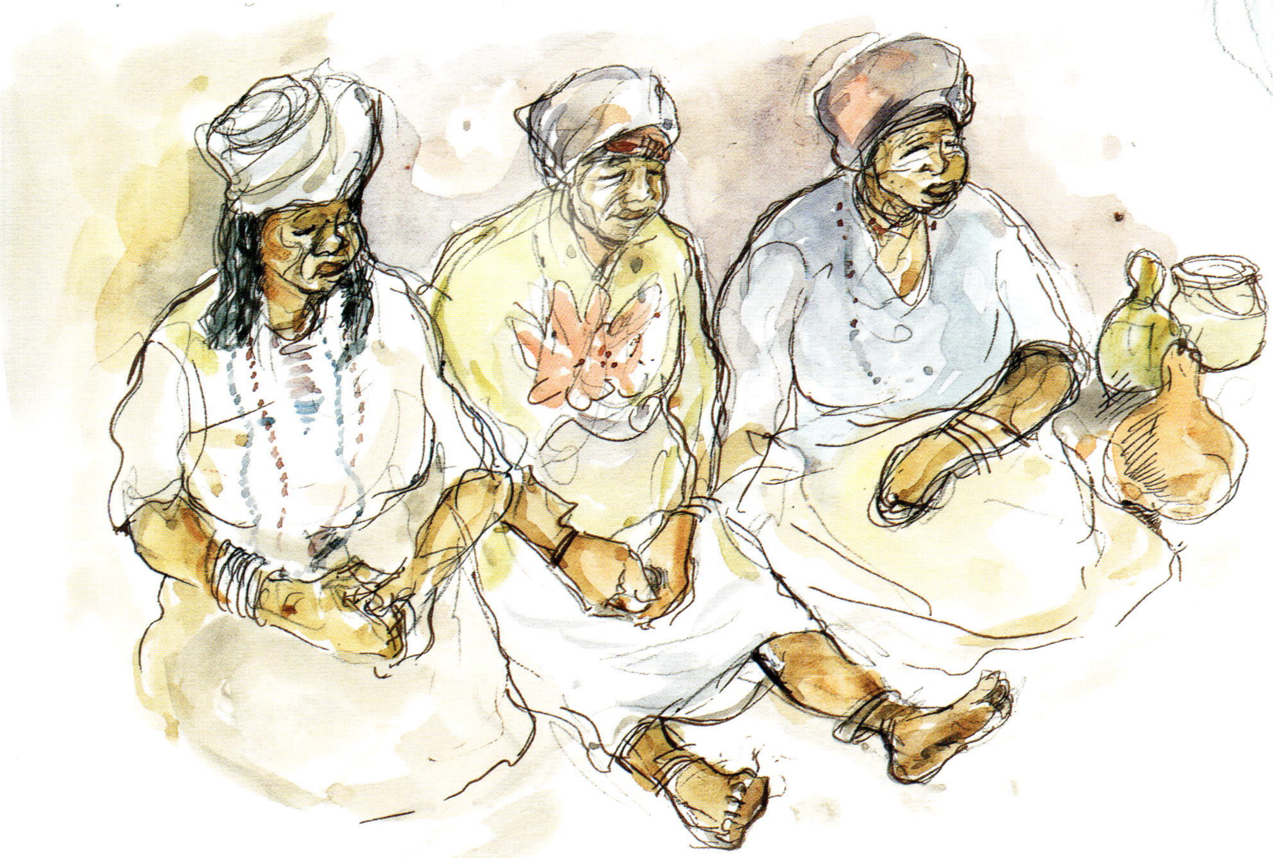

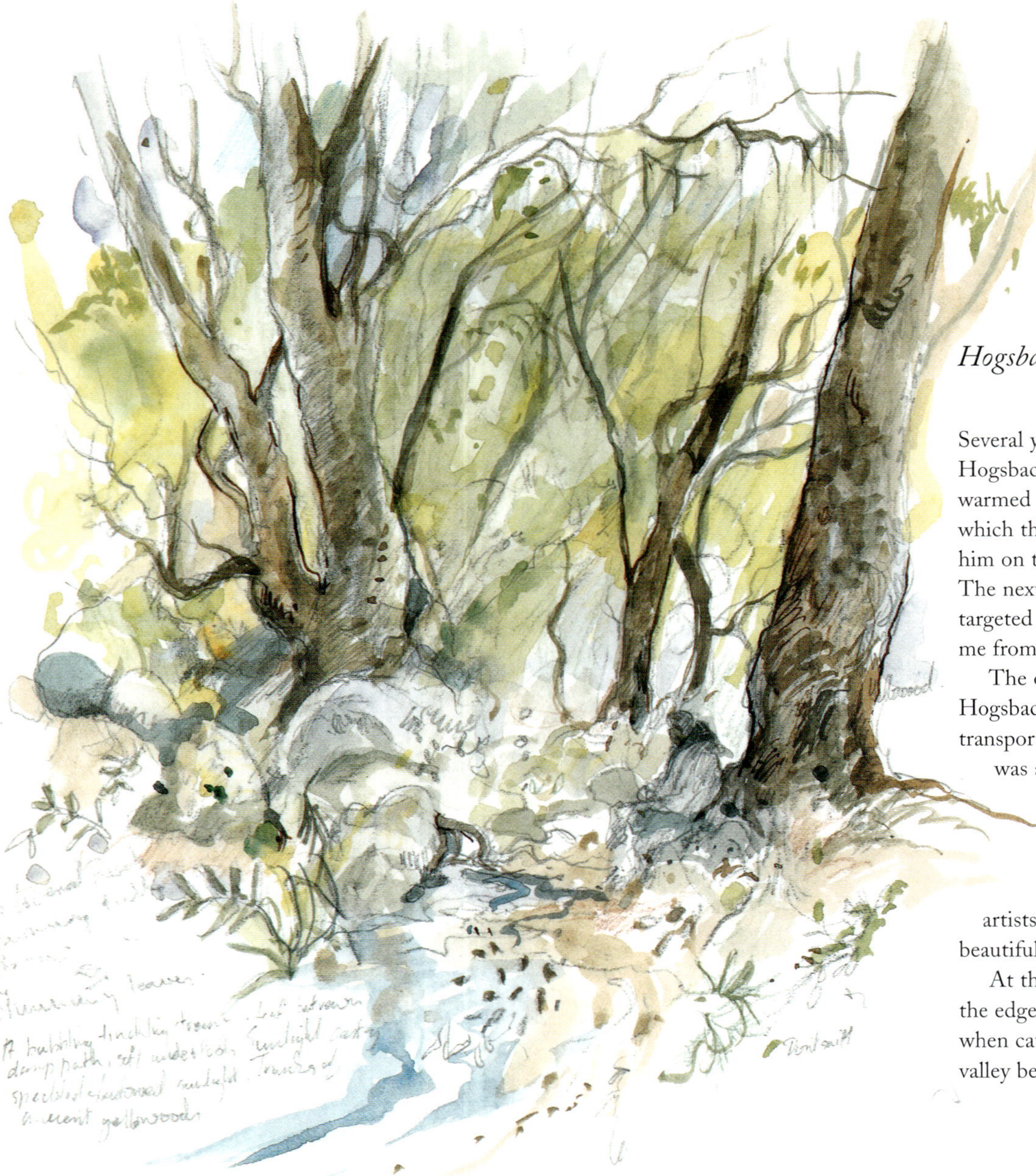

Hogsback

Several years ago we stayed overnight at the original Hogsback Inn. It was winter and a roaring log fire warmed the room. There were deep armchairs, in one of which the hotel cat was curled in languid luxury. I swept him on to the floor which marked me as a bitter enemy. The next day, walking through the garden, I was targeted by the cat's baleful, accusing glare directed at me from the shade of a juniper bush.

The owner of the hotel showed me pictures of the Hogsback as it looked over a century ago, with a transport wagon in front of a corrugated iron store. I was amazed that the hills were bare and grass-covered – there was no sign of the forests that were to be planted later on these heights and which have become so much a feature of the area. Today Hogsback is a quaint haven for artists, craftspeople and retirees seeking a quiet life in beautiful, tranquil surroundings.

At the Kettle Spout the thin stream cascading over the edge sometimes turns on itself and rises upwards when caught by a blast of wind surging up from the valley below.

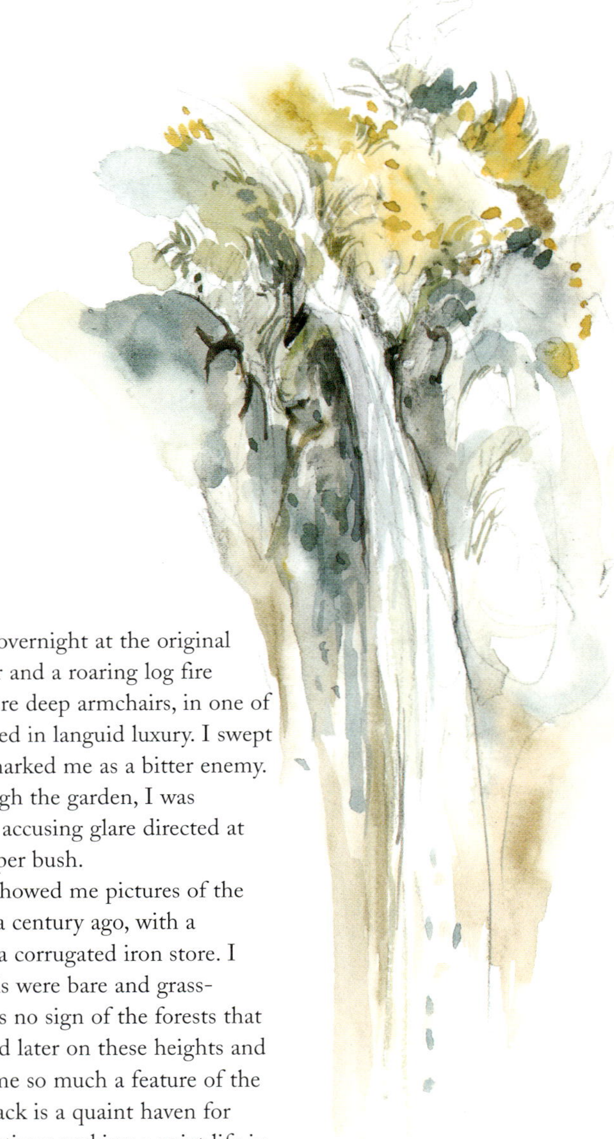

Gaika's Kop

We leave Hogsback and travel north on the road to Cathcart, passing a conical mountain named after the Xhosa chief, Ngika, but corrupted to give it the name 'Gaika's Kop'. We cross the Tyume River. The air is clear, fresh and bitterly cold at this time of the year.

A dog runs in front of the car and I swerve and brake but can't avoid hitting it. Fortunately, it doesn't seem to be hurt as it runs off yelping. We stop to collect our shattered nerves, have a cup of coffee and do these drawings of the river wending its way south before it plunges down the mountain to the Tyume Valley.

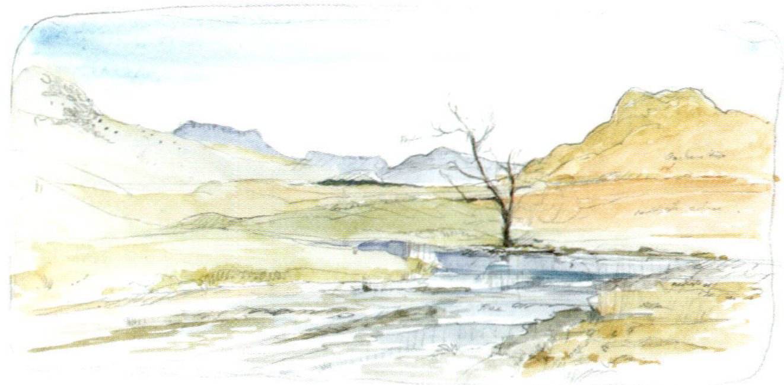

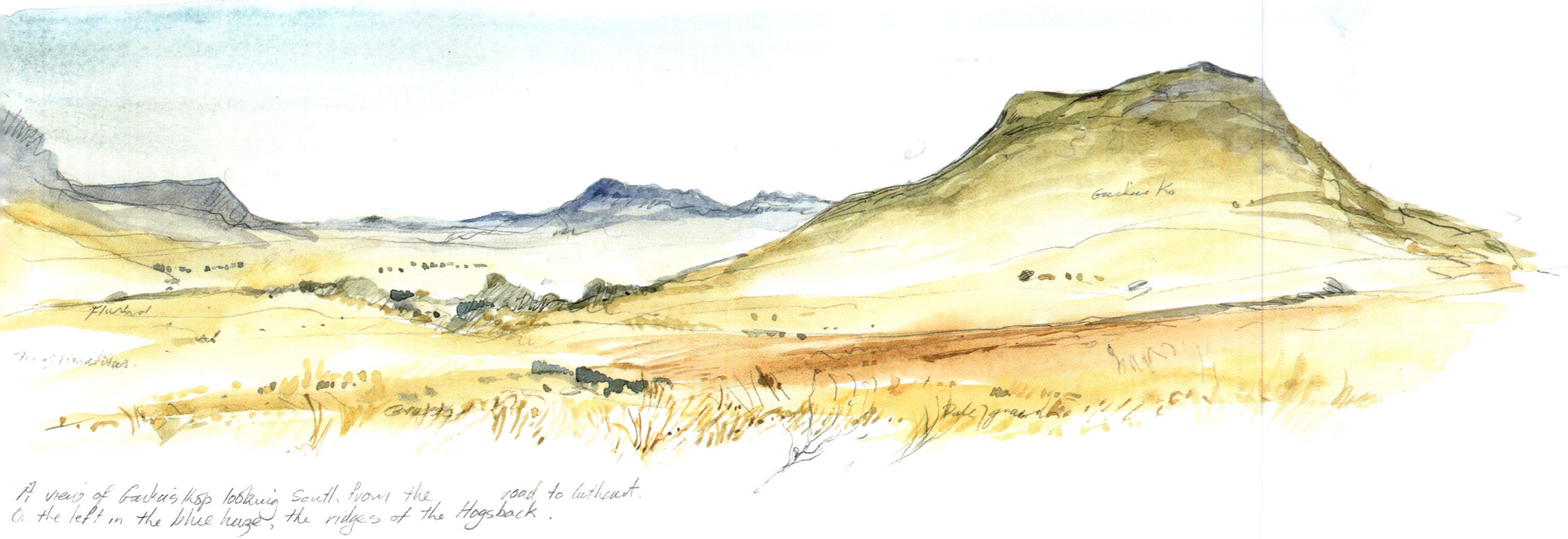
A view of Gaika's Kop looking South from the road to Cathcart.
On the left in the blue haze, the ridges of the Hogsback.

Sheep shearers

Sheep-shearing on a farm in the Cathcart district, owned by Lyndon Snelling. A team of sheep shearers from Whittlesea have been engaged to shear the Doonie merino. We are told they are among the best shearers in the country, amazingly skilled and swift, their shears snipping the fleece close to the skin so that the wool peels off the sheep like the skin of an orange. The shearers must have a good knowledge of the anatomy of the sheep and the curves of the body so that they cut close without cutting the skin and the wool is of even length. Within ten minutes the heavy fleece is removed in one piece and thrown on to the sorting table. Shorn of their heavy overcoats, the sheep are half their size and look strangely gawky, pale and vulnerable as they are guided off the shearing floor.

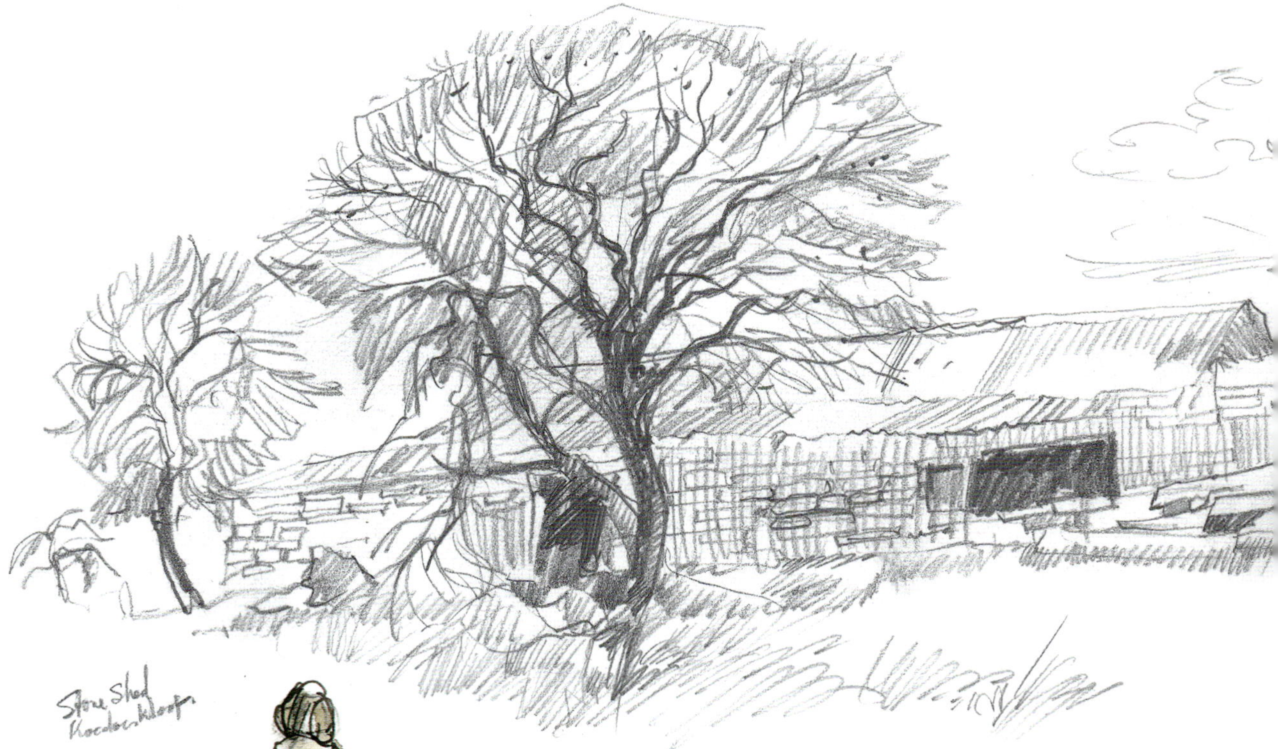

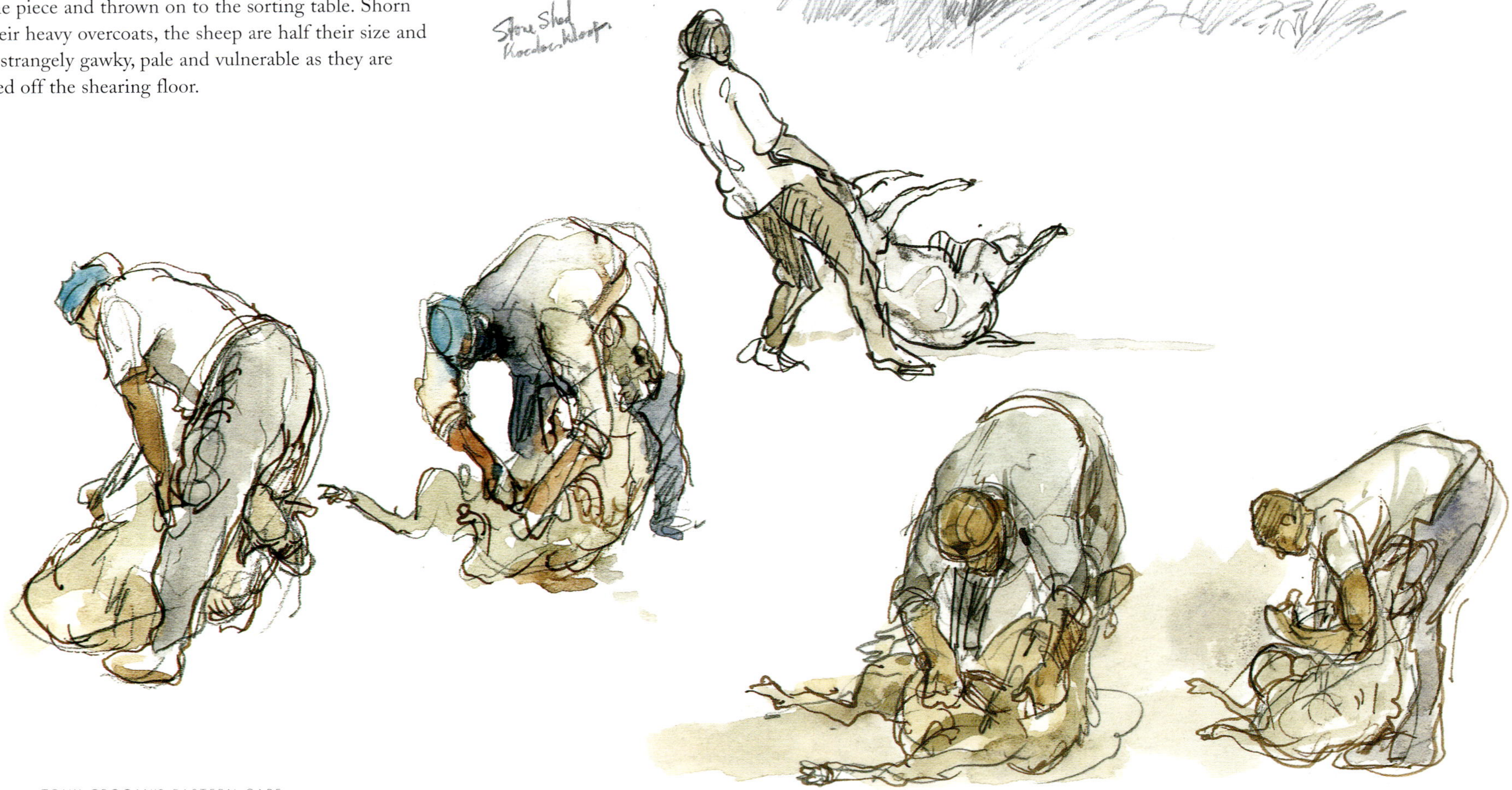

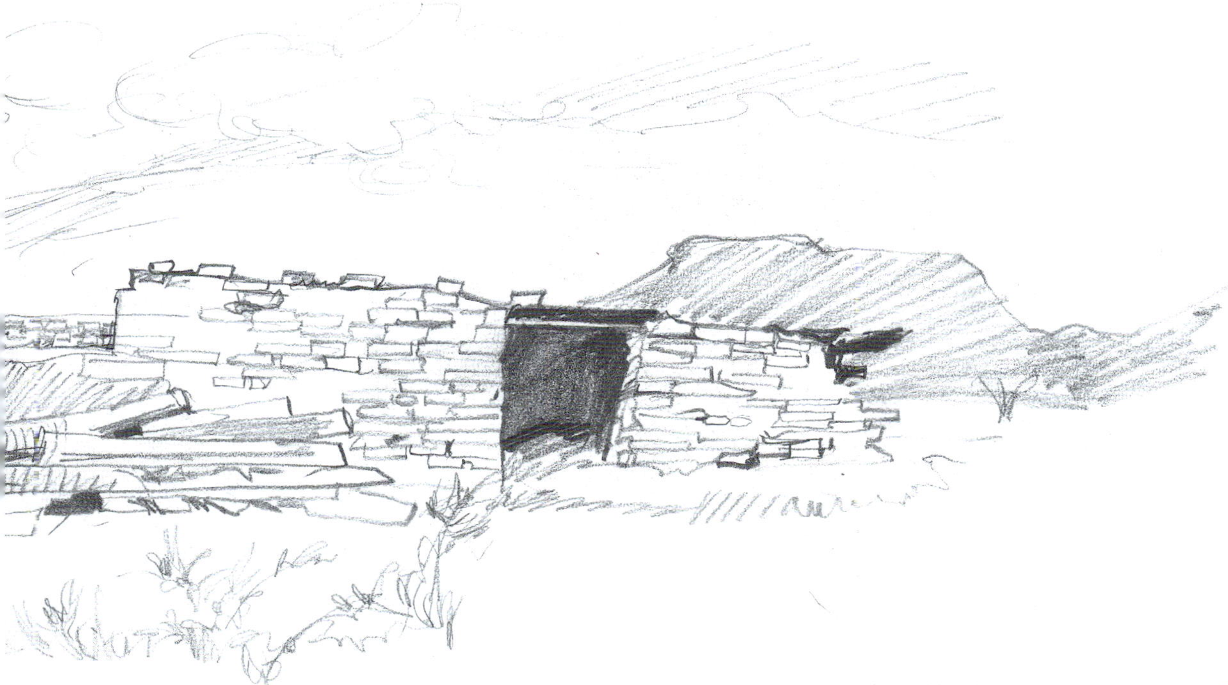

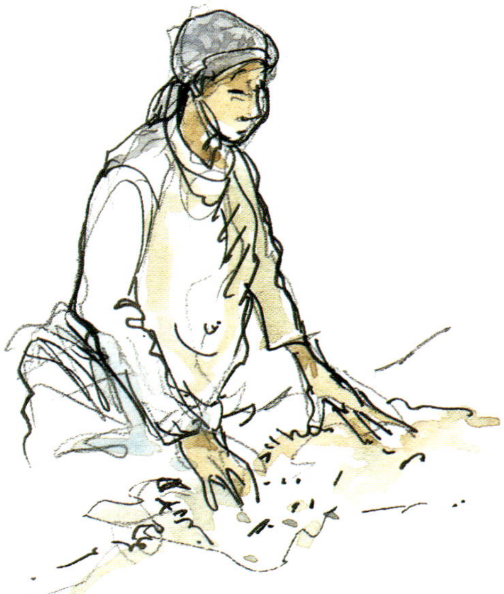

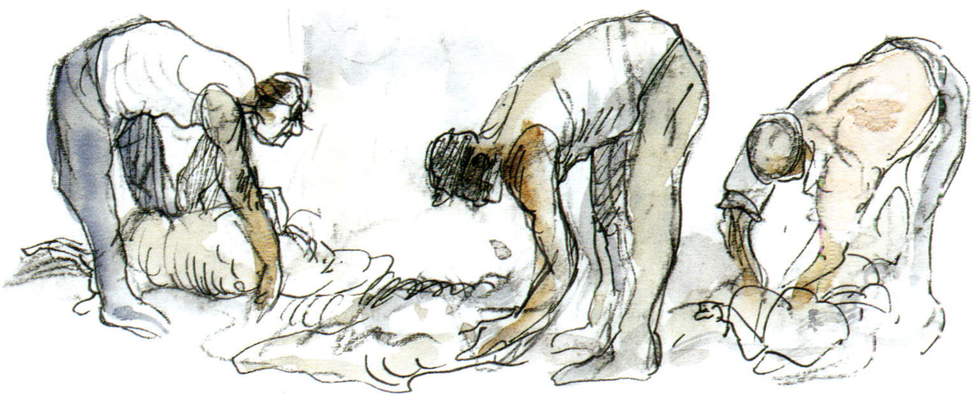

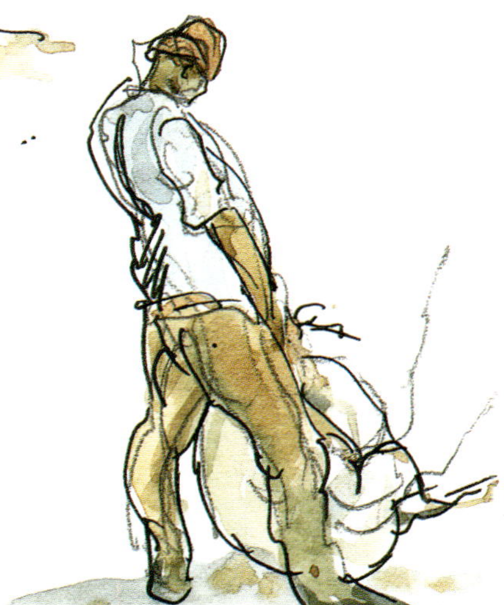

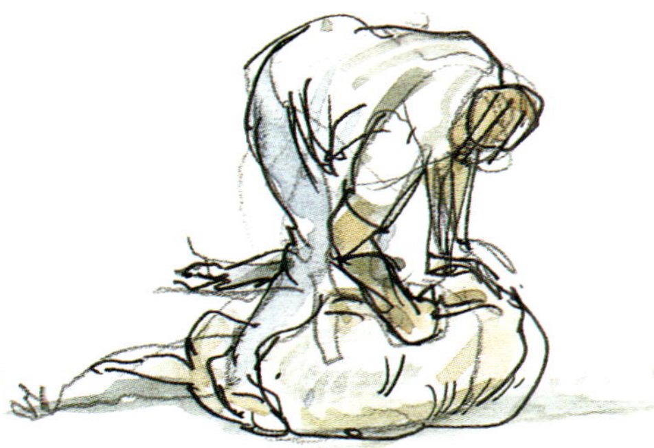

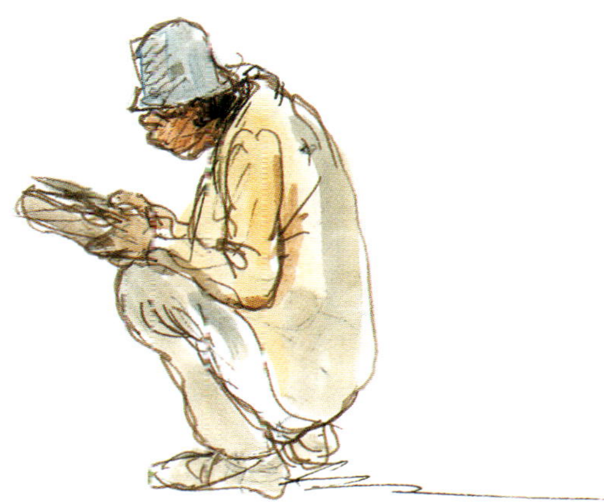

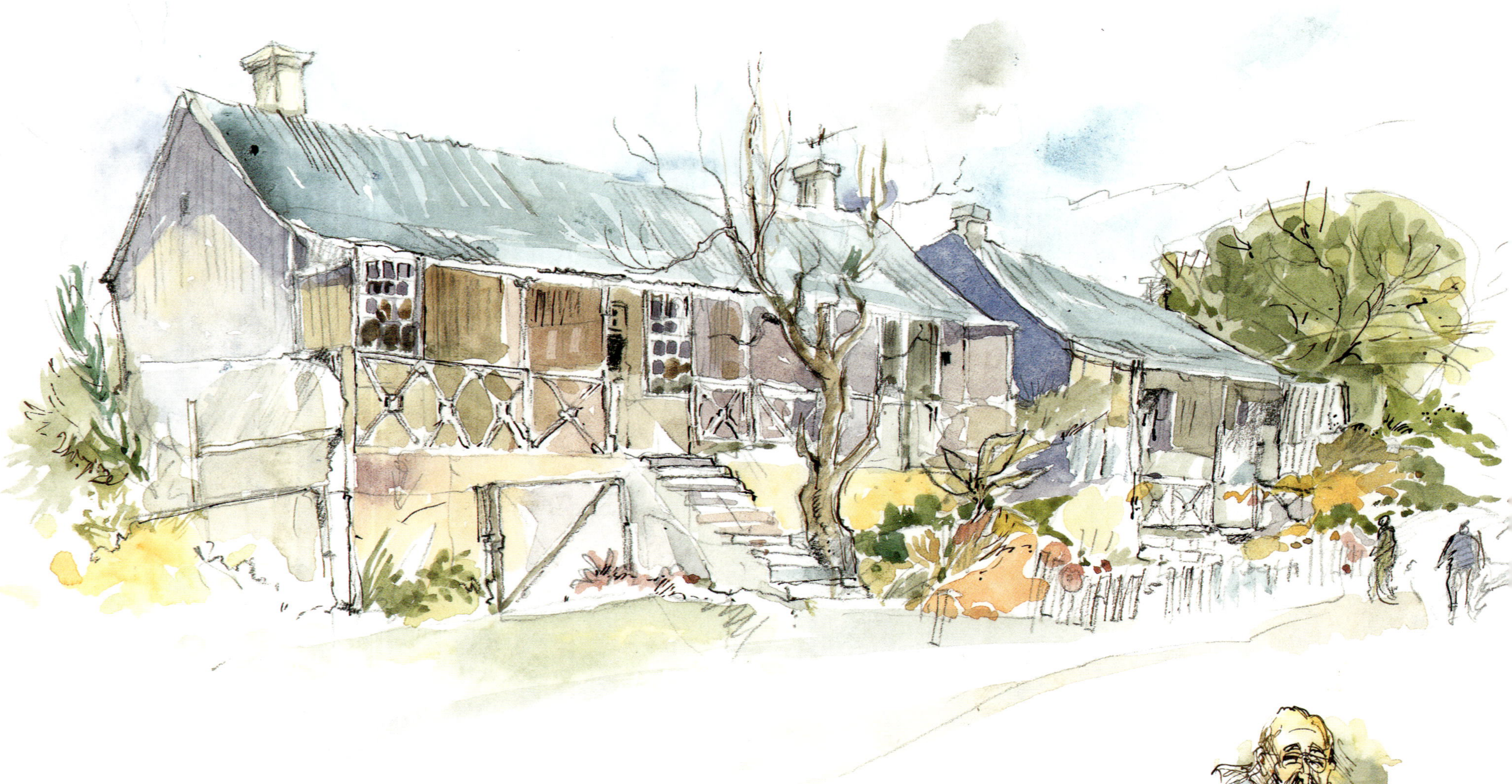

Cathcart

Cathcart, one of the old frontier towns, has a broad main street lined with some beautiful stone buildings. We relax in a small coffee shop and watch through the window a group of toy-toying, placard-waving municipal workers making their way down the street. It must be a commonplace event because nobody takes much notice.

We go up to the Kenya houses, so called because they were offered in a magnanimous gesture by the Cathcart Council to Kenyan whites dispossessed and rendered homeless by the Mau-Mau uprising in the 1950s. I knock on the door of one of the corrugated iron cottages and am admitted by an

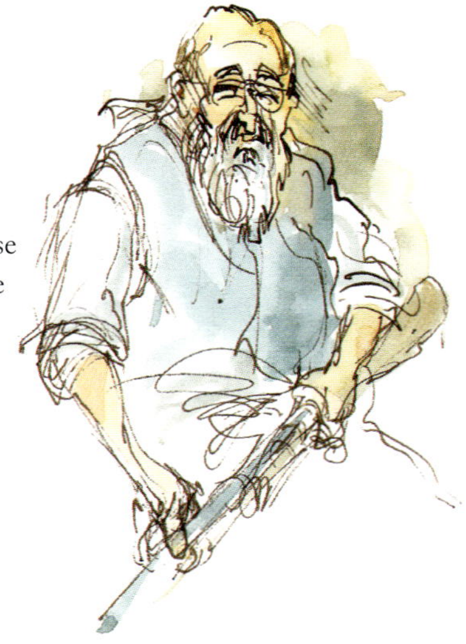

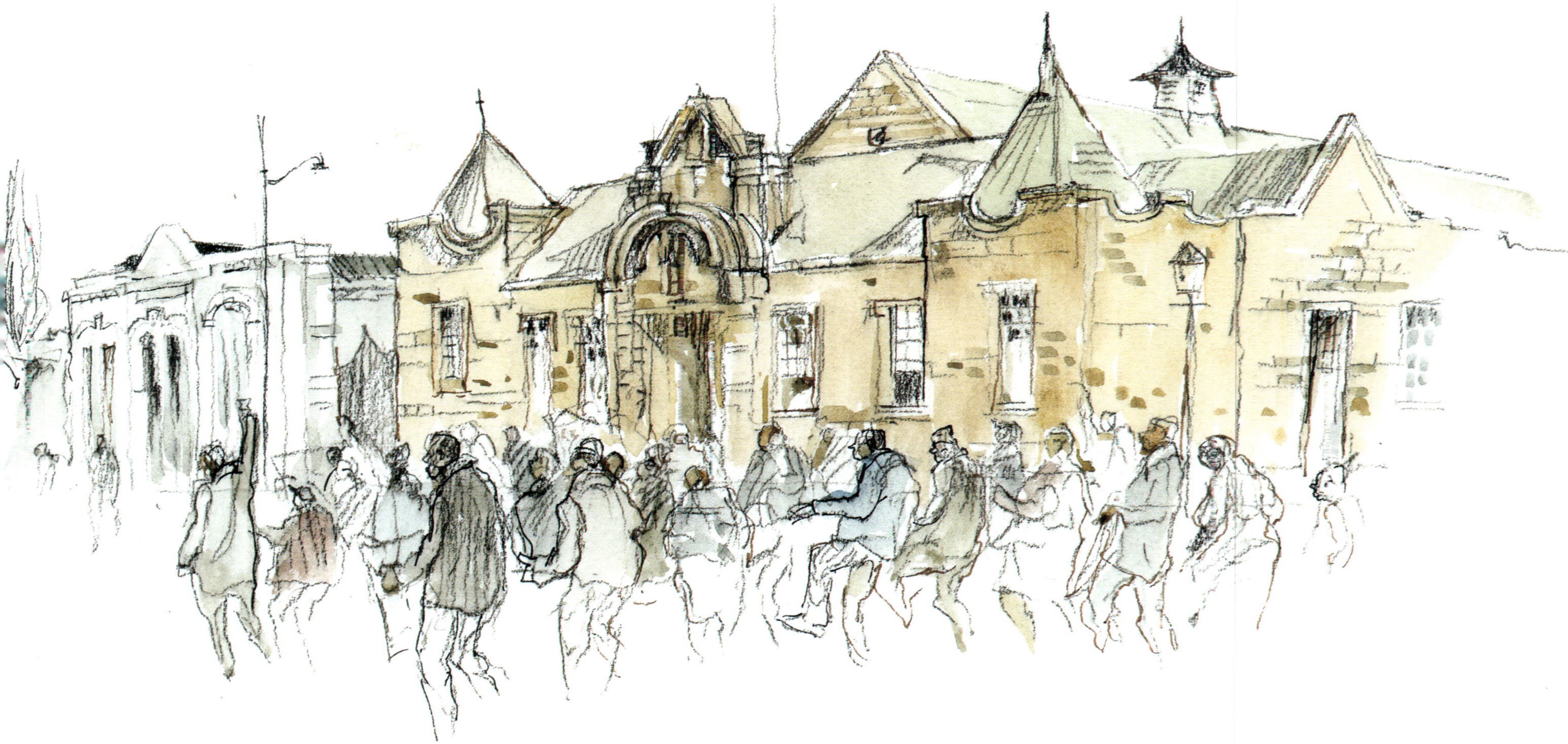

elderly woman, who introduces me to her husband, a bearded figure sitting in an armchair who, I am alarmed to note, is cleaning a rifle. He is chatting to the local fireman, who says he worked for the municipality in Komgha for years but has now transferred to Cathcart. He looks out of the window and sees a thin plume of black smoke rising in the clear morning air. It is probably a tyre being burned by the protestors we saw earlier.

"Ag," says the fireman, shrugging his shoulders, "let them get on with it."

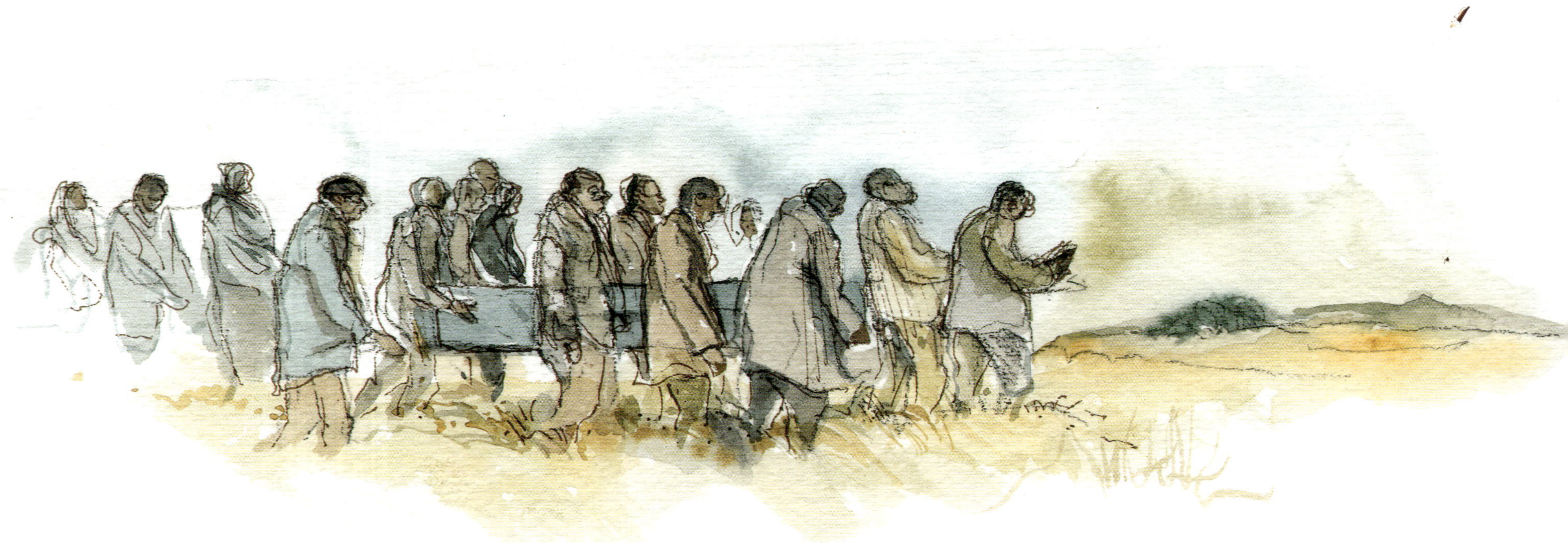

Across the Transkei

We travel north to Barkly East via Queenstown and Dordrecht, jolting our way over the most atrocious roads, determining that if we ever came this way again we would avoid taking short cuts. We pass through parts of the old homelands of Ciskei and Transkei, now the burden of the new Eastern Cape administration, and I imagine a cause of their now legendary financial woes. I buy a copy of the *Daily Dispatch* and read an article by Dr Trudy Thomas, in which she makes the point that it has become fashionable to criticise the Eastern Cape government for financial mismanagement and the general muddle that it is in, but for all its high-handed criticism, the national government originally underfunded the province, then insisted that it carry the burden of 18,000 supernumeraries (superfluous civil servants) inherited from the previous government, which each year cost it nearly a billion rand in salaries.

"The government insisted they be retained but sent no money to pay for this dead wood," she writes.

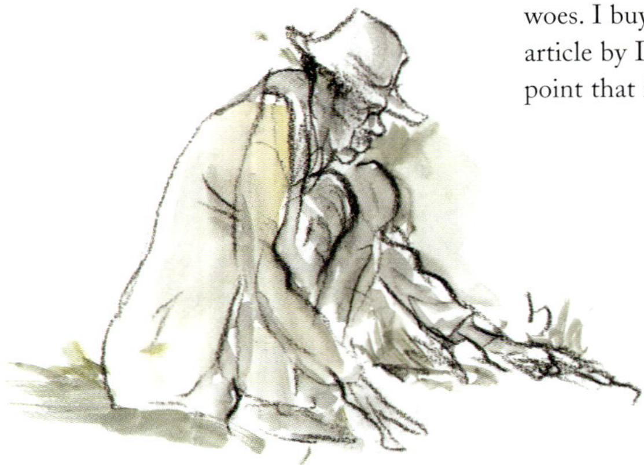

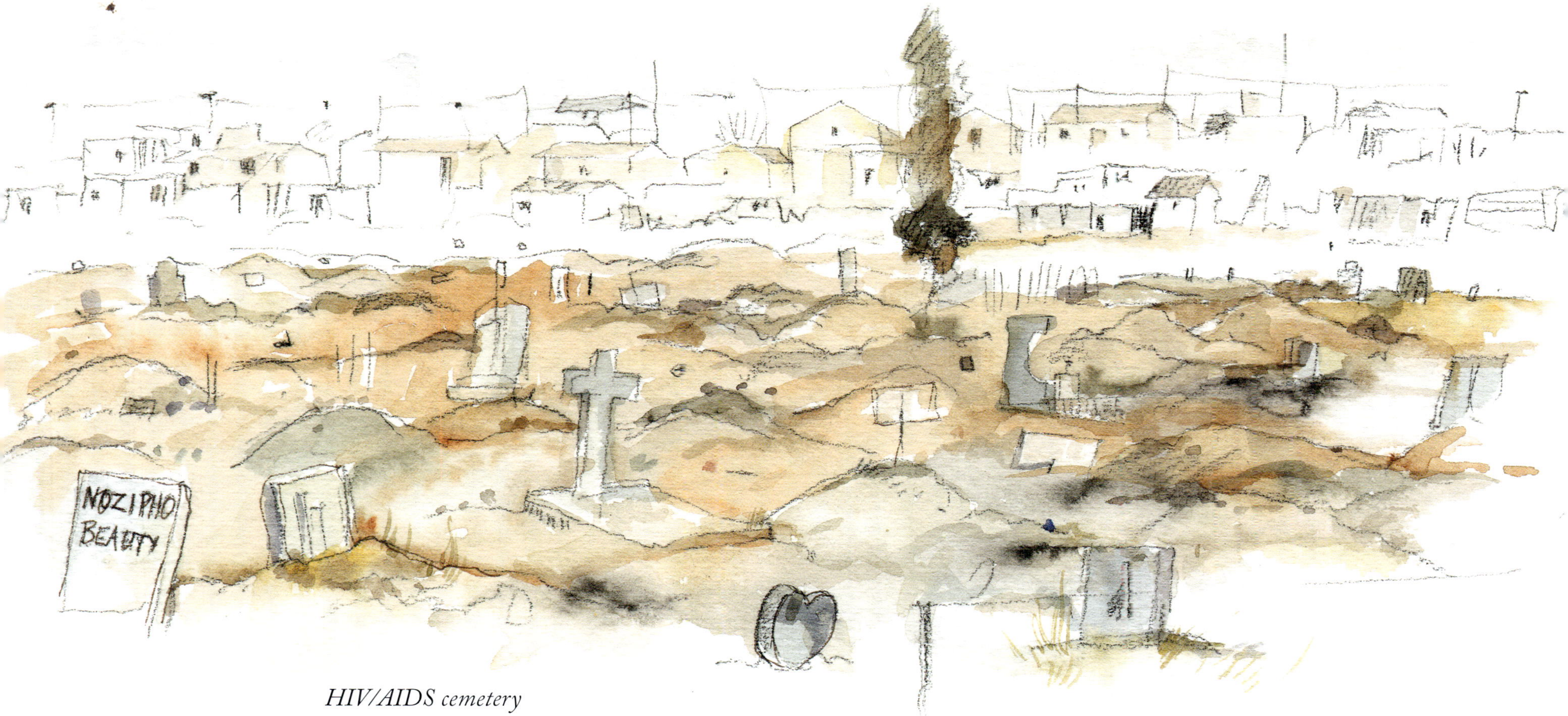

HIV/AIDS cemetery

The land in these previous, so-called national states is overgrazed, heavily scarred by soil erosion and overburdened by the weight of the population whose huts and dwellings pepper the hillsides and valleys. Pass through any village on a Saturday and you will notice the crush of people and minibus taxis. Kwaito music blares forth, and private enterprise is alive and well in roadside stalls, cell phone services and those businesses that thrive in poverty – loan banks and microlenders. More sinister are the tent hire companies for all too frequent funeral services over the weekends. On any weekend, you will see these sad processions wending their way to the graveyards. Anyone who doubts the cataclysmic impact of HIV/AIDS need only observe the cemeteries outside rural villages in the Eastern Cape. Below the hill of the township outside Barkly East, the red earth has been heaved up to cover hundreds of new graves. There are few headstones. Tender, loving inscriptions are painted on pieces of tin and wood – strangely, most of them in English. Wire and plastic wreathes, bottles of dried flowers and other poignant tokens of respect and remembrance adorn the simple graves. There is haunted despair in the voice of a man who observes, "The land is dying."

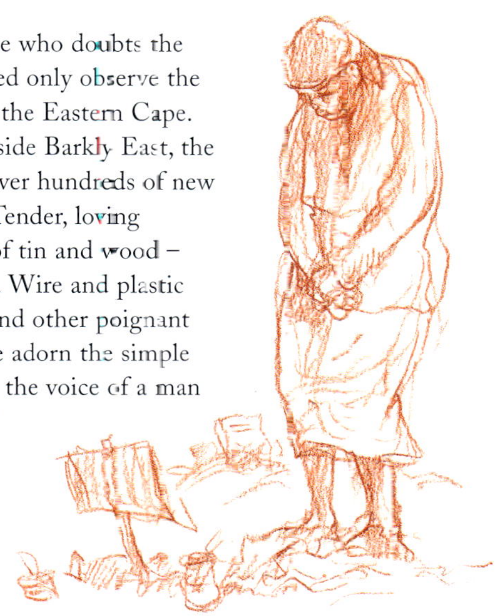

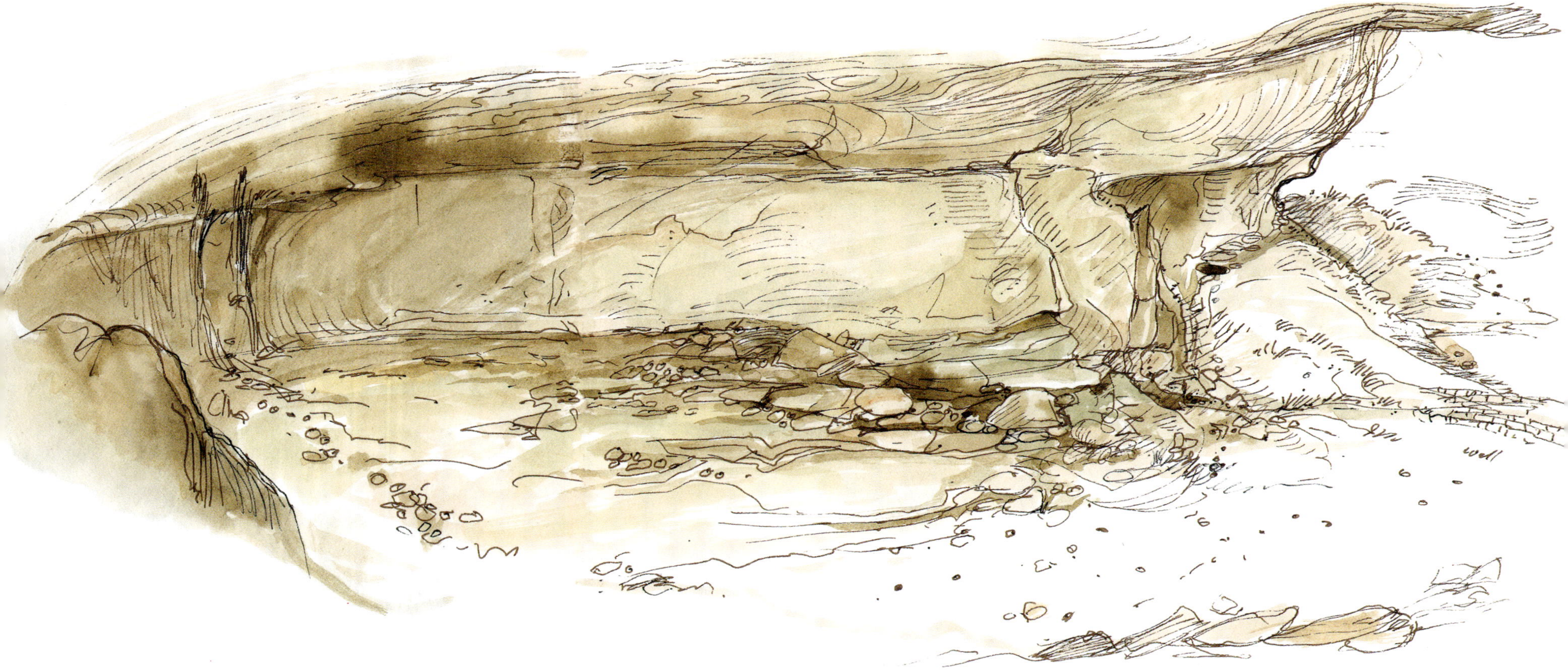

Bushmen paintings

Pitlochrie, the Sephton's farm north of Barkly East, lies in a spur of the Drakensberg called the Wittebergen. His forbears were 1820 Settlers from Salem in the Albany district, who came to this northern part of the province in 1867. The hills, covered in soft, tawny grass, are pallid in the haze of veld fires, which are common at this time of the year. Farmers light them to stimulate the growth of palatable grazing.

It was in these mountains, Paul Sephton told us, that another notable historical event took place. Donald Woods, the banned editor of the *Daily Dispatch*, made his escape from the country over these mountains, swimming 'a crocodile infested' river. Once he reached Lesotho he lost no time in cheekily phoning the then Minister of Police, Jimmy Kruger, to bid him a fond farewell.

Paul drives us through a stunning landscape where the the earth has slipped off the hills, exposing their bare stone flanks, and sandstone outcrops which have been eroded and sculpted into bizarre shapes. We bounce and jolt our way along an atrocious gravel road, over ridges of rock and potholes, which the little Toyota bakkie rattles over with ease. It has done a total of 300,000km on roads like these, Paul tells us.

We make our way down a kloof to a cavernous rock shelter in a promontory jutting into the valley. It formed a perfect shelter for the San, facing east into the sun, well protected from the prevailing wind with an extensive view of the winding river and plain below. Deep in the shelter on a perfect wall of sandstone, the little San hunters have exercised their art for centuries, creating a tableau of beautifully rendered animals, people and mythical figures. They are exquisitely painted, wonderfully observed and alive with graceful movement.

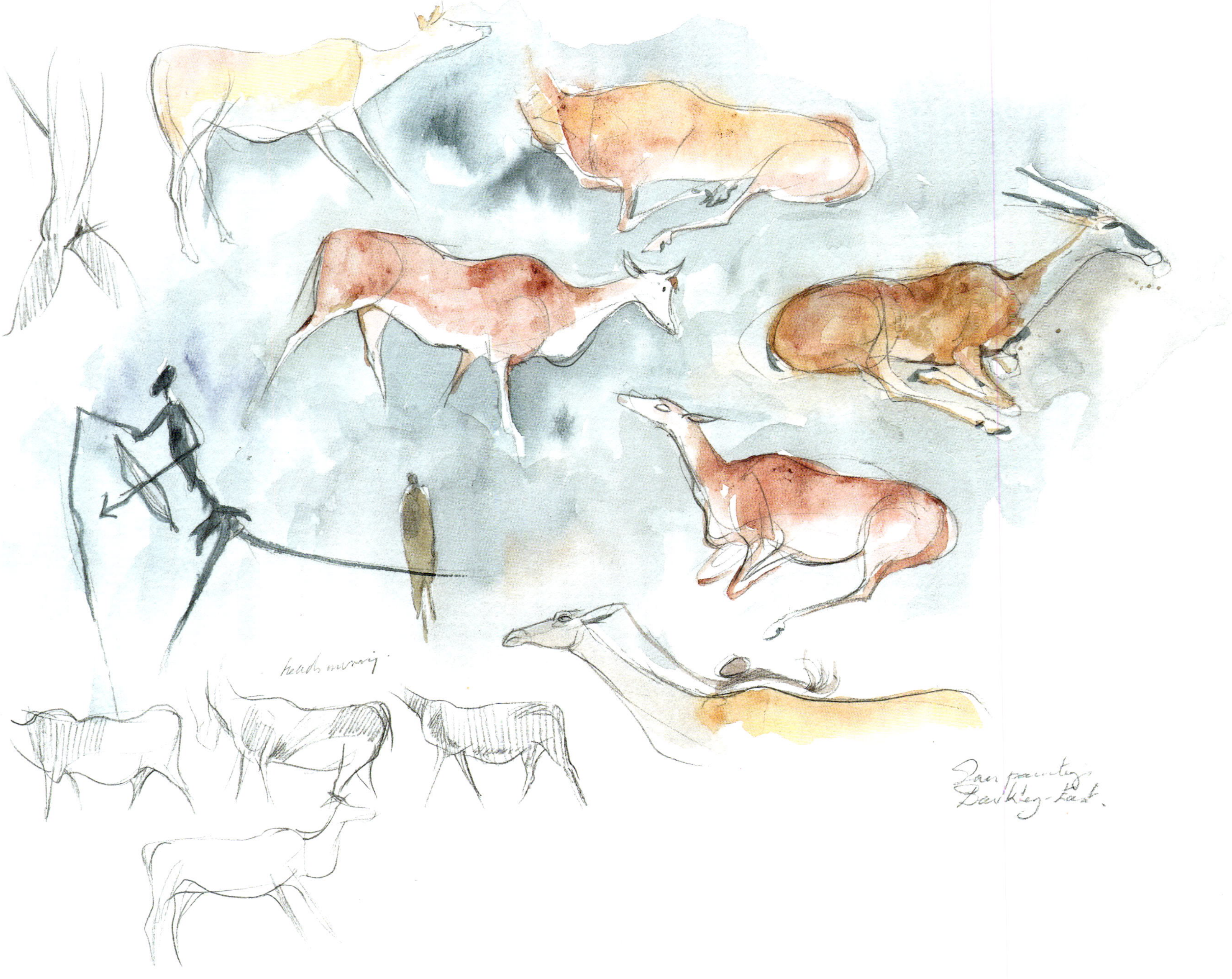

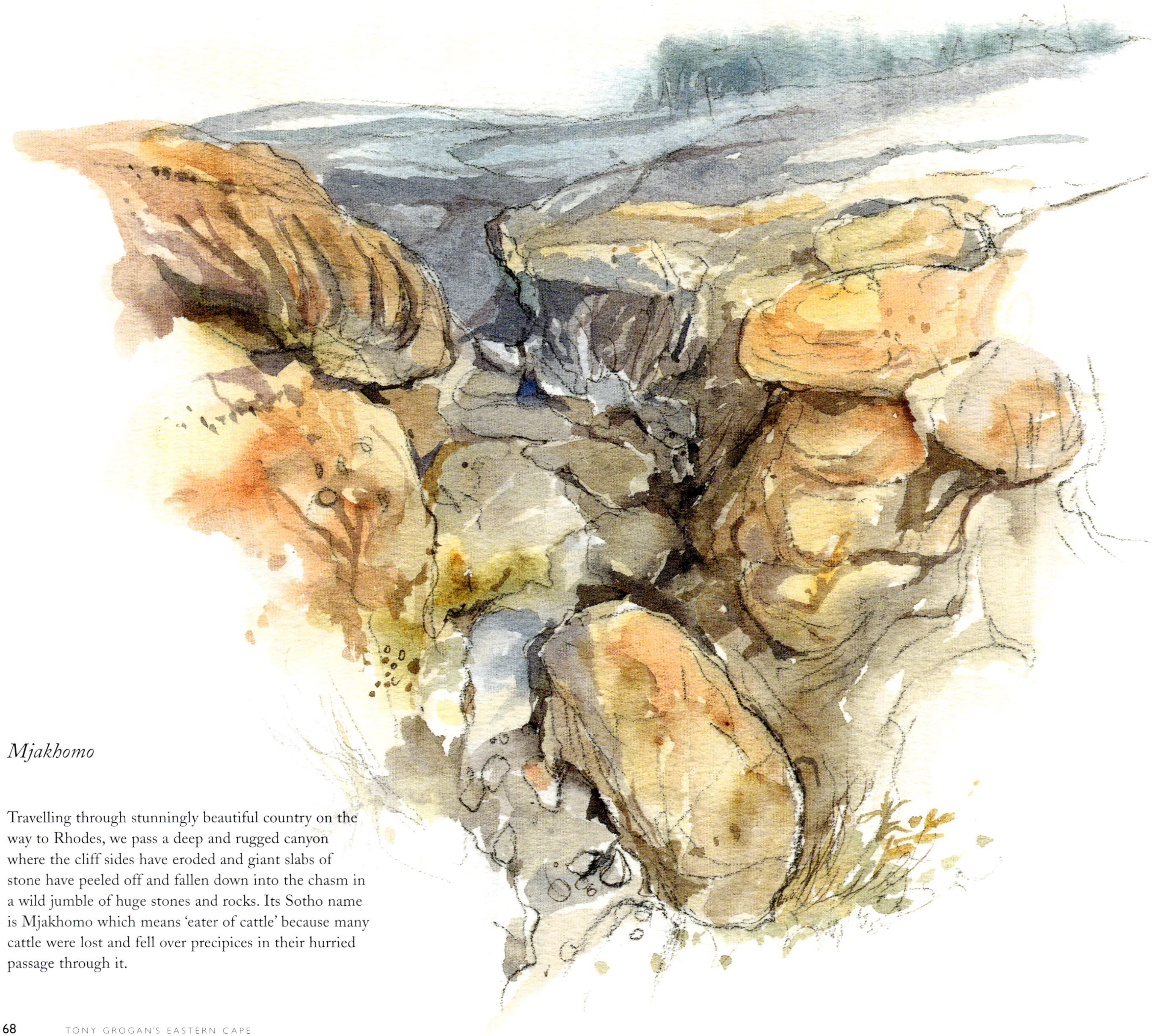

Mjakhomo

Travelling through stunningly beautiful country on the way to Rhodes, we pass a deep and rugged canyon where the cliff sides have eroded and giant slabs of stone have peeled off and fallen down into the chasm in a wild jumble of huge stones and rocks. Its Sotho name is Mjakhomo which means 'eater of cattle' because many cattle were lost and fell over precipices in their hurried passage through it.

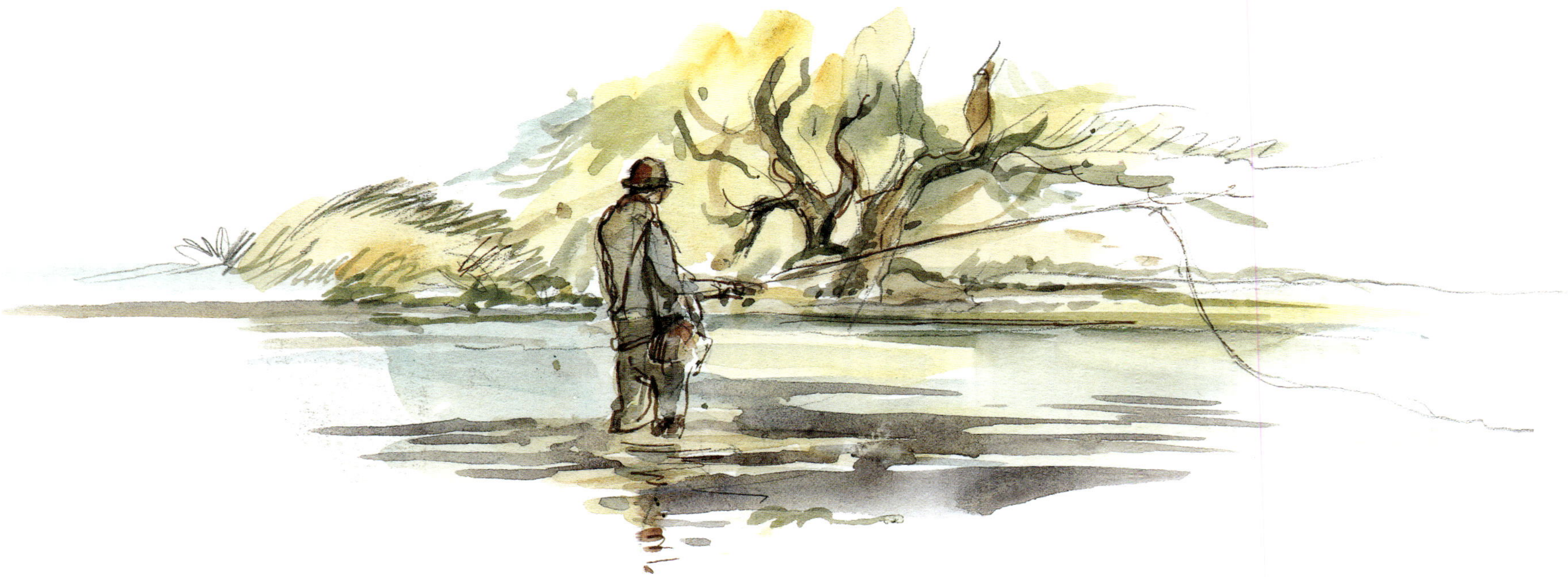

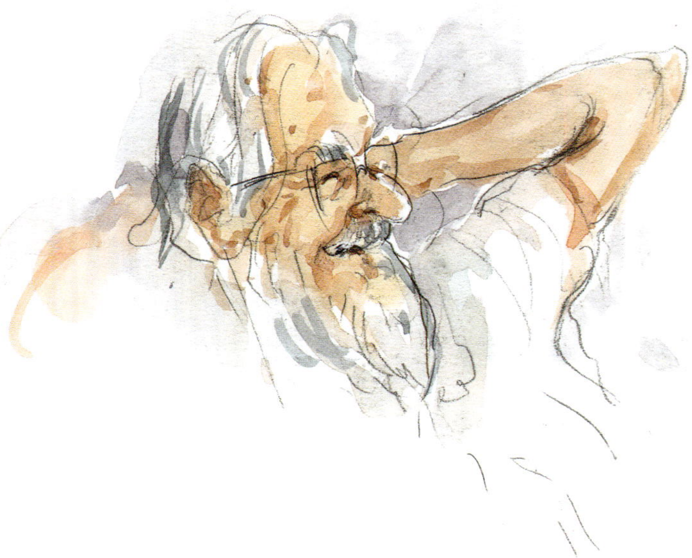

Rhodes

In the remote village in the foothills of the Drakensberg we have a beer and sandwich in the 'centre of the universe', Dave Walker's friendly pub in the Walkerbout Inn. Dave is a long-time resident of Rhodes. A precondition of living in a place like this, he tells us, is that you have to be mad, and having established that primary credential to survive you have to adopt a simple three-principled philosophy: time is irrelevant; distance of no consequence and never go anywhere without your own wheels. He has seen many changes. The hippies and various other alternative life-stylers, eager to escape the brash materialism of city life, came in the 1970s and early eighties, settled, then left when they discovered that Rhodes was bone-chillingly cold in winter and a hell of a long way from anywhere. Houses could be bought for a song then or sold to settle a small overdraft and the village languished. Now the yuppies have discovered Rhodes and property values have increased astronomically.

The last time I visited Rhodes they had just had the heaviest snowfall for 20 years. We drove to the top of Naude's Nek, one of the highest and most tortuous passes in the country and drove through a miraculous world of white as far as a bulldozer had cleared the road. Then we had to reverse most of the way back again before we could find a place to turn. People visit the area mainly for the skiing at Tiffindale or for the splendid trout fishing in the clear mountain streams.

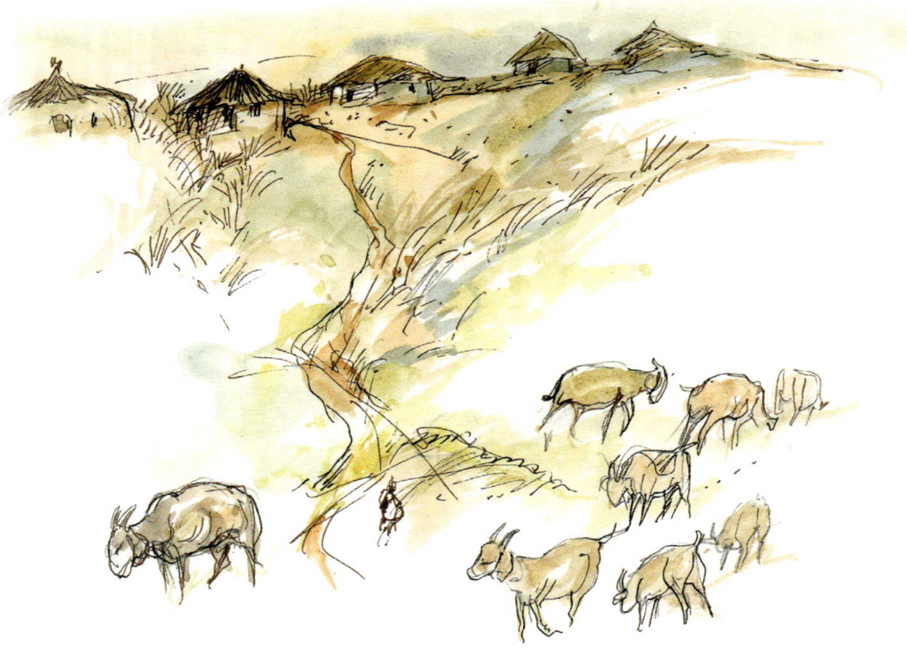

Barkly Pass

The northern Eastern Cape has some of the most spectacular mountain passes in the country, one of which is the beautiful Barkly Pass. From Elliot, it winds its way down the escarpment in broad, sweeping curves, affording entrancing views of weathered sandstone cliffs and great buttresses of rock eroded into weird and fantastical shapes. To the west, the precipitous rampart of the Drakensberg stretches away, ending in the soaring sandstone cliffs of the Xalanga (the vulture).

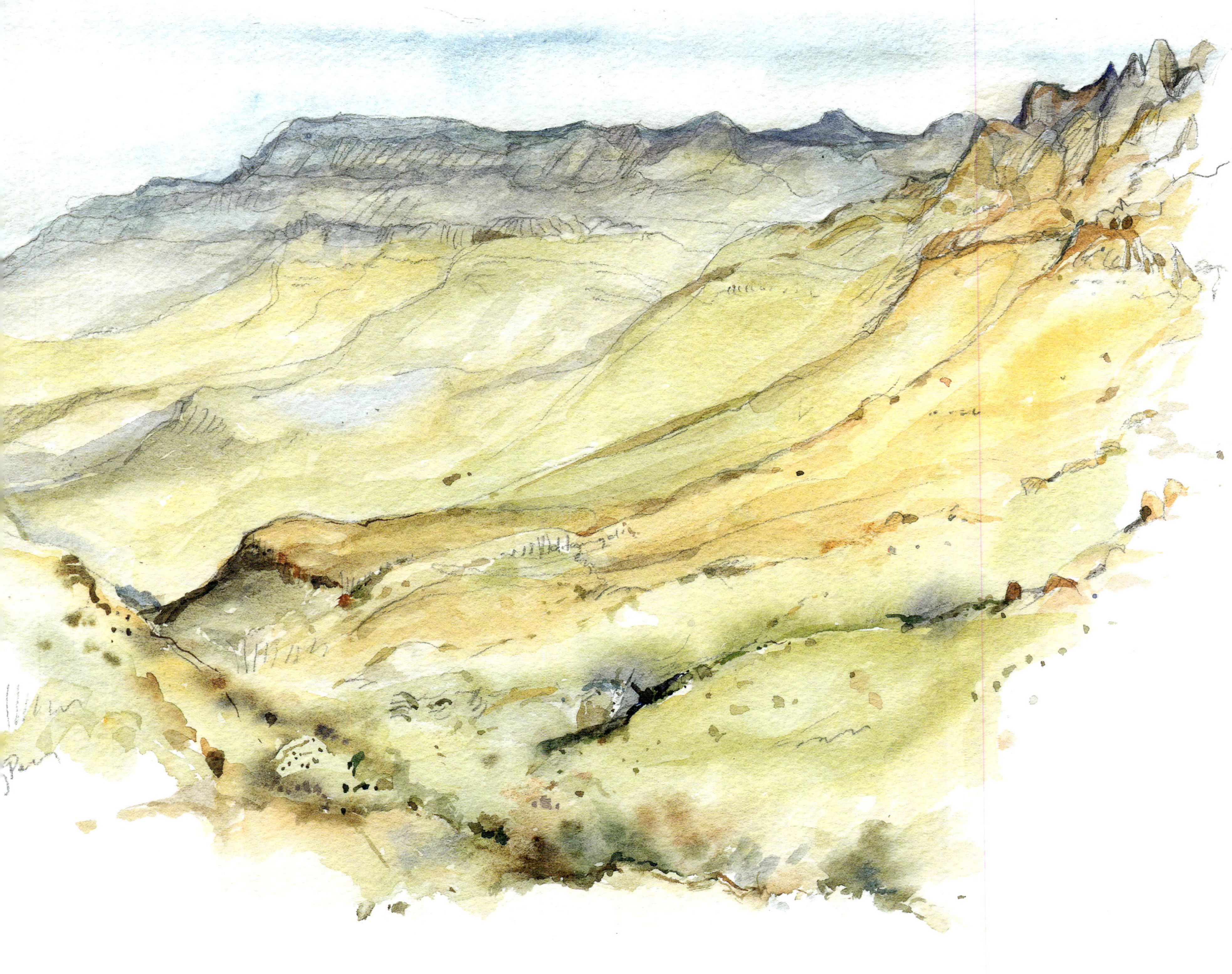

Hole-in-the-Wall

We spend a few days with friends in a seaside shack at Hole-in-the-Wall, a spectacularly beautiful stretch of coastline on the Wild Coast. It is a place where a quiet stream makes its way through dark green, thickly forested hills to enter the sea where somehow through a strange freak of nature, a great wall of rock has become separated from the mainland to create a barrier against the onslaught of the sea. The perpetual beating of the waves against the rock over the ages have found a flaw and carved a tunnel through the wall. It is an impressive sight to watch at high tide, when waves burst through this cavity and send radiating swells towards the shore across the calm lagoon on the landward side of the wall.

Local Xhosa legend tells of a Xhosa maiden who fell in love with one of the Sea People who emerged from the waves in the lagoon. Her father forbade her to go with her lover so one night the Sea People caused a giant fish to batter a hole through the rock with its head. As the Sea People rushed through, everyone fled except the maiden who joined her lover to return to the sea with his people and she was never seen again.

East of the wall is a large humpbacked, grass-covered hill called the 'Whale's back', which plunges precipitously into the sea where there are boiling chasms of white water. Here Jonny Lowe, my fisherman friend, tells me large kabeljou lurk in the foamy depths. Two young boys have taken the day off school, which takes a back seat when there is an opportunity to earn some money, scarce in this part of the world. Jonny gives them a couple of rods and they head off to the Whale's back. They return later in the day with a handsome kob of about 8kg, for which they are suitably rewarded.

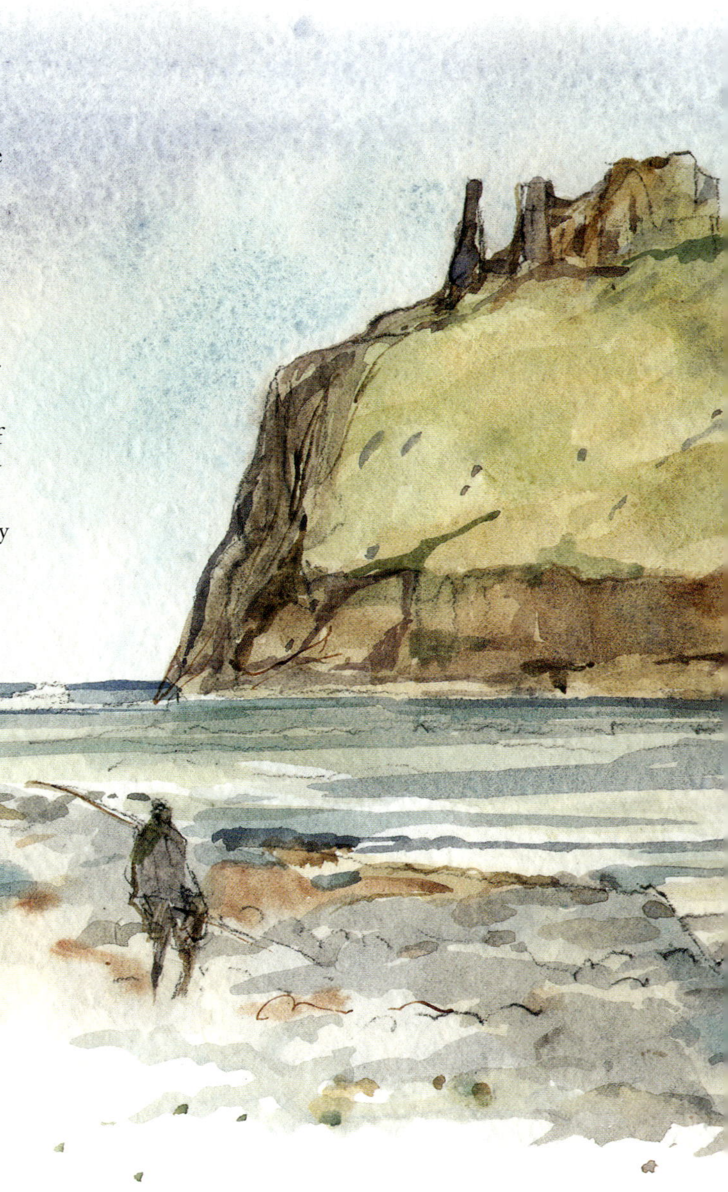

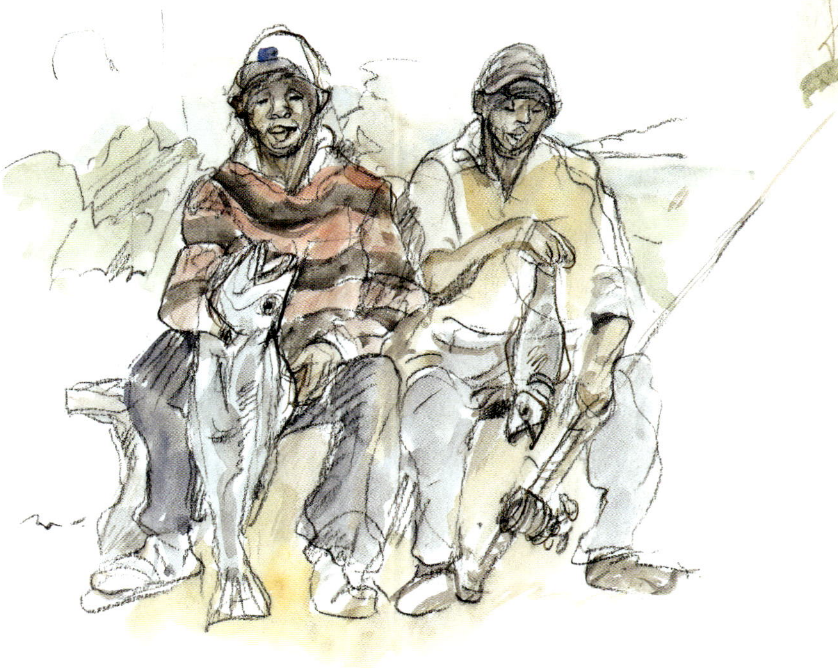

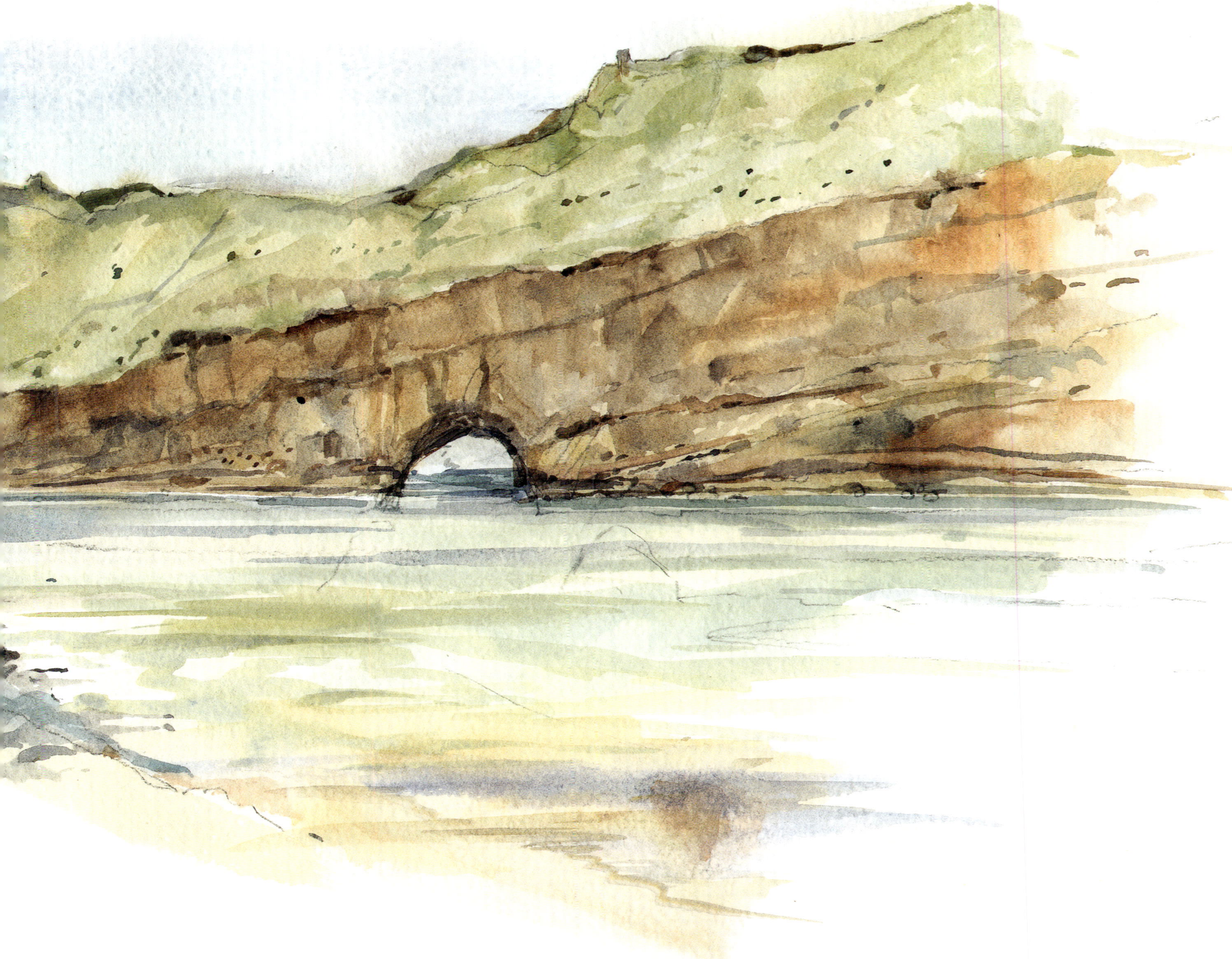

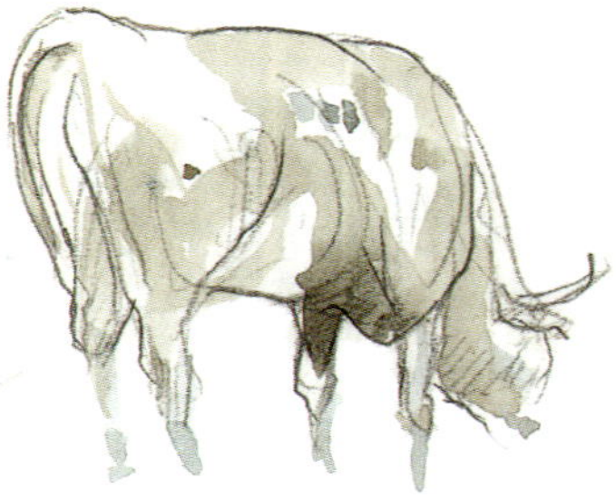

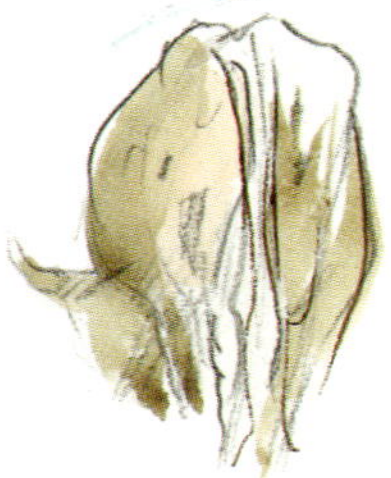

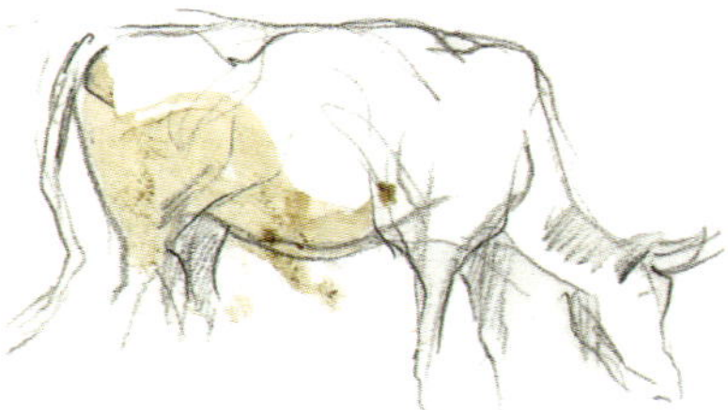

Gxarha River

We leave the main national road near Butterworth. I am fascinated by the legend which inspired the 1856 Xhosa cattle killing, and want to see the pool in Gxarha River where the young girl Nongqawuse experienced a vision in which she saw the spirits of the ancestors, who promised that the dead would rise, new healthy cattle would emerge from the sea, and the Xhosa people would enjoy a time of plenty if they killed their all cattle and destroyed their crops. It would seem that defeat in several frontier wars, land pressure, the missionaries' Christian message of salvation, and the fact that many of their cattle were already dying of lung-sickness all played their part in making the Xhosa receptive to this kind of millennial solution to their problems. Perhaps it is not surprising that an impressionable, possibly neurotic, adolescent girl, her mind inflamed by accounts of colonial injustice and persecution, fancied that she saw the ancestors arising from the depths of the pool to offer salvation to the sorely tried Xhosa. It is believed that her uncle, Mhlakaza, an embittered man, who had in fact been the first Anglican Xhosa convert, encouraged these delusions and conveyed their message to the paramount chief, Sarhili. Sarhili, whose own herds had already been decimated by cattle sickness, believed and duly instructed his people to carry out the ancestors' instructions. The cataclysm which resulted is well known. When the prophecies failed to materialise, disaster stared the Xhosa nation in the face. Famine stalked the land and ultimately 45 000 people are believed to have died from starvation.

Trevor Wigley, a tour guide in the area, shows us to the pool. He grew up in the old Transkei, speaks Xhosa fluently and knows the people well. I ask him if people remember and talk about the cattle killing. "No," he says, "It is a subject of shame and embarrassment to them."

The pool is a quiet flat stretch of dark water overhung by palms and thick bush. Dappled sunlight plays in its depths, reflections dance on the surface, the wind sighs through the trees and bird calls echo in the valley. In this atmosphere I suppose it's not difficult to fire the imagination and conjure up ghosts that lurk in the depths of the subconscious.

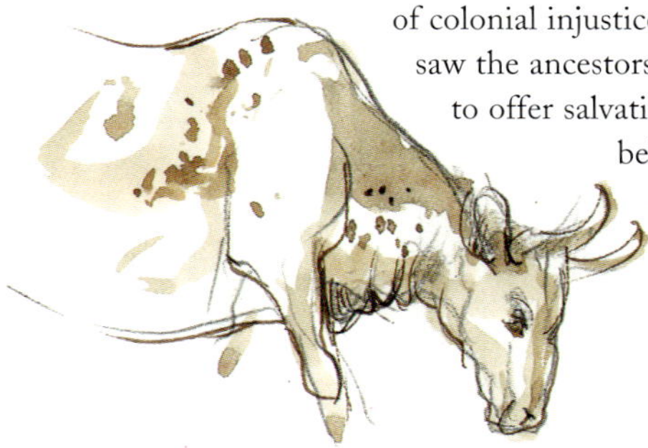

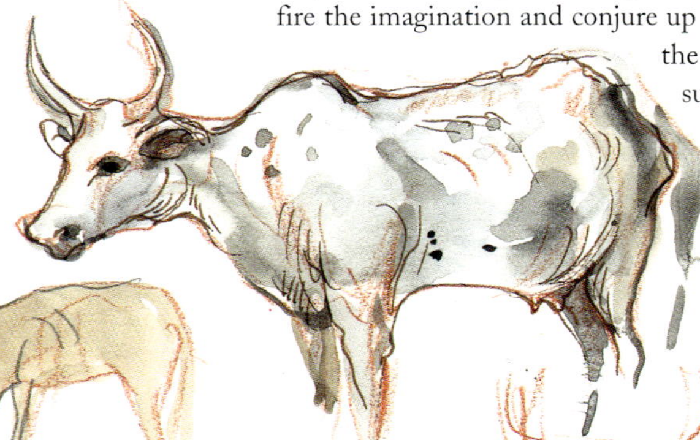

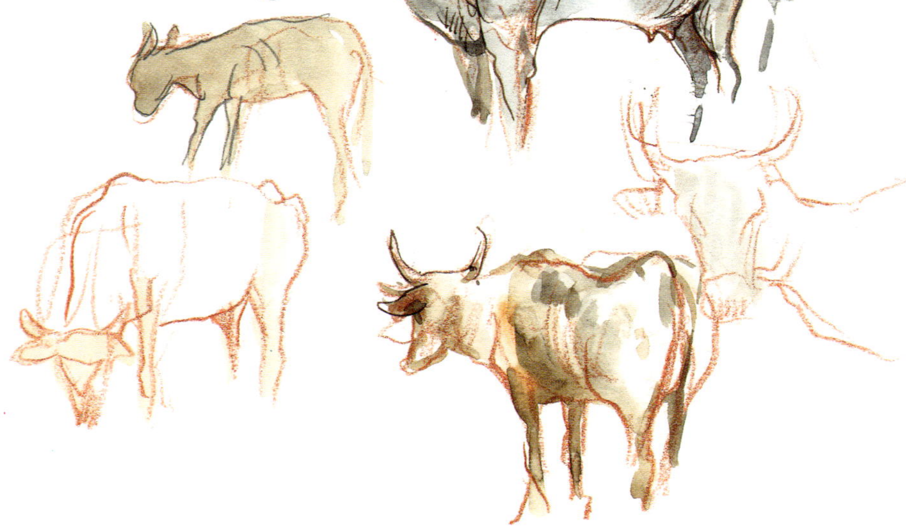

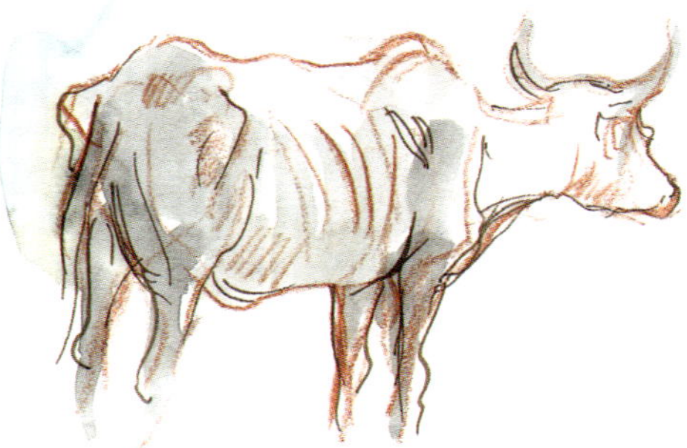

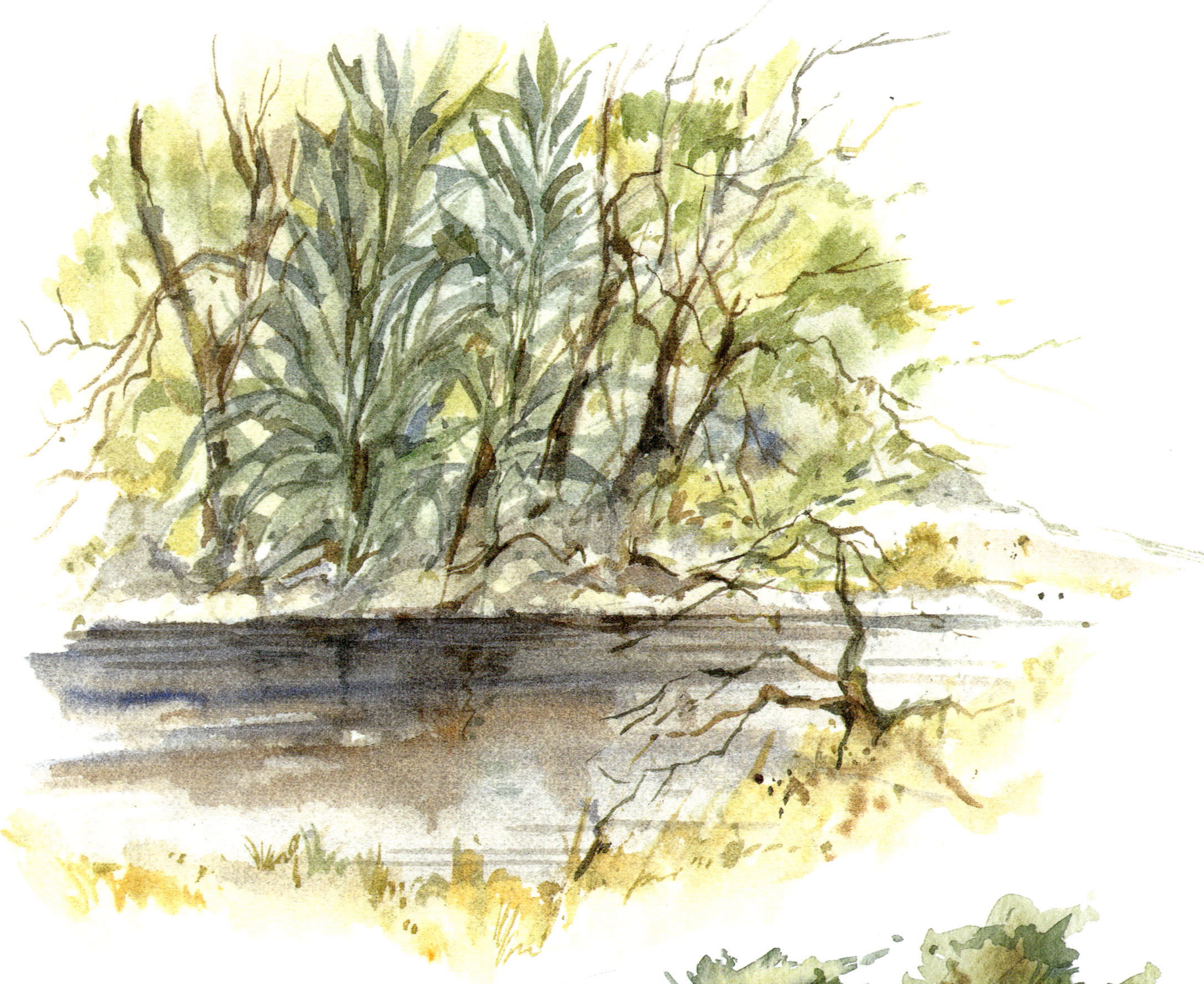

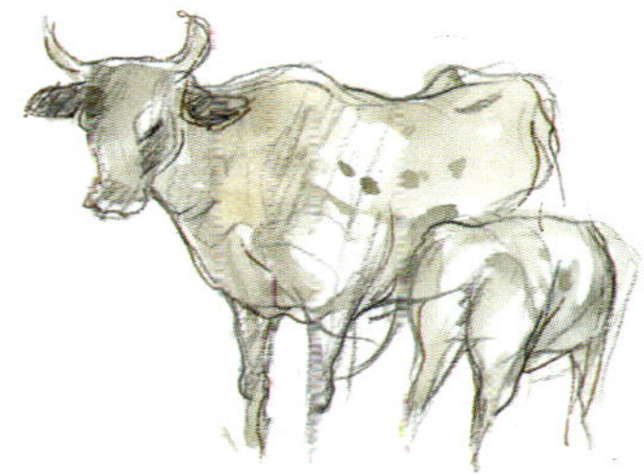

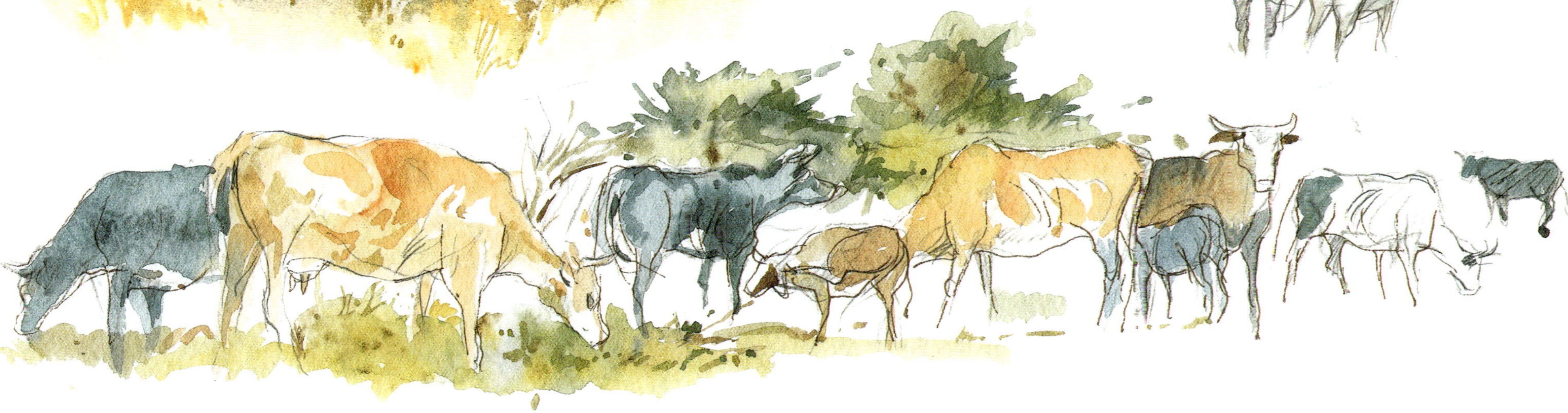

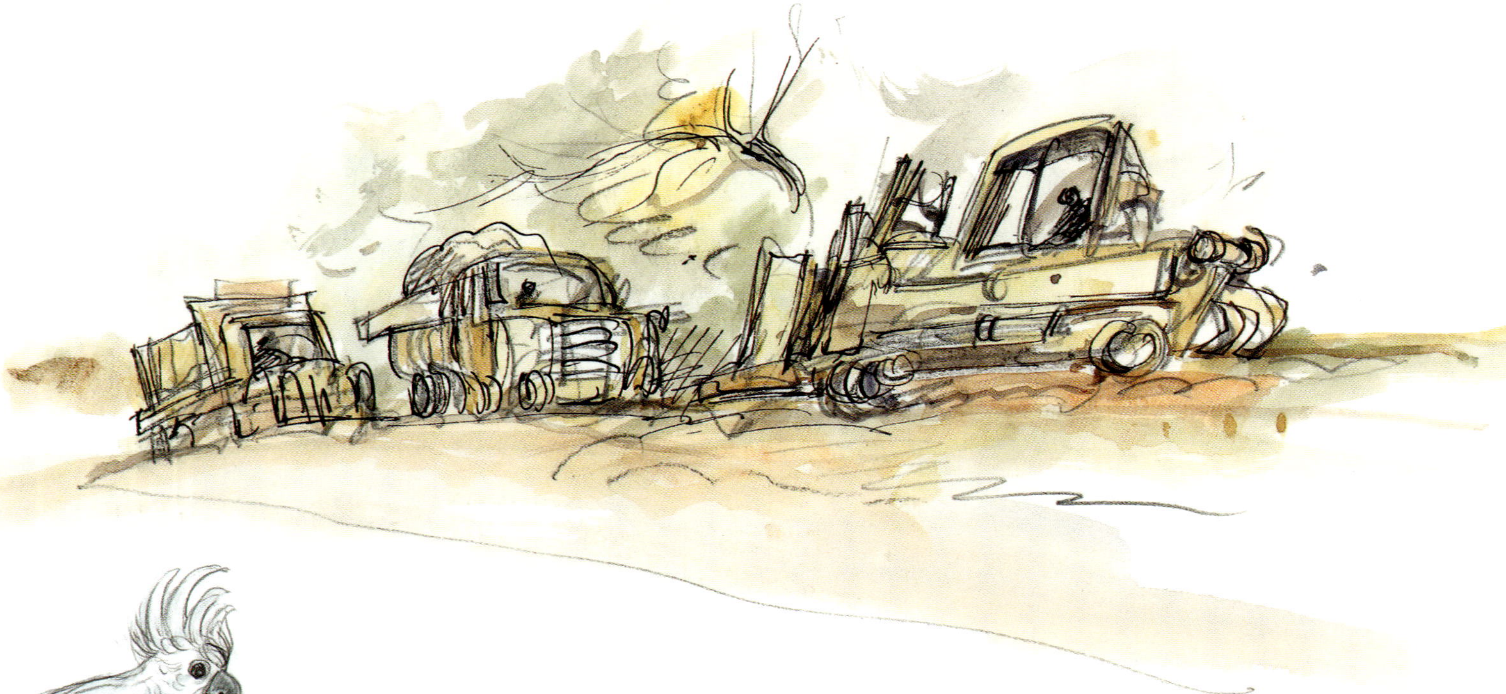

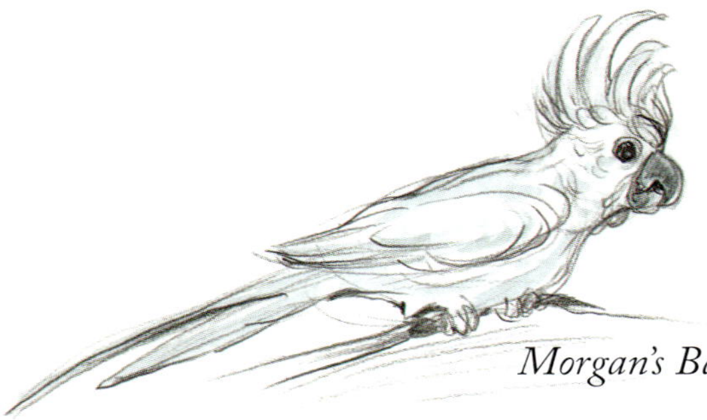

Morgan's Bay

There are many detours on the road to Morgan's Bay as a new road is being constructed, crossing valleys over infills and carving its way through hills. Bulldozers and heavy trucks belch smoke and raise clouds of dust. It looks as though the approval for the proposed new coastal road from Port Edward, at the time of my drawing still subject to environmental impact assessment, is regarded as a fait accompli.

I lunch in the courtyard of Morgan's Bay Hotel, entertained by Baldy the cockatoo doing twirling acrobatics on his perch. Afterwards, I stroll along the coast to do a drawing of an attractive and typical feature of the Wild Coast shoreline – a grass-covered headland ending abruptly in red cliffs plunging directly into the sea. Tumultuous waves, driven by a boisterous east wind, hurl themselves in a fury of bursting spray at this rocky wall.

Back at the hotel I re-encounter Baldy in the convivial pub, now parading up and down the counter whistling, cracking peanuts and raising his crest cheekily at customers. There is a black farmer from Peddie staring moodily into his beer. It seems his wife has left him because she couldn't abide country life. He watches me doing a sketch of Baldy and asks whether I could do a drawing of him. I oblige with a simple caricature of him herding some cows. It seems to cheer him up a little.

Another patron is a post-graduate student from the UK, drinking beer and doing sponsored research for a doctoral thesis on the communication skills of the red-billed hornbill. It occurs to me that his findings could be more interesting and less costly if he were to study the communication skills of Baldy, the cockatoo.

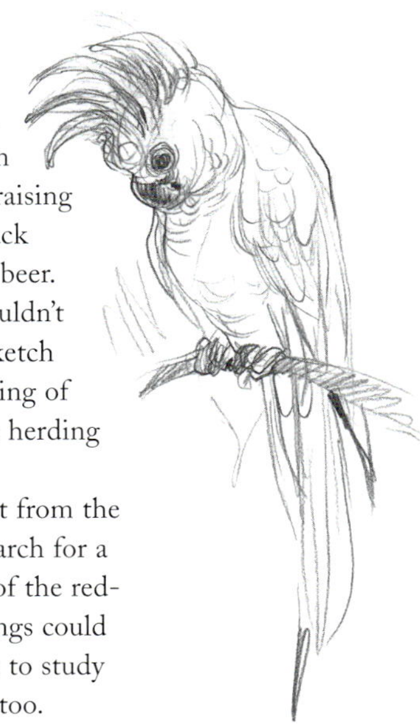

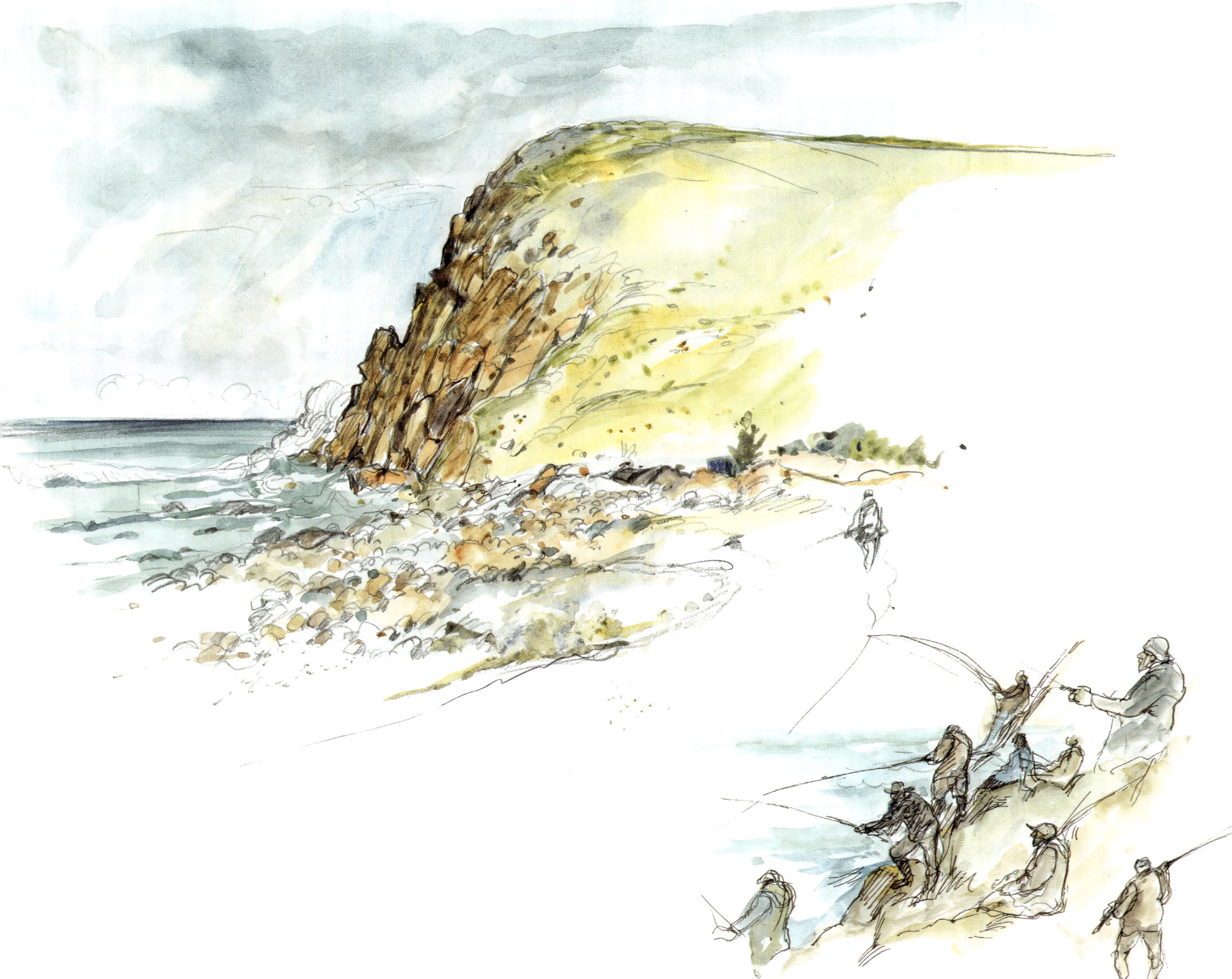

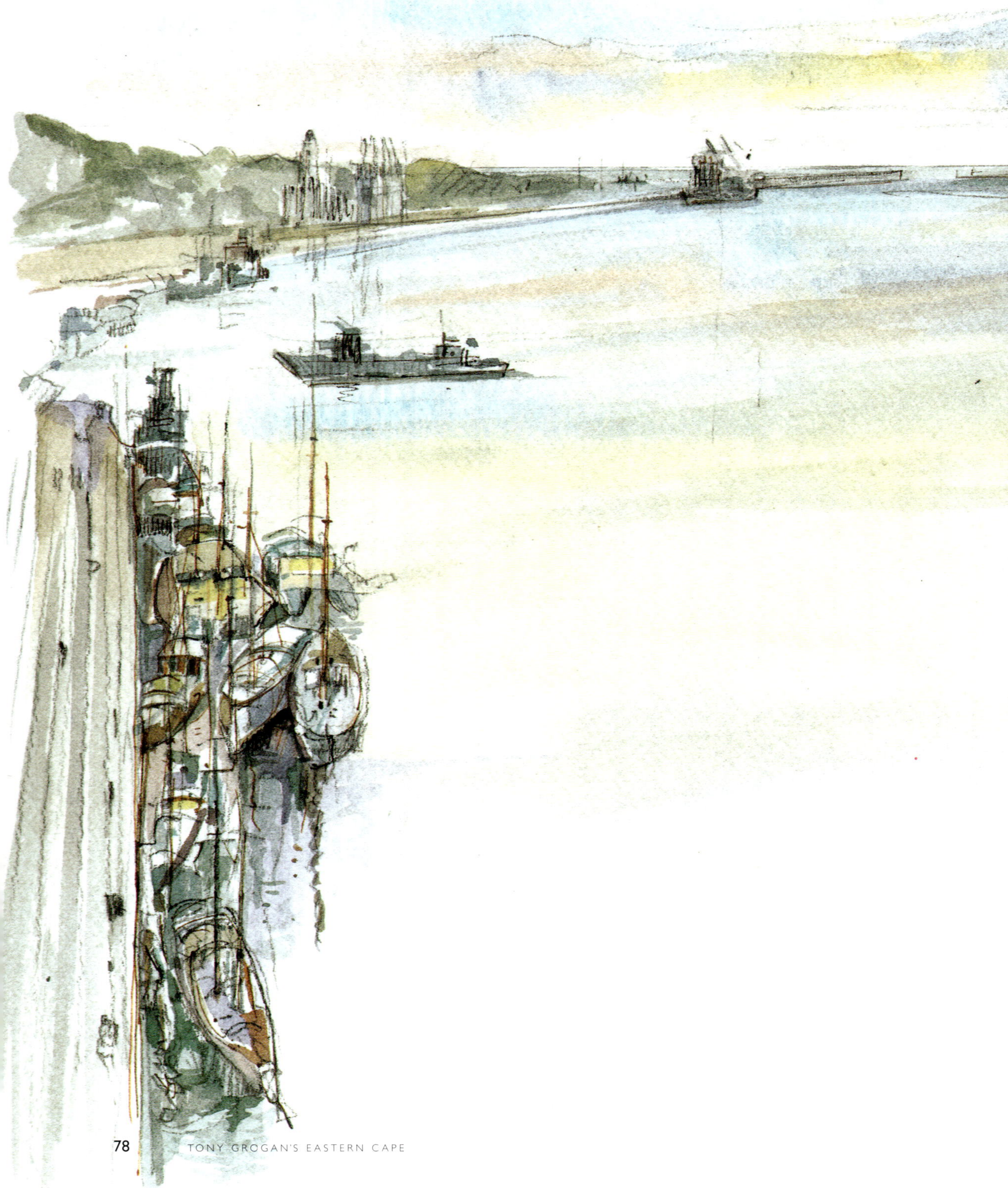

East London

East London is the only river port in the country. Viewed from the old bridge across the river, the harbour seems empty, unlike the old days when the wharfs were lined with boats and there was a lot of activity on the quaysides. But I am told that now boats come in, deliver their containers and off they go without mooring for the night or the number of days it takes to load and offload their cargo.

I grew up in East London and enjoyed an untroubled and happy childhood. We lived on the edge of town which was then Nahoon. Beacon Bay and the ribbon development along the coast to Gonubie and beyond was not even a distant dream. It was a good place in which to grow up. We had the 'bush', as we called it, on our doorstep, the broad Nahoon River, where there were always boats that had come adrift from their moorings upriver to mess around in, and lovely stretches of beach along that matchless coastline. My grandfather was Port Captain in East London. His house was where the turning basin of the harbour is and my father recalled the sea at spring tide spilling over the back garden wall. I remember the house before it was demolished. It had a blank, bricked-up window, which my father told me had been a sash, and on one unhappy occasion came down with a bang on my grandfather's bald head. My father said he thought it was very funny so he laughed loud, but not very long, my grandfather being an irascible sea captain who failed to see the humour. Sadly, the harbour is now off-limits and you can't meander happily along the wharfs and walk along the main breakwater as we used to.

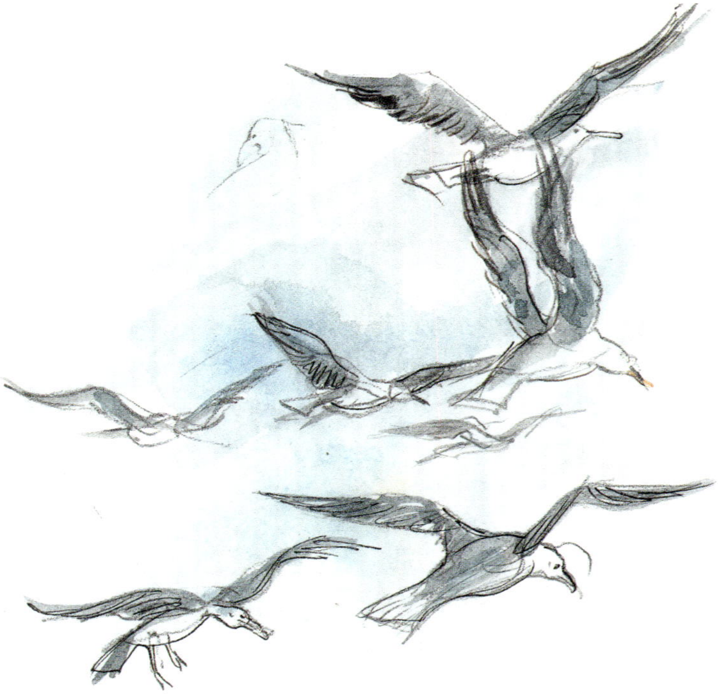

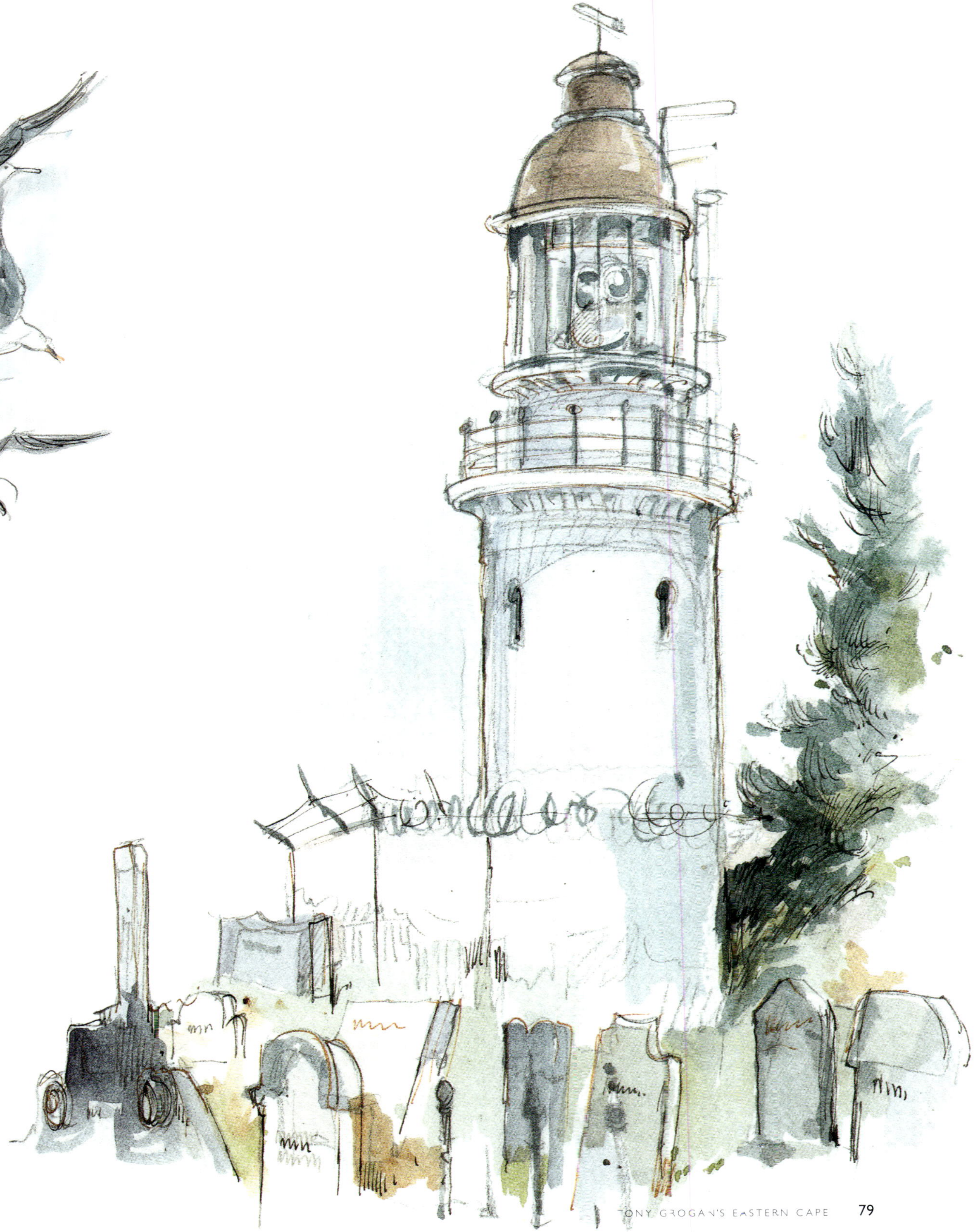

The Hood Point Lighthouse

The lighthouse has been a guide to shipping along this stretch of coast since 1895. The tombstones of the West Bank cemetery provide a gloomy foreground. Not all ships have been warned off the rocks by the light, because the *Stewart Star* came to grief in the 1930s a short distance offshore, almost immediately in front of the lighthouse. For years the rusted bow section was a well-known landmark on the coastal road before it was cut up and sold for scrap metal.

Marjorie Courtney

We visited Marjorie Courtney-Latimer at her East London home a few years before she died. She was 91 at the time, her mind as alive and clear as ever. I showed her the drawings of the coelacanth I had made in the museum and she approved of them, saying they captured the movement and character of the famous fish which she had found and brought to an astounded world's attention in 1938. This was a fossil fish thought to have been extinct for the past 50 million years. Until then, few outside Africa had heard of this little town on the Eastern Cape coast. Sitting in an armchair, a small fox terrier on her lap, she related how this incredible event had changed her life.

She had gone down to the fishing jetty to see if Captain Goosen's fishing trawler had brought in any specimens of interest. He told her that they had caught mainly sharks but among them was this odd-looking blue fish in which she might be interested.

Noticing the protruding pectoral fins, she immediately realised that here was something extraordinary. She and her assistant carted the fish around in the blazing heat of a December day, trying to find a place to keep it refrigerated and encountered one obstacle after another. A taxi driver refused to transport a smelly fish in the boot of his car and the local undertaker refused to have his clients keep company with a dead fish. She at last managed to persuade a cold storage company to keep it in their refrigerator until she could find a taxidermist to preserve the fish.

In the meantime, she had sent a letter with a drawing to Professor Smith who was holidaying at Knysna. He was at first sceptical as he had only seen the coelacanth in fossil form, and three weeks elapsed before he made his way to East London to make the announcement of this extraordinary scientific discovery to an astonished world. The fish was named *Latimeria chalumnae*.

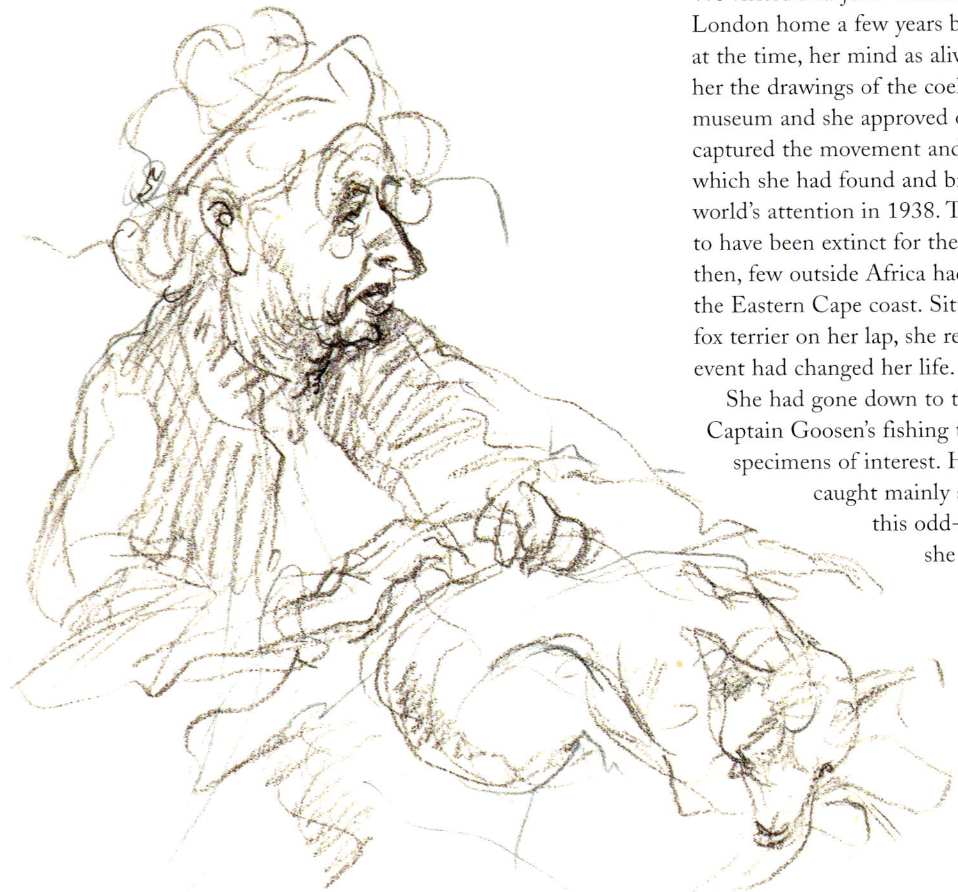

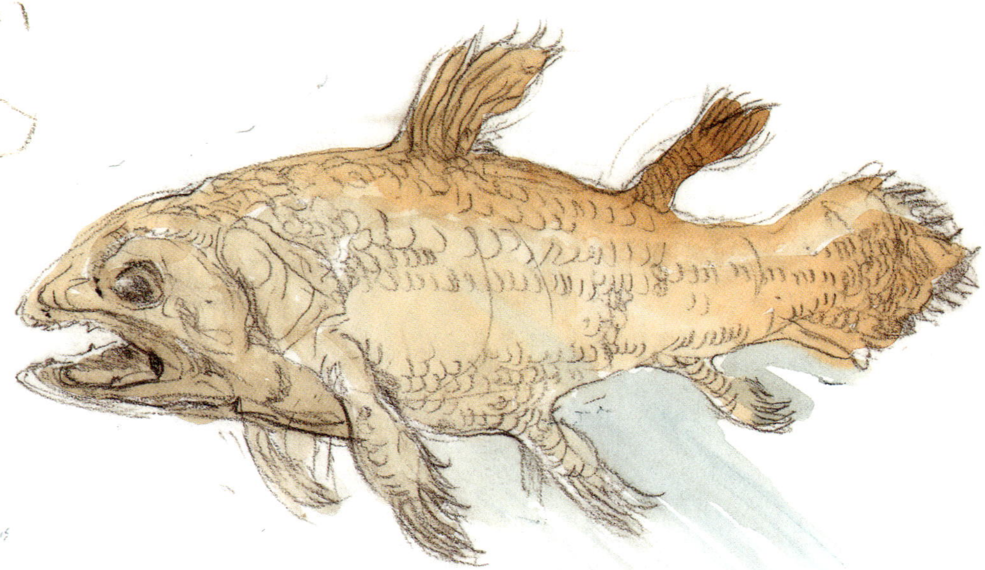

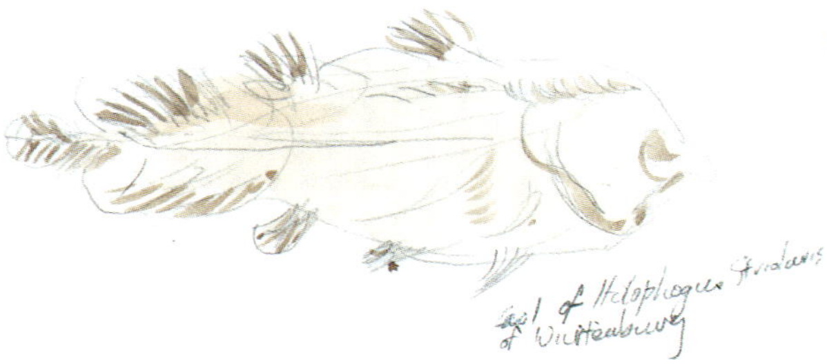

East London City Hall

The foundation stone of East London's elegant City Hall was laid in 1897. The tower was added to the original design to commemorate the 60 years of Queen Victoria's reign. There are two monuments, one a statue of the Black Conscious leader, Steve Biko, and the other an equestrian statue of a military scout scanning the horizon. There used to be two early field guns but these were apparently sold and ended up in a scrap metal yard, which caused the South African Gunner's Association to explode.

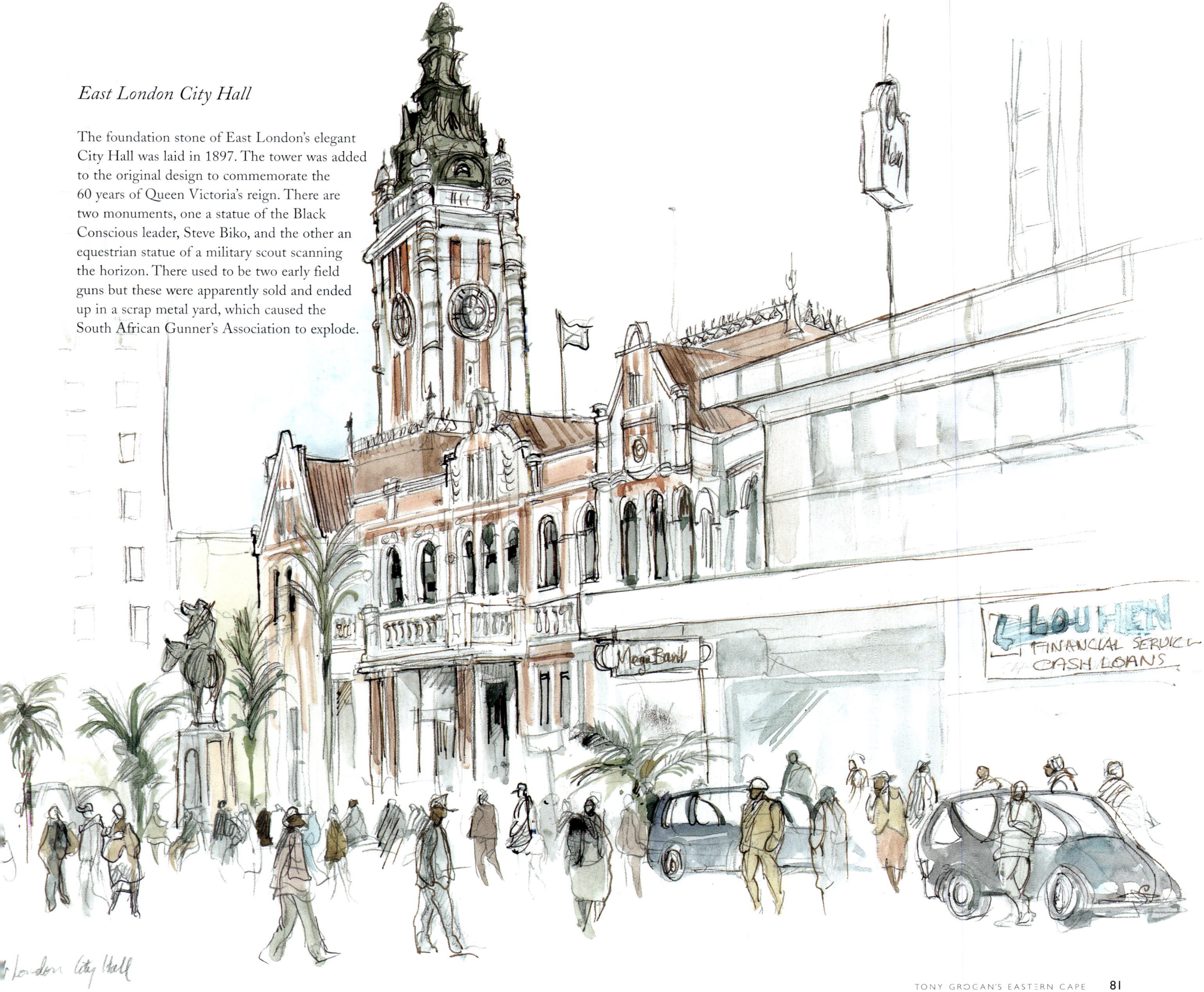

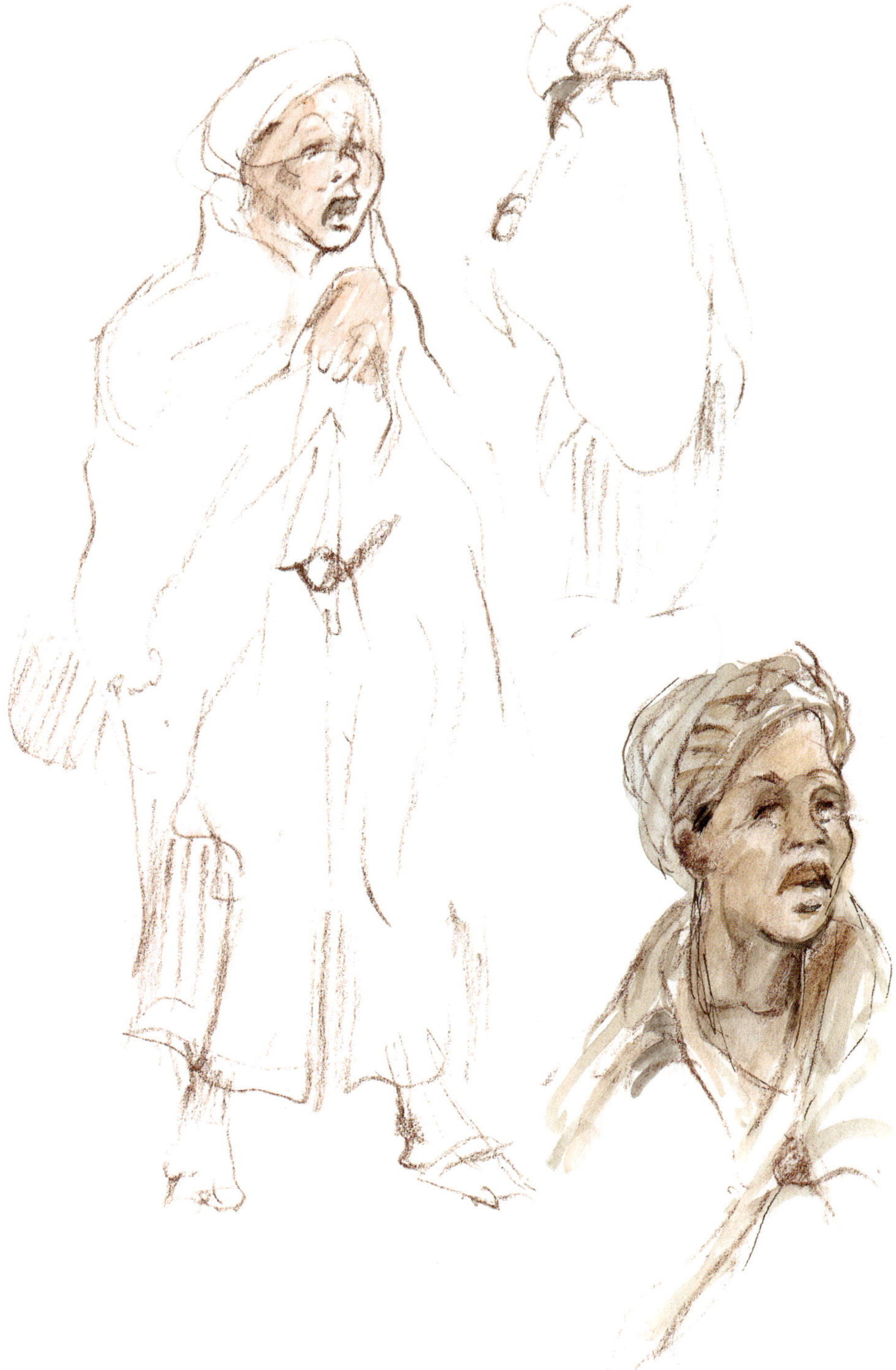

Cove Rock

I drive across to the west bank of the Buffalo River where the houses are still as shoddy and weather beaten as I remember them, but am surprised to see much new residential development further along the coast. There is a luxury housing development overlooking one of my old haunts, Cove Rock, that sinister, rocky eminence lying like a shrouded corpse on the bleak sandy waste, which marks that piece of coastline. The rock, which is cloven in two by a wide channel through which the waves boil and surge, is embedded in the mythology of the Xhosa who associate it with strange and mysterious forces. Noel Mostert describes how the great Xhosa prophet and seer, Makanna, who in 1819 had led the Xhosa in their thwarted attack on Grahamstown in a last act of desperation to rid the land of the white colonisers, sought the aid of the ancestors. In order to summon them, he said he was required to leap across the formidable gap in the rock. Whether his faith or his courage failed him we do not know, but he did not leap and the ancestors did not rise up from the foam, leaving him a lonely and disconsolate figure sitting on the height of the rock as night fell, while his disappointed followers abandoned hope and engaged in a dispirited feast on the beach below.

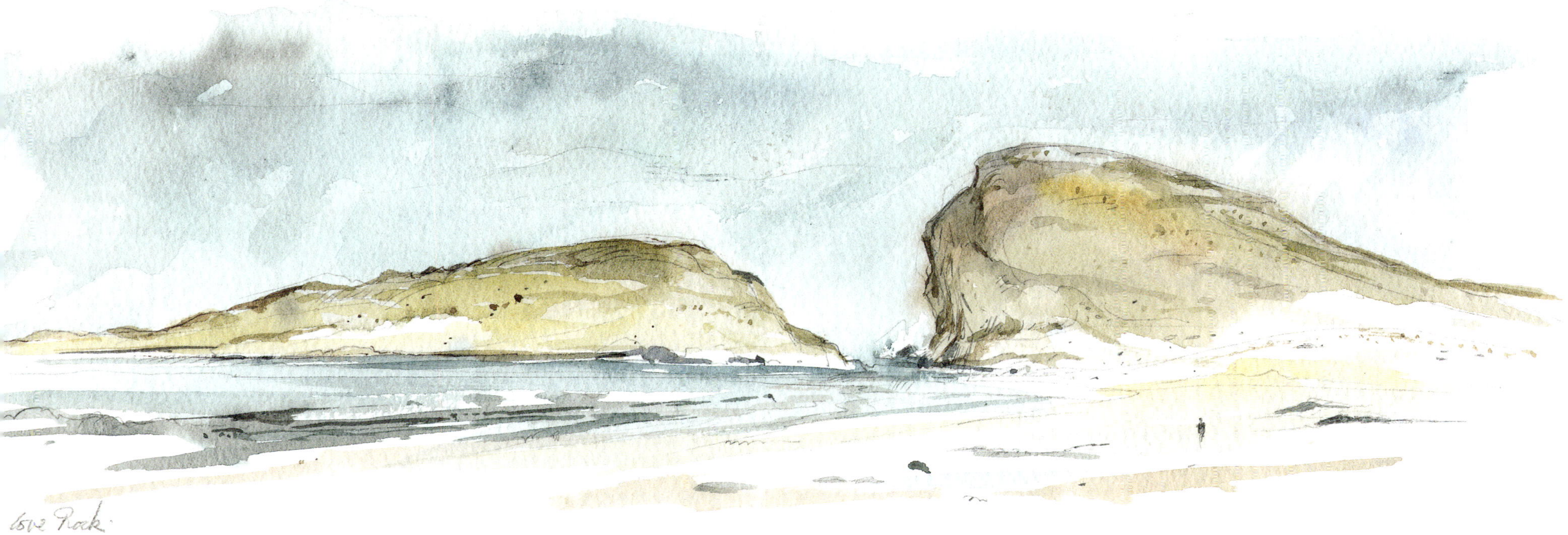
ove Rock

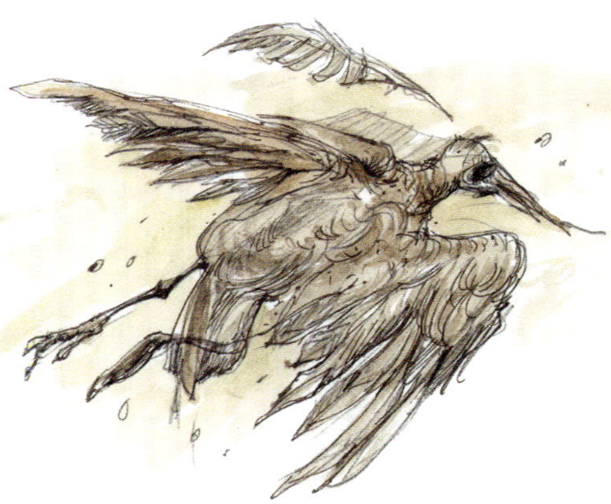

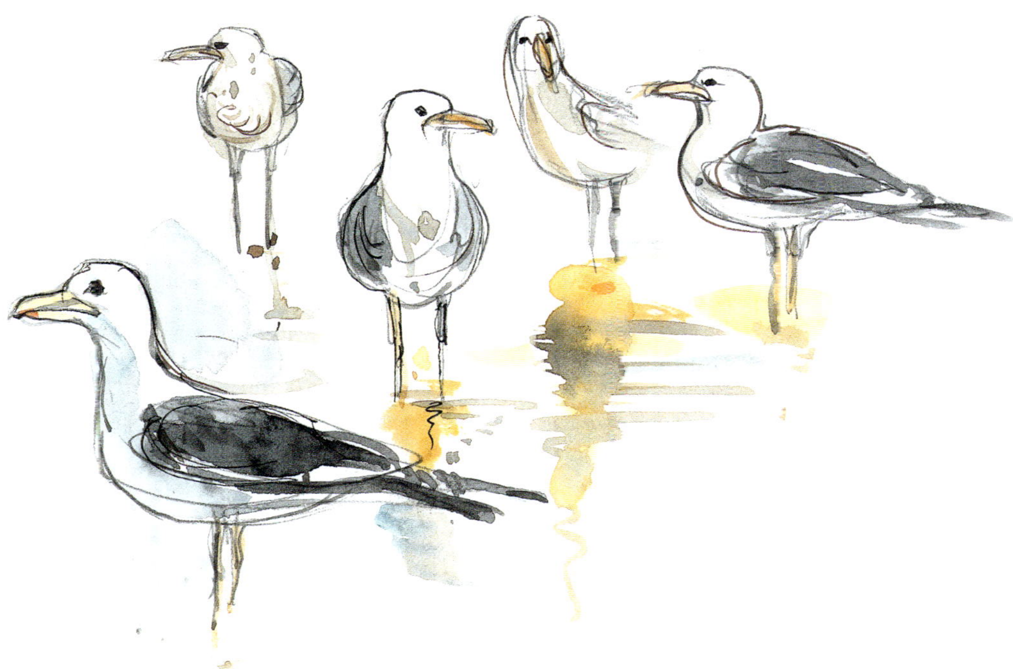

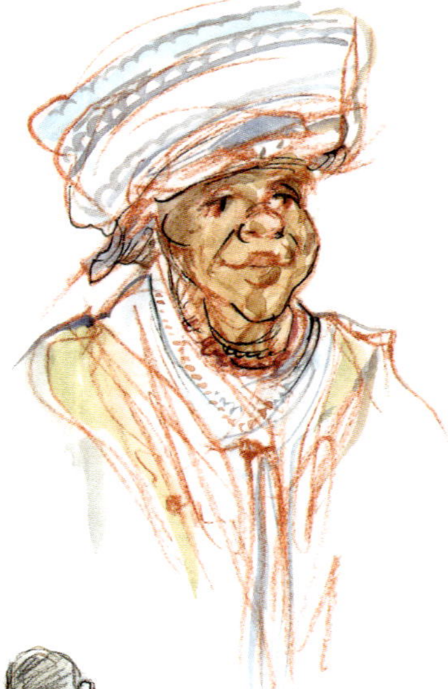

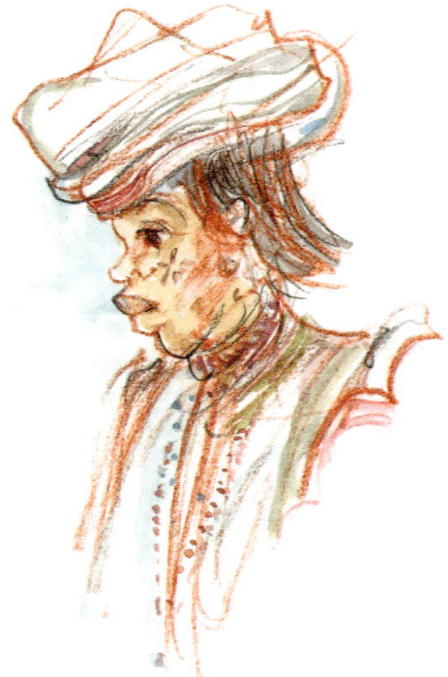

Initiation

We find Cynthia Stali and Joliswa Lumkile at a bus stop, spectacularly garbed in brilliant Xhosa traditional dress. Cynthia's son was initiated last year and they are going off to celebrate his coming out. I ask whether they would mind my coming along to record the event. "You are very welcome," they reply, just follow the minibus taxi when it comes to pick them up in two hours time. We follow the bus on the road to King William's Town and then turn off to a small rural hamlet. Pigs and chickens scatter before the taxi, which turns into a gateway of an enclosure where a large crowd of guests is already assembled. More are streaming in from all directions.

My idea is to be as discreet and unobtrusive as possible because we aren't invited guests. Perhaps mingle on the fringe and draw a few sketches and then quietly retire. But this isn't the idea of our warm-hearted and welcoming hosts who hail us, telling us to bring our car

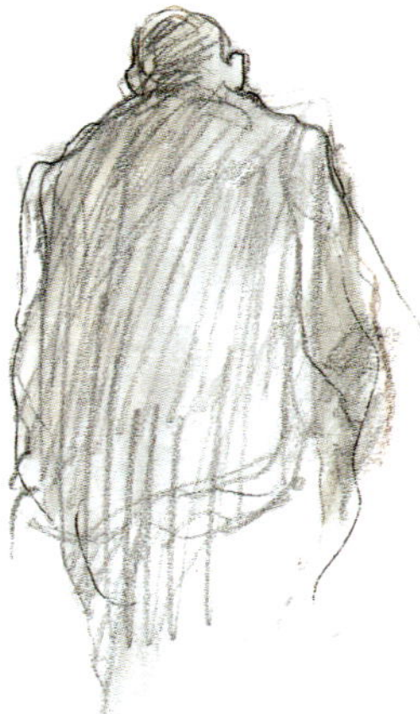

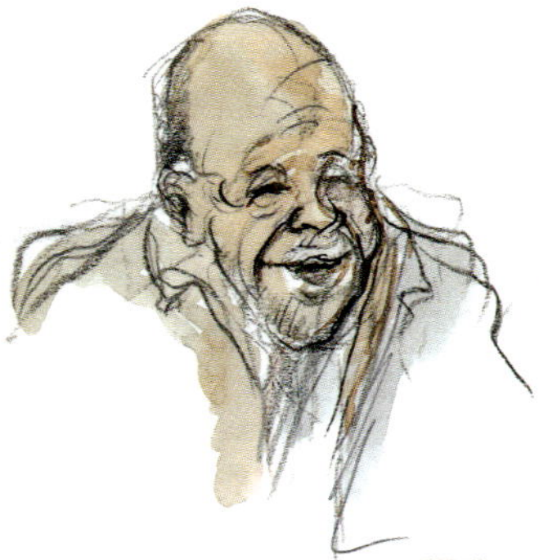

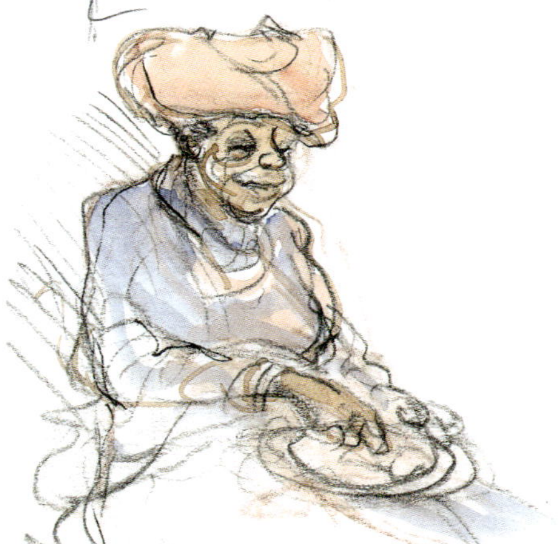

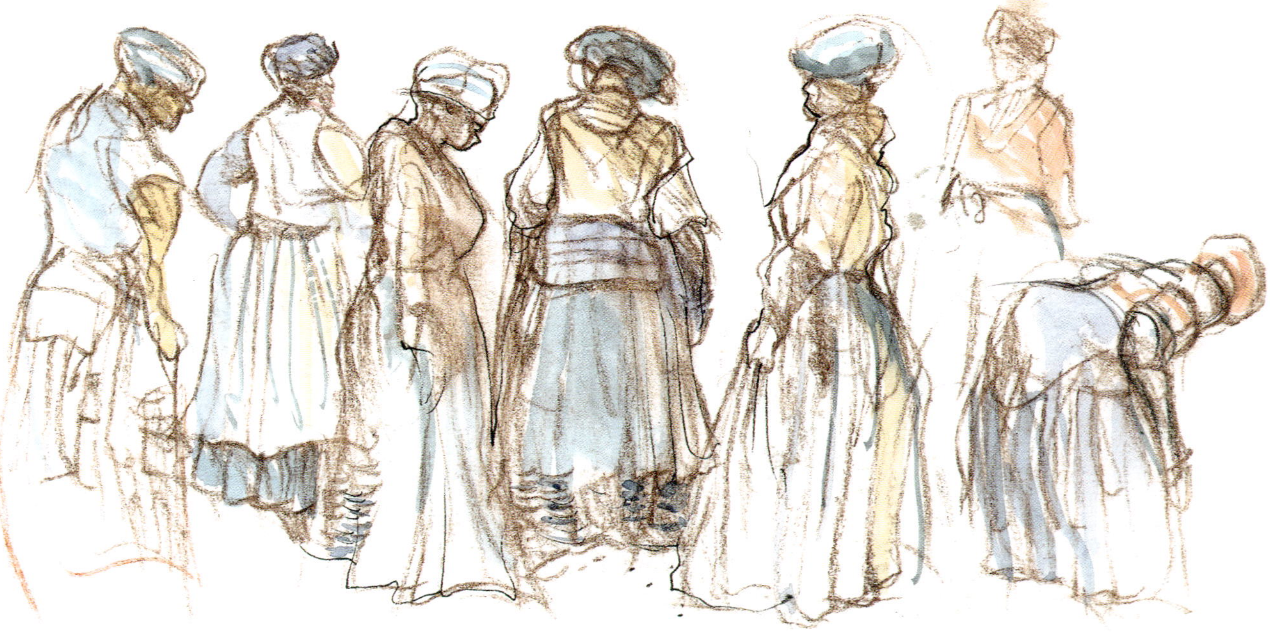

inside and "Press your hooter!" We do our bit to add to the cheerful noise. We are invited into a hut to meet the utatumkhulu, the grandfather and elder of the family, and plied with some Xhosa beer which we took turns to swig from a plastic jug.

"Did we have a camera?" we were asked. They didn't seem too impressed when I said I didn't have a camera, but I had a sketchbook and would do some drawings. Then a young woman arrived to save the day as she had a small camera and the occasion could be recorded more authentically. Our hosts insisted we pose with various members of the family, then with a group of lively, laughing women in brilliant traditional dress. Only then did they ask me to draw various people, each drawing greeted with pointing fingers and shrieks of laughter.

I had noticed that the older men of the group were sitting in a circle, no doubt quietly getting on with the serious business of drinking while the women in their colourful Xhosa dress with beads and bangles sang, danced and ululated, by and large setting the festive tone of the occasion. By now I had managed to jot down a few impressions of the action and some of the characters. Two of the women had decided to explain the details of symbolism and details of the initiation ceremony to their white visitors, but when they learned that Steve and I had grown up in East London they seemed a bit put out and said we probably knew about this already.

But we didn't really, especially one strange and puzzling item of the proceedings in which the women approached the men dancing, singing and waving aloft bottles of unopened Klipdrif brandy. "What did the bottles represent?" we asked. They represented breasts, we were told. We concluded that this must symbolise the initiate leaving behind the things of childhood, like mother's milk, and graduating to something stronger.

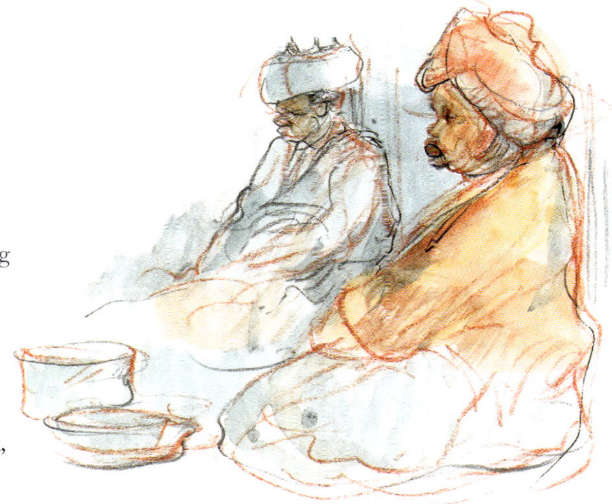

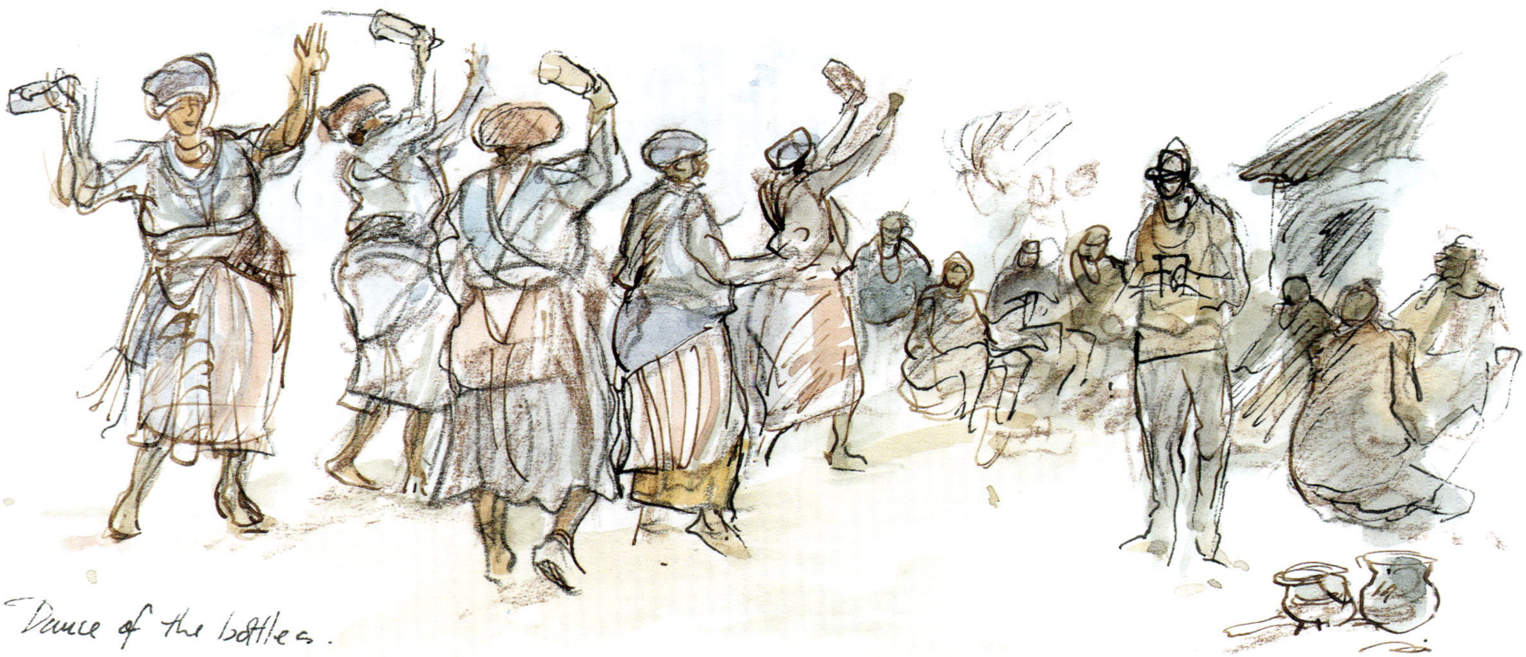

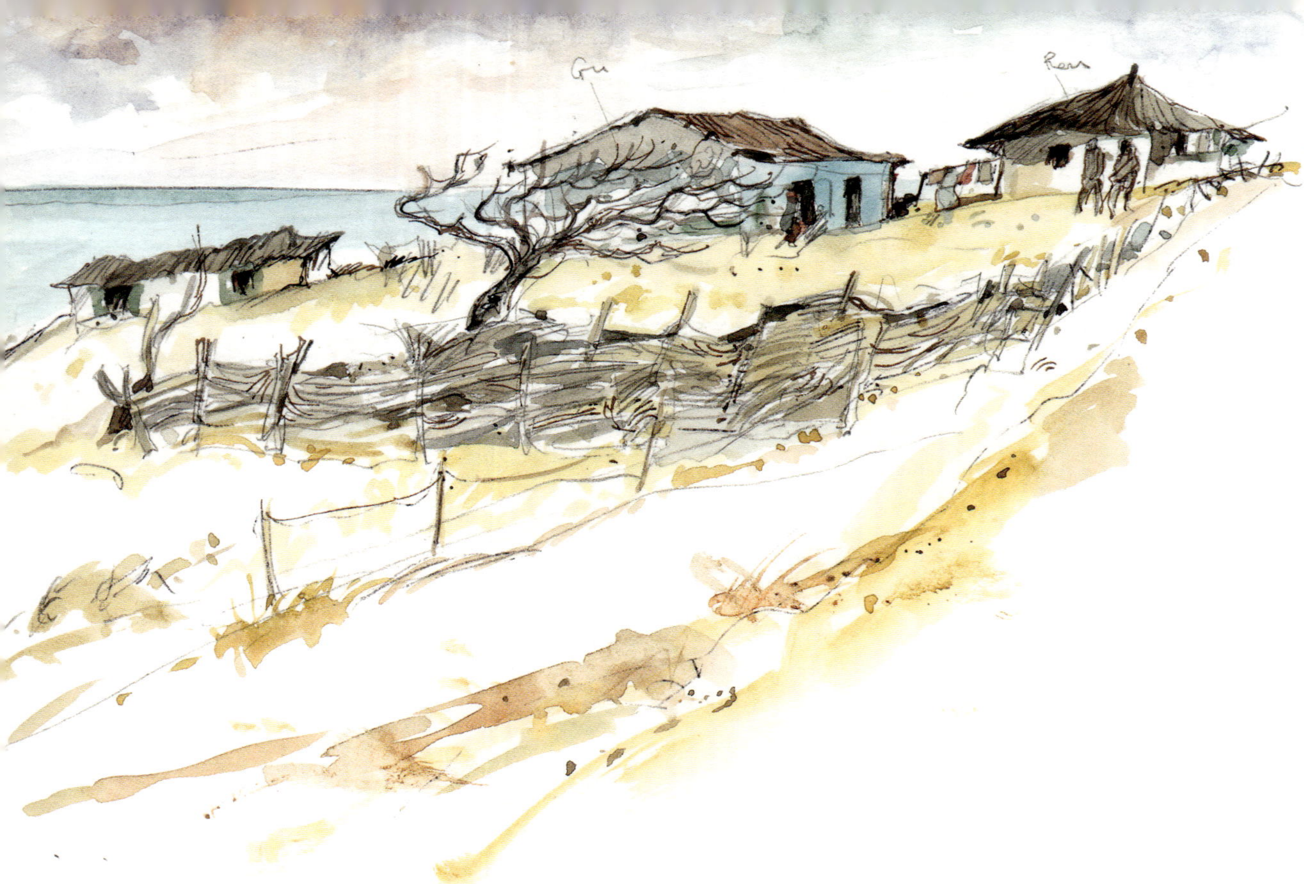

Hamburg

A small holiday hamlet at the mouth of the Keiskamma River. Like most of the large ancient rivers of the Eastern Cape, it approaches the sea near the mouth across a flat plain with reed banks and mudflats on either side. I remember it as a famous fishing spot where some of the biggest cob were caught. I don't know how good the fishing is these days – not very, if we judge by the testimony of a group of bleary-eyed fishermen partaking of beer and breakfast around their 4x4, who shrugged their shoulders and said they'd caught "bugger-all" all night.

The old Hamburg Hotel, with its homely pub and dartboard, is now a bed-and breakfast breakfast establishment run by a lady from Scotland, but old

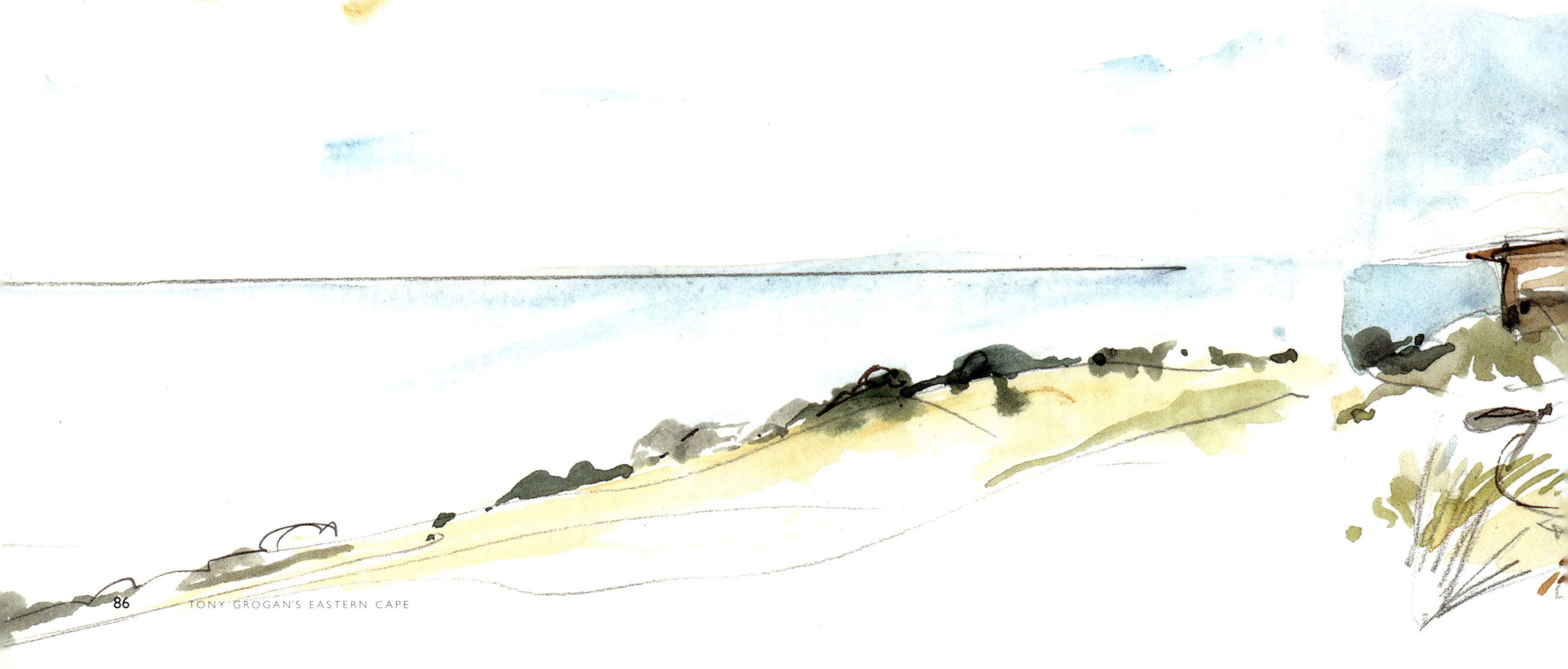

faded photographs of triumphant fisherman with prize catches still adorn the walls.

We order beers and sit outside on the terrace, languidly enjoying the warm spring sunshine and the view of the broad, placid river and the distant green hills. "Life's tough in the Eastern Cape," someone observes.

Like elsewhere along the coast, the cost of plots is rising all the time. One of the premier positions is further along the hill where a few ramshackle dwellings command spectacular, panoramic views of the broad expanse of the sea and the coastline. Another has a cattle kraal, a black pig tethered to a stake and a few scruffy fowls scratching in the dirt.

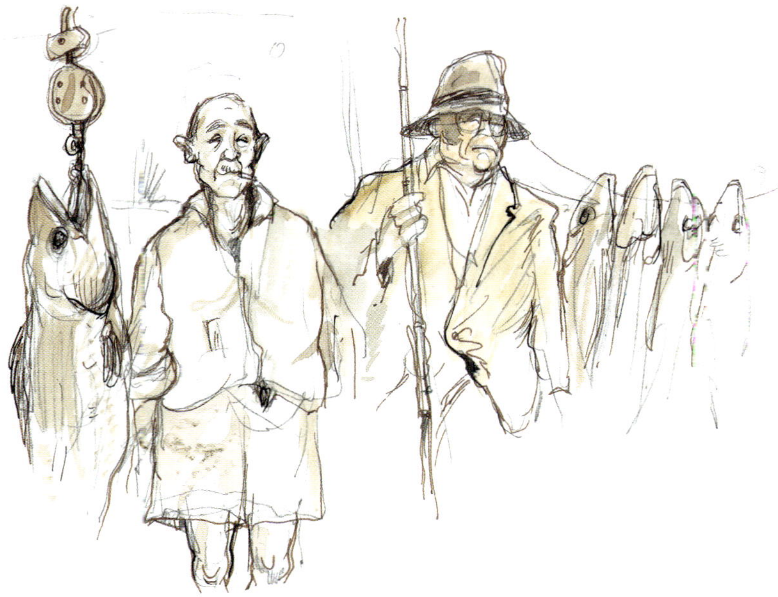

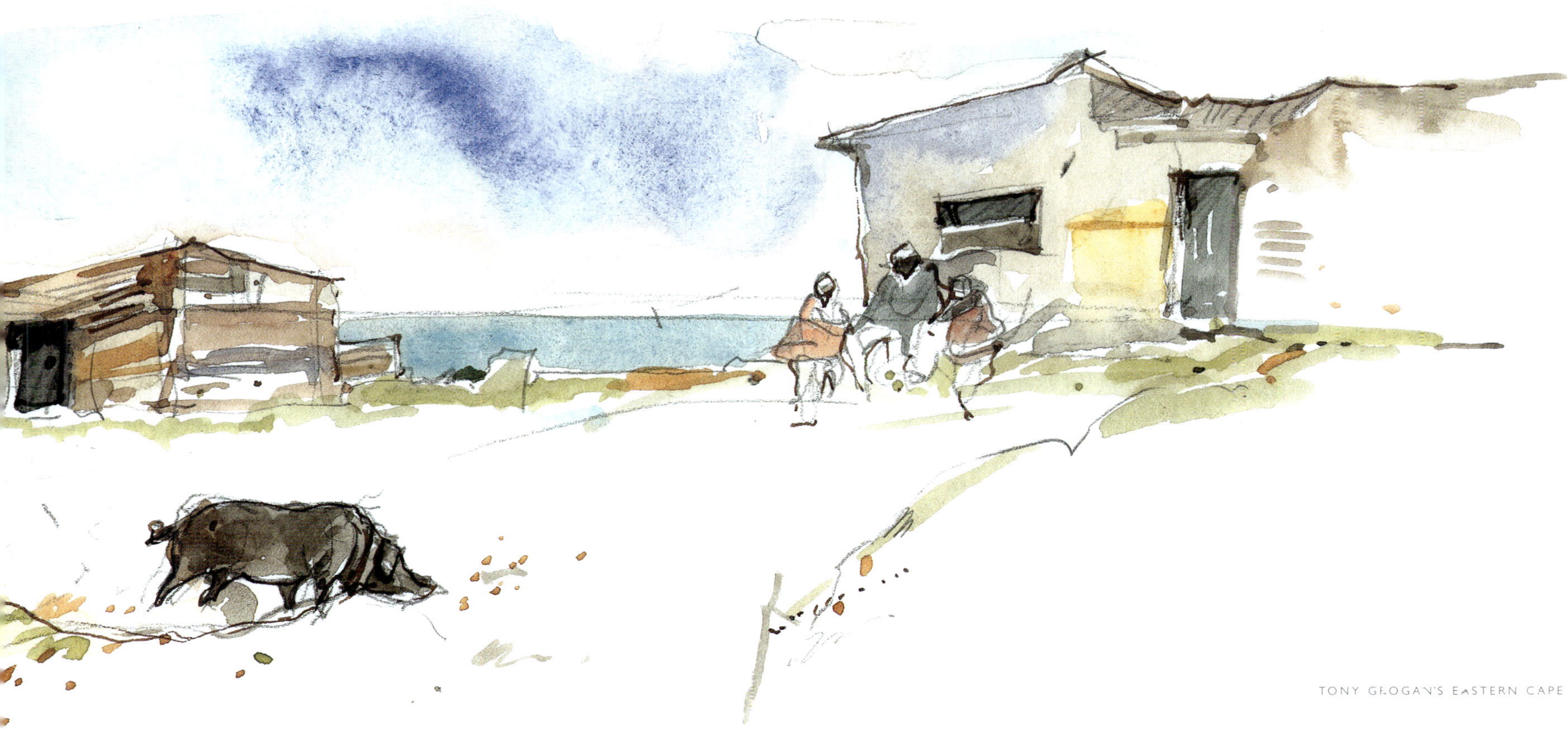

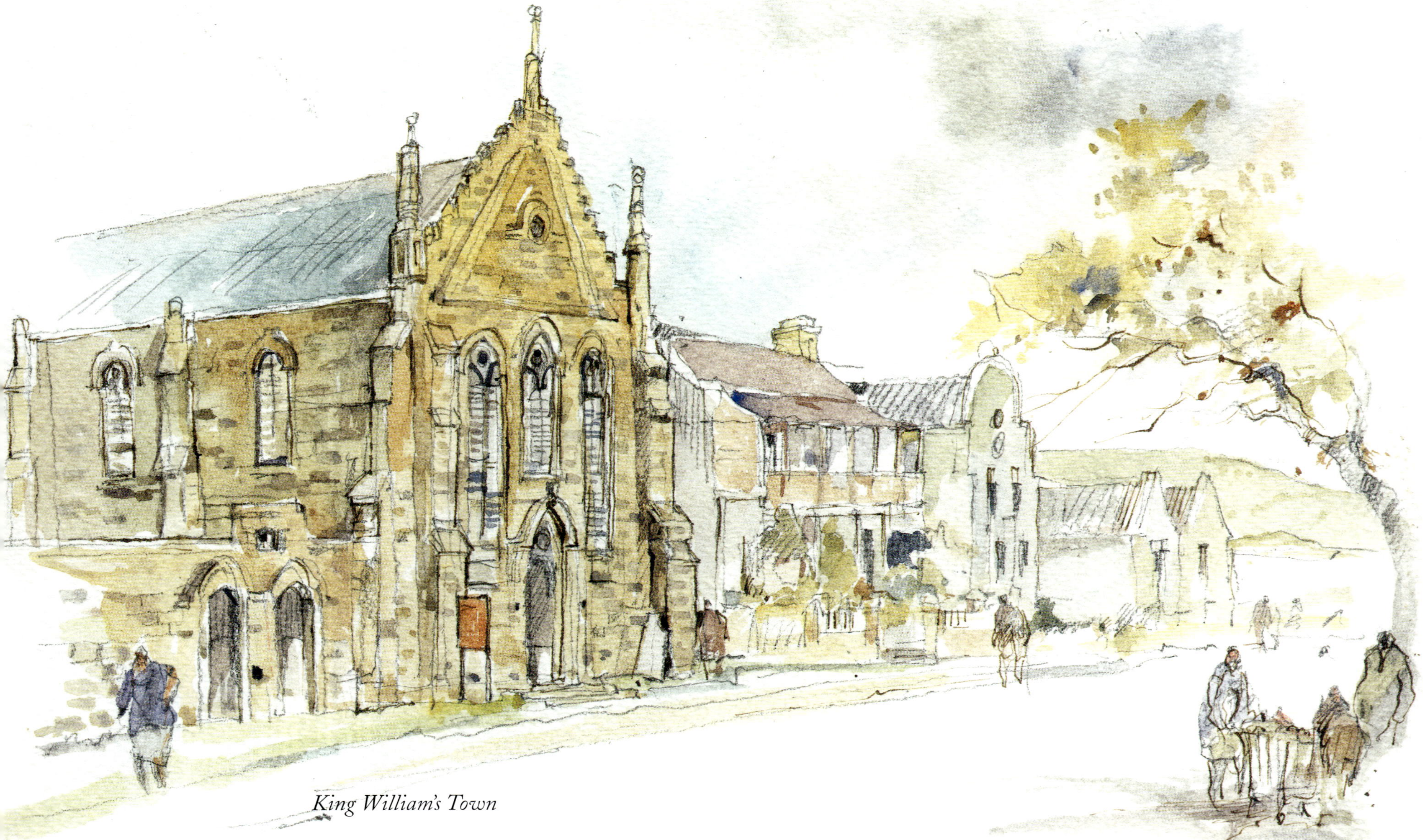

King William's Town

This early garrison town was located on the mission station of John Brownlee on the upper reaches of the Buffalo River. It was declared the capital of the short-lived province of Queen Adelaide which only existed for seven months before the proclamation creating it was repealed in 1835. In 1846 it was again occupied by British forces during the War of the Axe, and the Governor of the colony, Sir Harry Smith, proclaimed the Crown Colony of British Kaffraria with King William's Town as its capital.

The Methodist Church, built in 1842, and next to it the manse and the synagogue. It was near here that Governor Sir Harry Smith indulged in one of the theatrical flourishes for which he was renowned. At the end of the 1846 War of the Axe, surrounded by serried ranks of troops and cannon, he castigated an assembled group of Xhosa chiefs and their followers. He presented to them individually two staffs, one a sergeant's halberd and the other a staff with a round brass knob, apparently an old door knob, and they were

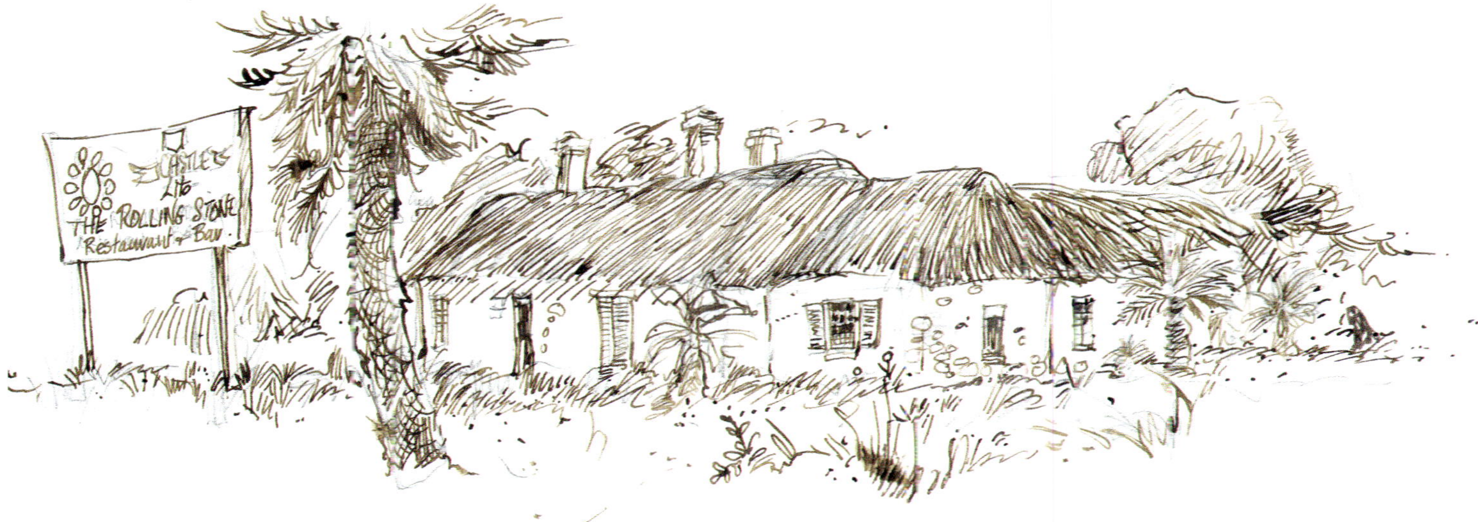

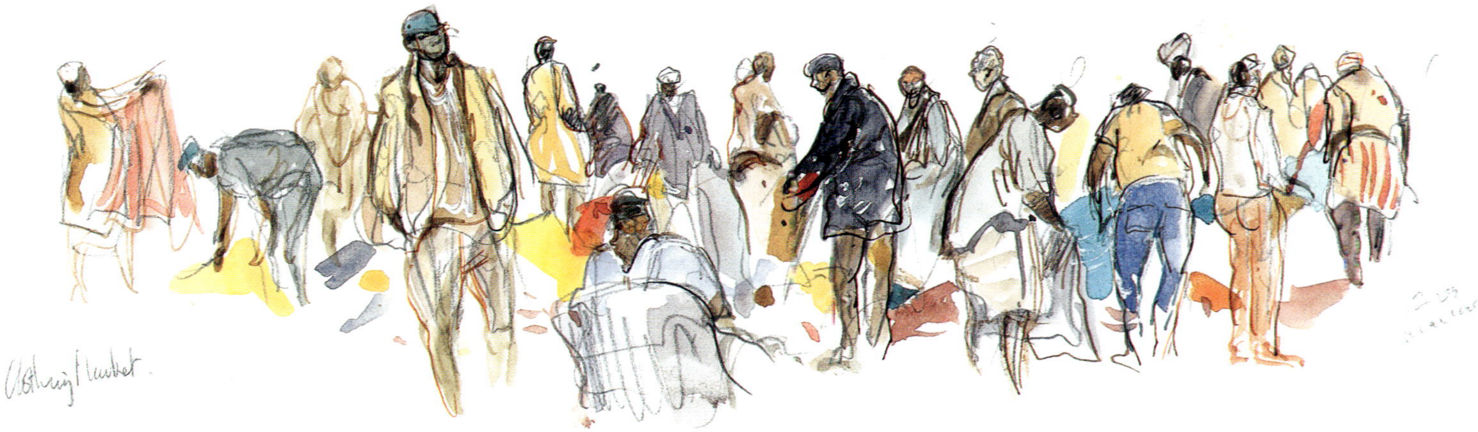

told to choose between war and peace by touching one of the staffs. Under the circumstances they naturally chose the staff of peace. He then declared himself Inkosi Inkulu (Great Chief) over all of them, threw shredded pieces of paper into the air with the words, “There go your treaties” and hurling the staff of war to the ground, he concluded the ceremony by leading three rousing cheers for peace. What the bemused chiefs made of this performance is difficult to surmise but it didn’t work too well, because within four years the country was again in flames with the outbreak of the Eighth Frontier War, the War of Mlangeni.

Across the road the old governor’s house is empty and the previous lush garden a wilderness of grass and weeds. The last time I was here it was a restaurant. There is a notice at the gate saying ‘No entry’, but I go in anyway. The only person who accosts me is a shabby person asking for bus fare. What the place has been used for since I don’t know, but there is an oddly worded sign leaning against the trunk of a giant blue gum tree proclaiming ‘The MAIC will sweep away the lies.’

There is a lot of informal trading with street stalls selling fruit, vegetables and cheap commercial wares, and a clothing market where people are measuring and making their selections from piles of garments on the ground.

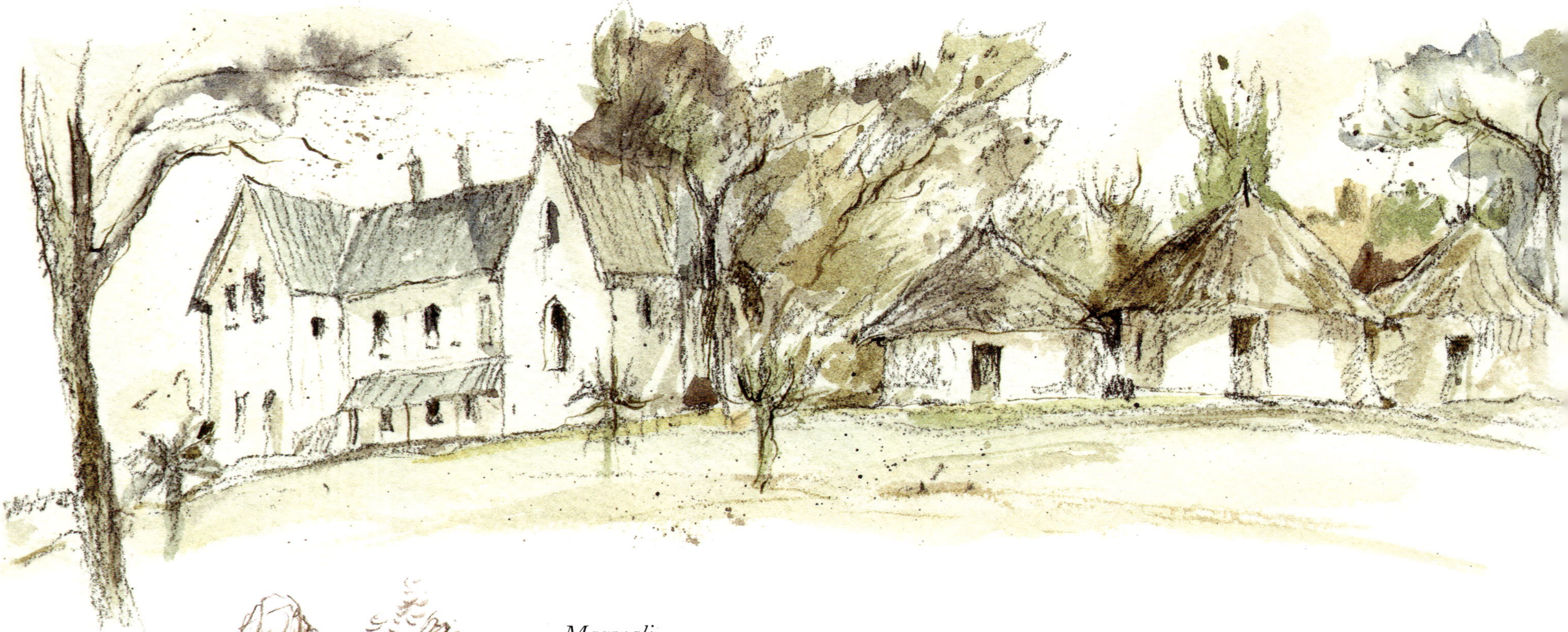

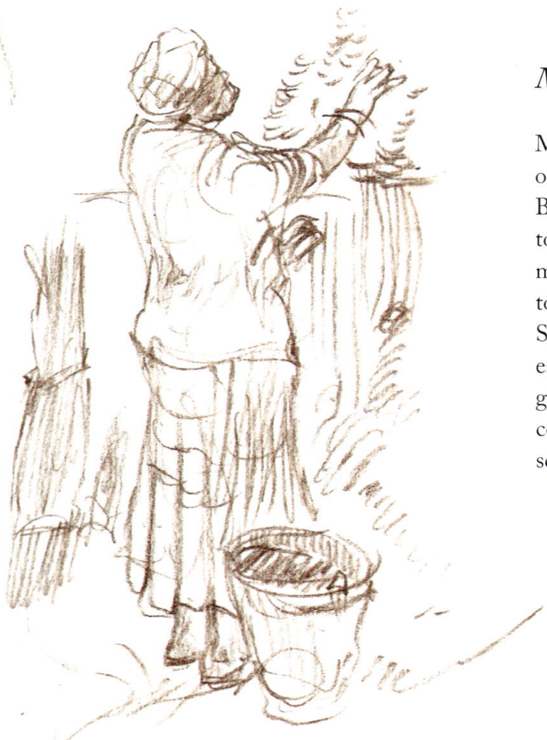

Magwali

Magwali near Stutterheim has a long history. It was one of the early mission stations established in 1820 by John Brownlee. One of Brownlee's converts, Tiyo Soga, went to Scotland and trained as a teacher and minister. He married a Scottish woman, Janet Burnside, and returned to Magwali to continue his work among his people. Soga went on to become one of the most famous of the early African ministers of the church. A well-known girls school was established in Magwali in the late 19th-century, and three Scottish ladies came out to run the school. The school building, now unfortunately in disrepair, and the three huts in which they lived can still be seen under the blue-gums on the hill.

The countryside is lush, greener and more fertile than regions quite close by, possibly because it is frequently dampened by thick mists. Even today in late November it is cold, there is an intermittent drizzle and low clouds blanket the landscape.

I am greeted by Tjhilelwa Bolana who is my guide around the village of Magwali. She shows me a craft shop with women at work, weaving mats and sewing traditional garments. Like most of the rural settlements,

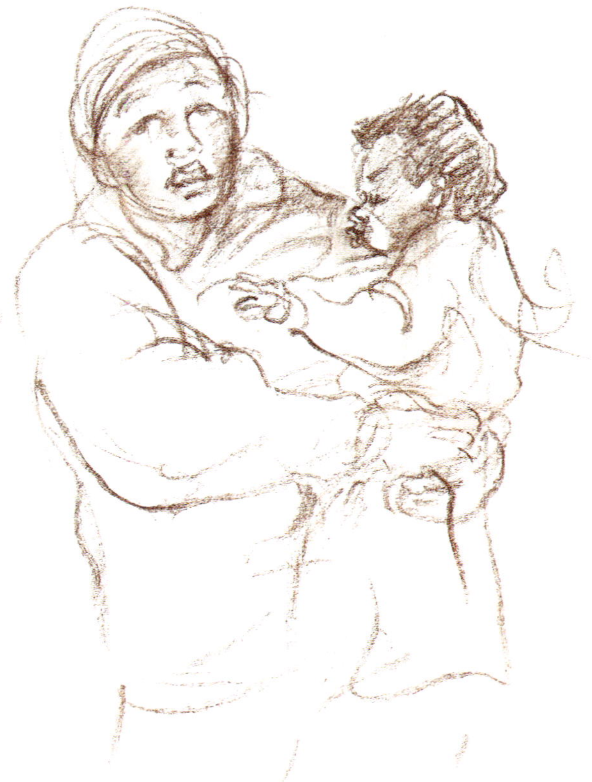

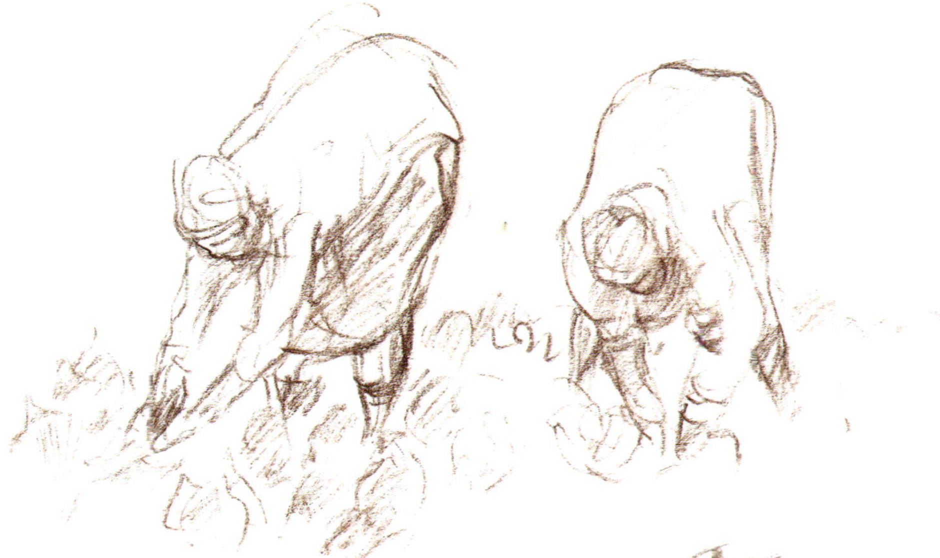

unemployment is high – 90% here, Tjhilelwa tells me – and people plant their own food to subsist. A group of women are weeding a cabbage patch. Tjhilelwa insists that I make a full record of everything. I traipse after her, sketchbook in hand, stuggling to keep pace. I must draw members of her family – her sister Nosipho, who is busy making a bead necklace, and her 'Umakhulu', a very old and dignified lady sitting upright in bed in her hut. She sits quite still as I finish my drawings. I do two drawings from different angles, and she professes herself more satisfied with the second.

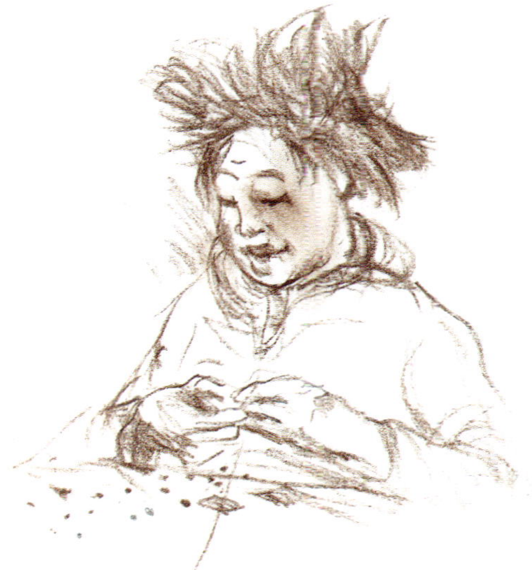

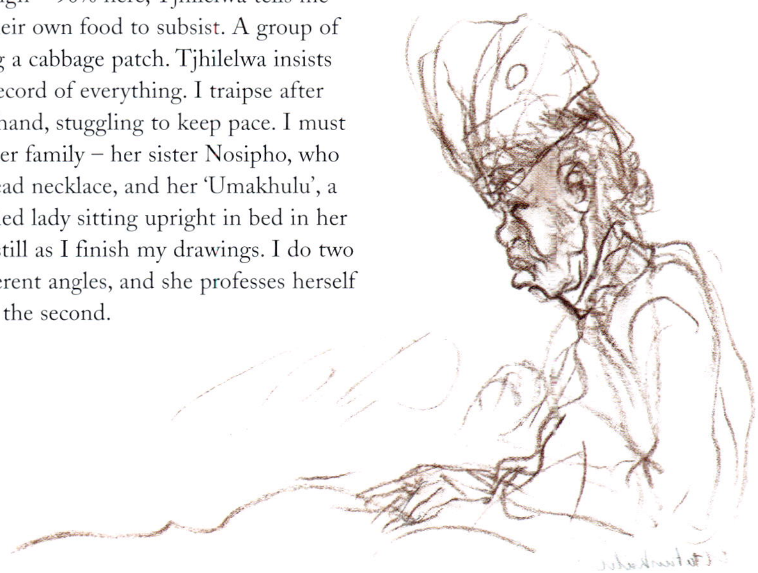

Grahamstown

Grahamstown is at the heart of Settler Country, a city of quiet, shaded avenues and dreaming spires where history peeps through every hedge and garden fence. Like Graaff-Reinet, its early buildings have been retained and beautifully restored so that it has kept much of its original character. Mainly an educational centre with its distinguished schools and university, it has remained largely free of industrial development which is both a blessing and a curse, as employment is high and the township continues to sprawl and expand out of sight over the hill, east of the city. It is blessed with a large number of churches which gives it the sobriquet 'The City of the Saints' – unless we believe the old urban legend that the title was bestowed when a requisition for a vice was sent to the regimental supply depot and met with the response, "We regret, we have no vices in Grahamstown."

The most impressive of the churches is the Gothic-style Cathedral of St Michael and St George, which dominates the centre of the town. It is a beautiful building, the soaring lines of the interior architecture and the soft light inspiring a mood of reverence and spiritual upliftment, largely lost on St Andrews schoolboys in the gallery, I remember as a student, shuffling and yawning their way through interminable sermons.

The cathedral has many historical momentos, tablets and memorials, including one to Colonel John Graham, founder of Grahamstown, who, while sitting under a thorn tree that once grew on a spot close to the cathedral's entrance, decided to establish a garrison town here in 1812.

Rhodes University has grown enormously since I was there as a student, but the city has largely retained its charm and historical character. Grahamstown was a quieter place in those far-off days. Few students had cars and those that did parked them on hills so they could be easily push-started. There was only one traffic policeman by the name of Archer, who rode about importantly on a large motorcycle to keep the limited traffic under control and the pavements free of loiterers. His sense of his authority was as high as his English was fractured. He once told a group of students, lounging on the steps of the Magistrates Court, to "stop lying the steps full" or he'd give them "a kick from after".

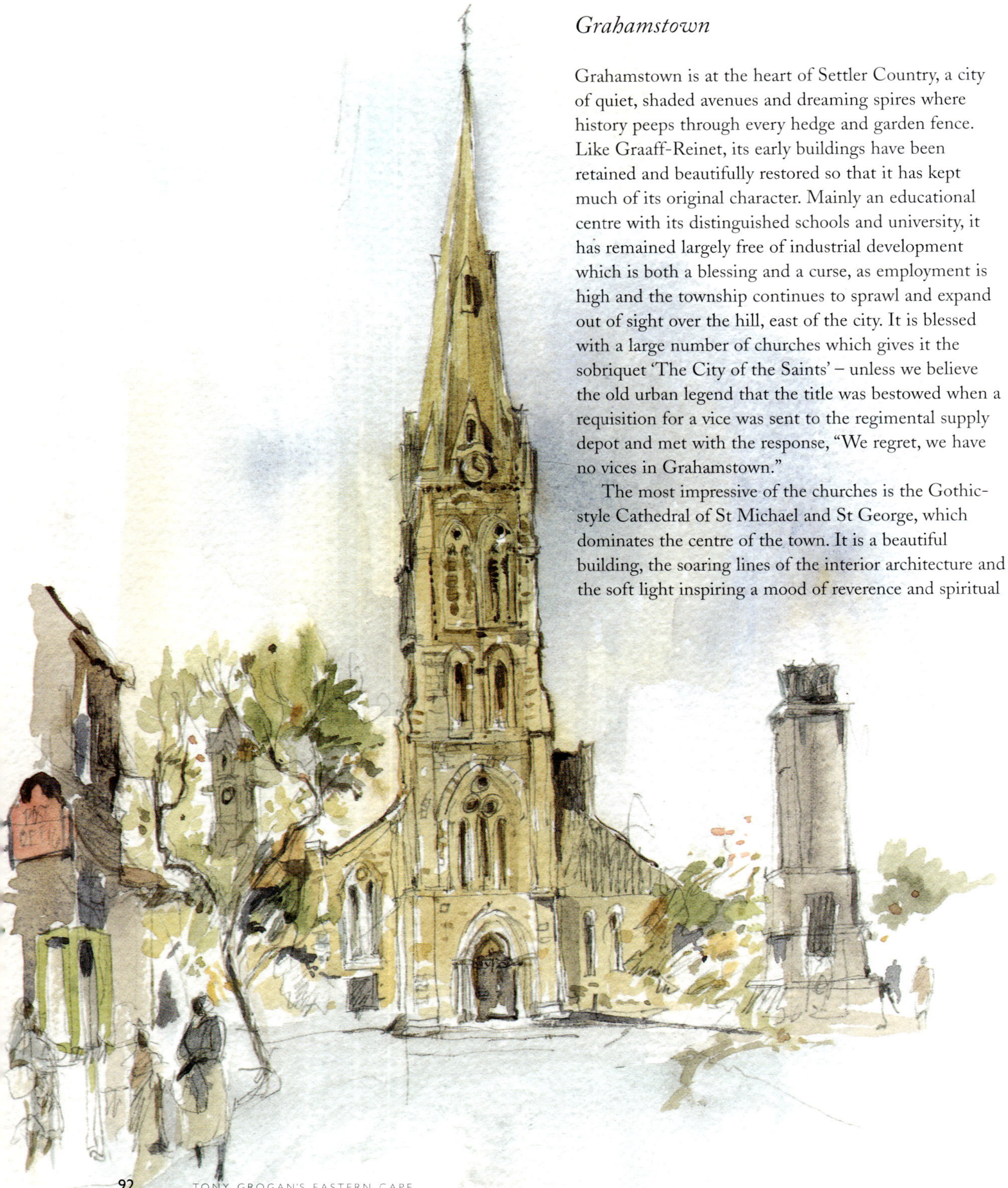

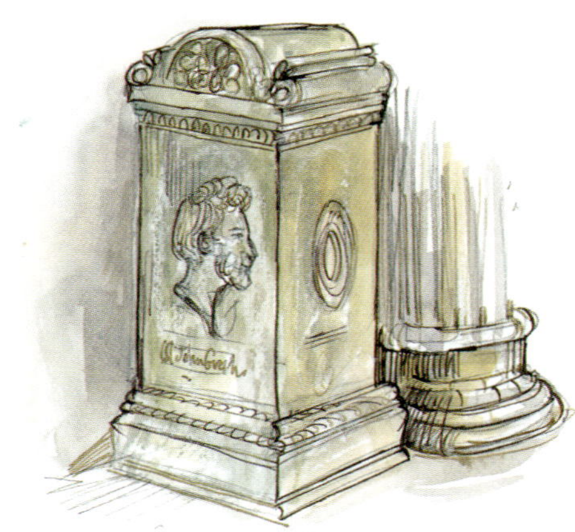

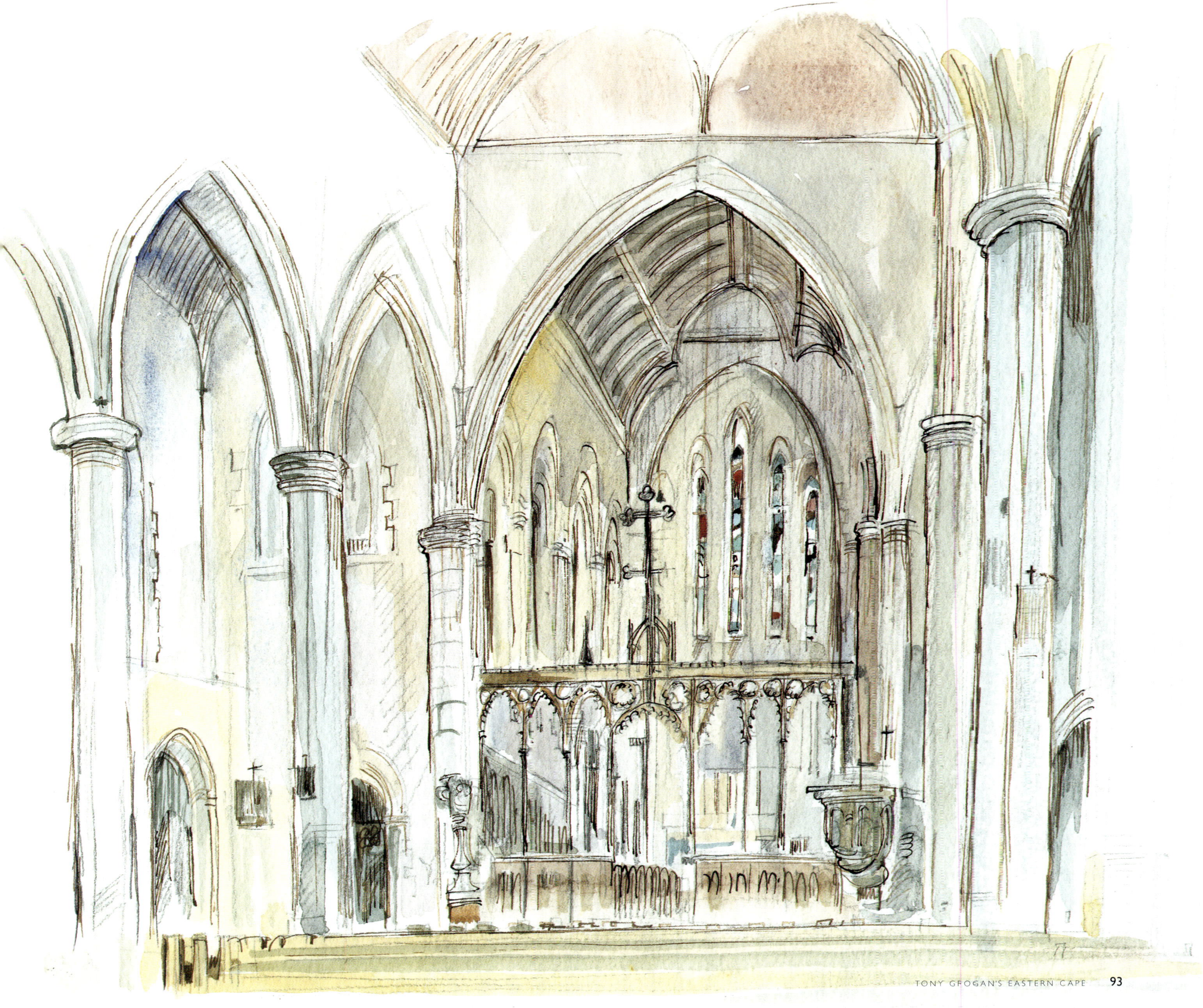

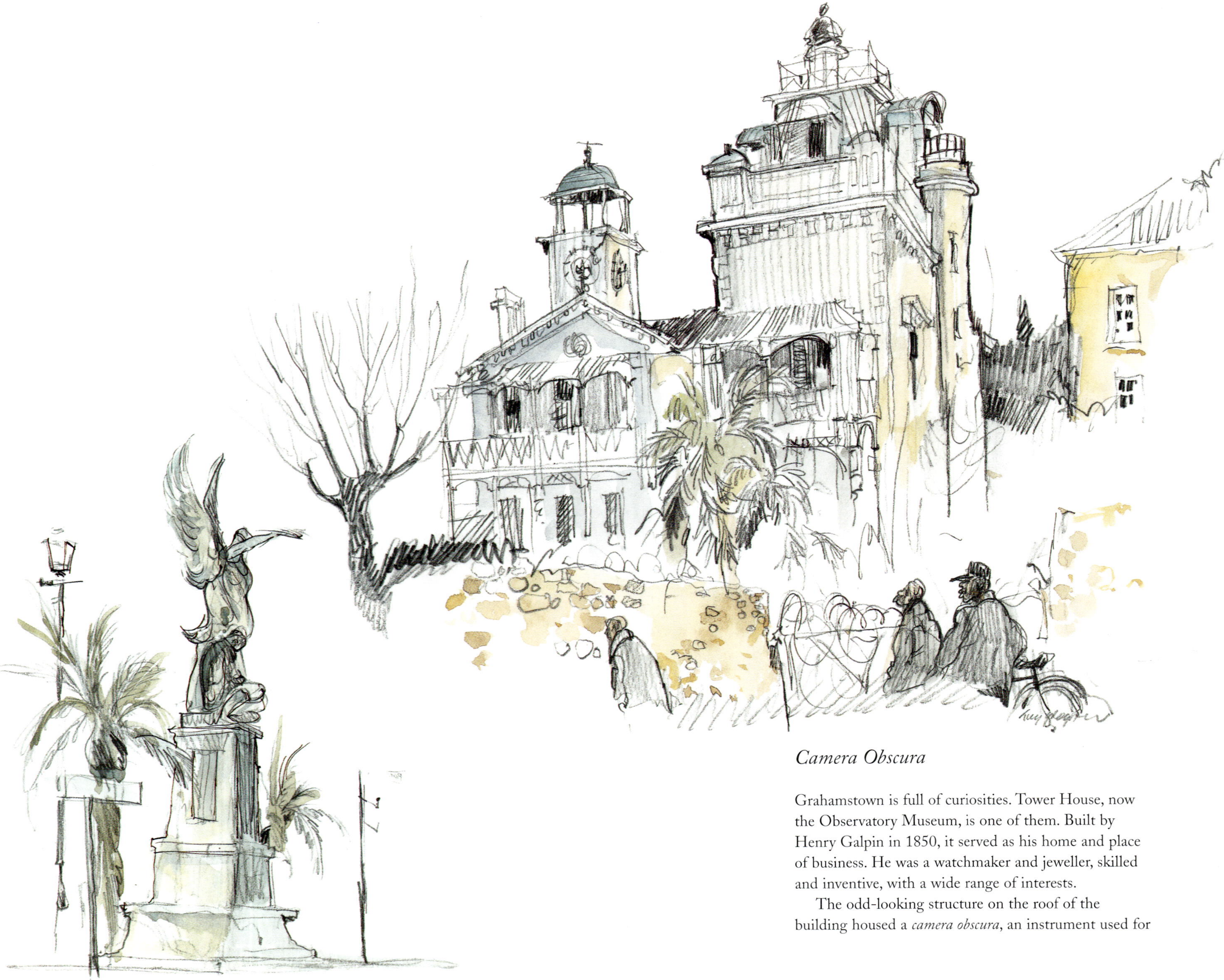

Camera Obscura

Grahamstown is full of curiosities. Tower House, now the Observatory Museum, is one of them. Built by Henry Galpin in 1850, it served as his home and place of business. He was a watchmaker and jeweller, skilled and inventive, with a wide range of interests.

The odd-looking structure on the roof of the building housed a *camera obscura*, an instrument used for

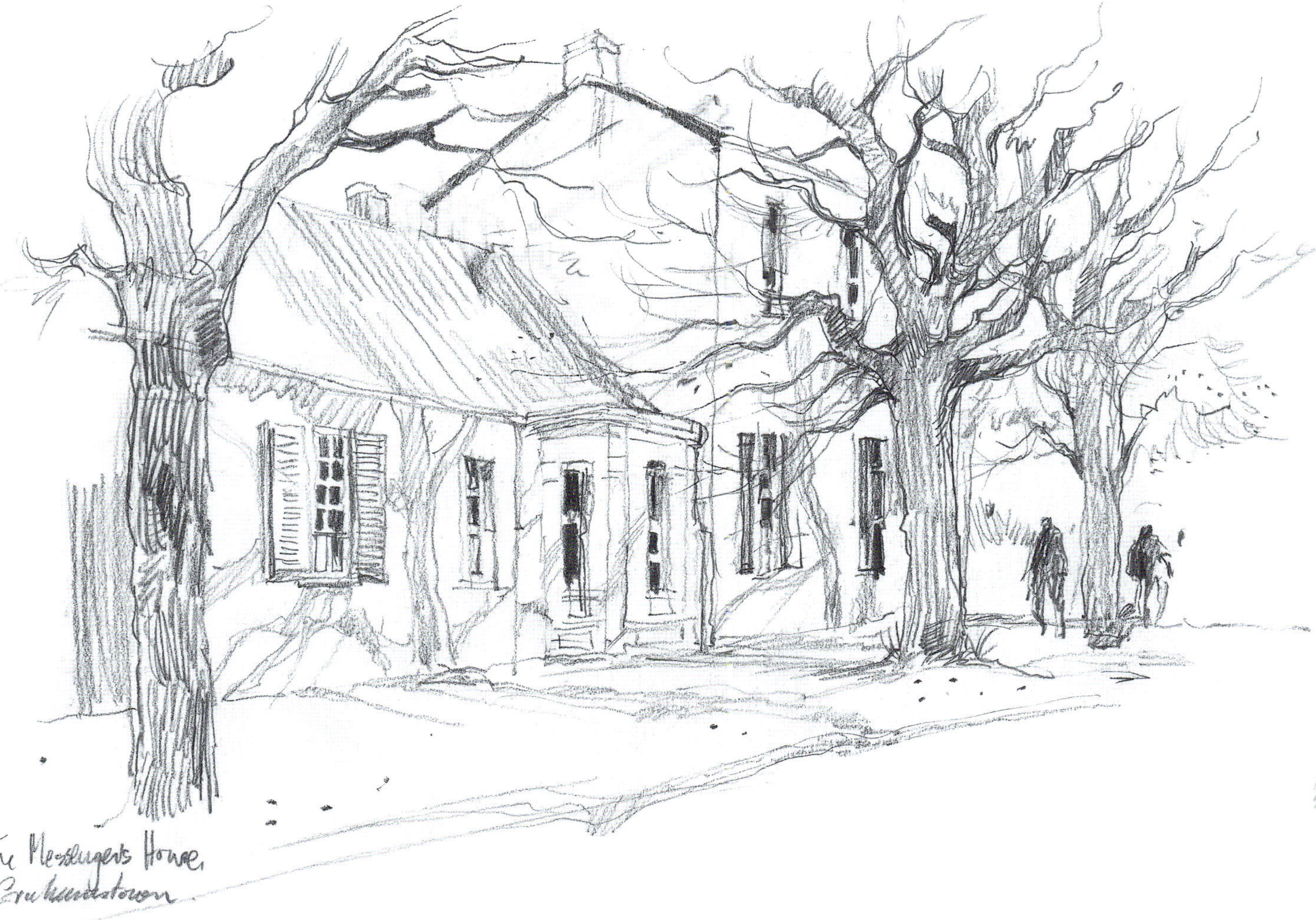

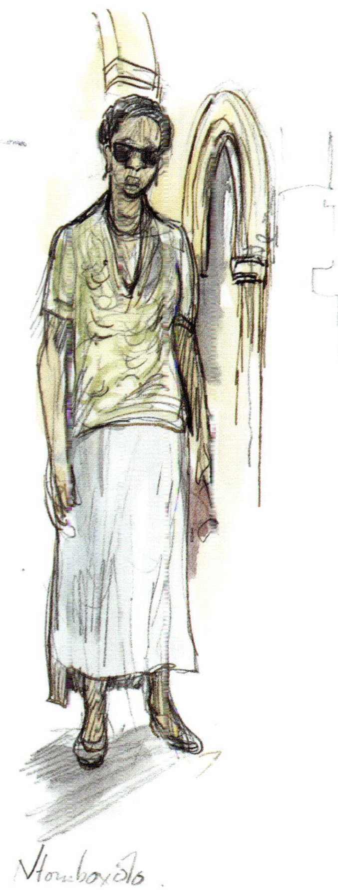

projecting views of the city and surrounding countryside on to a screen. I have not been able to fathom what the purpose of this elaborate device was for, as you can see the same views by simply looking out of the window. In an adjacent, circular chamber he kept a telescope and instruments for calculating the time from the sun each day. His roof clock was the timepiece by which all clocks and watches in Grahamstown were regulated.

The House of the Messenger of the Court is the oldest house in Grahamstown. Its frontage with that of the old gaol was used to define the building line of the High Street.

A passing student notices what I am doing, boldly stands in front of me and challenges me to draw her.

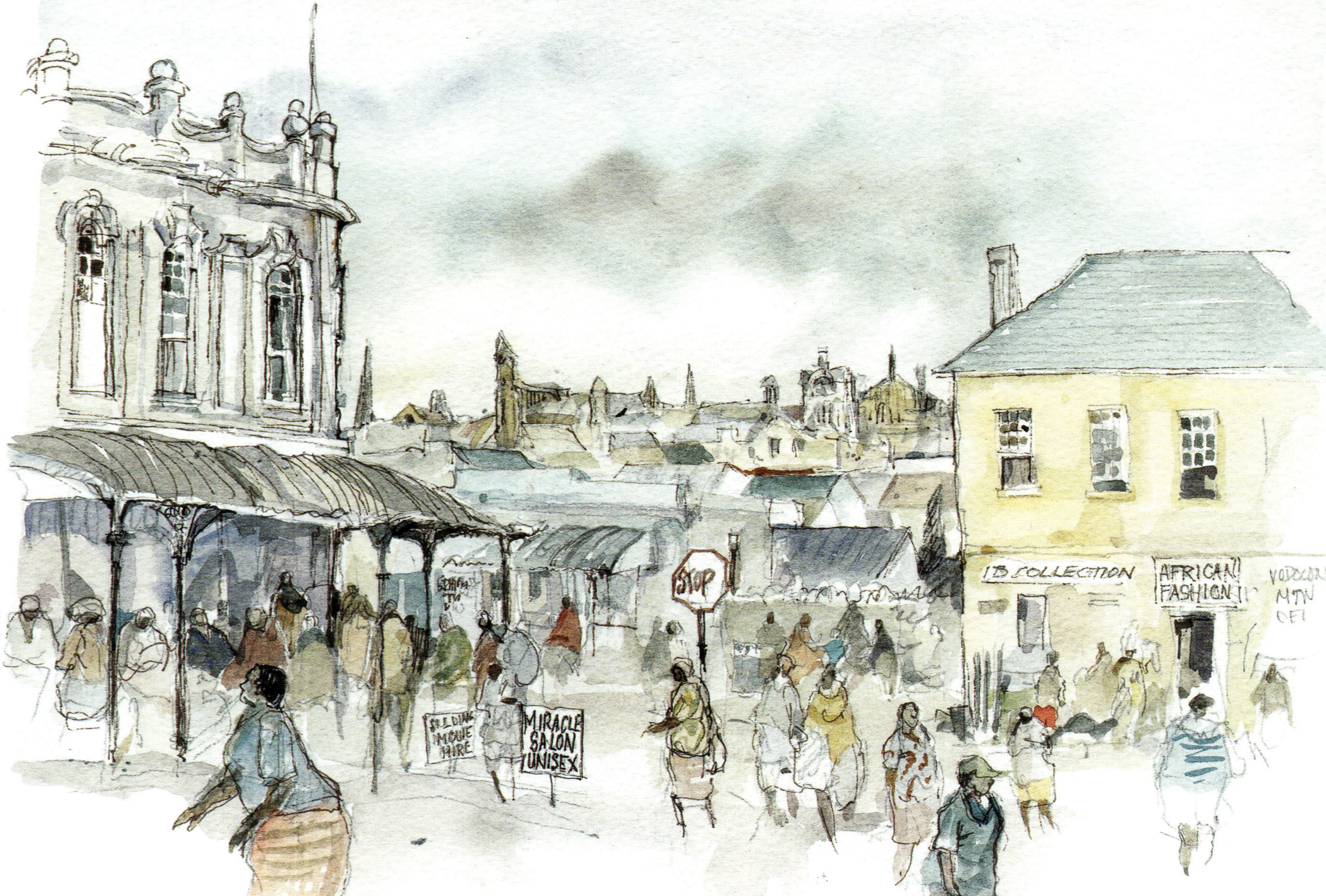

Beaufort Street

Mid-morning in Beaufort Street. There is a seething mass of people going about their business. Music is in the air. It blares forth from portable radios and thumps like a giant drum in passing taxis. The towers and spires of the city can be seen in the skyline.

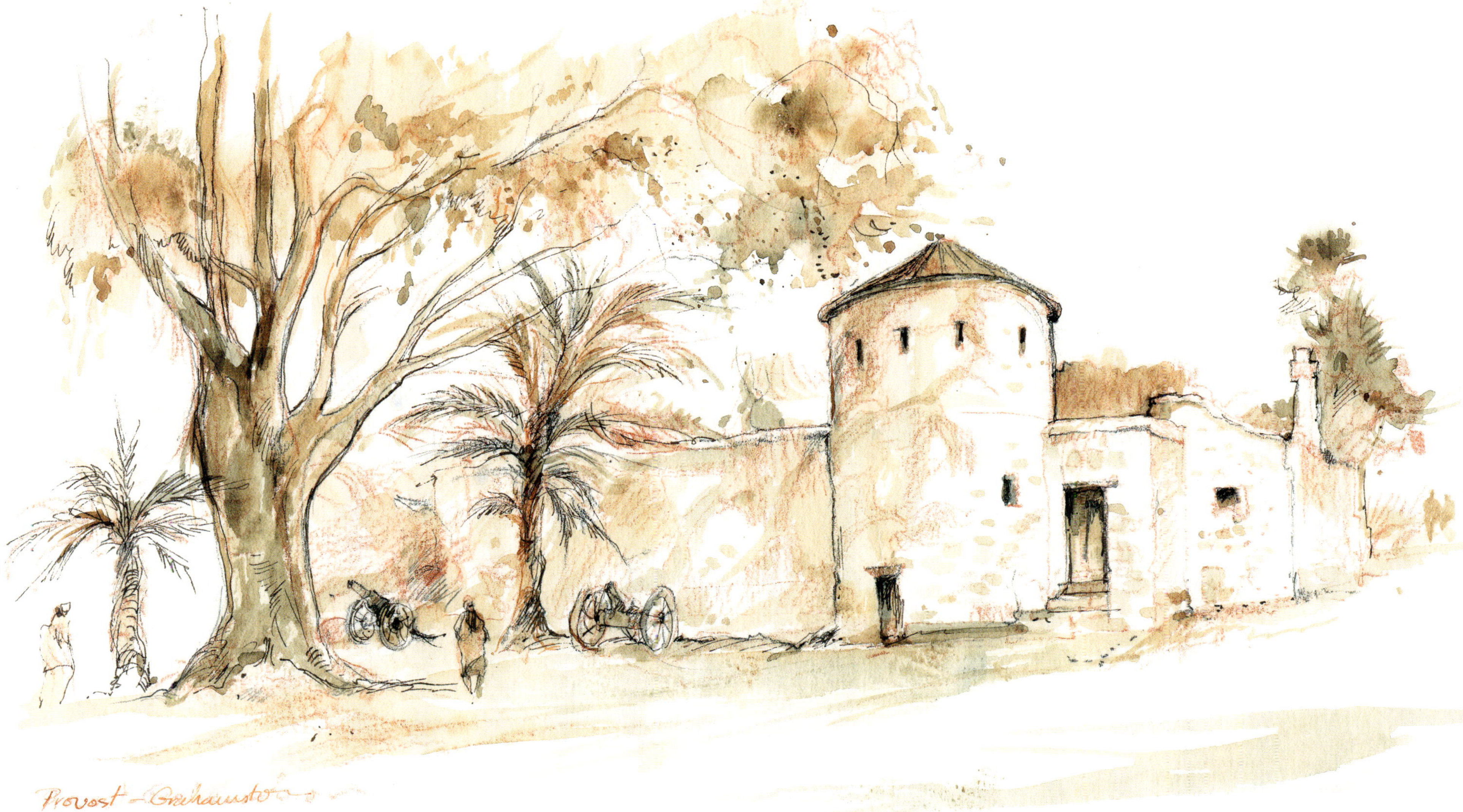

Provost

The ingeniously designed Provost, the old military prison in the botanical gardens in Grahamstown, was built by the Royal Engineers in 1836. The prison is planned so each window of the guardroom commands a view of two of the eight cells and its exercise yard. Life was rough, justice cruel and entertainment scarce in those days, so for diversion you could watch a military flogging near the Provost or for a grand finale, a public hanging in front of the old jail. The excessively harsh punishment administered by the military on their own soldiers, which often so demoralised the recipient that he was ruined for life, or by the white penal system on criminals, puzzled and shocked the Xhosa who seem to have had in place systems and traditions which allowed far more opportunity for repayment to victims of crime and redemption for the culprits. It is interesting to speculate whether it was this traditional spirit of reconciliation which infused the hearings of South Africa's Truth and Reconciliation Commission.

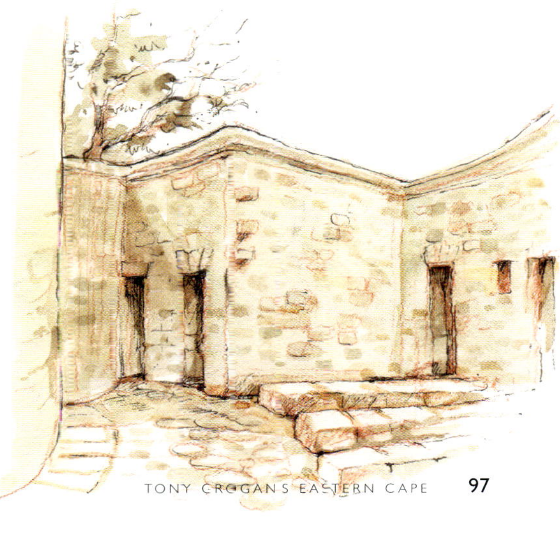

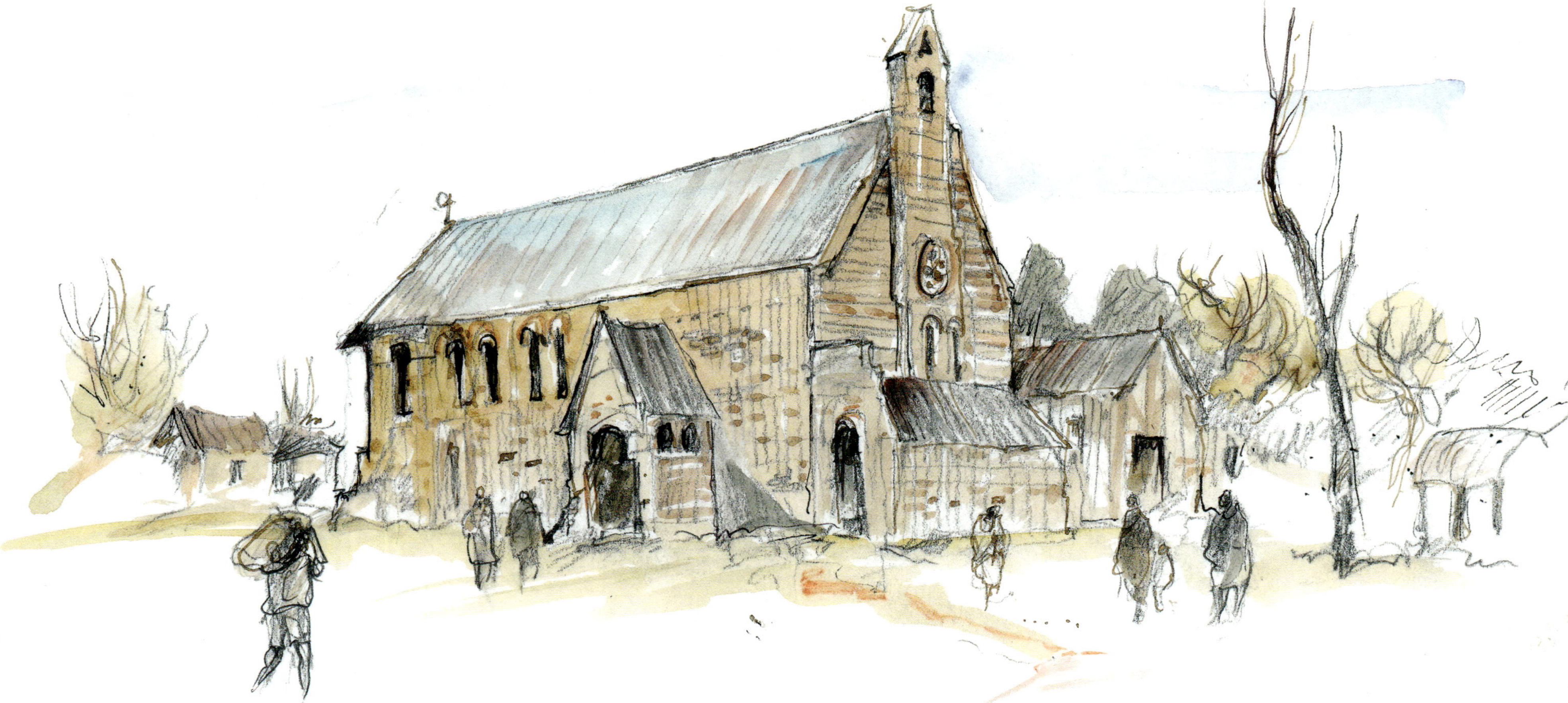

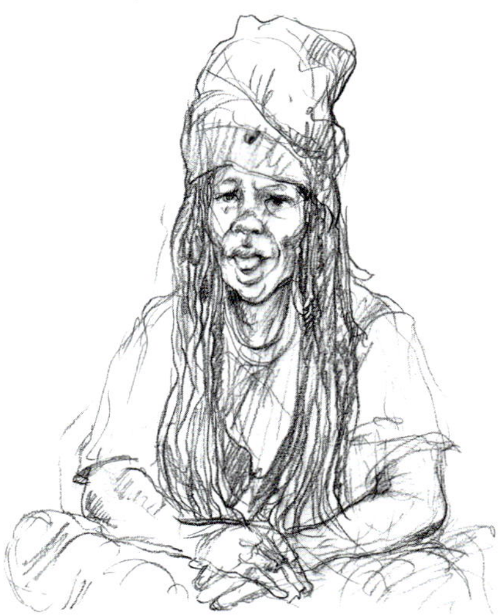

Fingo Village

Fingo village is the oldest township in Grahamstown and the closest to the city. Controversy surrounds the identity of the Mfengu. One view is that they were refugees displaced by Zulu invasions, living as vassals among the Xhosa. The story goes that when a British military force crossed the Kei River in 1835, the Mfengu took the opportunity to escape from serfdom to the Xhosa, threw themselves on the mercy of the troops and accompanied them back to the colony. They were granted title to the land in 1855 for their loyalty in supporting the British and colonial forces in many frontier wars. This didn't deter the Nationalist government from declaring Fingo village a 'coloured' area in 1957 as part of their bizarre plan to carve up urban areas into exclusive racial zones, but years of resistance by Grahamstown citizens and the city council prevented

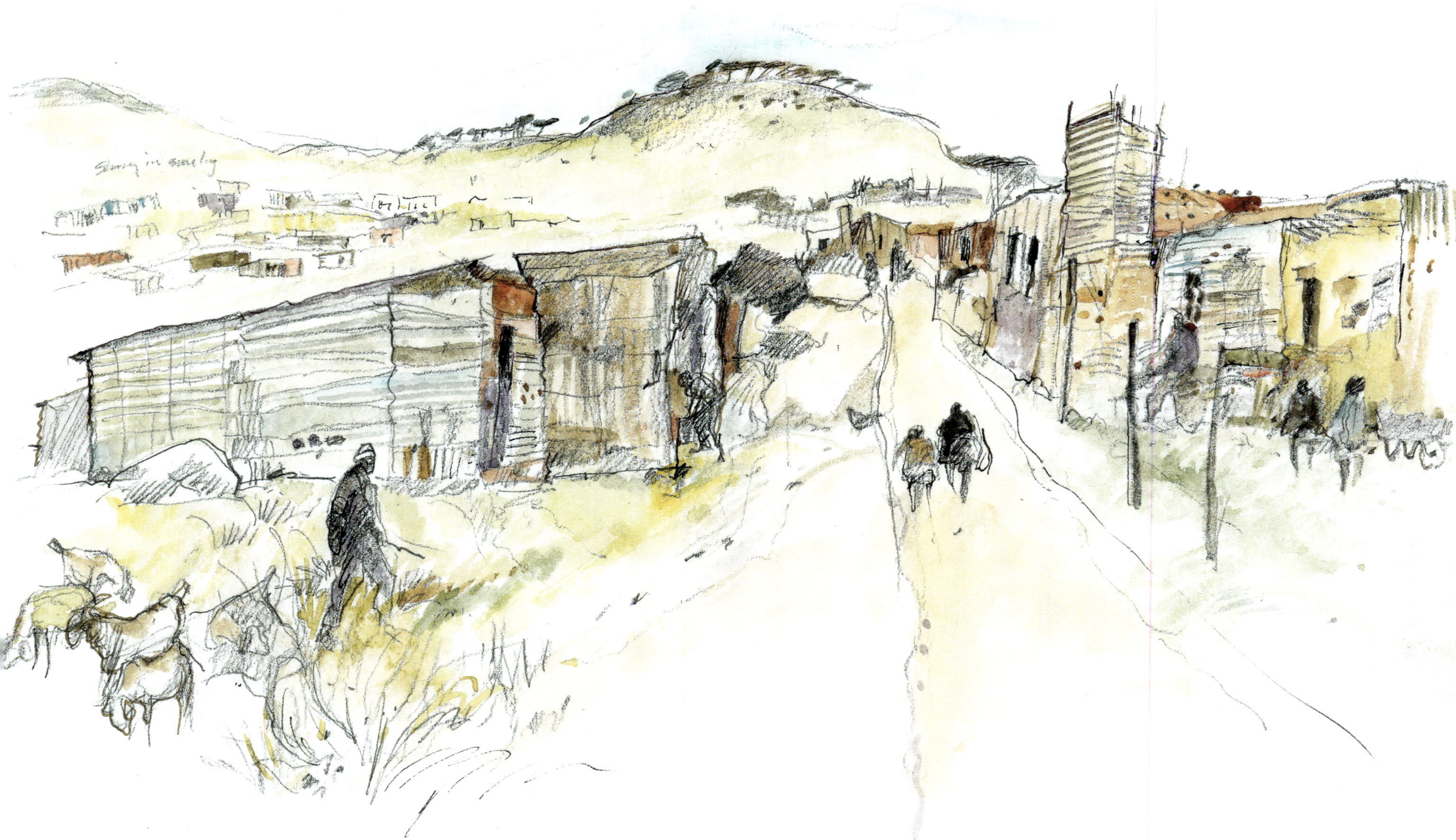

the planned removals of the residents and freehold title was finally restored in 1980.

The red-brick St Philip's Anglican Church, pictured here, was built in 1860.

The woman who poses for the drawing has an expression of melancholy wistfulness, her beauty fading with years of hardship and poverty.

The sprawling squatter camps, where makeshift shacks jostle for limited space on the slopes of Makana's Kop, show the other face of Grahamstown from that presented by the beautiful churches and genteel cottages and mansions. Reflecting the squalor and poverty of this place is its name, 'Dead Horse Kloof', a title straight from the pages of a seedy Western. Apparently carcasses used to be dumped nearby in a stream, which could not have been very hygienic.

It was from this hill that in 1819, thousands of Xhosa warriors, encouraged by the prophet Makanna, launched an abortive attack on the small military village of Grahamstown.

Trappes Valley

Trappes Valley station was once a busy siding serving the local farmers. Now it is abandoned, the station buildings vandalised and falling into ruin. The rusted railway line is overgrown with grass and weeds. It is a forlorn spectacle. If only some enterprising individual could resuscitate the steam train which used to ply the line between Grahamstown and Port Alfred – I remember it as a very pleasant 90-minute trip, but that's history.

There was a store here once, and a petrol pump. In the yard of a house nearby, a bored individual is engaged in that time-filling Saturday afternoon task of washing his car. "Man," he assures me, "When this line was open, this place was as busy as Jo'burg central." Those were the days.

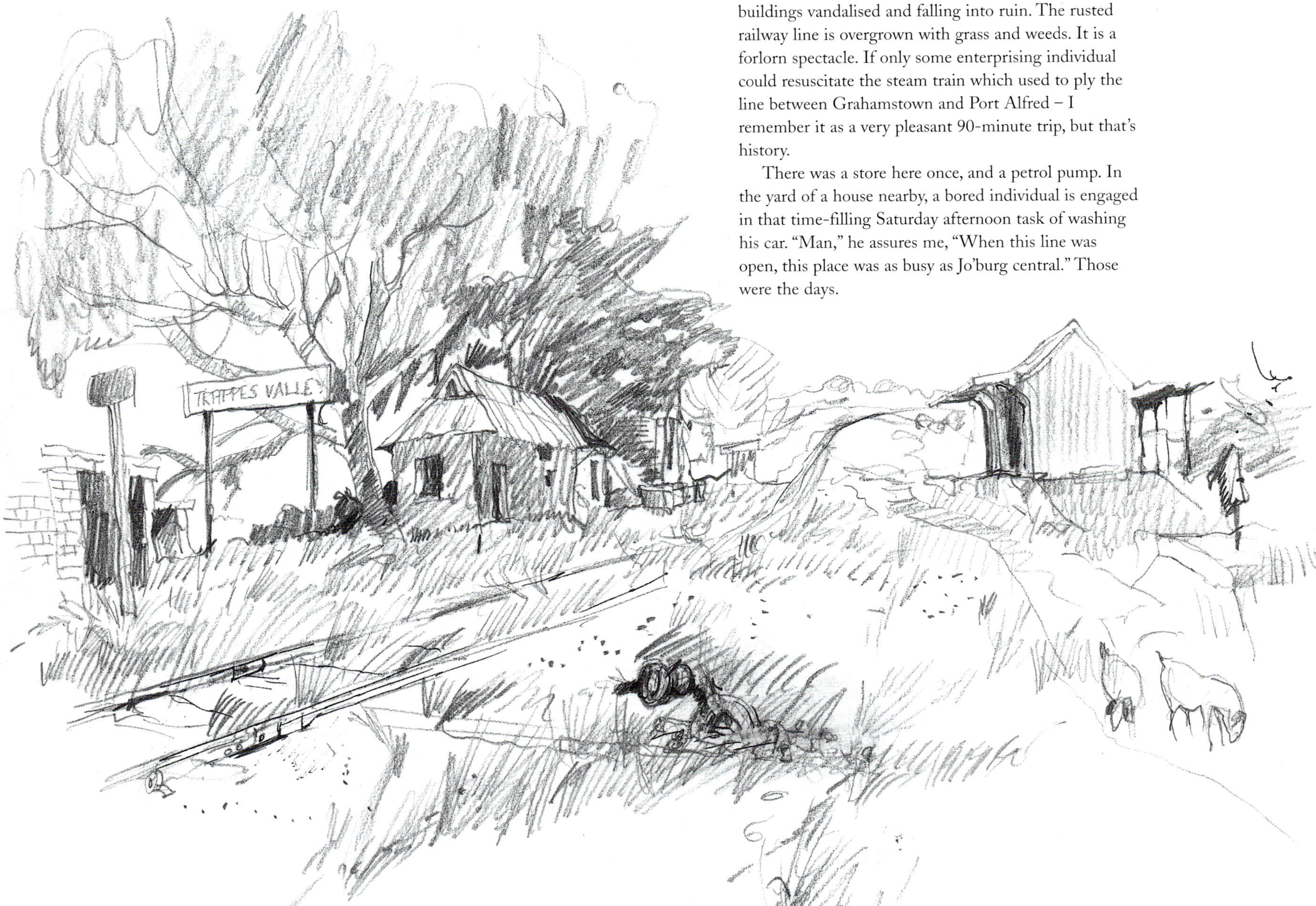

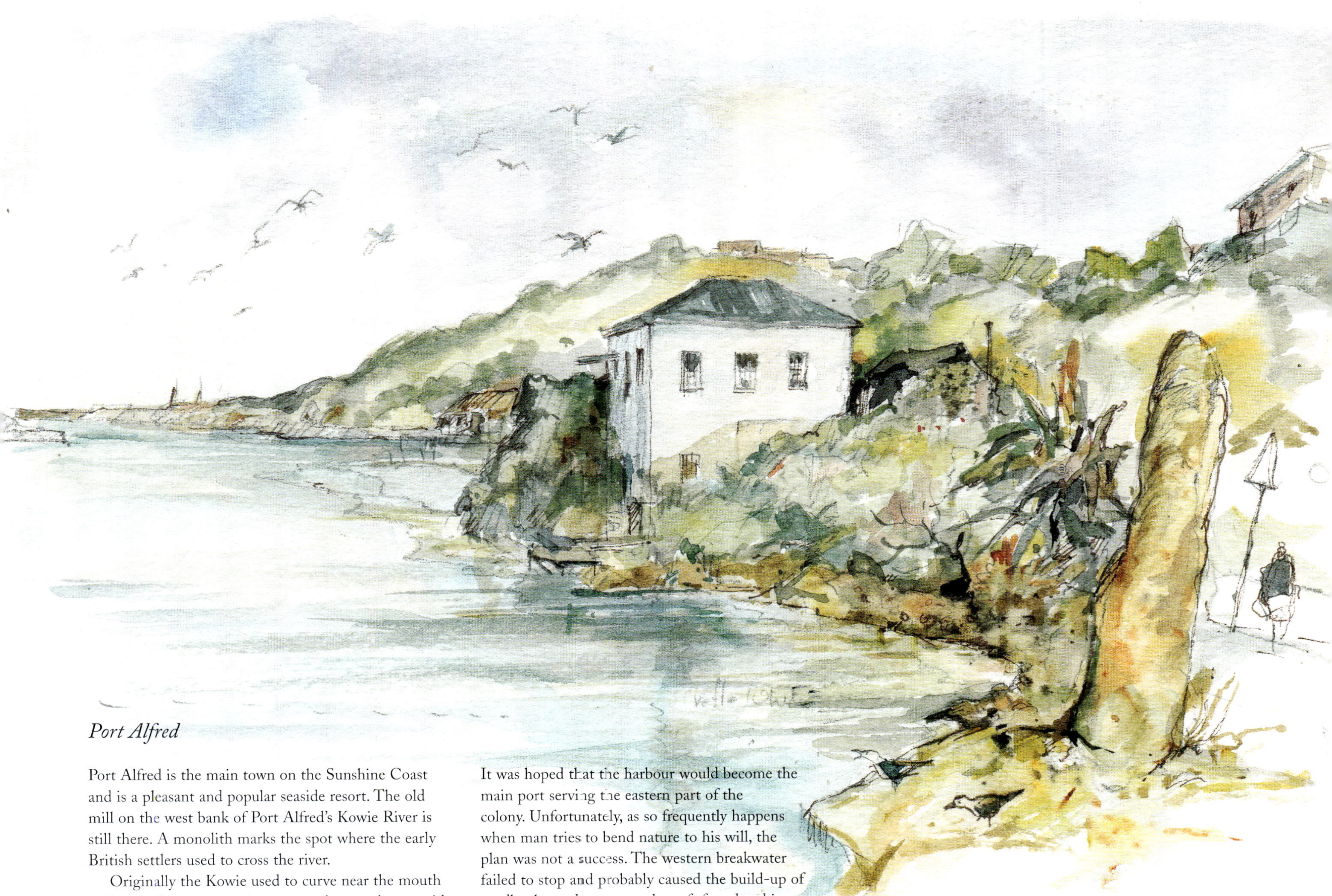

Port Alfred

Port Alfred is the main town on the Sunshine Coast and is a pleasant and popular seaside resort. The old mill on the west bank of Port Alfred's Kowie River is still there. A monolith marks the spot where the early British settlers used to cross the river.

Originally the Kowie used to curve near the mouth and enter the sea at a point more or less on the east side of the present marina. The course of the river was altered to its present position by building a retaining embankment of sand along the east side of the river, held in position with interlaced branches of trees, the port thus becoming known as 'the basketwork' harbour.

It was hoped that the harbour would become the main port serving the eastern part of the colony. Unfortunately, as so frequently happens when man tries to bend nature to his will, the plan was not a success. The western breakwater failed to stop and probably caused the build-up of sandbanks, and many sturdy craft foundered in the narrow inlet of the river. Full-masted ships did dock at the wharf further up the river where the warehouses can still be seen, but too many came to grief and eventually the harbour was closed to shipping at the end of the 1800s.

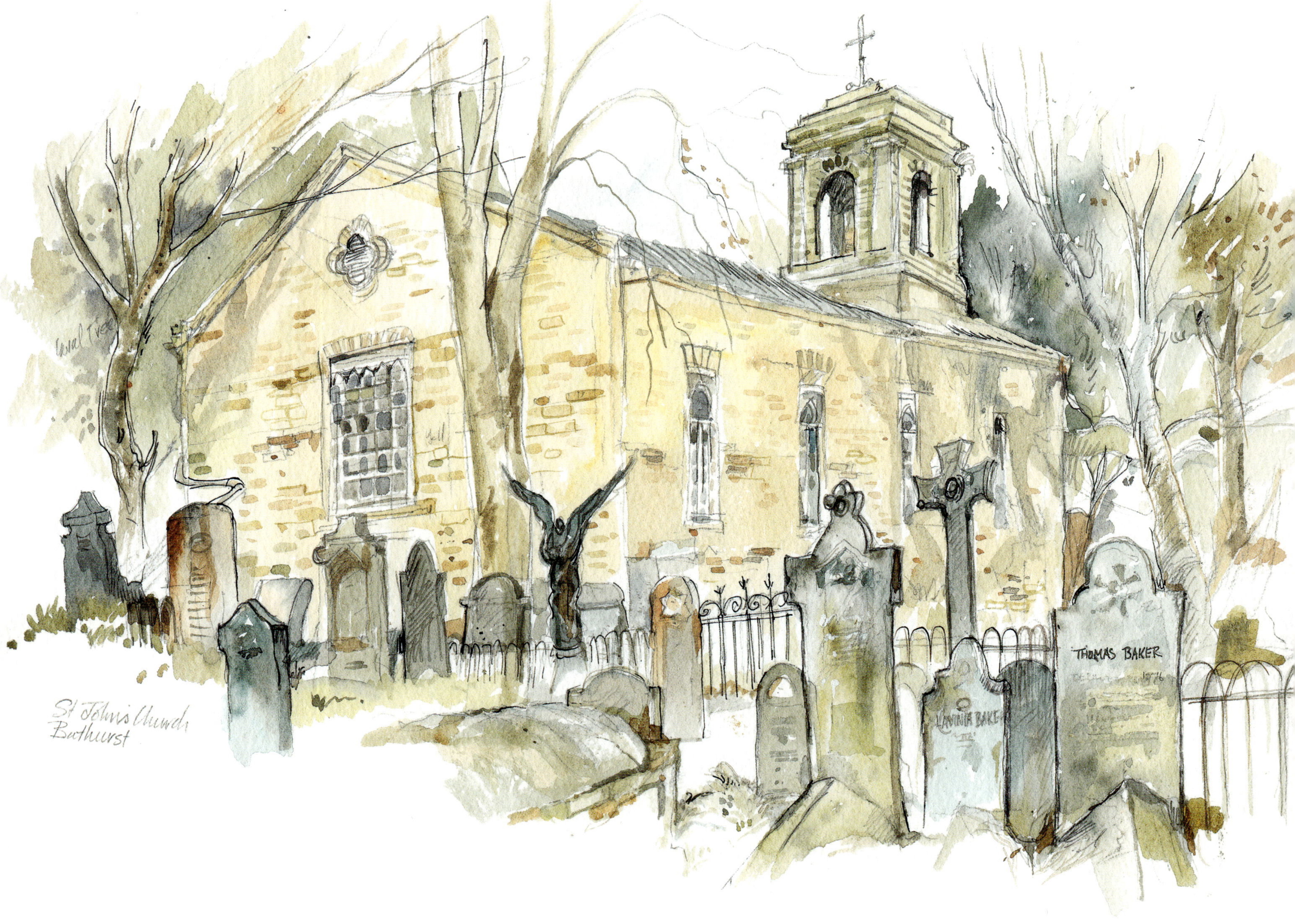
St John's Church
Bathurst
THOMAS BAKER

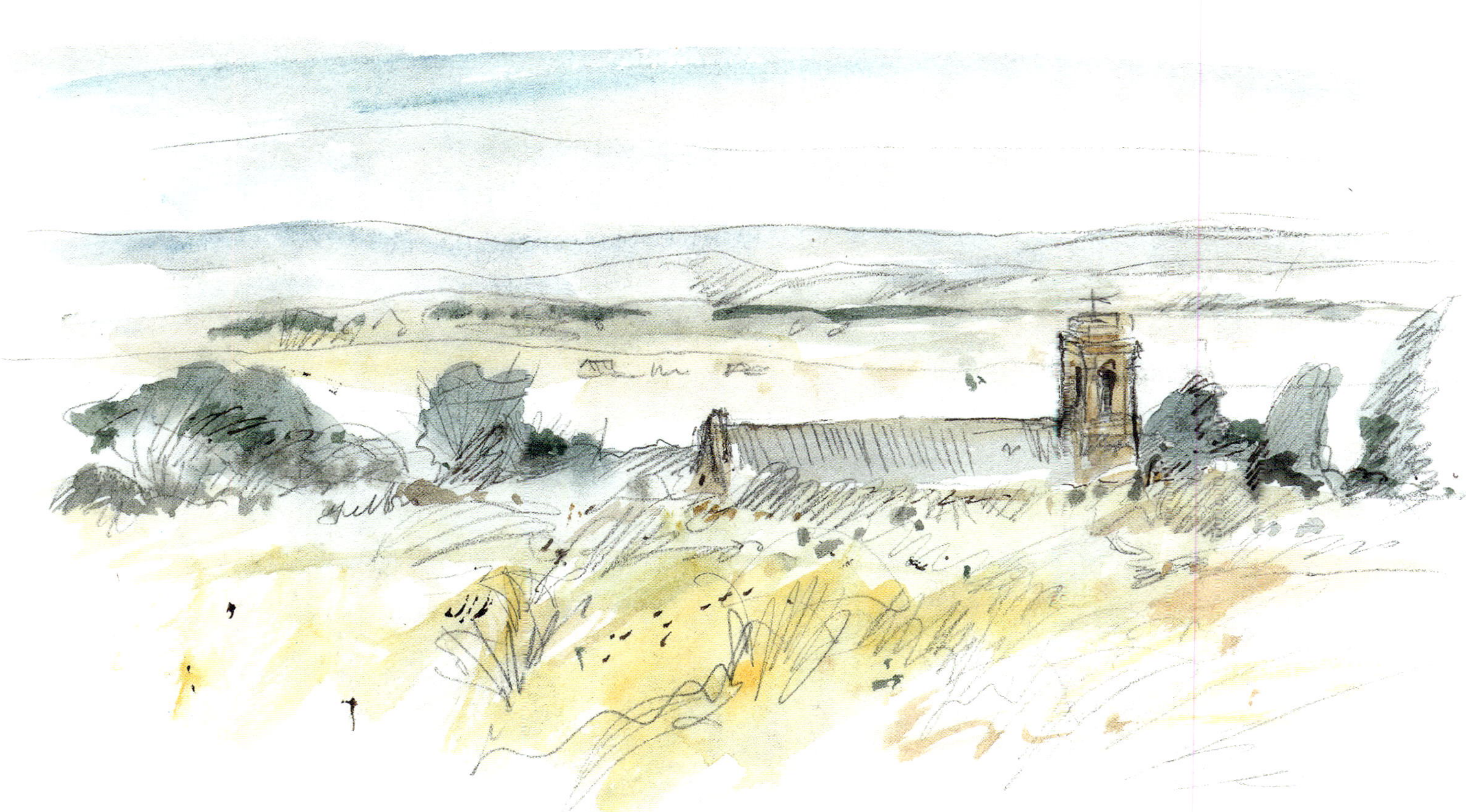

Bathurst: St John's

The fortress-like St John's Church in Bathurst, the oldest Anglican church still in use in the country, is a testament to the faith and endurance of the early British settlers. While still unfinished, it served as a refuge during the Sixth Frontier War in 1834 when Xhosa warriors poured over the border, plundering farms and putting many homes to the torch. It was a particularly traumatic and embittering experience for many settlers, who had only just managed to find their feet and had everything swept away in a few hours. The Xhosa themselves had reason to be angry as they felt the effects of steady colonial encroachment on their land.

Miles Bowker, quoted in Guy Butler's *The 1820 Settlers*, described the scene of the terrified settlers sheltering in the church:

"Found a number of people at Bathurst in the church which they had fortified. Not a gun worth a sixpence among the whole of them. Most of the people armed with pitchforks and bayonets... Never saw so many cattle before with so few hands to protect them."

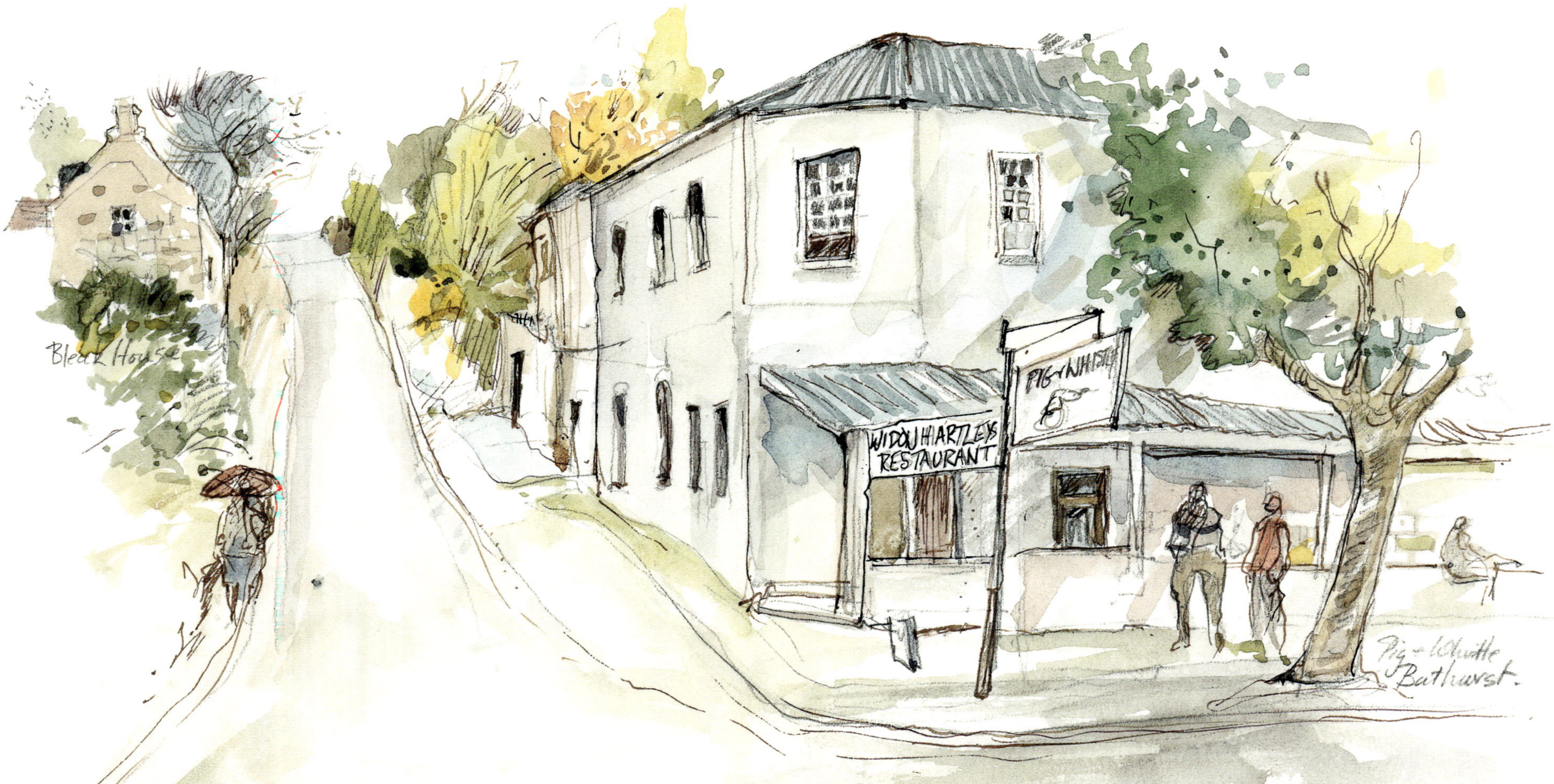

Bathurst

Bathurst's Pig & Whistle is the oldest pub still in use in the country. It belonged to the widow Hartley in the early days of the settlement when it was known as the Bathurst Inn. Sir Rufane Donkin, the acting governor at the time, originally intended Bathurst to be the primary town, as it was central to where the main body of settlers lived, but like many of his decisions, it was overruled when Lord Charles Somerset returned, so Grahamstown became the capital of the Eastern Province. This upset settlers like Jeremiah Goldswain who complained in his journal that to get married he had to walk to Grahamstown and traipse around the countryside trying to find the minister. By the time the ceremony was over and he and his new bride had arrived home, he relates in his diary in his quaint phonetic spelling, "It was past eight o'clock at night and I had not travled less then 40 miles and the gratest part on foot and from the time we left home to go to Grahams Town to pass the Matremonel Cort I had travled upwords of 160 miles." Not the ideal start to his honeymoon.

I spent the night at the Pig & Whistle some years back. The owner then owned a small black pig that snuffled and snorted its way around the hotel. Out of sensitivity to the pig, breakfast was fried eggs but no bacon.

On the left-hand side of the road en route to Port Alfred, a short distance from the Pig & Whistle, is one of the original simple settler houses, obviously added to and sporting a sign reading 'Fab fudge'.

I wander up to Bathurst's very interesting agricultural museum. It's a weekday and there are no other visitors so I have the undivided attention of the

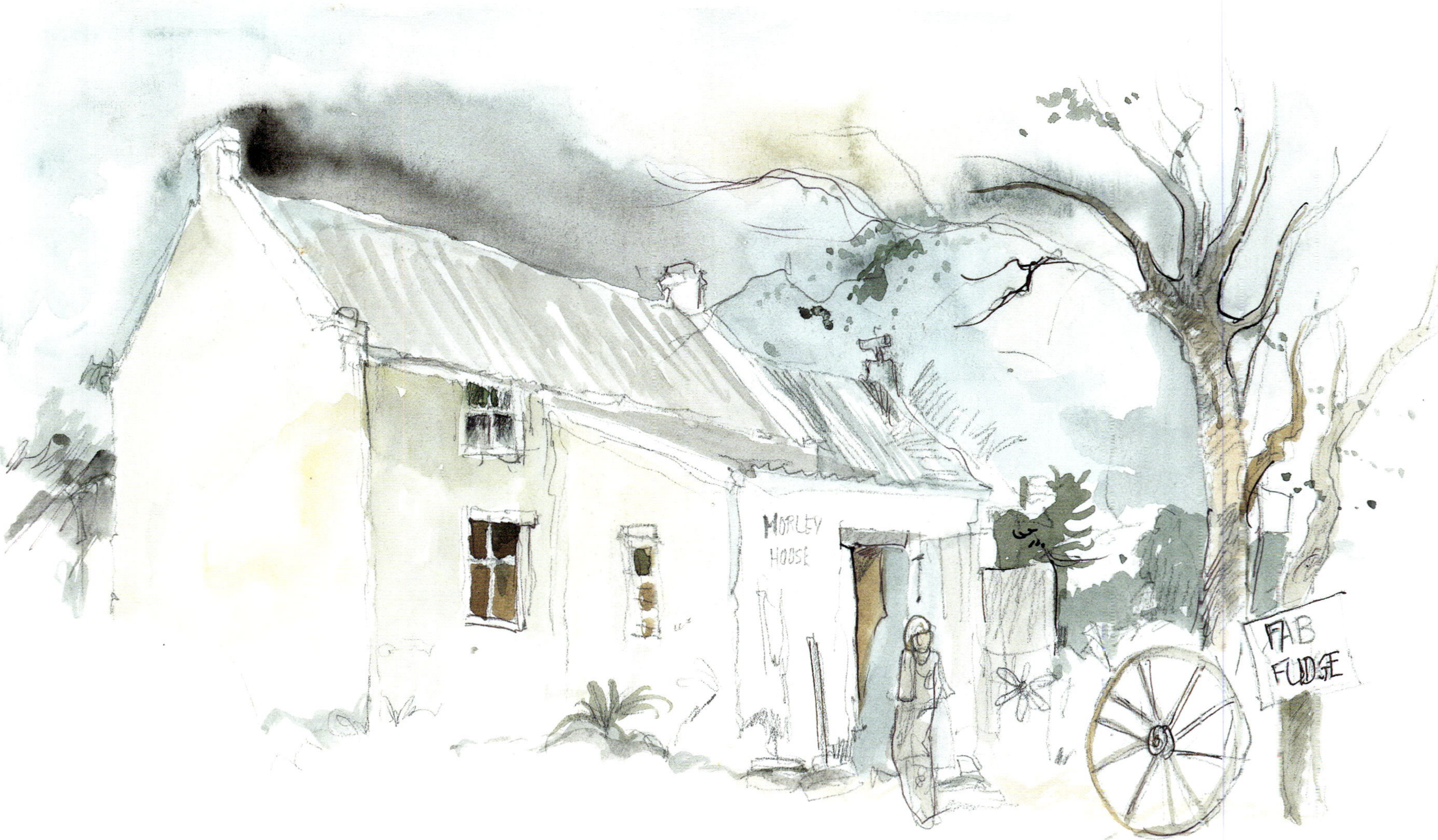

caretaker, John Killian, who conducts me on a tour, explaining with infectious enthusiasm the functions of the various machines in the collection. There is a fascinating array of old farm implements, machines, contrivances for every purpose and none is newer than 75 years, says John.

"In fact," he says with awed respect for the ingenuity and skill of these early inventors who devised these machines, "they are as effective as modern inventions that replaced them, and what's more they still work." Which is more than I can say for many modern machines designed for early obsolescence. Here we have a paraffin-heated incubator, a clockwork car you can still wind up, butter mixers, seed dispensers, a selection of ponderous early tractors and a diabolical device for opening a patient's jaw and keeping it that way while the dentist gets down to work.

"You know," says John, "We think everything is new, but it's not really new." It's true, but I am nevertheless happy that the dental jaw-opener has been consigned to the dustbin of history.

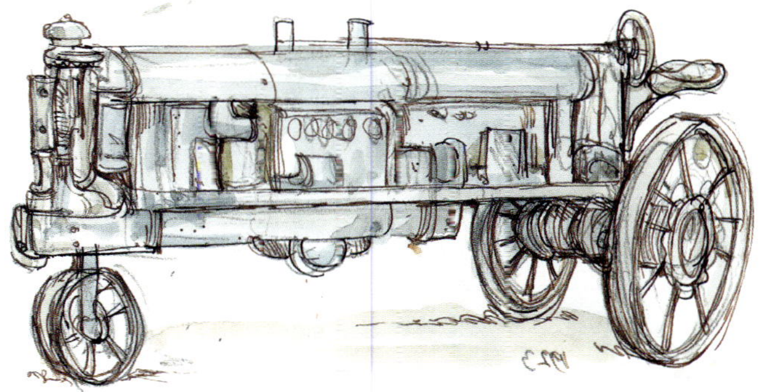

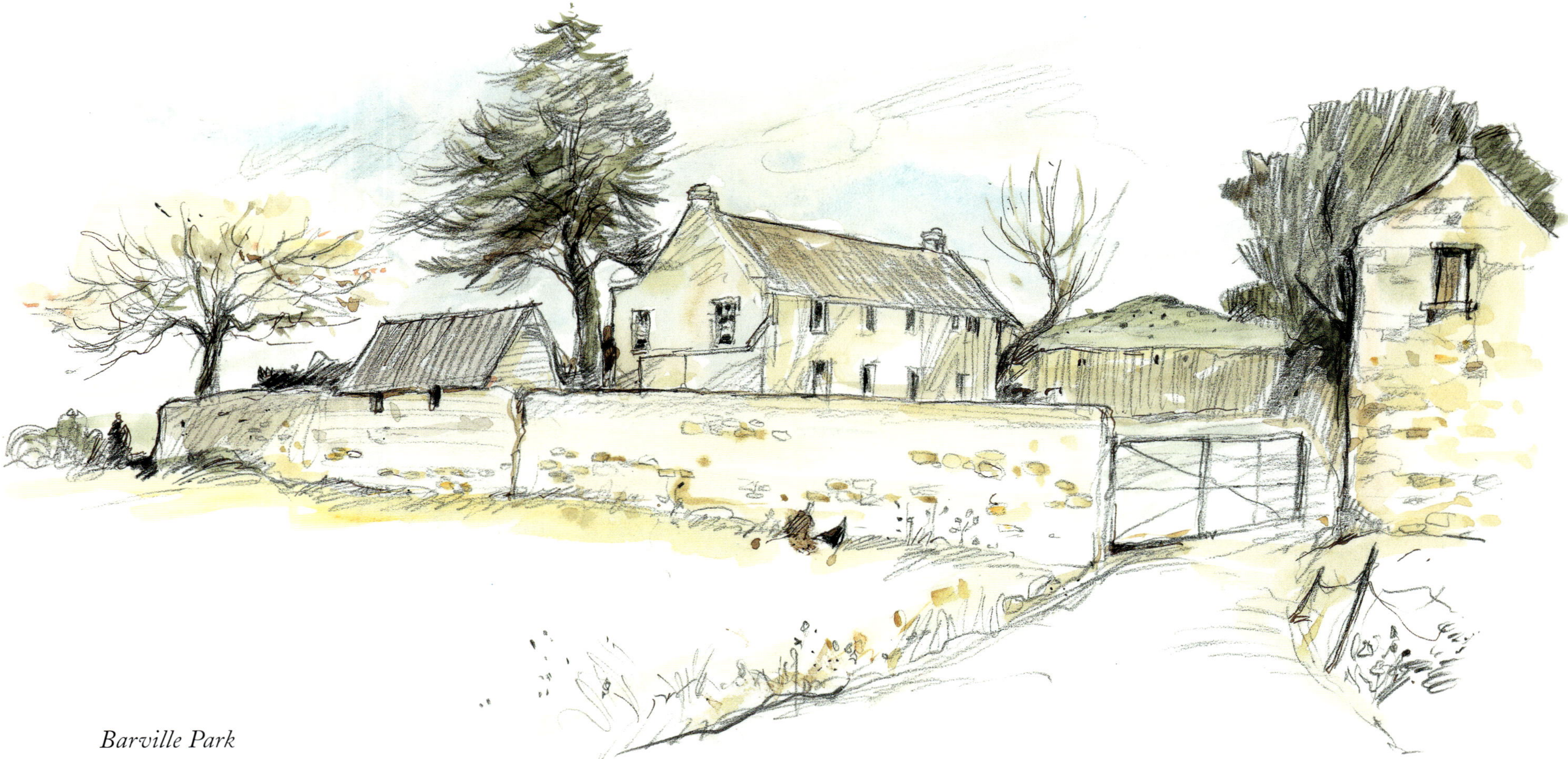

Barville Park

Barville Park is an excellent example of an early fortified farm in the Eastern Cape. Surrounded by a loopholed defensive wall, it gave shelter to the families of early settlers and their cattle in times of war. I discovered the last resting place of the owner, General Campbell, among the graves behind the Provost, the old military prison in Grahamstown. Alas, he didn't live to enjoy life in his new abode near Southwell. He was killed when he was thrown from his horse while riding there from Grahamstown.

His bailiff, Cyprus Messer, sent ahead with fourteen of the party to prepare the general's house and kraals, described the setting in rapturous terms: "I like this part of the country very much. All things seem to thrive well. I never saw in England so much good land together. I have here huts completed and a well that I sank at the top of the garden. Which has plenty of excellent water. I have felled sufficient timber to build General Campbells's house and the men are digging stone for the walls. I have made a large kraal for the cattle; all that have seen it say there is not its equal in the colony."

His enthusiasm might have been a little premature, because early attempts at agriculture weren't propitious – the soil was poor, water was scarce and the allotments too small to sustain the number of people settled on them. Added to this, they had to suffer the depredations of wandering bands of Xhosa helping themselves to their stock, alternative spells of drought or devastating floods – feast or famine seems to be the history of weather in the Eastern Cape – and wheat rust which destroyed their first crops. The ignorance of matters agricultural didn't help much either, and we read of instances of these sturdy yeomen planting potatoes two feet deep in the soil and carrots upside down in trenches with their points sticking up in the air.

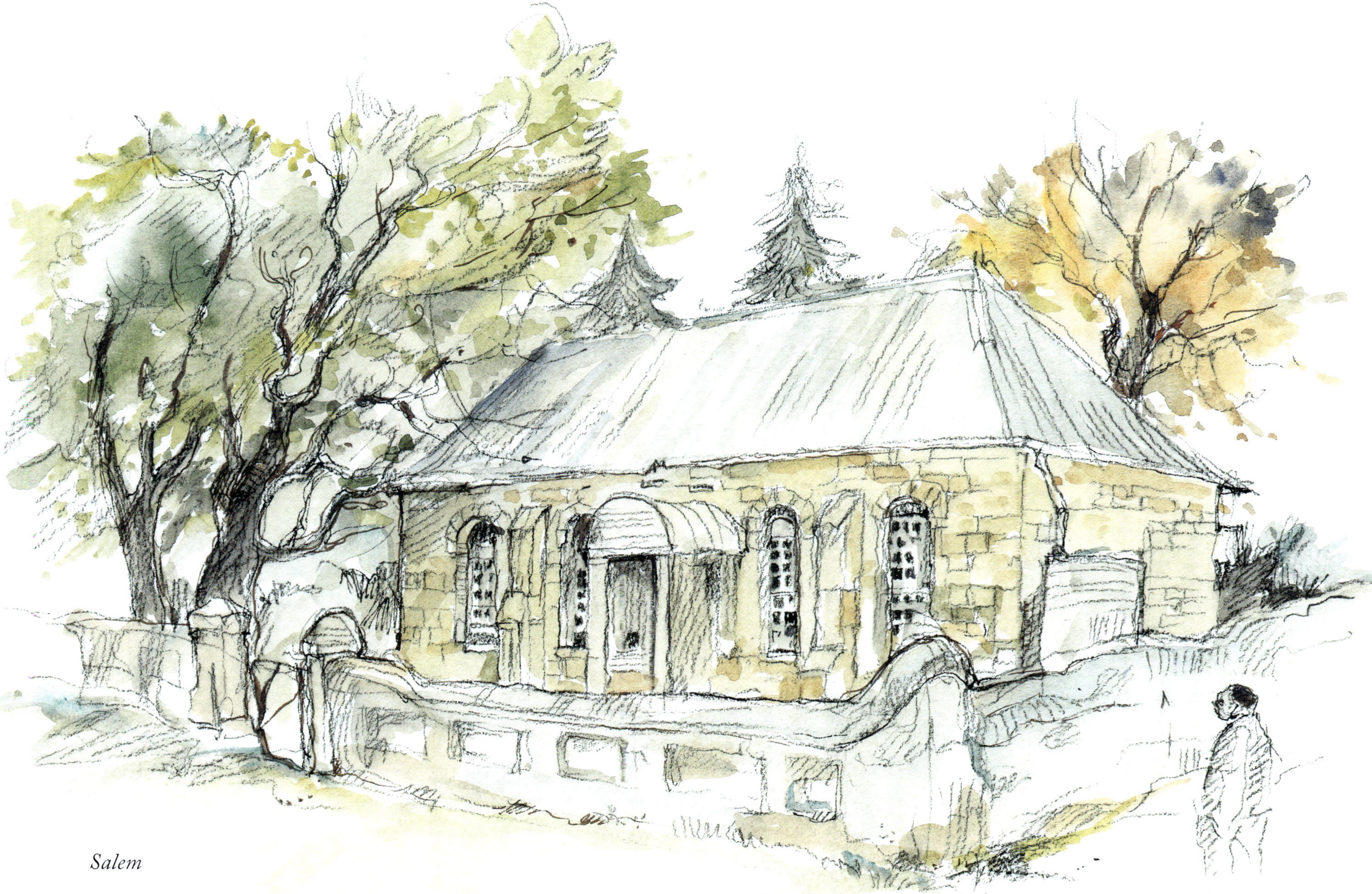

Salem

Founded in 1820 by Hezekia Sephton and his party of 344 settlers, Salem is a scattering of small houses in a shallow valley and is probably not much changed since those early days. The central feature of the village is the cricket ground and next to it, the Methodist Church built in 1850. The earlier church, now a school, dated 1832, is the subject of this drawing.

Salem is remembered for the story of Richard Gush, the Quaker, who saved the settlement when it was in danger of attack by a large party of Xhosa during the war of 1835. He went out unarmed to remonstrate with them and ask them why they were terrifying women and children out of their wits. Disarmed by his courage and frankness, the warriors said they wanted bread as they were hungry. Gush collected bread, pocket knives and tobacco which he gave to the Xhosa and they departed, leaving the village in peace.

More recently, Salem has come to public attention as the setting for JM Coetzee's novel *Dusklands*. I doubt that his gloomy prognostications will cause a rush of eager investors to the village.

Today there are few people around. I chat to a disenchanted and bored policeman, who tells me he has had enough of working for the police and is leaving to seek his fortune elsewhere

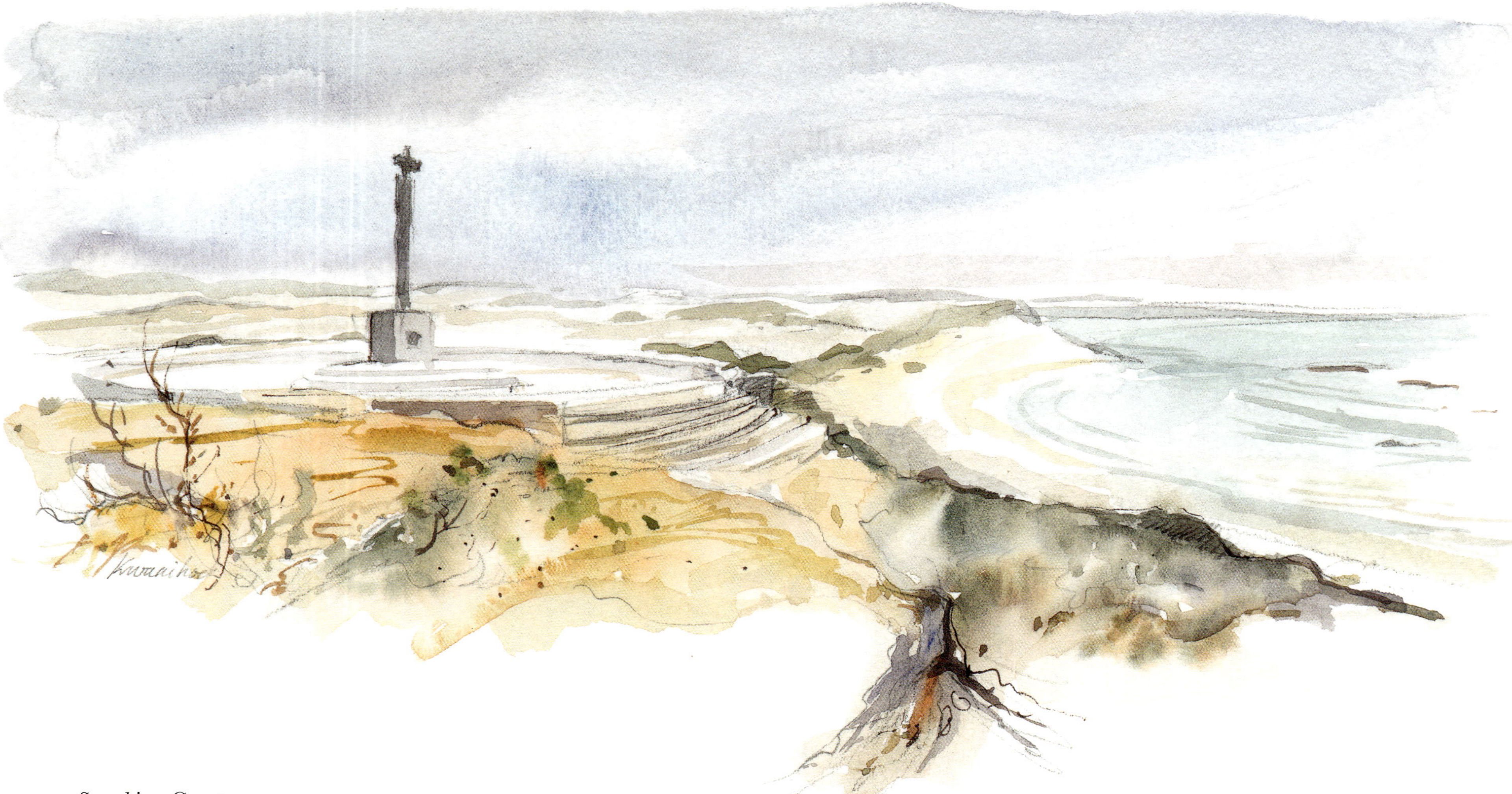

Sunshine Coast

A stretch of the Sunshine Coast near Bushman's River, an endless vista of white sand and bush-covered dunes sweeping down to the sea. It's exhilarating to walk along this lonely coastline, particularly as the smooth surface of the soft sand is no longer scarred and criss-crossed by the wheel tracks of 4x4s since the banning of these vehicles from the beaches.

If you continue further along the coast towards Port Alfred, you will come to the site where Bartholomew Diaz reached the furthest point of his exploration and planted a stone cross on a lonely outcrop of rock on the shore. In 1938, following the most exacting academic sleuth-work based on early maps, ships log books and drawings of the coastline, Professor Eric Axelson worked out that the location of the cross was a rocky promontory at Kwaaihoek. The discovery of crystalline fragments of the cross confirmed the correctness of his research.

As we walk along the beach we are mystified to discover a dead steenbok, obviously drowned, washed by the incoming tide. My friend Peter Anderson, with whom we are staying at Kasouga, tells us that it is not the first time he has discovered a buck in the water. On a previous occasion, he pulled the limp body of a bushbuck out of the waves, laid it on the sand, then proceeded to give it artificial resuscitation by pumping its ribs, until to his delight he felt a flutter of life as its heart started beating and it was soon on its feet and tottering into the bush.

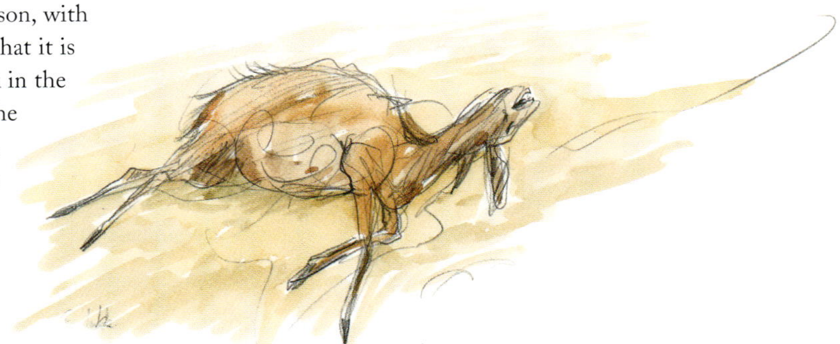

Drowned grysbok on Kasouga beach

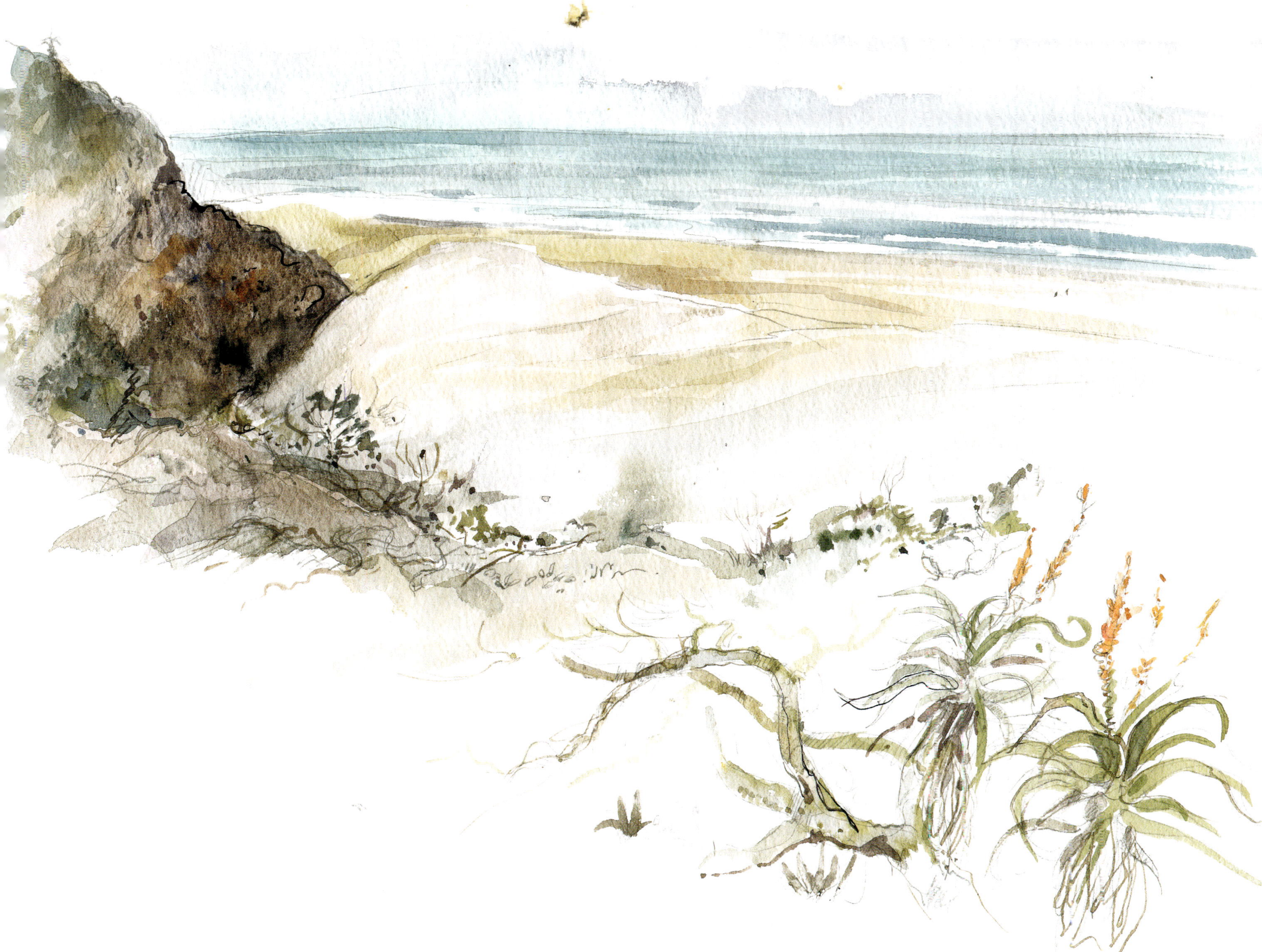

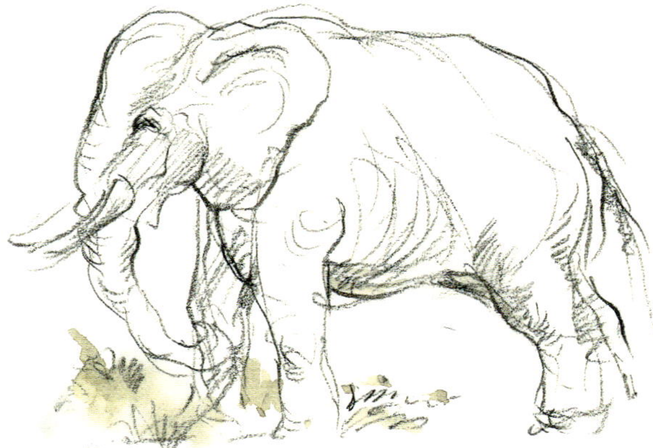

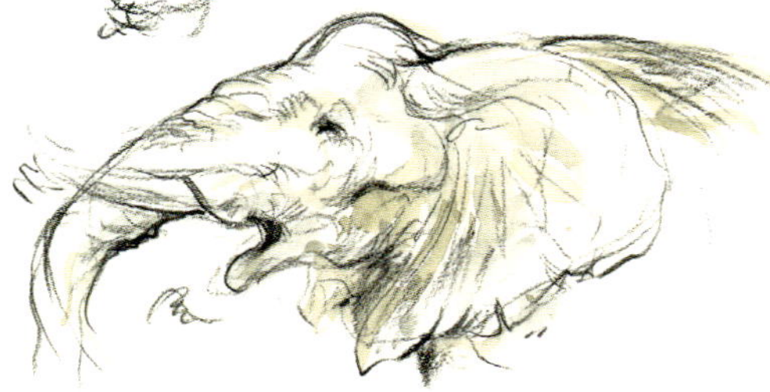

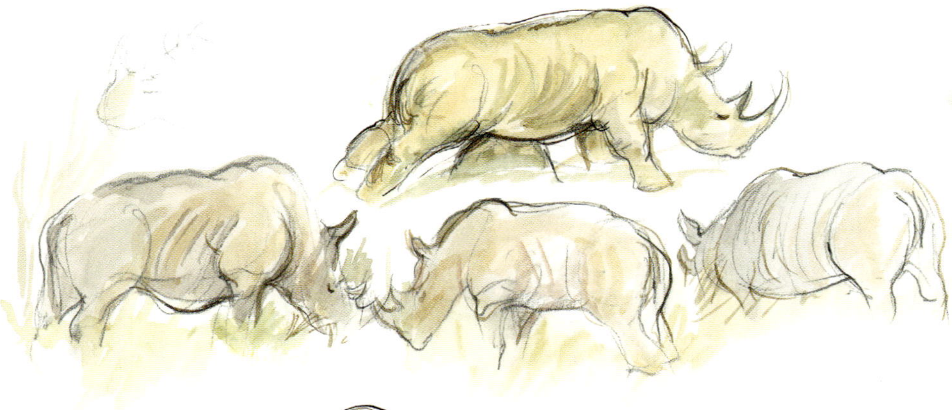

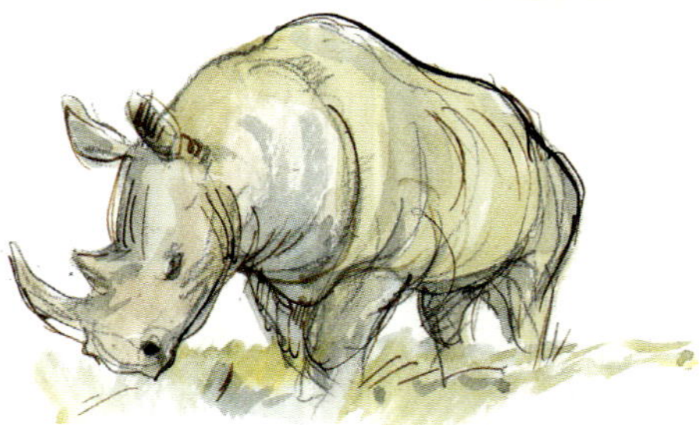

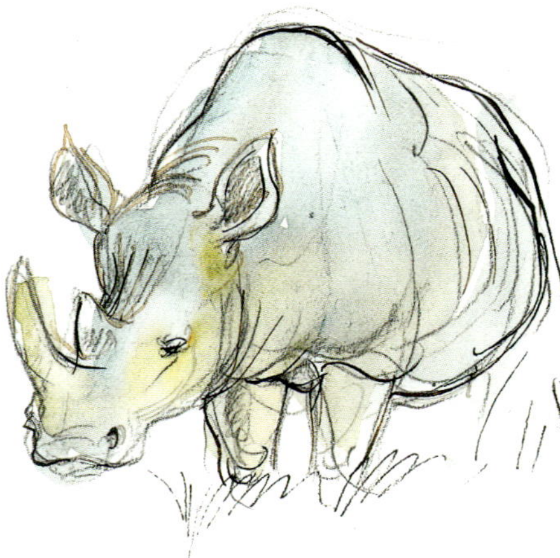

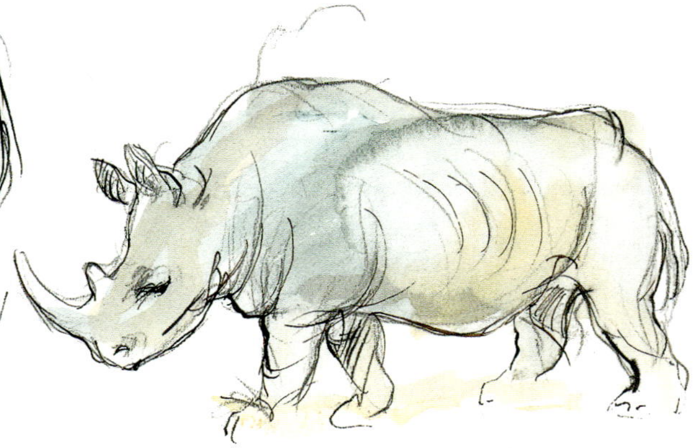

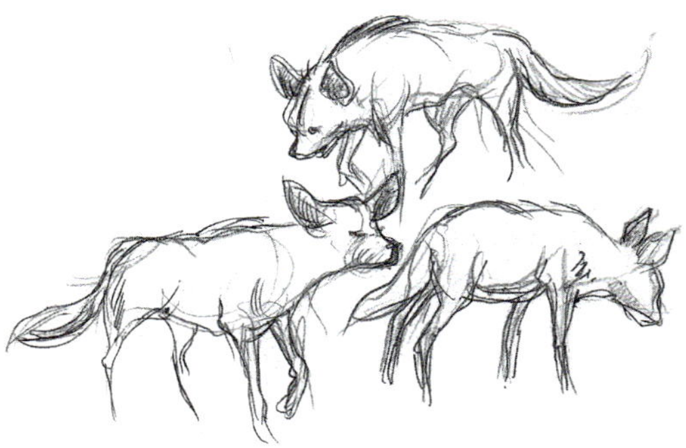

Shamwari

Shamwari is one of the largest and finest of the private game reserves in the Eastern Cape. While we were there, we saw all the game we wanted to see and I was able to make some very satisfactory drawings from close up, guided by a well-informed ranger who managed to track down in the course of the afternoon elephants, lions and rhino in that vast tract of virgin bush. We also saw a black rhino in the distance and the remains of a large buffalo which had irritated one of these irascible animals by crossing its line of vision.

Previously confined to a camp, lions now roam free in the reserve. We came across a large male lion ambling along the road. He had apparently left his harem at the bottom of the valley. When there was a roar from another lion and an answer from his own females, he turned his great shaggy head to look

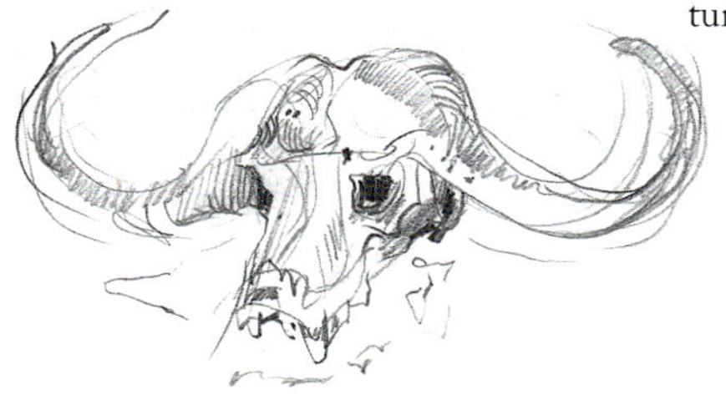

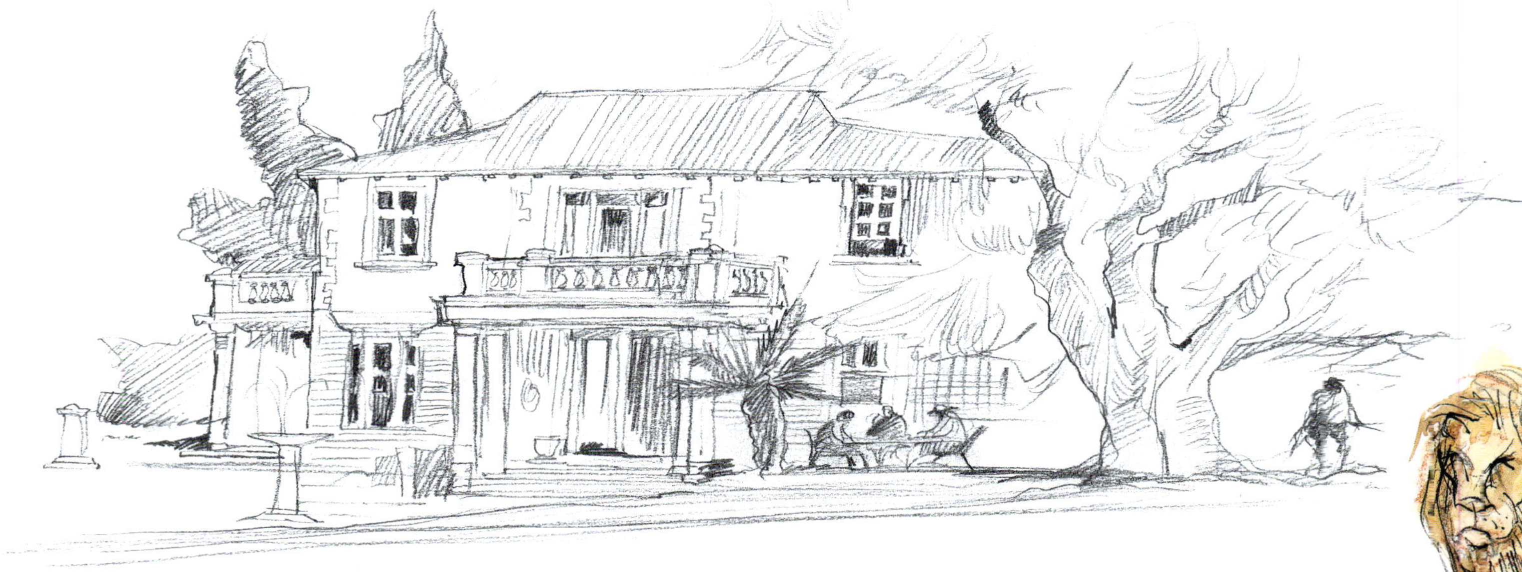

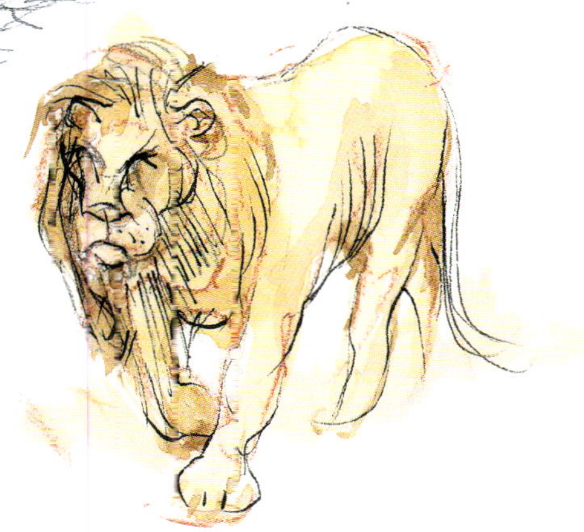

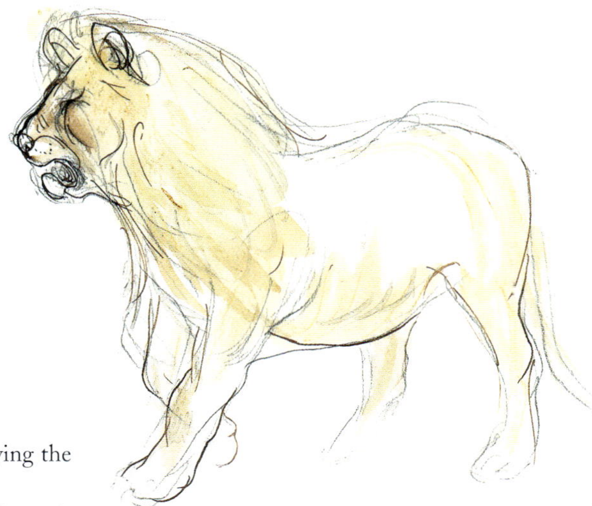

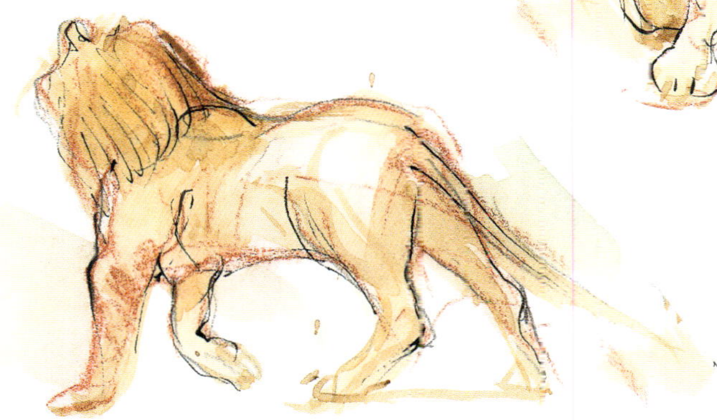

back indignantly, as if querying the nerve of these females to communicate with another lion, then sent out a challenging roar which reverberated across the hills. I had never seen a lion roaring up close and it was an impressive sight, his great chest heaving like giant bellows to produce a sound to make the earth tremble.

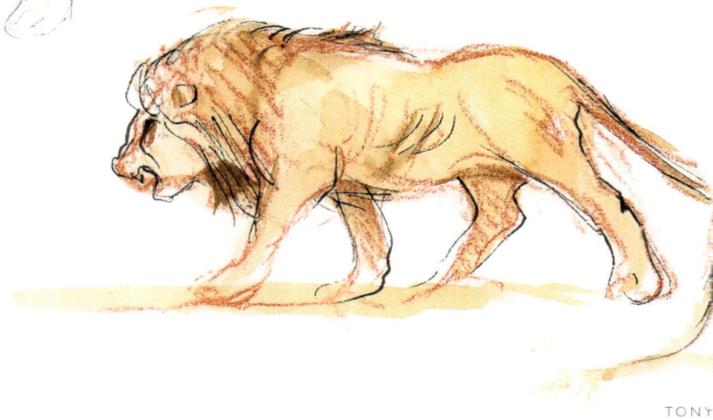

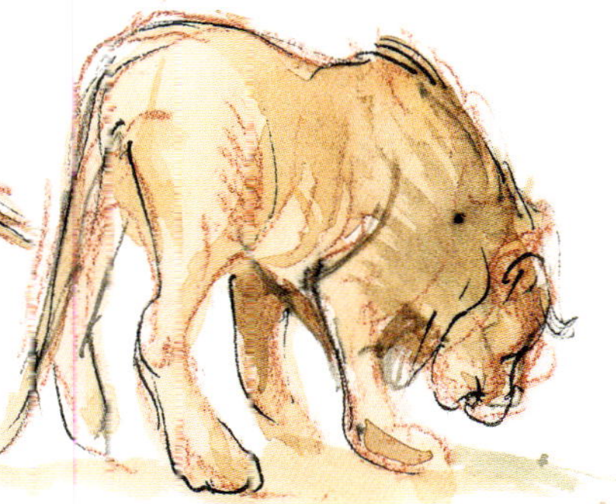

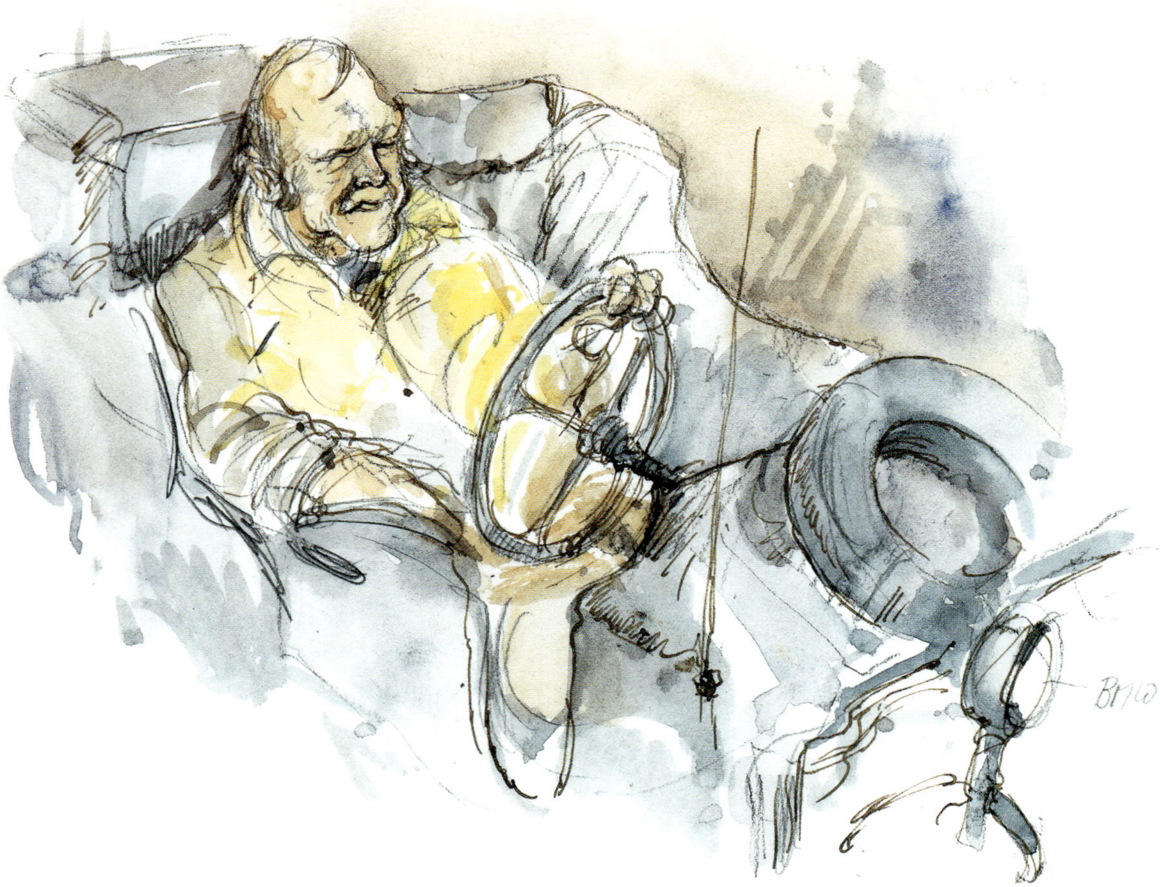

Dudley Fowldes

Perhaps the most unforgettable character I had the good fortune to meet was Dudley Fowldes, the quintessential rural Eastern Caper. Here was a man with a sense of roots and continuity that we find among so many farmers of this region whose families have been on the land for five and six generations. Dudley's forebear was a wheelright whose workshop was at Rautenbach's Drift, the crossing of the Bushman's River on the road to Grahamstown.

Dudley was a man of simple tastes, unconcerned with wealth and status and the small matters that fretted the mind of the average man. Weeds grew cheerfully from the gutters of his house, paint flaked from the walls and the lawn grew rank and untended. He was a man who exuded calmness of mind and goodwill. While we chatted on that warm windless day, a few cows wandered into the yard and joined us to hear what we were talking about – which was MacIver the remarkable vehicle, with large back wheels and an extended chassis, that Dudley had lovingly fashioned from an old Volkswagen Beetle. With all the weight on the back wheels and hardly any on the front, it was designed to mount any obstacle and grind its way through dongas and over rocks, anthills and tree trunks.

Least of Dudley's worries but of particular concern to Adrian Gardiner, owner of Shamwari Game Reserve, was the fact that his farm protruded like a sore thumb into the reserve. A contented man, Dudley refused to sell even though offered several million rands for the farm. Ever-pragmatic, he gazed into the distance when the offer was made, ruminated slowly and reflectively then gave his answer: "Man," he said in that slow and thoughtful way of speaking they have in the Eastern Cape, "a million rand is a hell of a lot of money... but I'm over 60 so I won't have time to spend it... so no thanks."

Alas, Dudley died a few years ago. He didn't have children. The farm was in a pristine state with much of it beautiful thick Eastern Cape bush and riverine forest, so it is perhaps appropriate that it was added to the greater Shamwari Reserve and its natural beauty preserved for posterity.

Alicedale

Alicedale, on the main line from Port Elizabeth to Johannesburg, was once a junction of the line to Grahamstown and generations of past pupils have fond memories of the high jinks they got up to at the station while they waited to change trains. When the train no longer stopped at the station, the little village became a neglected backwater, marooning a community of railway workers who were paid off and retired.

Now the village has been given a new lease of life with its redevelopment as a tourist venue in a combined government and private initiative. The old railway college is being converted into a hotel, the station itself into a craft centre and they are busy laying out a golf course. Local skills and labour are being used to build some traditional Xhosa huts.

As is usual with rediscovery of these neglected dorps, not everyone is excited by the revived interest, particularly those who moved there in the first place to seek peace and quiet. A charismatic church has established a renewal centre and loudspeakers fill the morning air with loud, rapturous gospel music. One of the local characters, a bearded, crusty individual, shuffles down the road to see what I am up to. He is a man of faith, he tells me. God cured him of his addiction to alcohol. His peace, however, has been shattered by the worshipful racket going on.

"Must they make such a noise to worship God?" he asks. "He's not deaf, you know."

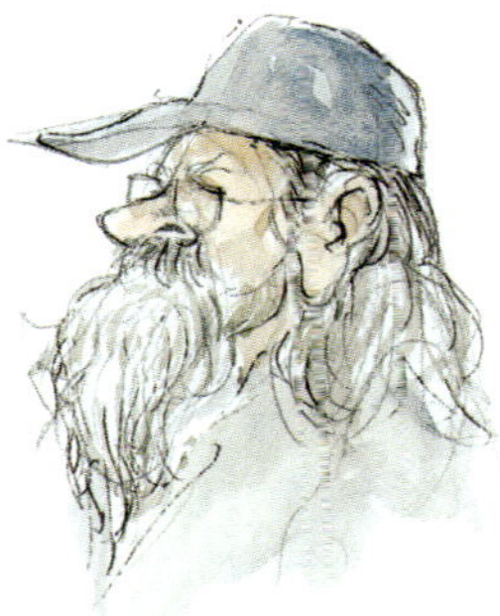

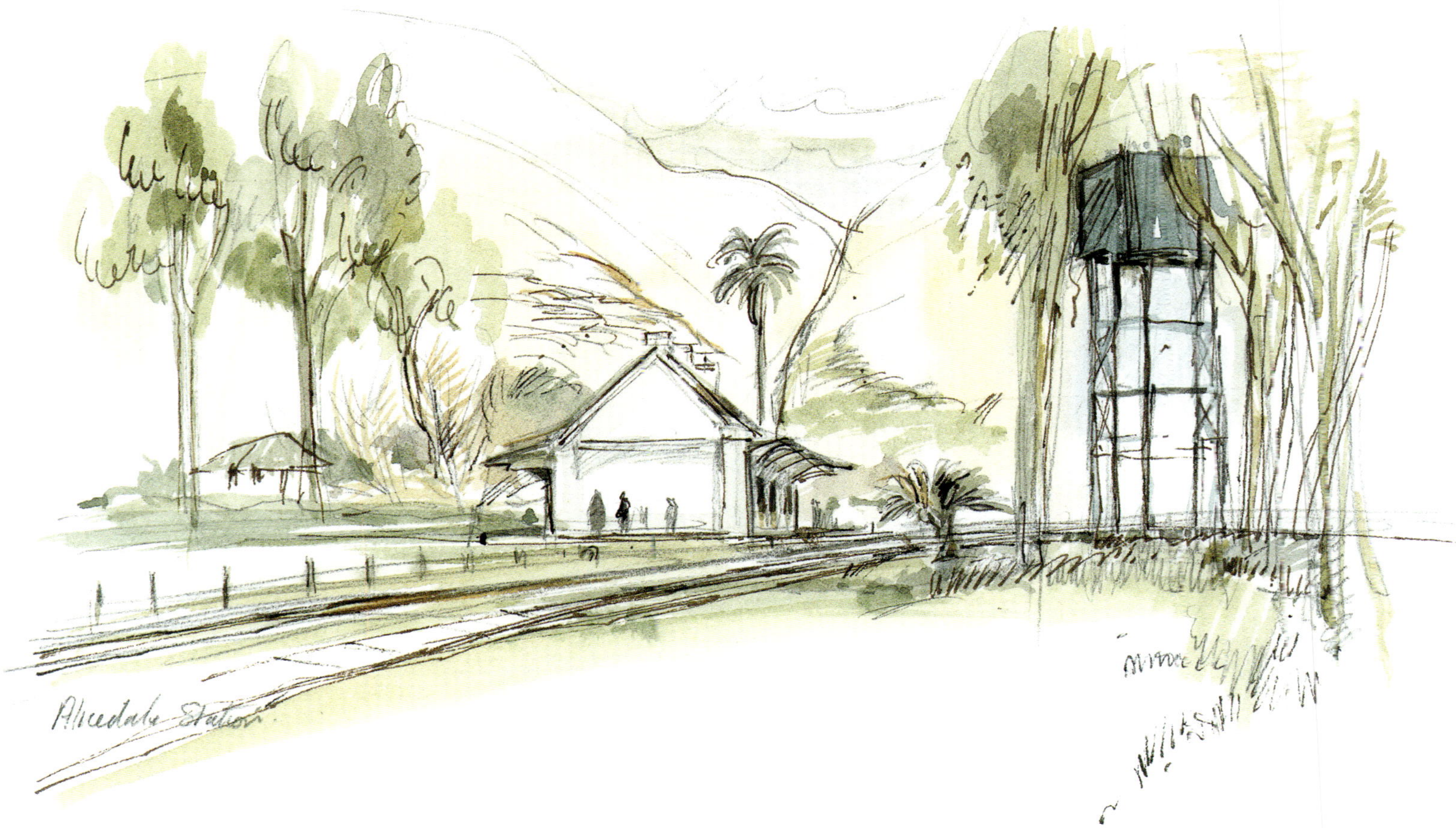

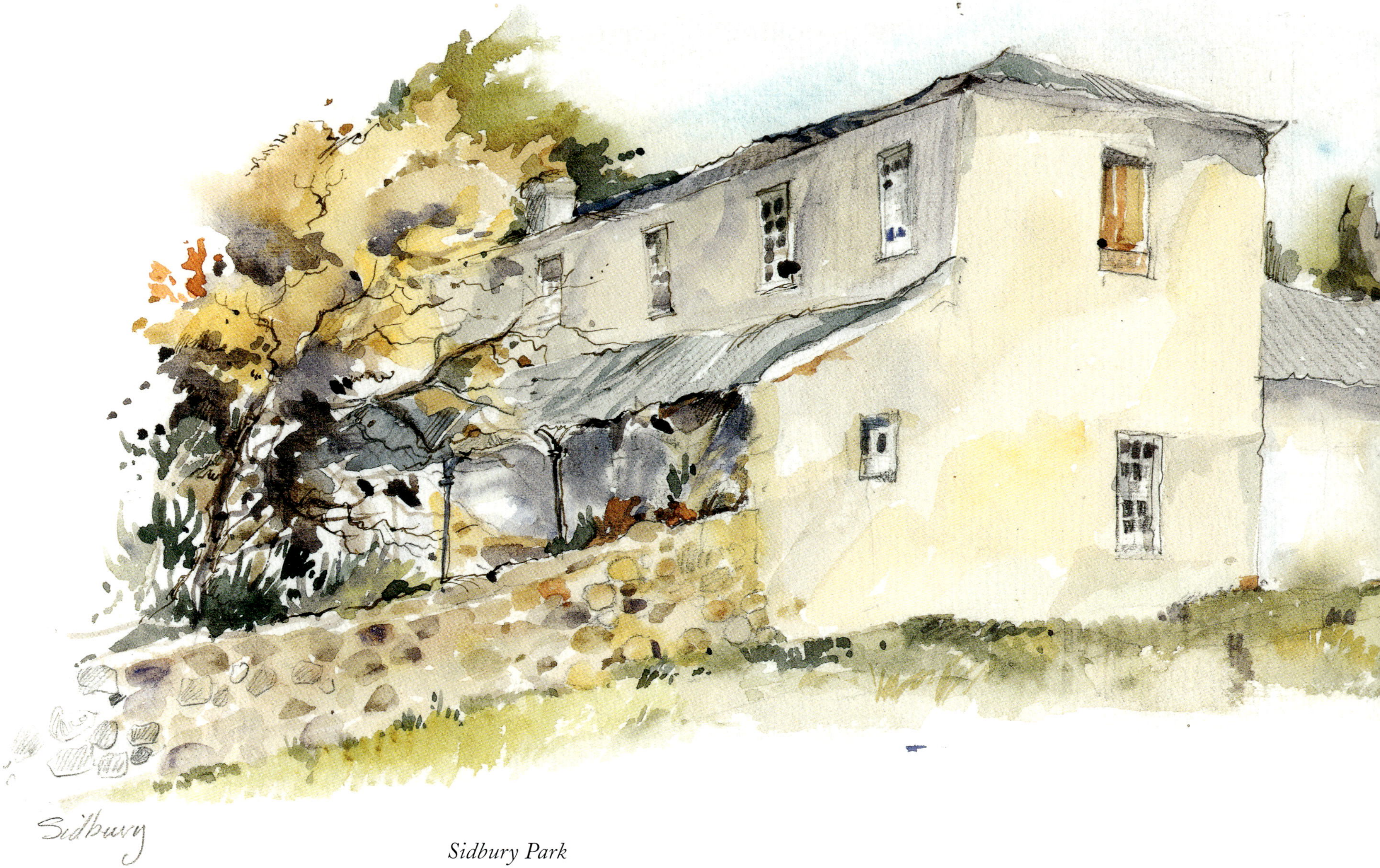

Sidbury Park

Lieutenant Daniell founded the small village of Sidbury on the old main route to Grahamstown from Port Elizabeth. He was one of the first breeders of merino sheep in the colony and obviously believed in investing in good stock – in 1829 he paid one hundred pounds for four rams and six ewes, a considerable sum in those days.

His descendent, Roy Berrington, received us in the old homestead, Sidbury Park. He was very proud of the manor house and spent years scouring the Eastern Cape to recover items of furniture and fittings that had left the house over the years. Some years before he had suffered a major robbery. He suspected that the burglars had been helped by one of his workers, who revealed that the valuables had been taken to a house in the township of New Brighton in Port Elizabeth.

"I blackened my face with shoe polish," Roy told us, "and, you know, I speak the language so well that in the dark a Xhosa wouldn't know that it was a white man

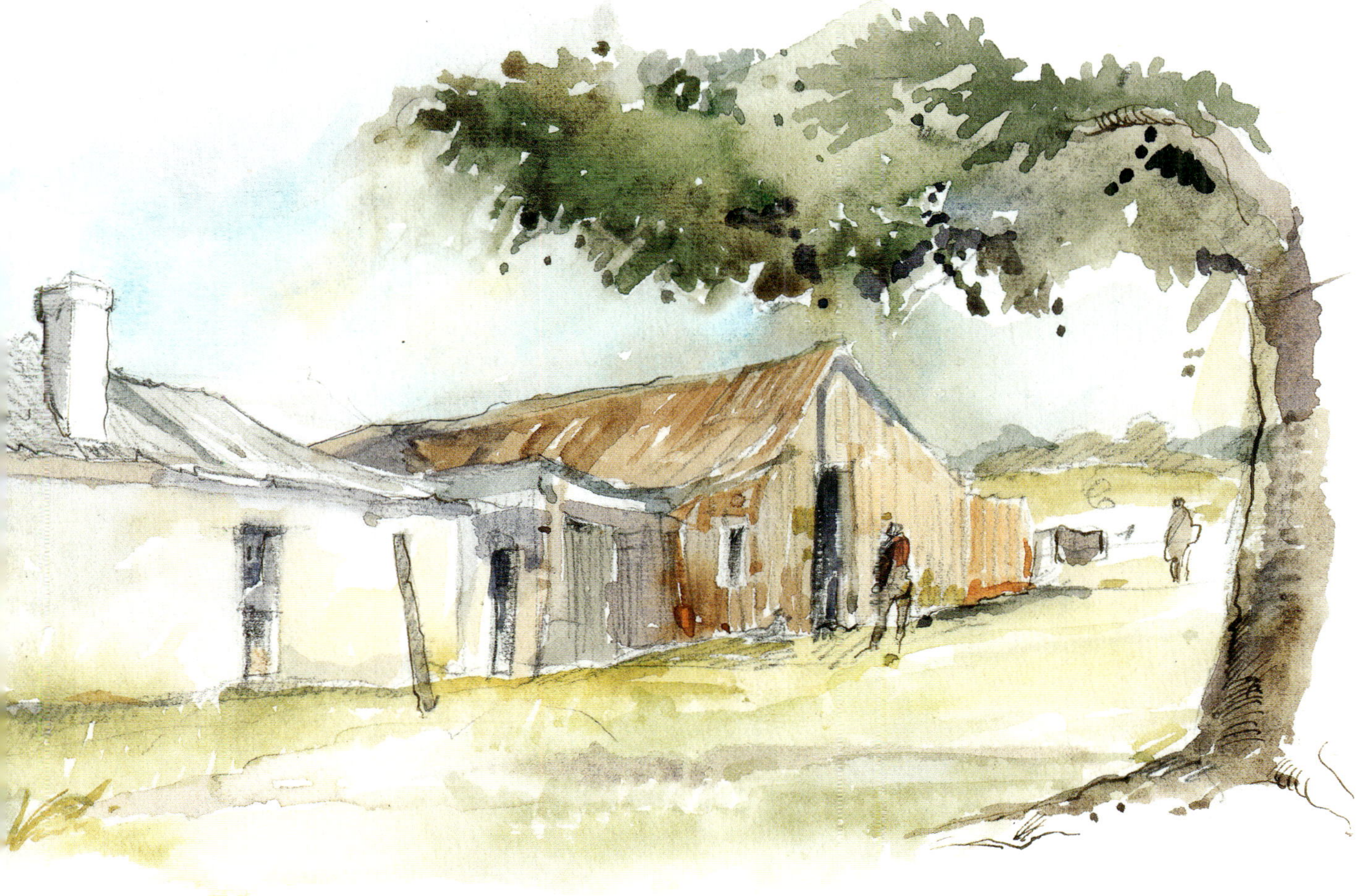

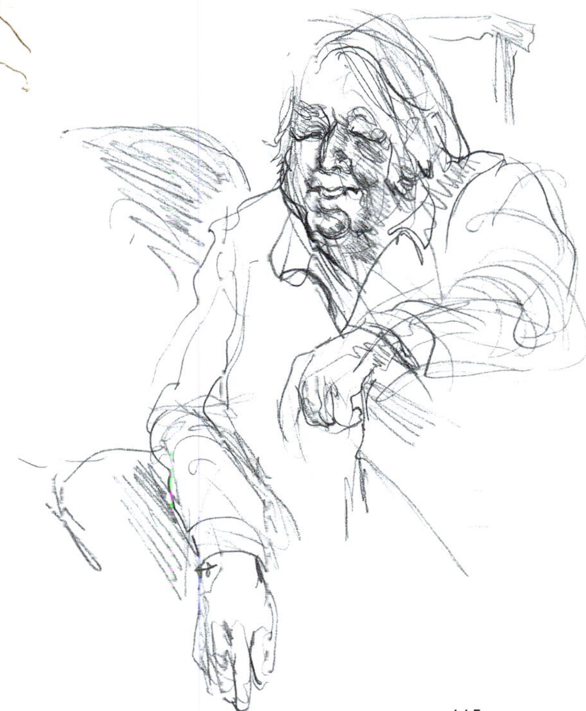

speaking. Then I got in my bakkie and went and fetched my things back."

They are an intrepid lot, these Eastern Cape farmers. The story reminded me of Dick Bladen, another farmer in the district, who, surprised one night by two robbers and forced into his car with orders to drive them to Fort Beaufort, simply turned off the road in the dark and drove them down the precipitous Woest Hill just outside Grahamstown. Dick recalls the car bouncing over boulders and crashing through trees and bushes to cries of "Hau!" and 'Tyini!" from his passengers until it came to a rest at the bottom, probably against one of those immovable sneezewood fence poles. Dick had still not lost his presence of mind, nor for that matter his sense of humour. "Sorry," he apologised in Xhosa, "I must have fallen asleep". After tying Dick to the wreckage of the car, the two dazed would-be hijackers staggered off into the night.

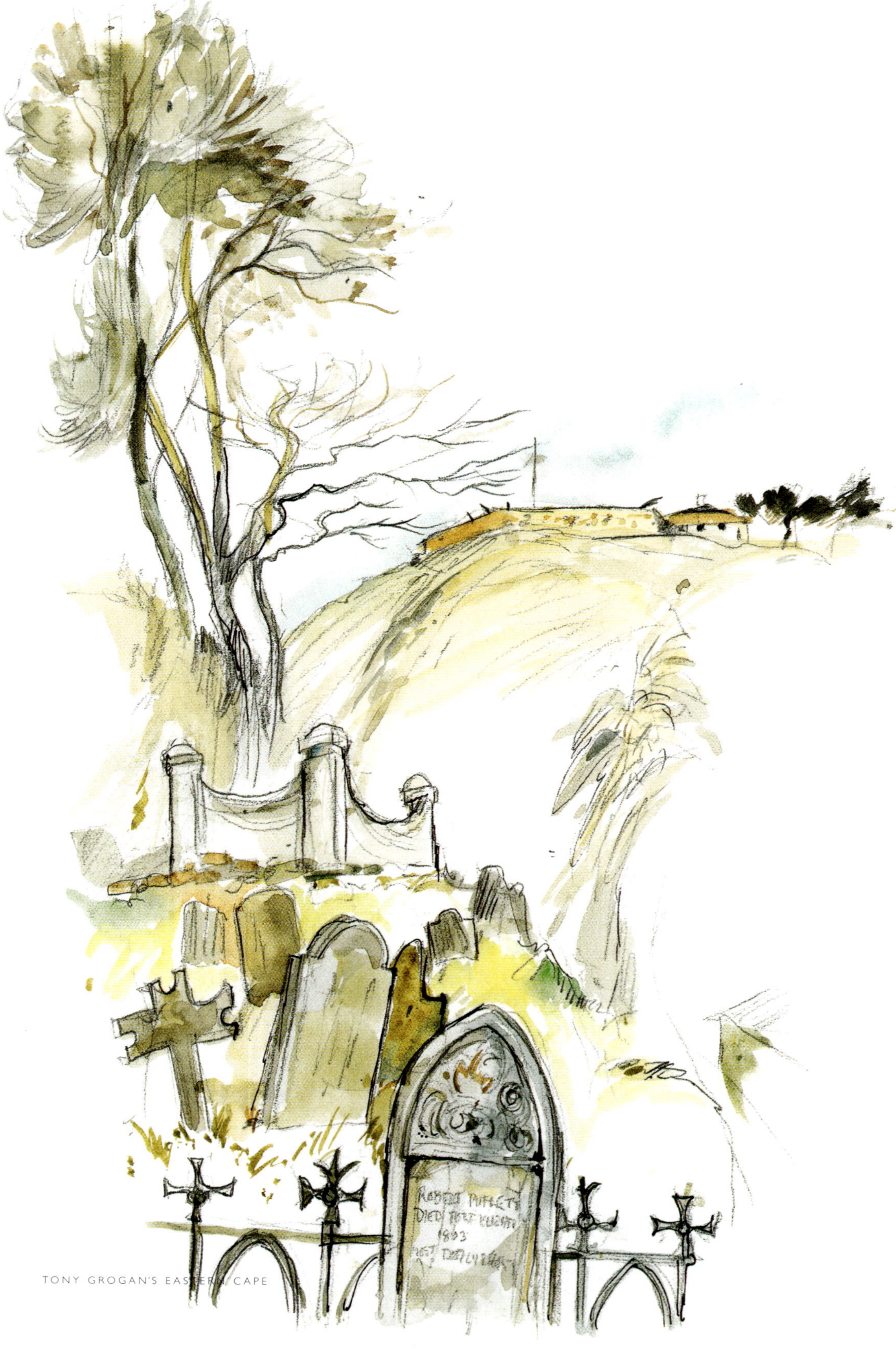

Port Elizabeth

Early paintings of Port Elizabeth show a huddle of small buildings on a barren hill rising above the shore. You can see Fort Frederick, the earliest structure, No. 7 Castle Hill, which is still there and the Donkin memorial, the stone pyramid that Governor Sir Rufain Donkin dedicated to the memory of his wife Lady Elizabeth Donkin after whom the city is named. One wonders what must have gone through the minds of the 1820 settlers when they were disembarked on the beach with their possessions on this bleak and desolate shore, having been enticed to emigrate by romantic visions of 'rolling parkland' as the travel brochures of the time described the new country. A sprawling city has grown on this shore with many reminders of its Victorian history in its architecture, parks and memorials.

I do a drawing of a view up the Baakens valley with the old Southend cemetery in the foreground and Fort Frederick built in 1799 on the crest of the hill. The cemetery is about all there is left of the old Southend where I spent many hours with my sketchbook before, like District Six, this vibrant, historic part of the city was obliterated on the orders of the master social planners in Pretoria at the time.

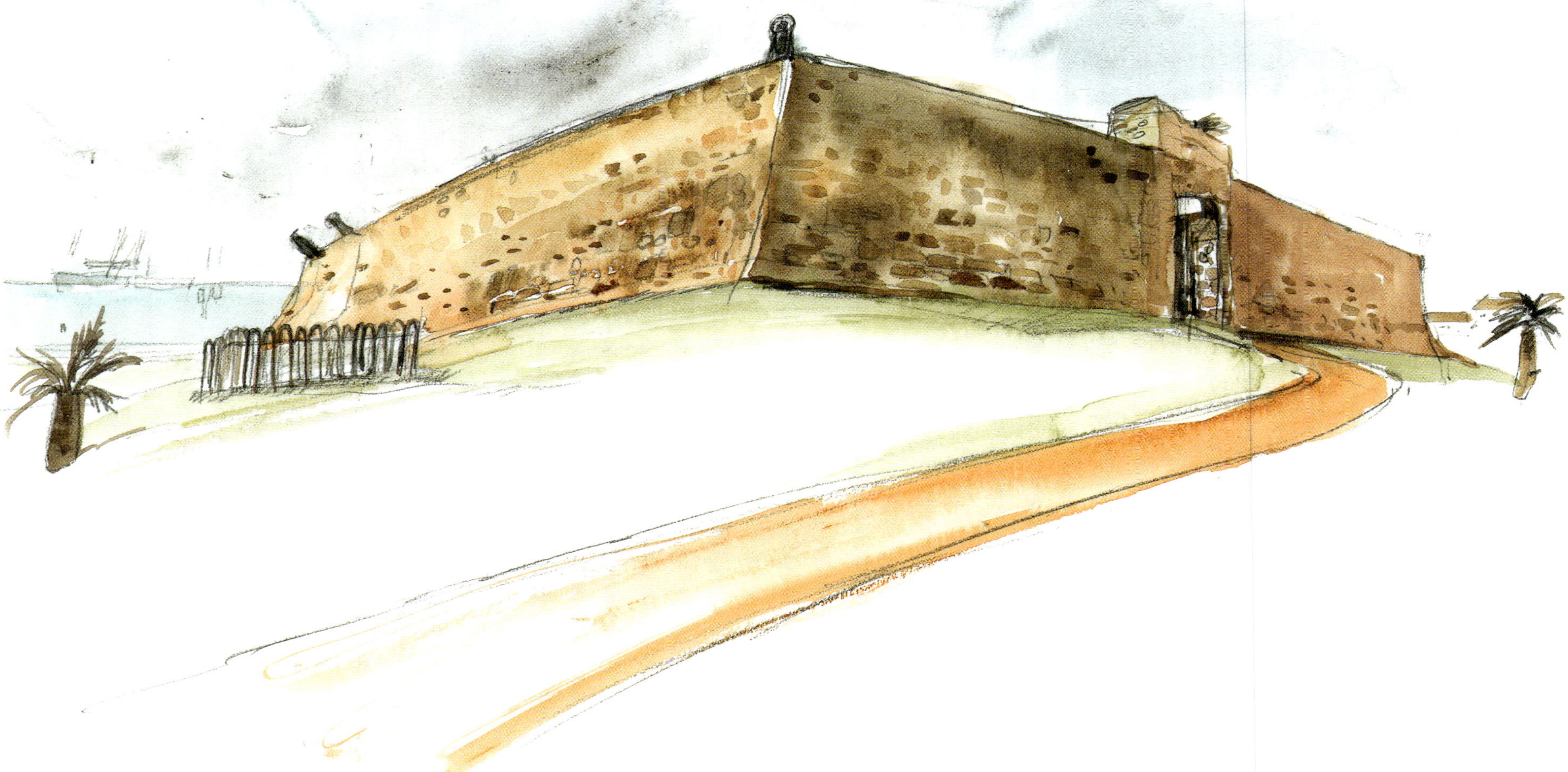

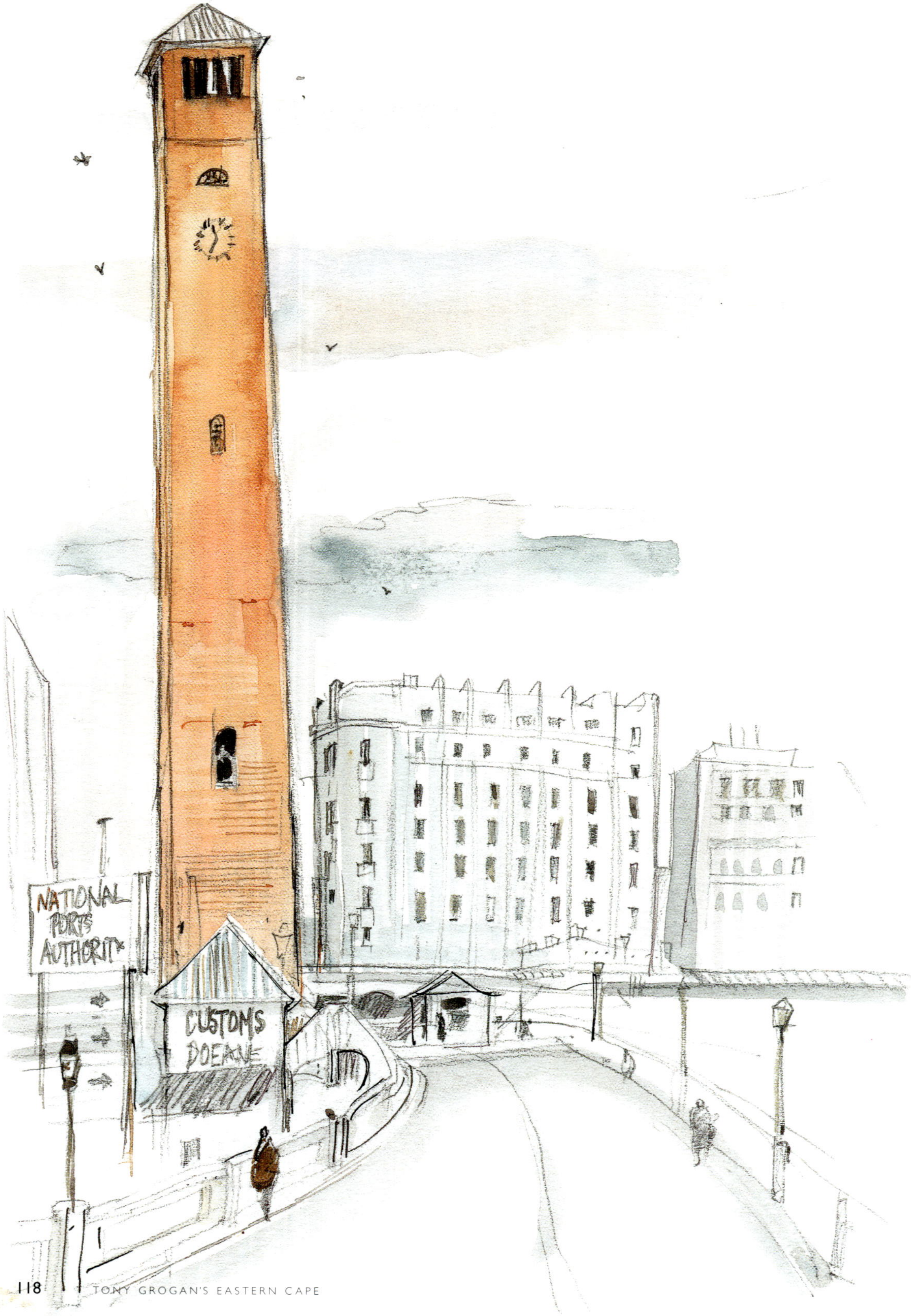

Port Elizabeth Towers

The central business district, as I remember it when I lived in Port Elizabeth, has changed. Many businesses have moved to the suburbs and Main Street, now Govan Mbeki Avenue, is a colourful mecca for informal trading and minibus taxis.

The Mayor's Garden in front of the City Hall is an interesting place to sit and watch the passing parade. The buildings in the vicinity are fascinating reminders of the city's Victorian past.

The City Library, with its elaborate façade and towers, is fronted by a statue of Queen Victoria in full regalia, holding a sceptre in her hand like a bowling ball. The terracotta façade of the building was manufactured in England and sent out in numbered pieces to be assembled here.

Towers are a feature of the surrounding buildings. There is the clock tower of the imposing City Hall and behind it the tower of the old Post Office, capped with an interesting conical spire. Another soaring edifice is the red-bricked Campanile built in 1923 to commemorate the landing of the1820 Settlers on a beach just south of this spot. The old familiar view of the Campanile down Jetty Street on the town side is now obscured by an overhead freeway, which cuts off the lower third of the tower, so I draw it from the harbour side.

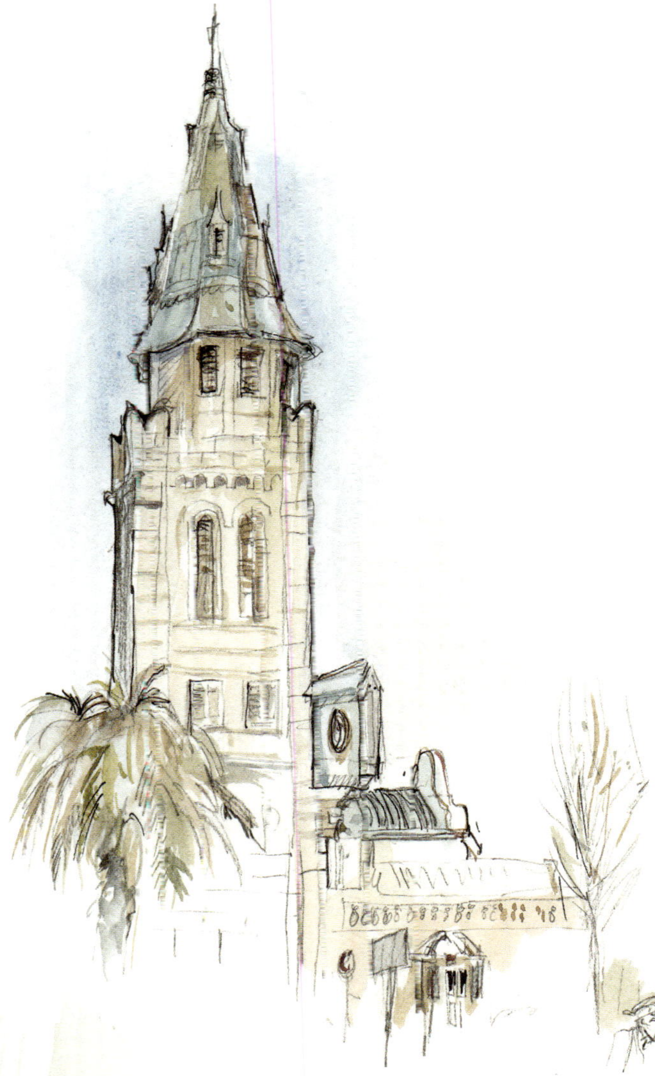

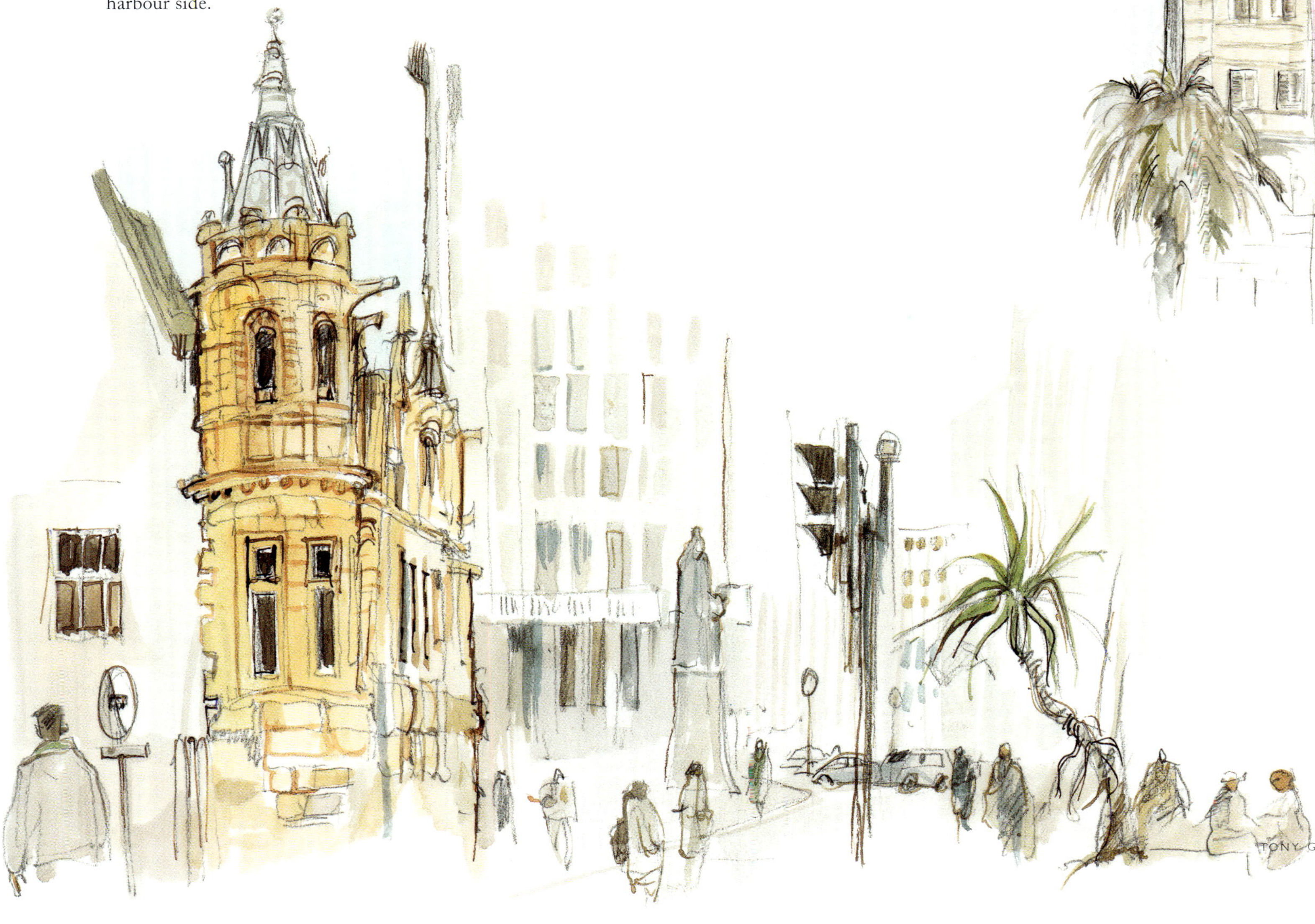

Ivor Markman, photographer and keen amateur historian with a passion for Port Elizabeth, conducts me on a tour through the central city. We toil up the steep hill past the Feather Market Hall where ostrich feathers were traded during the halcyon days of the ostrich feather boom.

Walking along pleasant, shaded streets in the older historic part of the city, we pass several fine church buildings. The Holy Rose Convent in Western Road is particularly beautiful, built of warm, honey-coloured sandstone. Ivor snaps away energetically, getting the right angles as I sketch.

We meander up to Rink Street to see the horse monument. PE is known as the 'friendly city', and this monument is testament to its kindly heart. It honours the animals that died in service during the South African War. It is the only monument I know of which commemorates the heroism and suffering of animals pressed into service to assist man in his insane passion to slaughter his fellows.

Then we wander along to St George's Park, past the cricket ground, and find in the shade of the trees the theme of compassion to animals continued in the daily feeding of the St George's Park feral cats. Sarah and David Edgecombe are pouring cat pellets into bowls for a

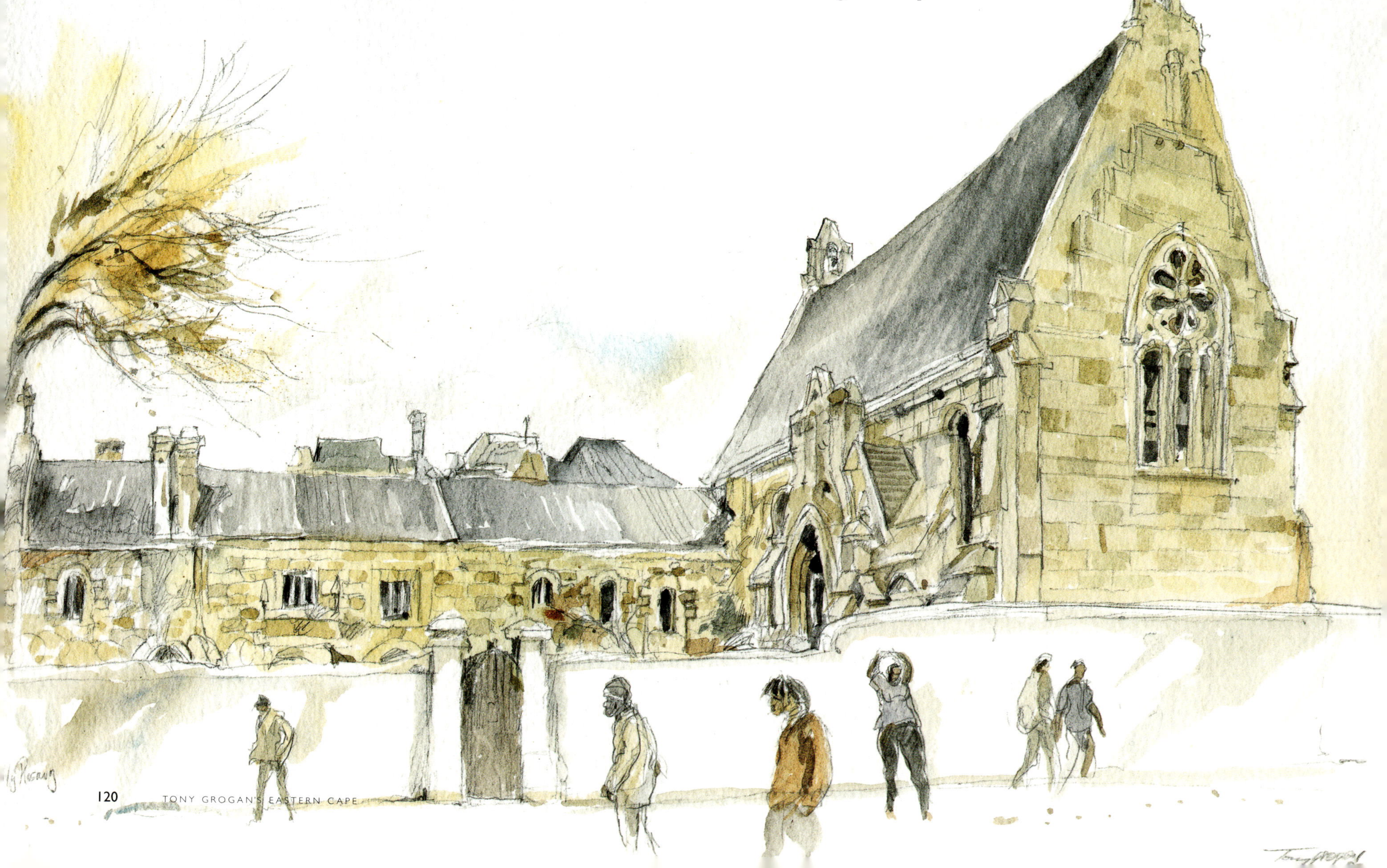

seething mass of cats that swirl eagerly around their ankles with their tails in the air. All have their names: Tom, Jerry, Ginger-Pop, Cauliflower, Debbie and Jet.

We spend a few reflective moments sitting in the now empty St George's swimming pool café, once managed by Athol Fugard's mother and the setting of one of the playwright's greatest plays, *Master Harold and the Boys.*

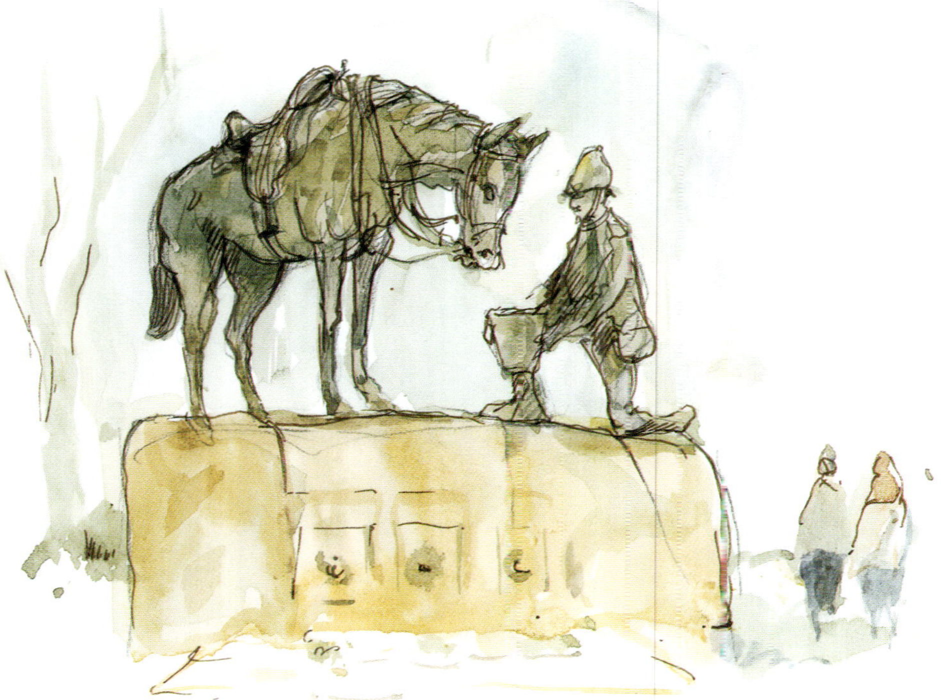

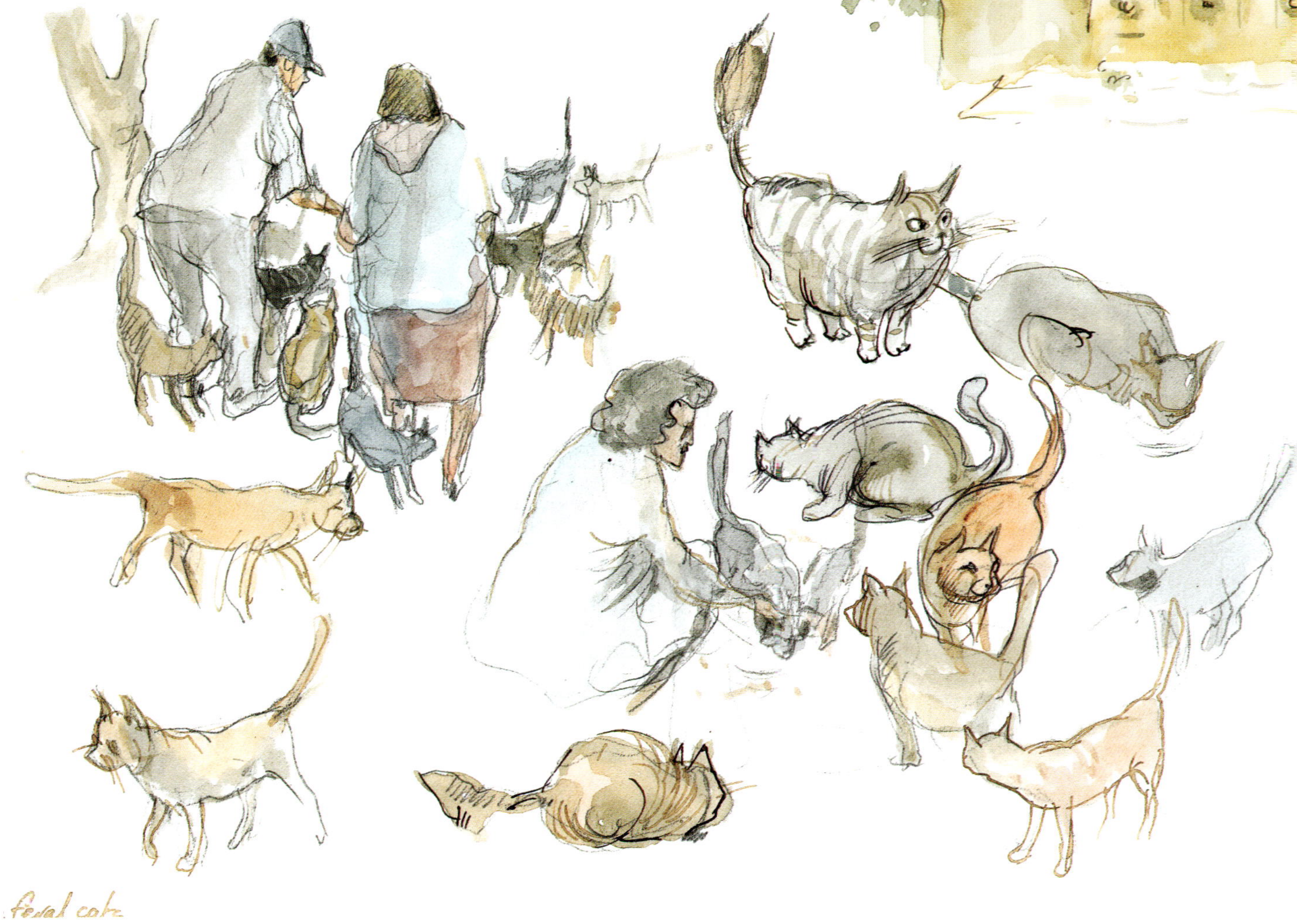

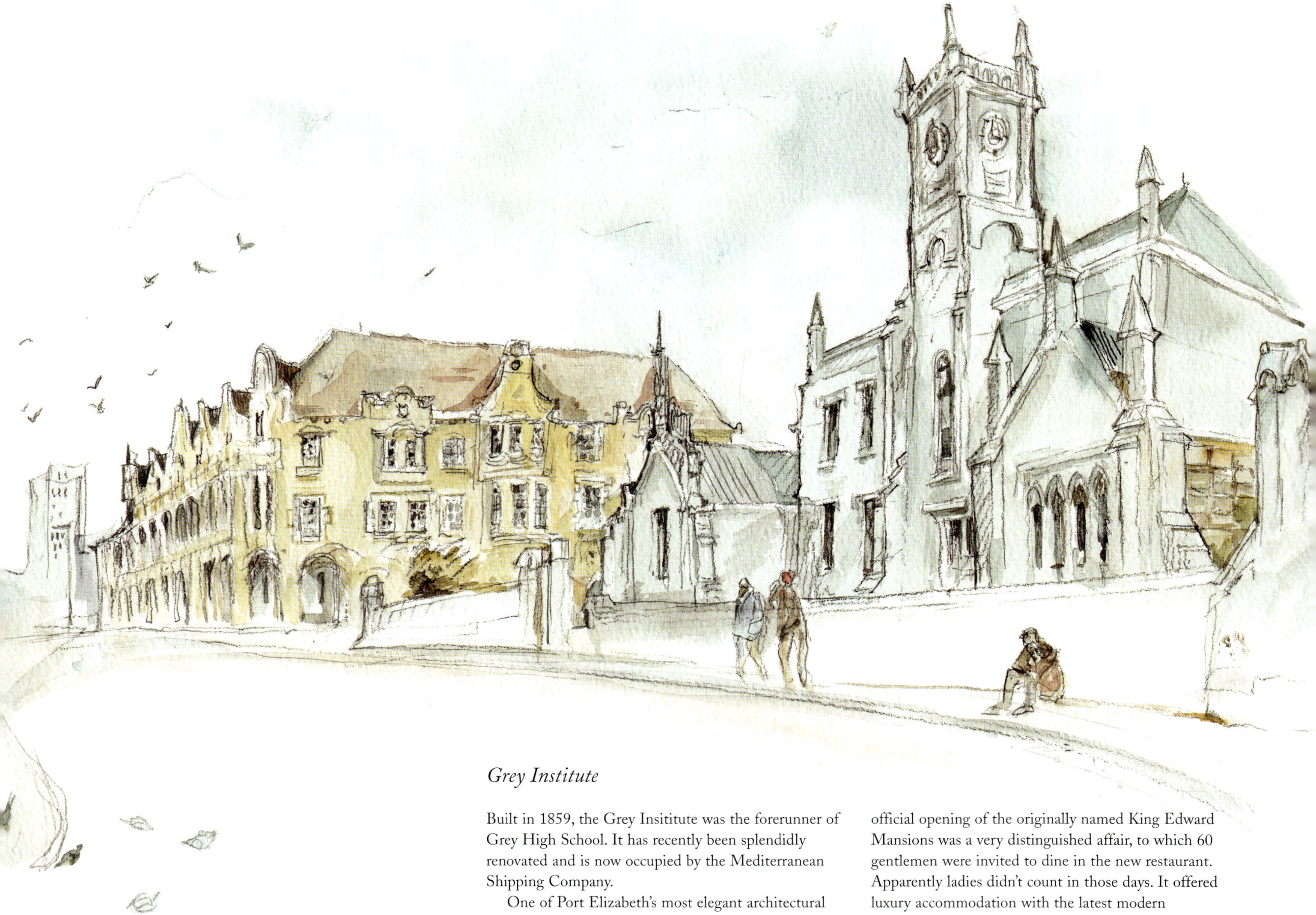

Grey Institute

Built in 1859, the Grey Insititute was the forerunner of Grey High School. It has recently been splendidly renovated and is now occupied by the Mediterranean Shipping Company.

One of Port Elizabeth's most elegant architectural relics from the past is the Edward Hotel, delightfully art nouveau in style and decoration both inside and out. Notes in the Donkin Heritage Trail tell us that the official opening of the originally named King Edward Mansions was a very distinguished affair, to which 60 gentlemen were invited to dine in the new restaurant. Apparently ladies didn't count in those days. It offered luxury accommodation with the latest modern conveniences, including incandescent gas lights and an electric bell in each room.

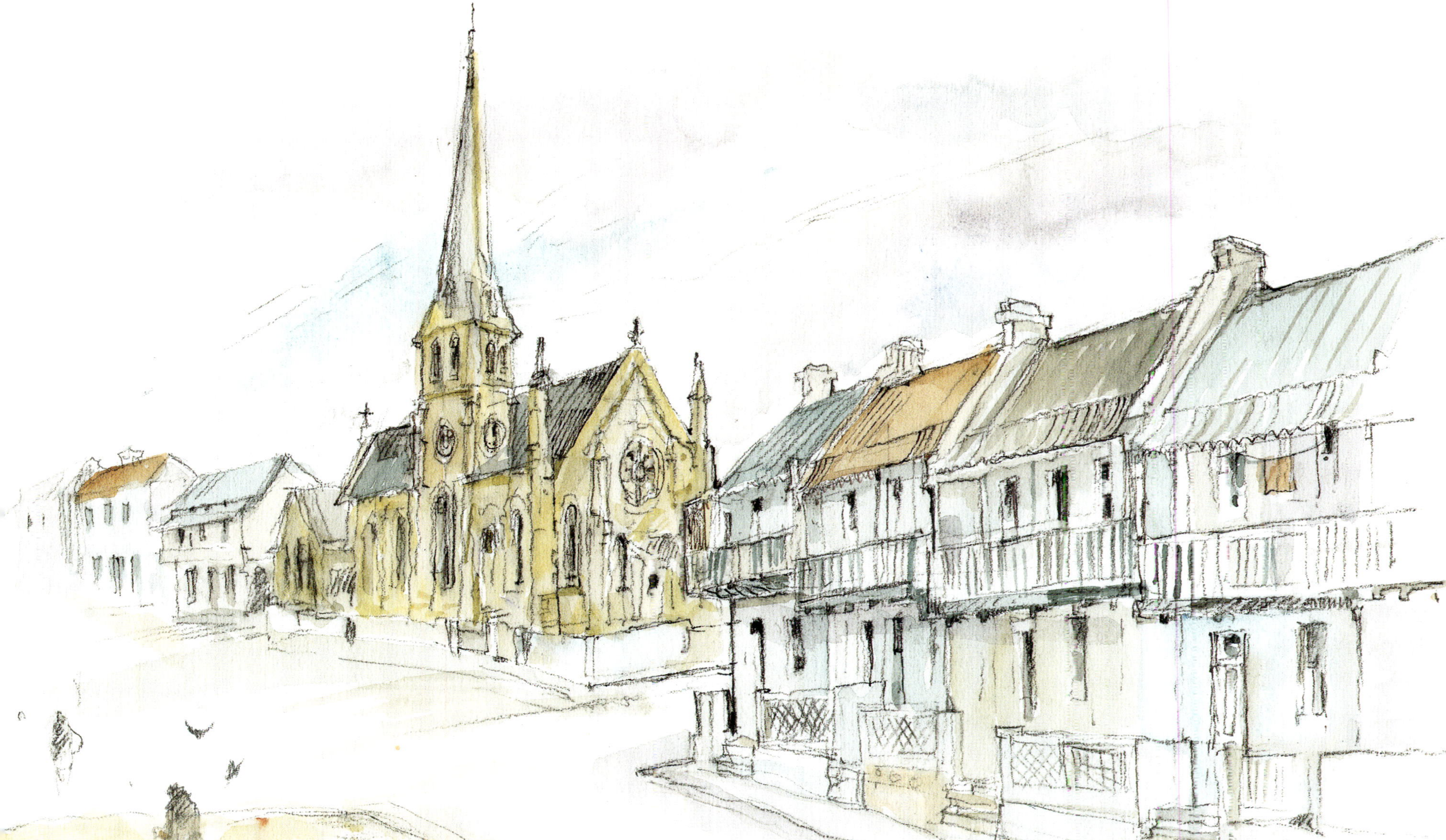

Donkin Reserve

The sweeping view of Algoa Bay across the Donkin Reserve has been preserved because of the height restriction on buildings below the reserve. It is a good place to sit on a park bench and absorb the atmosphere of the city – the sun shines brightly and people walking across the common lean into a strong east wind buffeting in from the sea. The lighthouse was built in 1861 and the stone pyramid is in memory of acting governor Sir Rufane Donkin's beloved wife Elizabeth, who died in India in 1818 without setting foot in the city which bears her name.

The building of the terraced houses in Donkin Street in the 1870s resulted in the covering of a stream, which was lamented by an early ecologist, one William Selwyn, in a poem, feelingly and ponderously titled, *The Lament of the Donkin Street streamlet, on being entombed by an unpoetical municipality*.

Port Elizabeth docks

A trawler undergoing repairs on a slipway in the Port Elizabeth harbour. I am interrupted in my drawing by one of those aimless people you find hanging around harbours. He offers me a flick knife which he tells me is made by an 'Oom' in Uitenhage. I buy it in a moment of madness, because I think my wife might find it useful in kitchen, but mainly because I feel sorry for him. Predictably Jen is not keen on it and also, predictably, it breaks after a short time.

Behind the Irvine & Johnston jetty is the gaunt framework of the iron ore conveyor which carries ore from the boats to the dumps near King's Beach. People living near the beachfront will not be disappointed to see the removal of the badly sited dumps, as they have complained for years of the east wind blowing clouds of ore dust off the mounds of ore and covering everything with a fine red film.

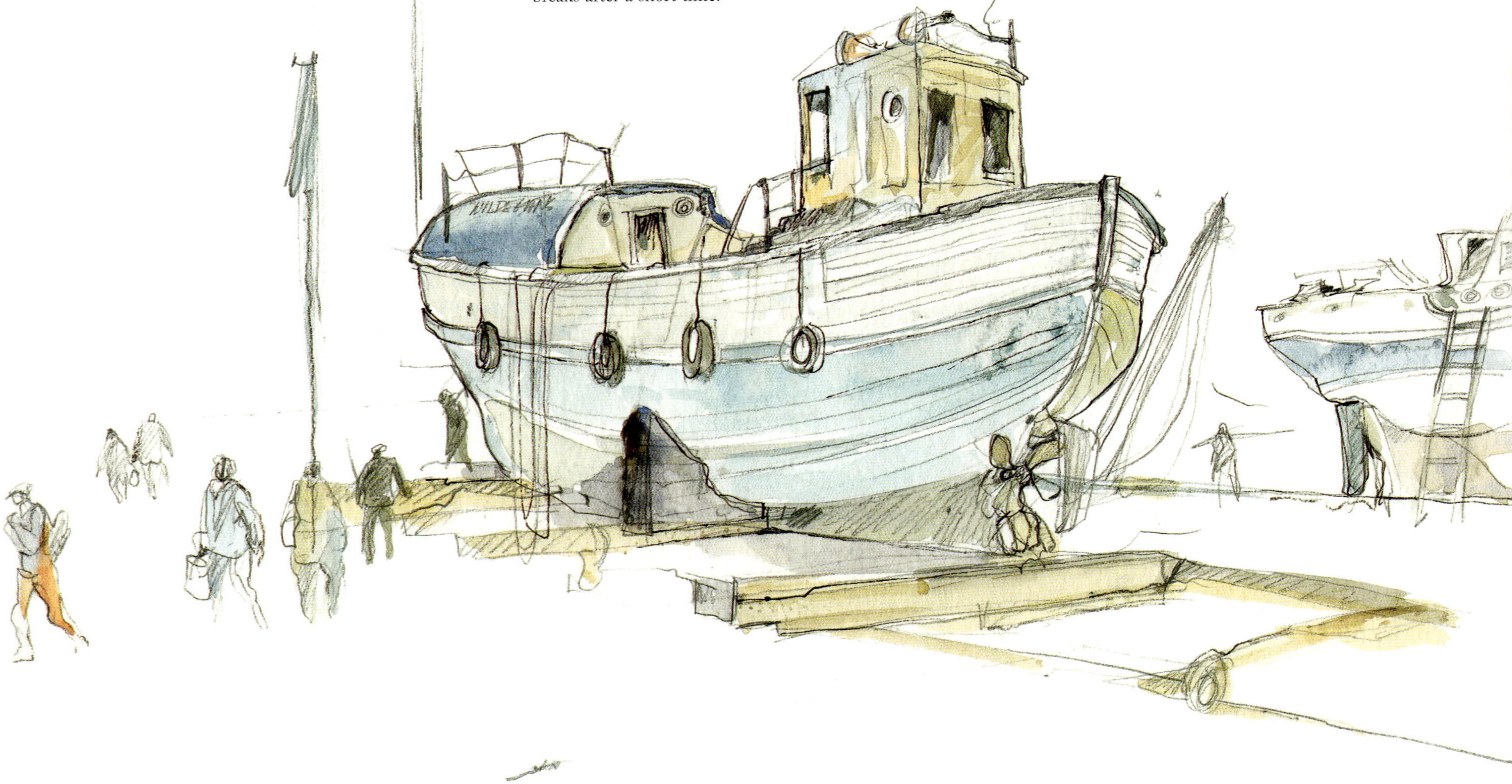

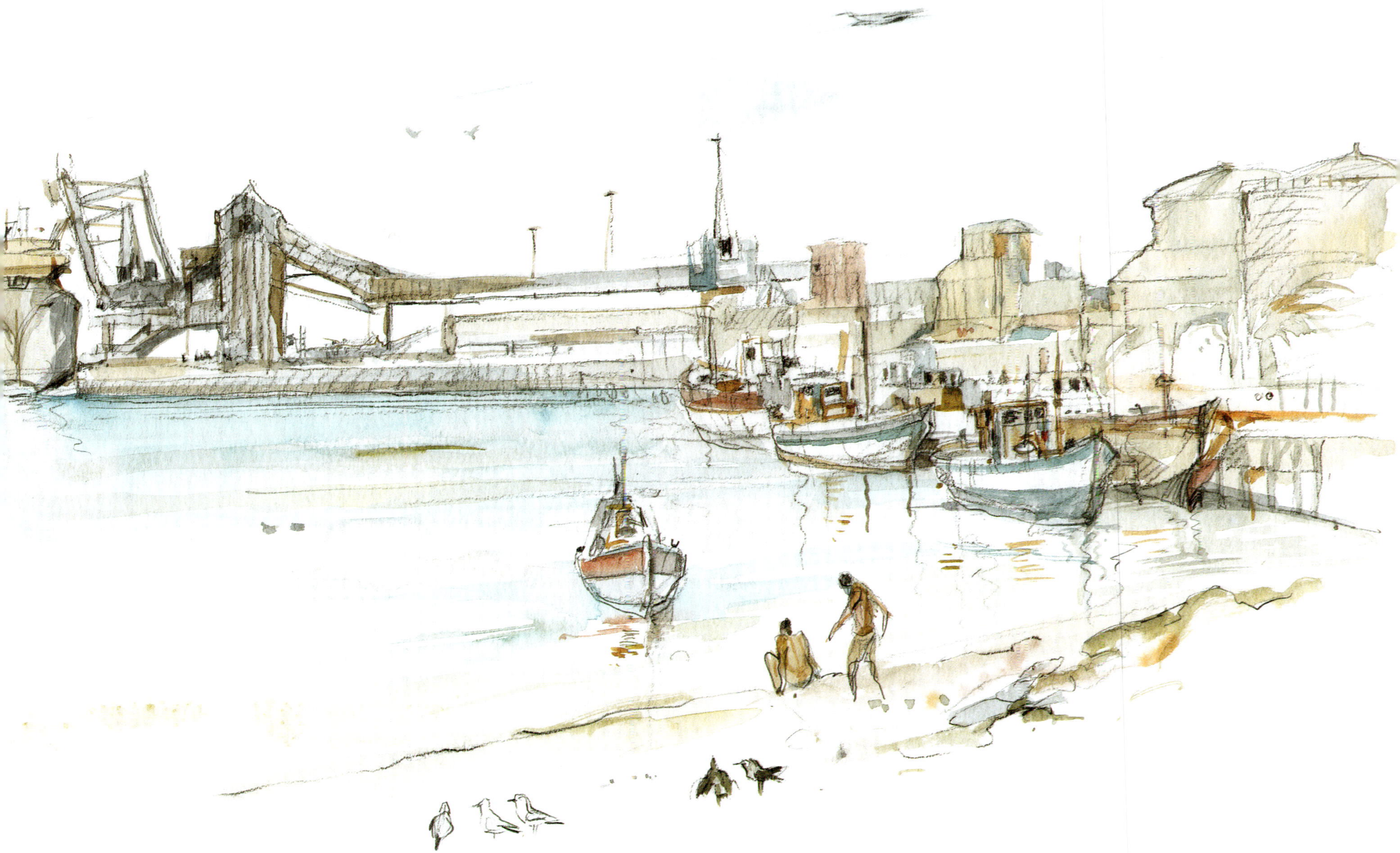

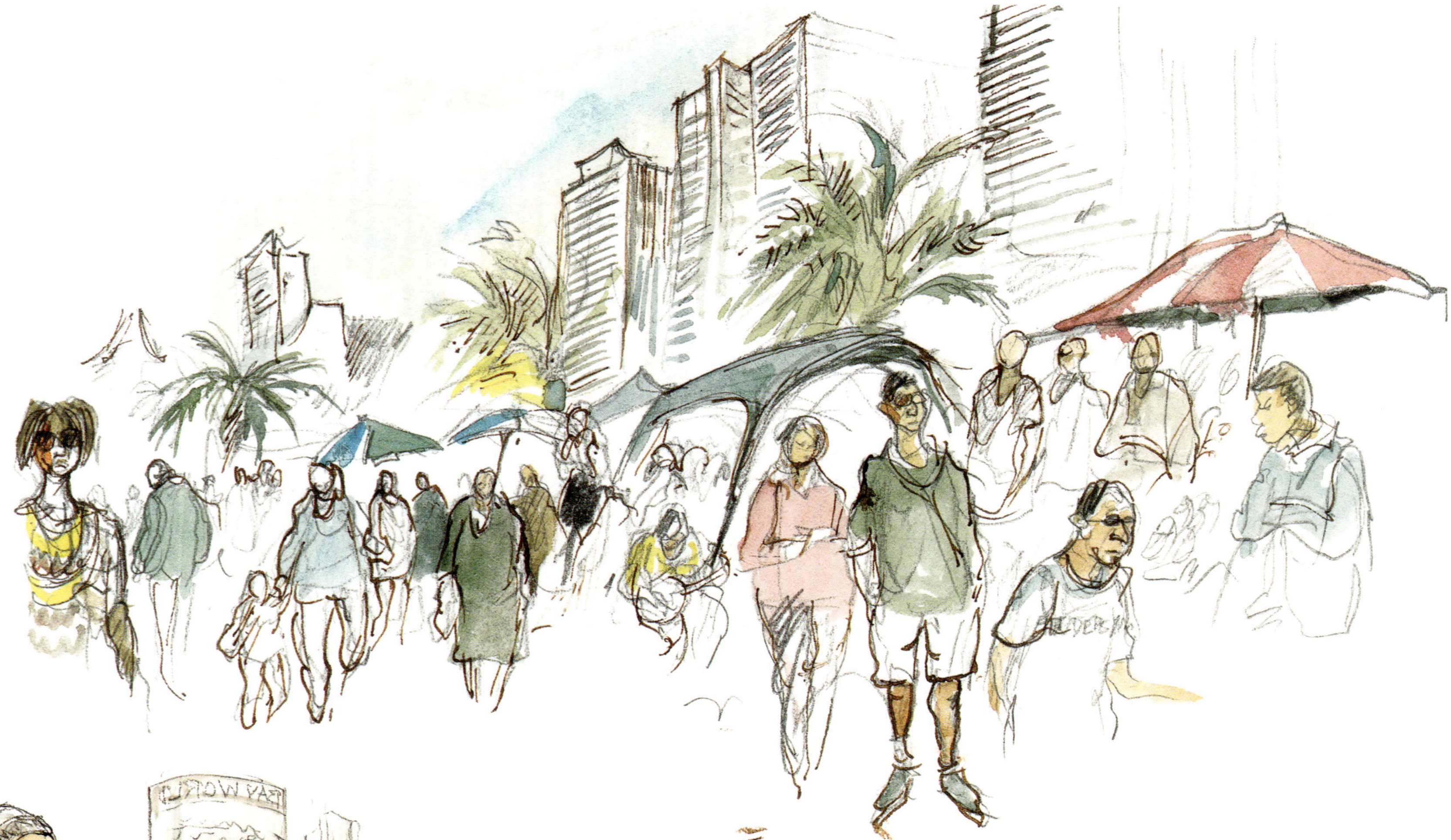

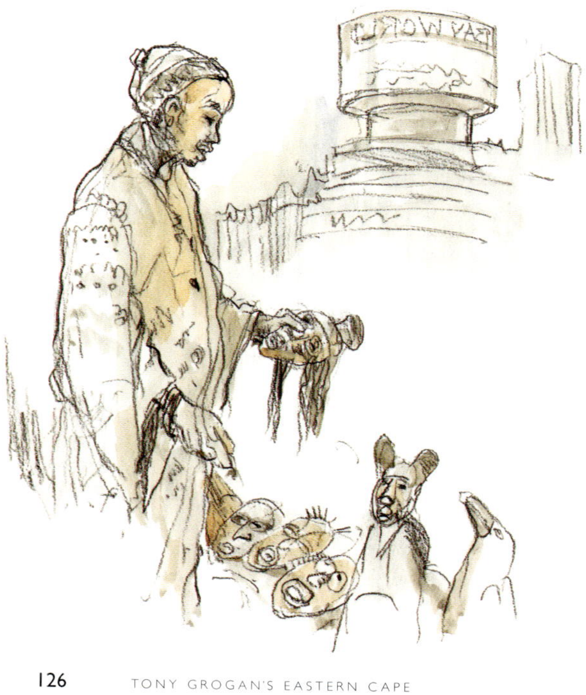

Port Elizabeth beachfront

The Port Elizabeth beachfront offers much in the way of recreation and entertainment – safe swimming in a calm, crystal sea; curio sellers and flea markets; the popular Oceanarium and Snake Park; the pier which juts far out to sea and is a wonderful place to promenade; and a swathe of lawn from the pier to Pollock Beach on which to jog, stroll and exercise.

The dolphins are a special feature of the Oceanarium and have entertained, charmed and fascinated spectators with their intelligent antics and aquatic acrobatics for many years. The guide's engaging instructions and encouragement to the dolphins is accompanied by information about the animals' habits and special qualities. The dolphins are rewarded for their antics but they seem to genuinely enjoy showing off, particularly when one of them in an energetic manoeuvre manages to splash a sheet of water out of the pool, drenching several spectators and eliciting wails of distress from a little boy sitting in the lower seats. Sadly, since I did these drawings, Dolly, the oldest dolphin, has died.

The curio seller from Senegal is a persuasive salesman, but unfortunately he is dealing with two impecunious locals who haven't the money or the inclination to purchase, even when the price drops dramatically to levels which they should have been in the first place.

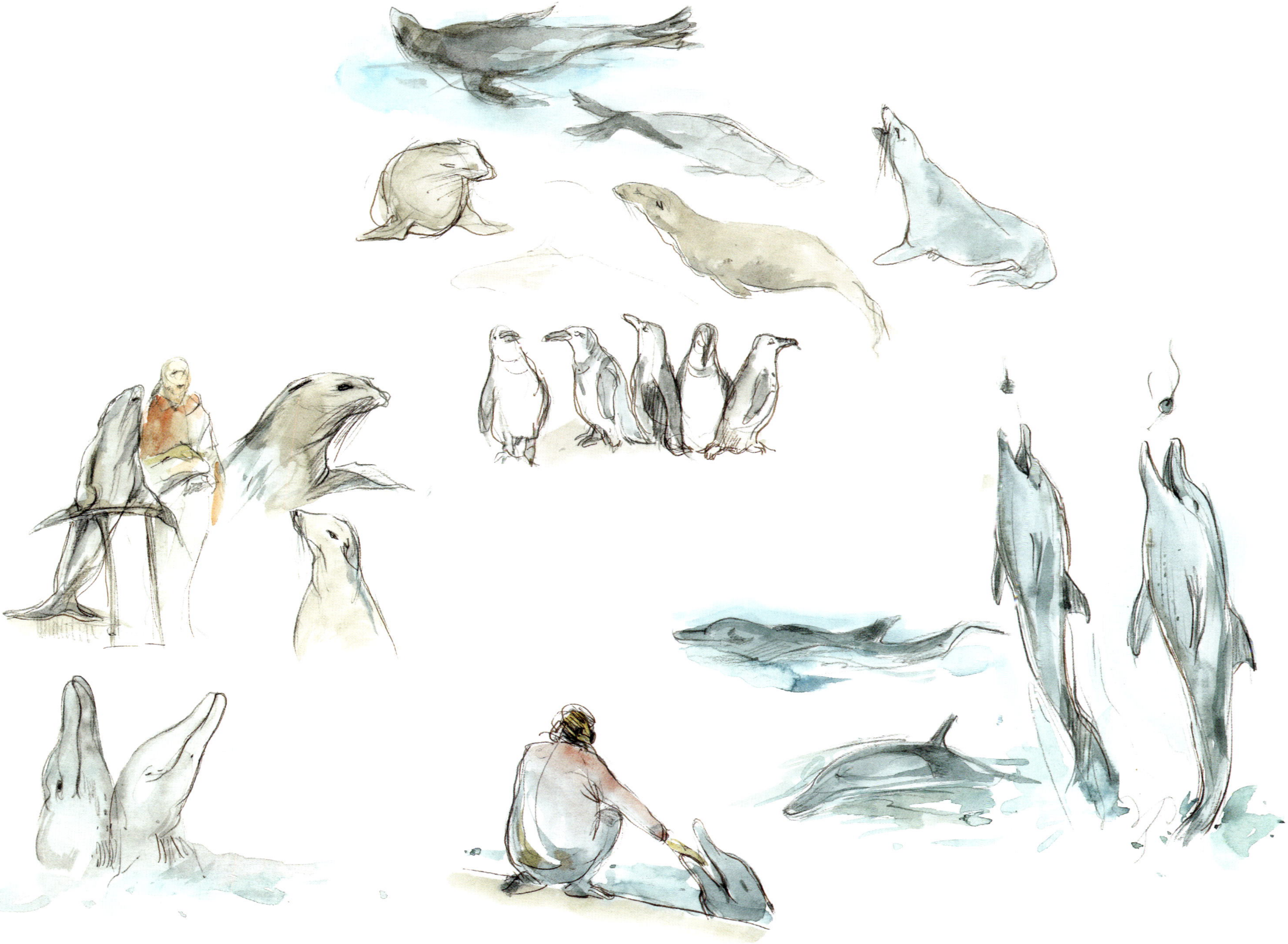

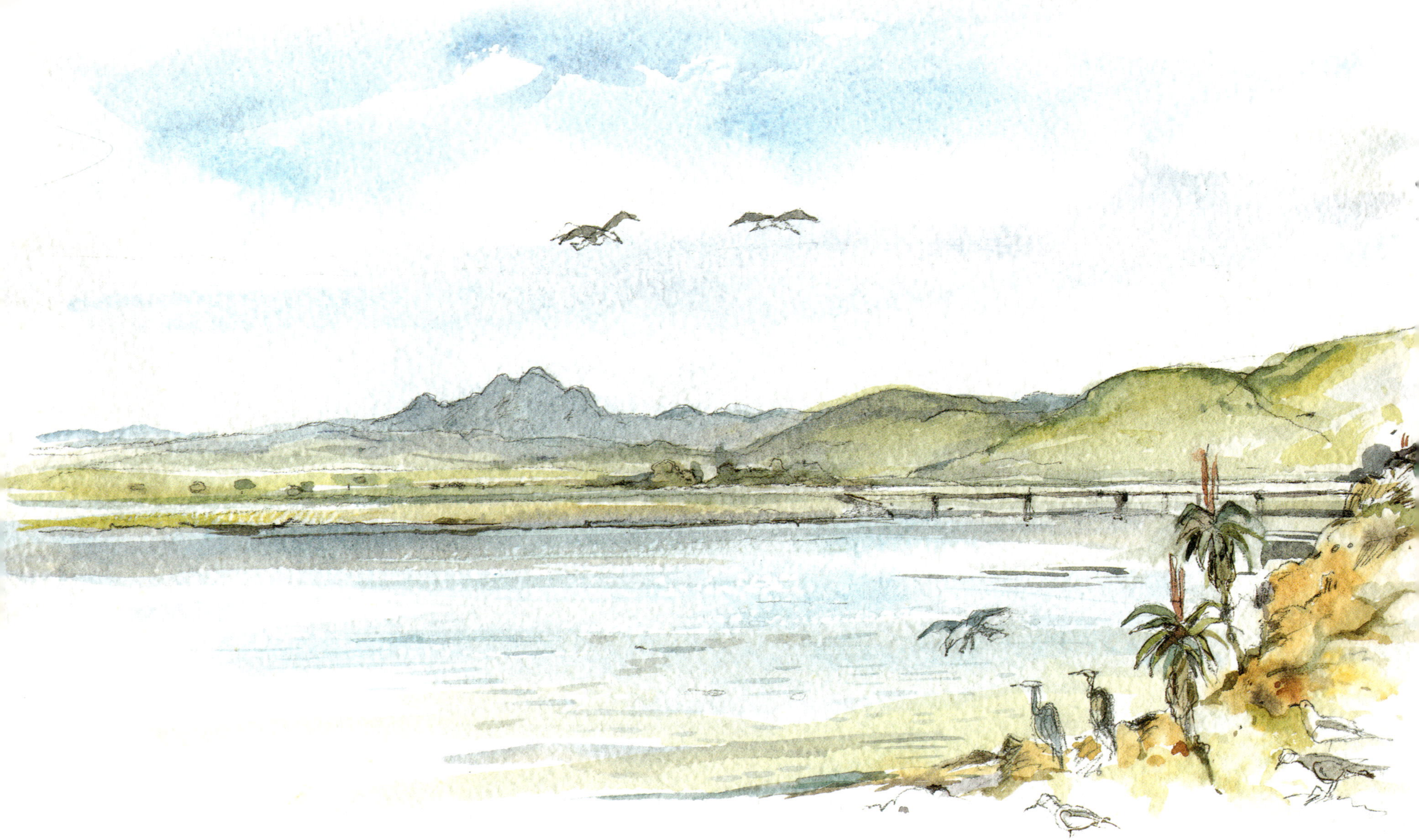

Gamtoos River

Travelling west on the N2, I always regard the last glimpse of the typical Eastern Cape as that of the aloes and thick, scrubby bush growing on the long hill that slopes down to the Gamtoos River. The Gamtoos follows a meandering course over an ancient flood plain on which farms have been developed to take advantage of the richly nutritious soils that have been deposited over eons. In recent years, extremes of weather familiar in these parts have seen the plain inundated several times in the wake of torrential rains.

The Khoikhoi lived here long before the colonists arrived. It was from here in 1810 that Sara (Saartjie) Baartman came, and from here that she was taken into humiliating captivity and exhibited around Britain as 'The Hottentot Venus'. And it was to this place that her remains were finally brought back from France in 2004 and reinterred in her last resting place at Hankey.

A tributary of the Gamtoos called the Groot River winds a tortuous course through deep kloofs towards the Cockscomb, the highest peak in the Groot Winterhoek mountains. I have fond boyhood memories of carefree and adventurous holidays spent on a lonely farm called Hadley situated in these mountains.

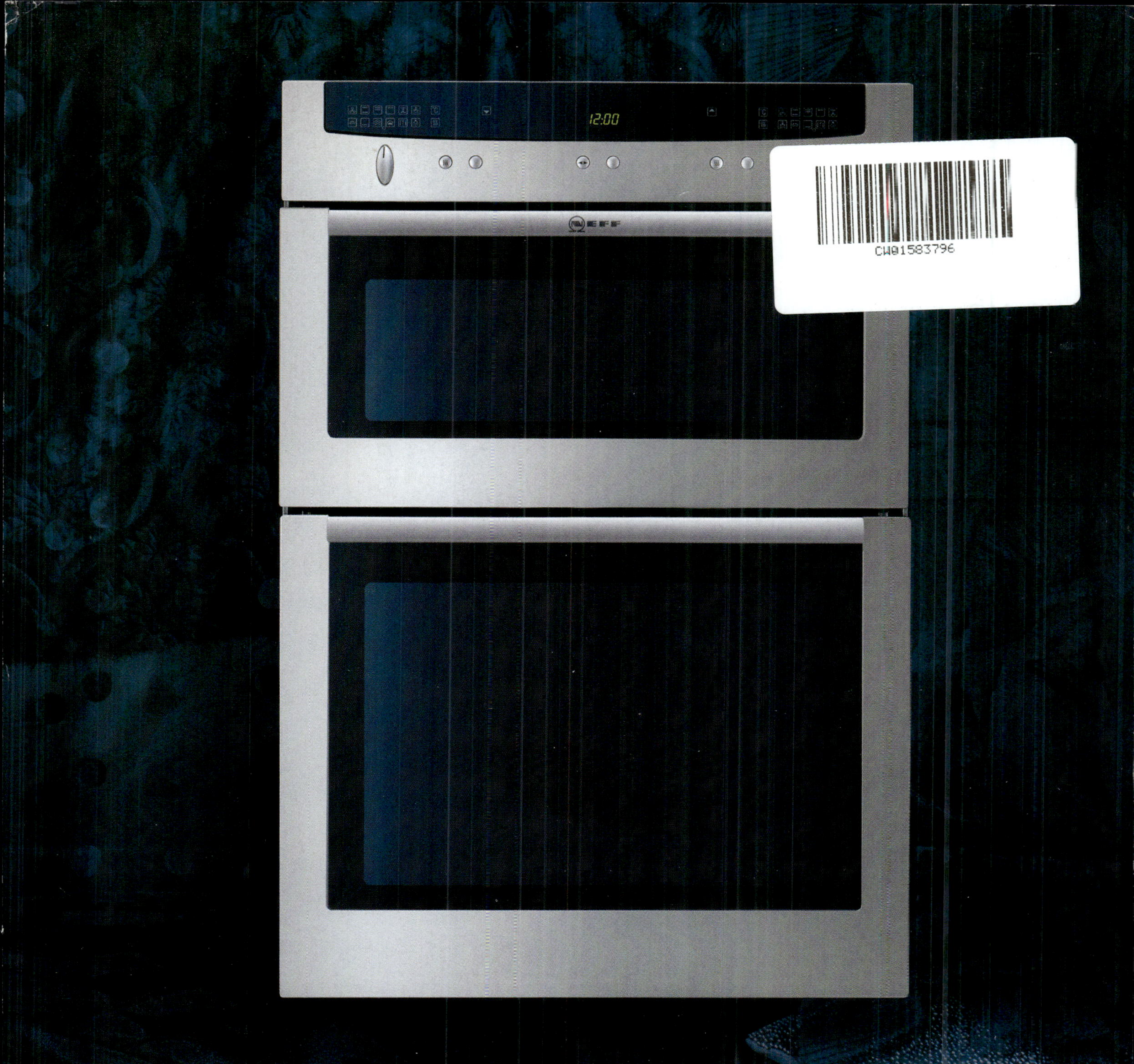

NEFF

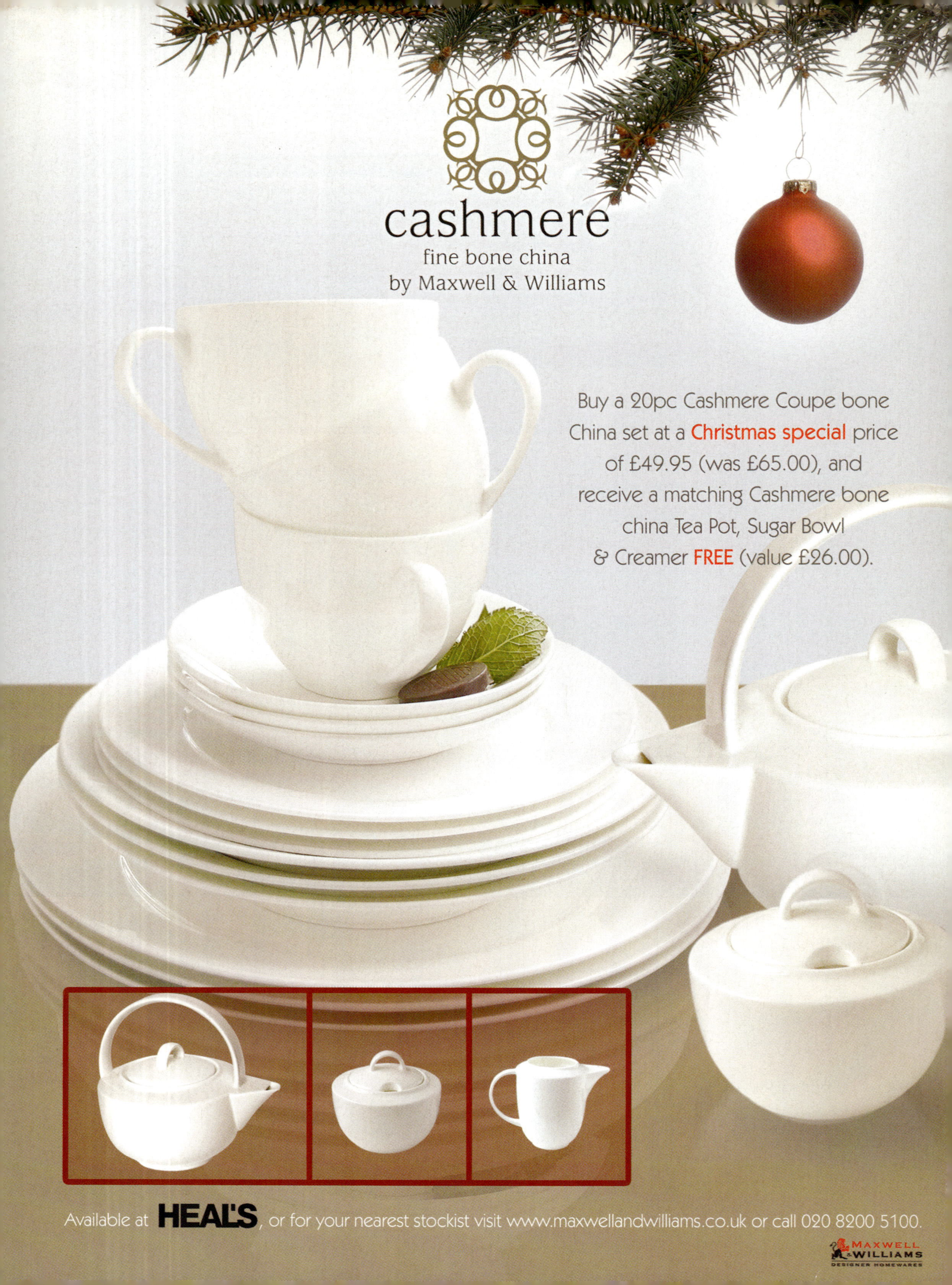

cashmere
fine bone china
by Maxwell & Williams
Buy a 20pc Cashmere Coupe bone China set at a Christmas special price of £49.95 (was £65.00), and receive a matching Cashmere bone china Tea Pot, Sugar Bowl & Creamer FREE (value £26.00).
Available at HEAL'S, or for your nearest stockist visit www.maxwellandwilliams.co.uk or call 020 8200 5100.
MAXWELL & WILLIAMS
DESIGNER HOMEWARES

Happy Christmas

The pressure to dish up the perfect Christmas lunch can be overwhelming, as I know only too well. For some reason best known to myself, the first Christmas after I got married I decided to invite both my family and my husband's to our house to celebrate the big day in style which meant a gathering of 12. This, despite the fact I had never cooked for more than eight people before. The pressure was on… I visualised myself mingling with my guests, topping up their champagne flutes and popping into the kitchen every now and then to prod the turkey and stir something. What a fabulous break it would be for the parents…

Things started to slip early on in the proceedings when I realised the turkey wouldn't fit in the oven and from then on the problems escalated by the minute, compounded by simple things I had overlooked, like the fact I didn't have enough pans or chairs and, more importantly, the corkscrew had gone walkabout. By mid-morning, I had thrown in the cloth and locked myself in the bathroom, praying for some sort of divine intervention and hoping this disaster of my own making would somehow go away.

If only I'd had this fabulous collection of Good Housekeeping Christmas recipes to help me... Somehow I think my first Christmas lunch would have been a different story. Needless to say, the parents stepped in and seamlessly took over, while I sheepishly hovered in the background before eventually being banned from the kitchen altogether.

Whether you are a novice or an experienced cook, this is the time of year when you want to serve great food everyone will love, while still managing to enjoy the celebrations yourself. From Christmas Eve supper to Boxing Day tea, we have come up with some stunning ideas to guide you through. This is the ultimate Christmas collection – look inside for 192 pages of inspirational recipes and terrific ideas to make sure you have your best and most stress-free Christmas ever. Each recipe has been tested at least three times to take the worry out of Christmas cooking – they really work and taste incredibly good, too. Now you can relax and enjoy the whole experience as we've covered everything you need to know to produce the perfect feast on the big day.

Happy cooking!

Sarah

Editor

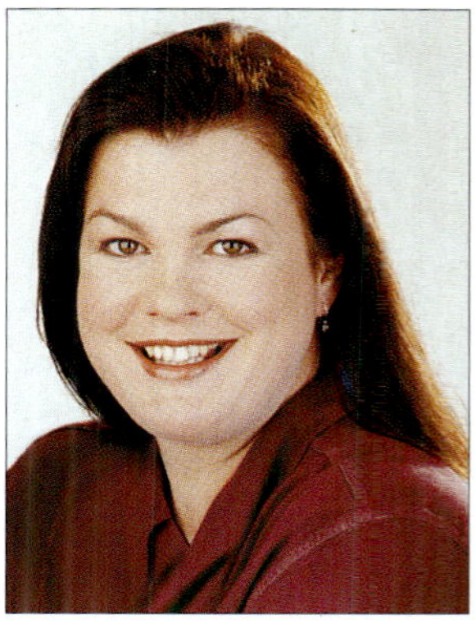

A special publication from **Good Housekeeping**

Executive Editors Karen Barnes, Ingrid Eames

Editor Sarah Wilson

Art Director Clare Shedden

Chief Sub-Editor Juliet Pospielovsky

Creative Director Denny Barnes

Consultant Cookery Editor Emma Marsden

Designers Della Rees, Penny Stock, Jane Tetzlaff

Sub-Editors Dawn Chapman, Julie-Anne Cosgrove, Diana Galligan, Wanda Hunter, Sally Jones, Alison Willmott

With special thanks to Kerry Fowler

Editor-in-Chief LINDSAY NICHOLSON

Production Manager Sandra Mysal

Associate Publisher Caroline Herbert

Advertisement Manager Rebecca Richardson

Business Development Manager Jill Maxwell

Senior Sales Executives Helen Maughan, Louise Wise

Executive Group Publishing Director LIZ KERSHAW

Photographs Marie-Louise Avery, Steve Baxter, Martin Brigdale, Jean Cazals, Graham Kirk, Sandra Lane, Jonathan Lovekin, James Murphy, David Munns, Lis Parsons, Michael Paul, Bill Reavell, Roger Stowell, Clive Streeter, Martin Thompson, Philip Webb, Tim Winter, Elizabeth Zeschin

BEFORE YOU BEGIN: notes for the cook

- Both metric and imperial measures are given for the recipes. Follow either set of measures, not a mixture of both, as they are not interchangeable.
- Please note that some recipes contain raw egg. The young, elderly, pregnant women and anyone with an immune-deficiency disease should avoid these, because of the slight risk of salmonella.
- If you are vegetarian and are looking for a vegetarian cheese, visit www.vegsoc.org for more information.

The National Magazine Company Limited.
Member of the Audit Bureau of Circulations.

Repro by Argent Colour. Printed and bound by New Jarrold Printing Ltd, Norwich.

Contents

Best-ever Starters 12-26

Starters

Christmas Lunch 28-63

Roast Turkey

Seasonal Roasts

Sauces

Stuffings

Side Dishes

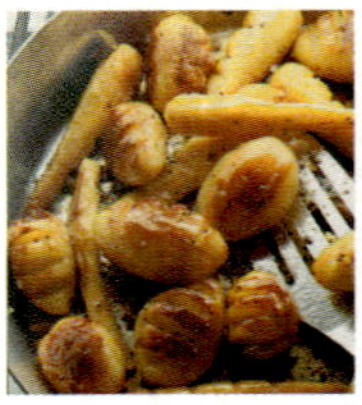

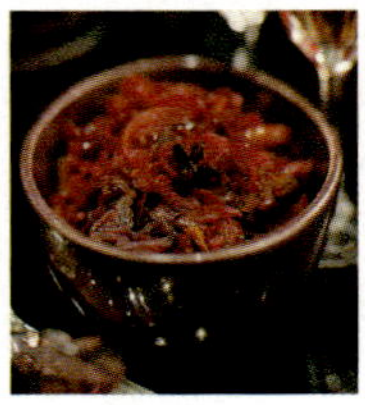

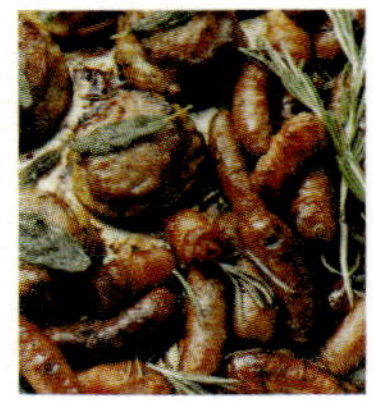

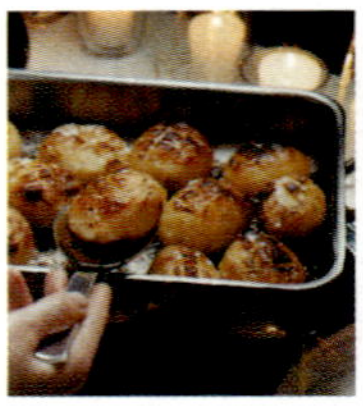

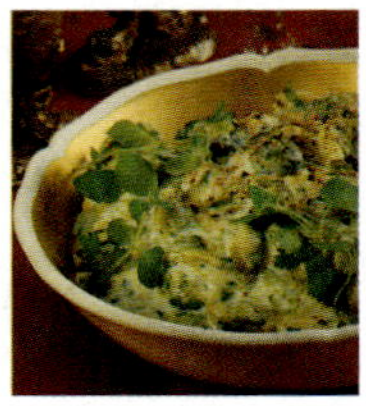

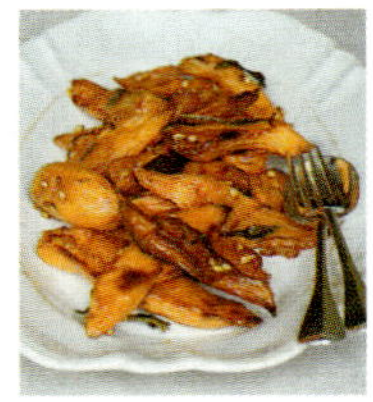

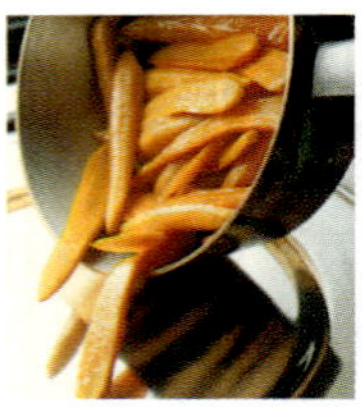

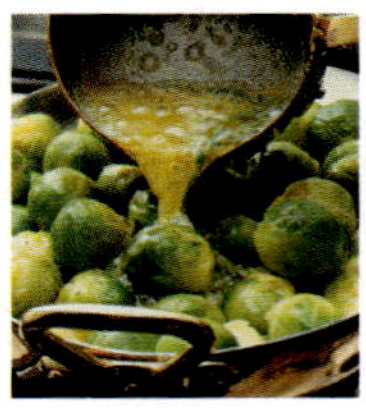

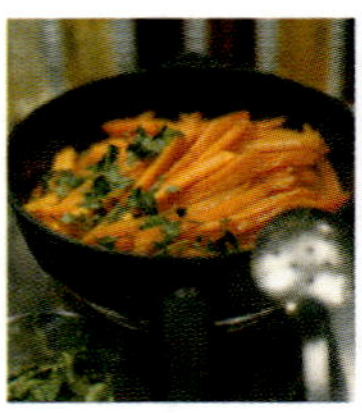

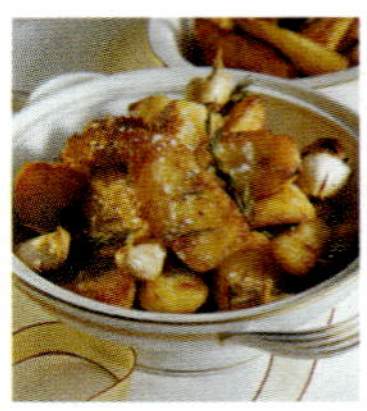

Special Dishes 64-99

Food for Friends

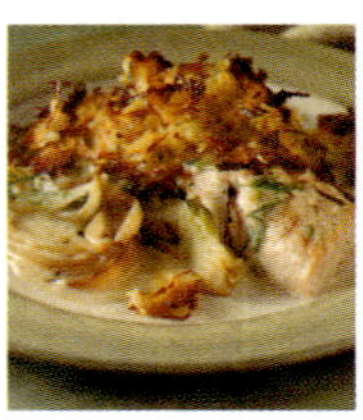

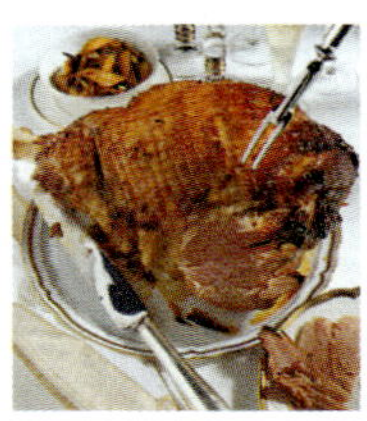

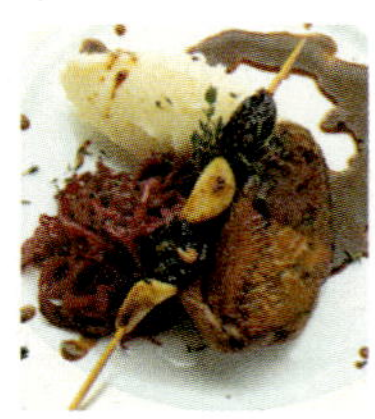

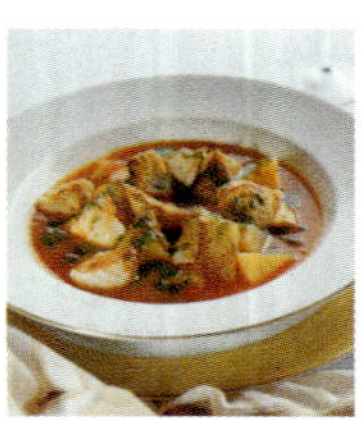

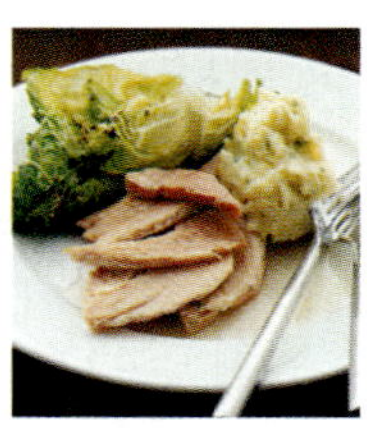

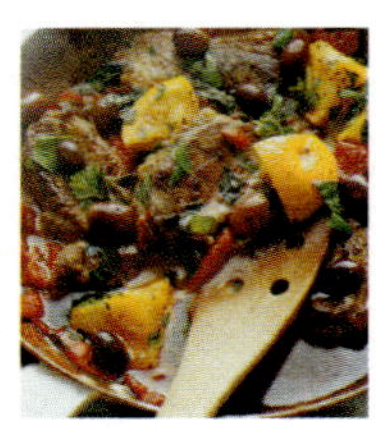

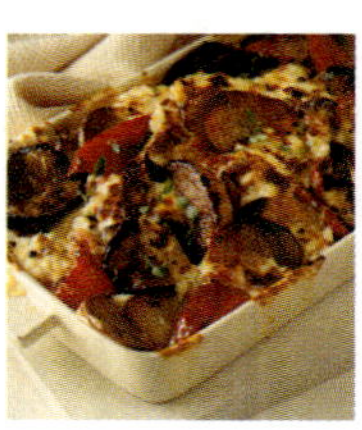

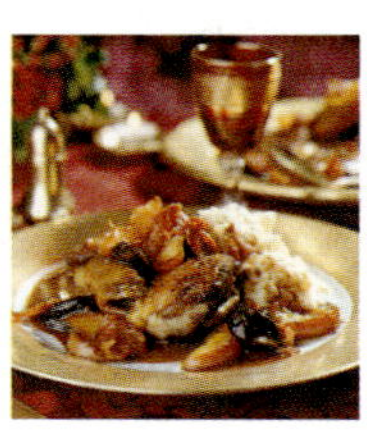

Vegetarian Courses

Leftovers

Irresistible Desserts 100-125

Christmas Puddings and Sauces

Desserts

Festive Baking 126-170

Mince Pies

Christmas Cakes

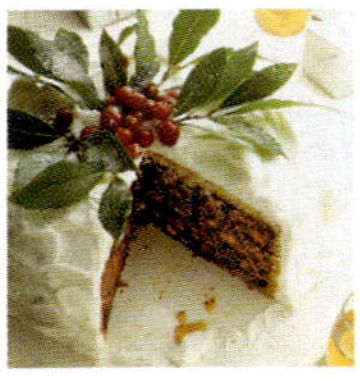

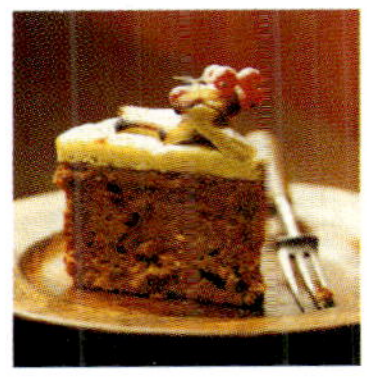

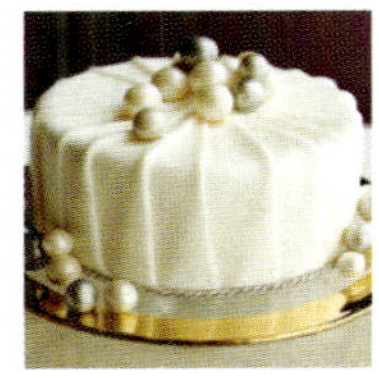

Cake Decorating Ideas

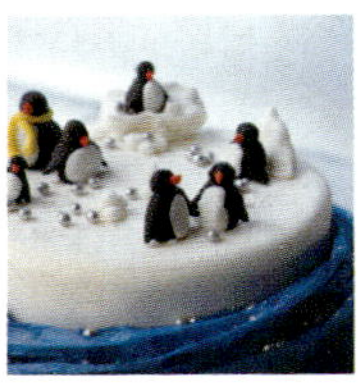

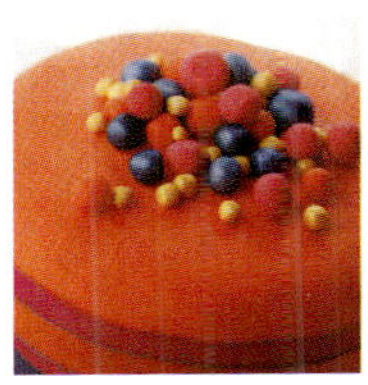

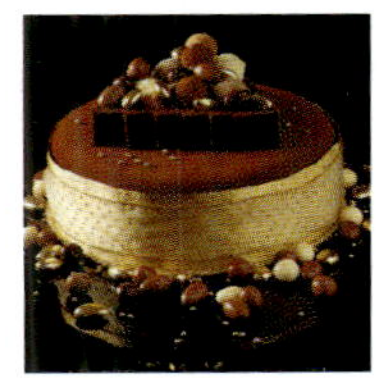

Alternative Christmas Cakes

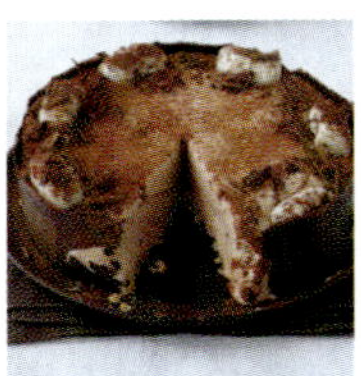

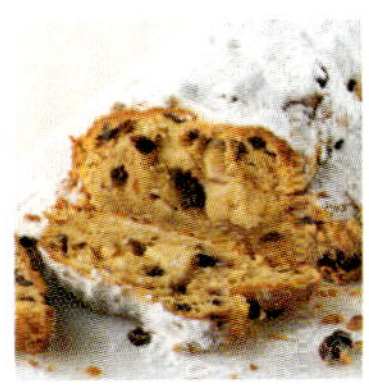

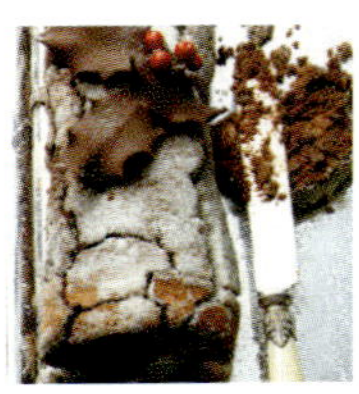

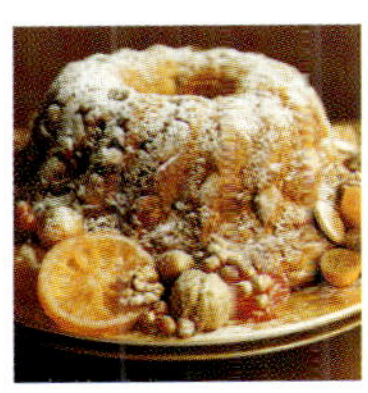

Sweet Treats

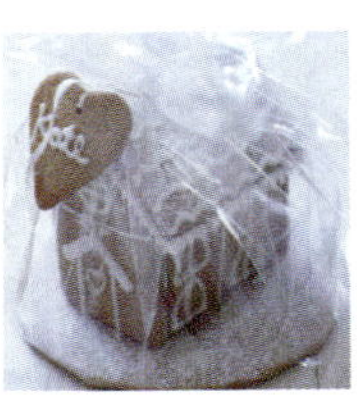

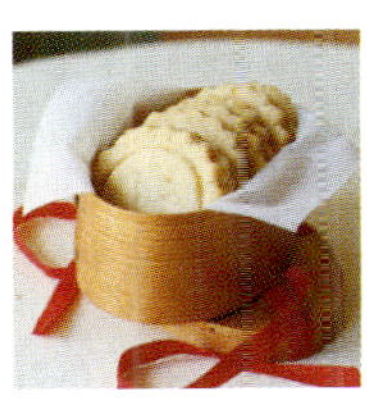

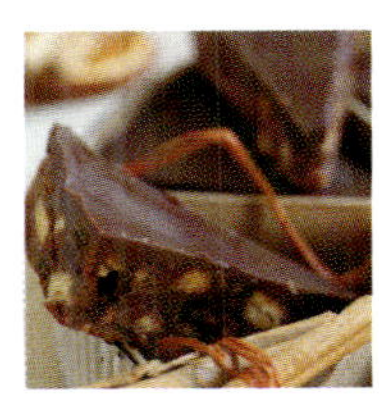

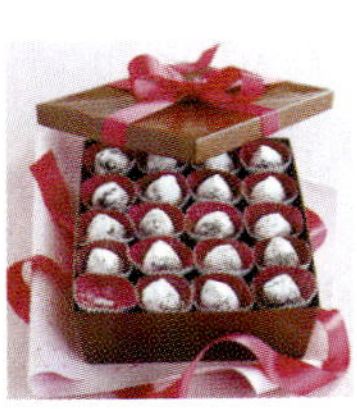

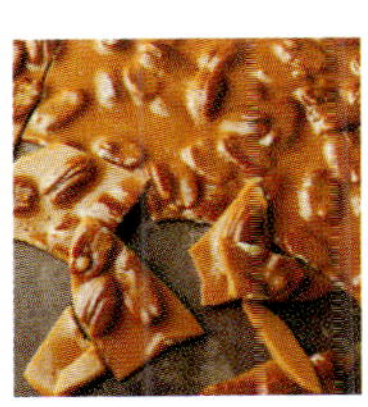

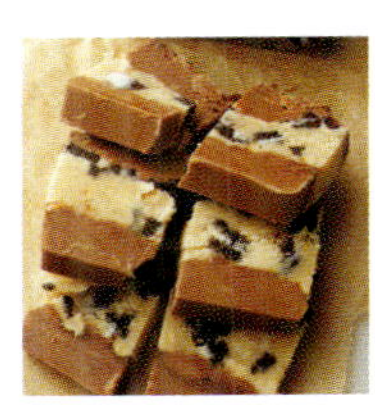

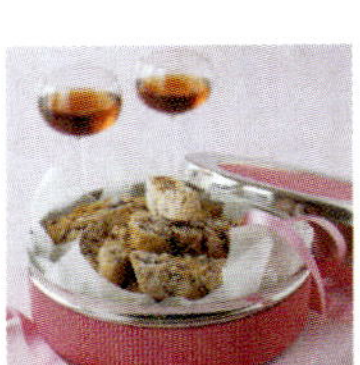

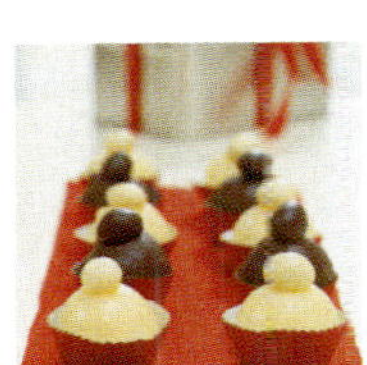

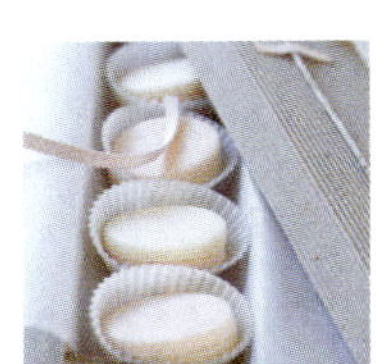

Seasonal Celebrations 172-186

Party Snacks

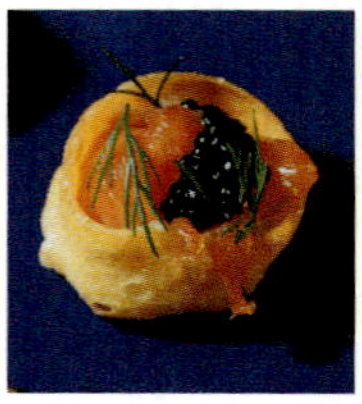

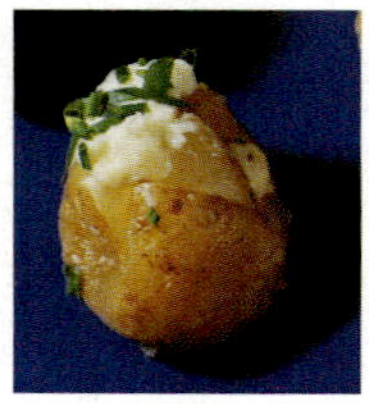

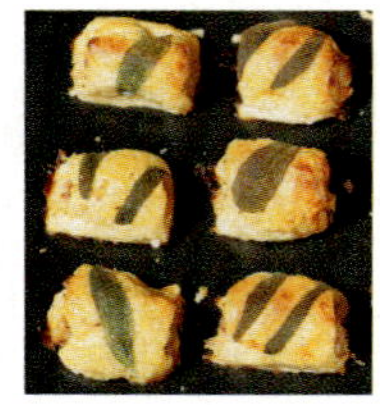

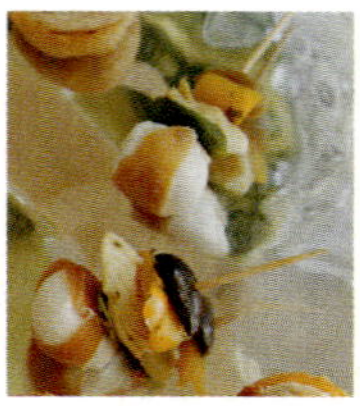

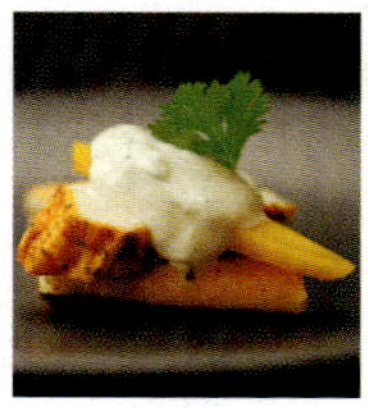

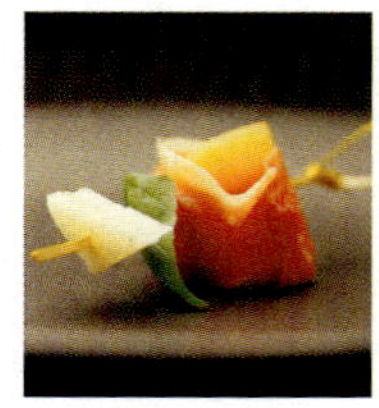

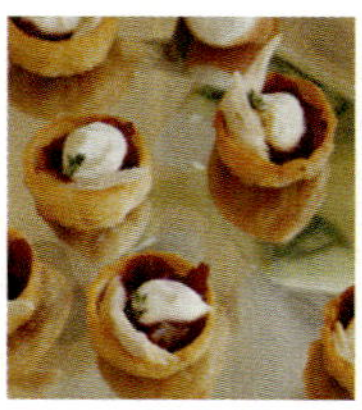

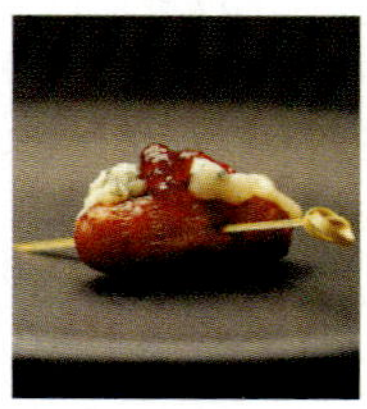

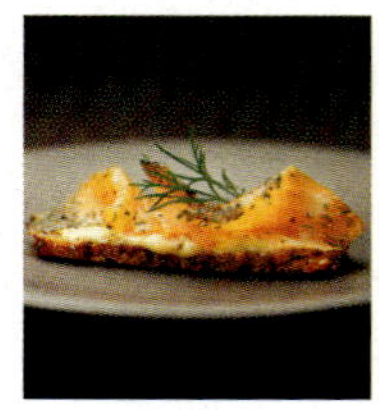

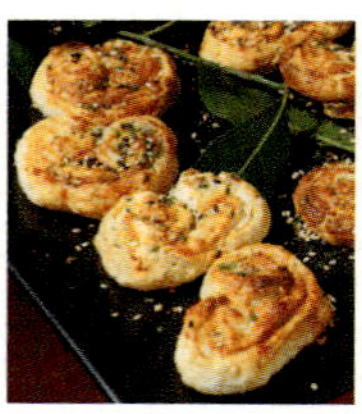

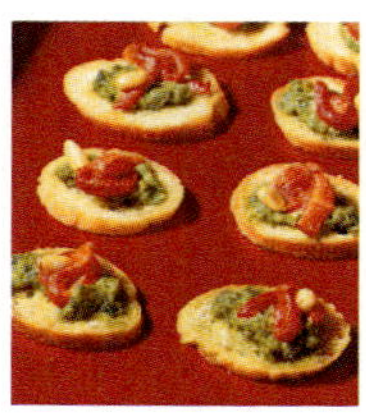

Party Drinks

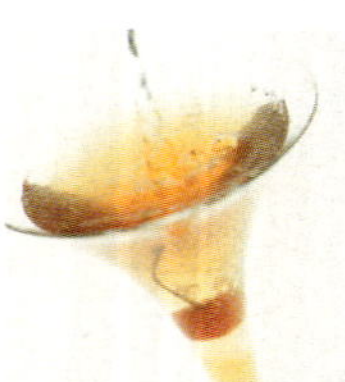

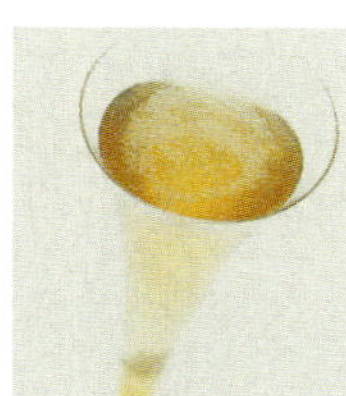

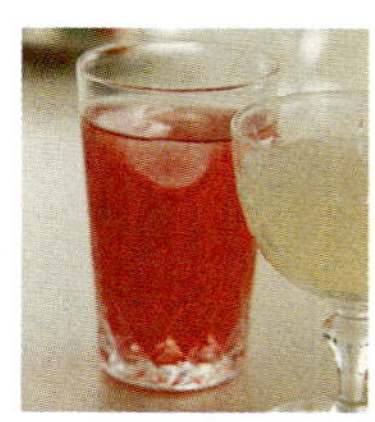

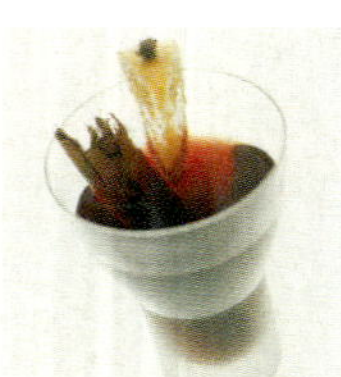

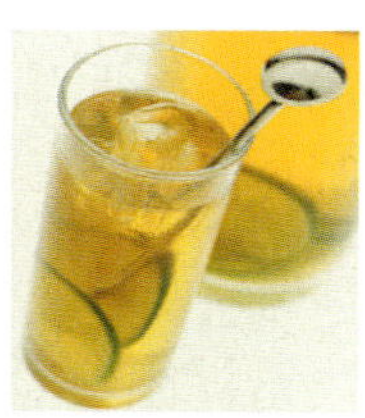

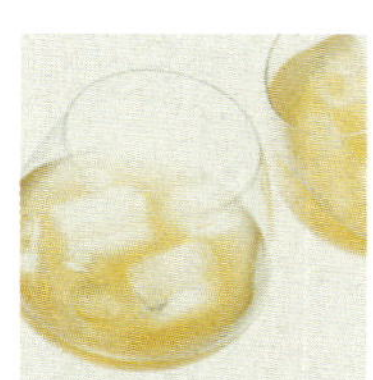

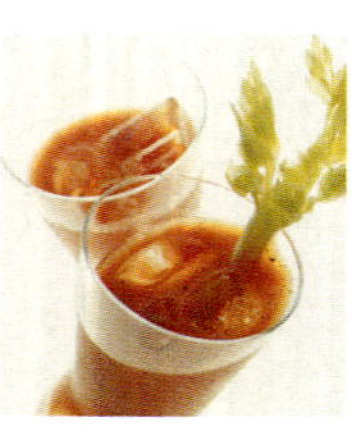

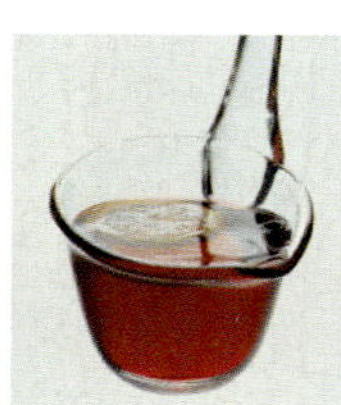

Reference

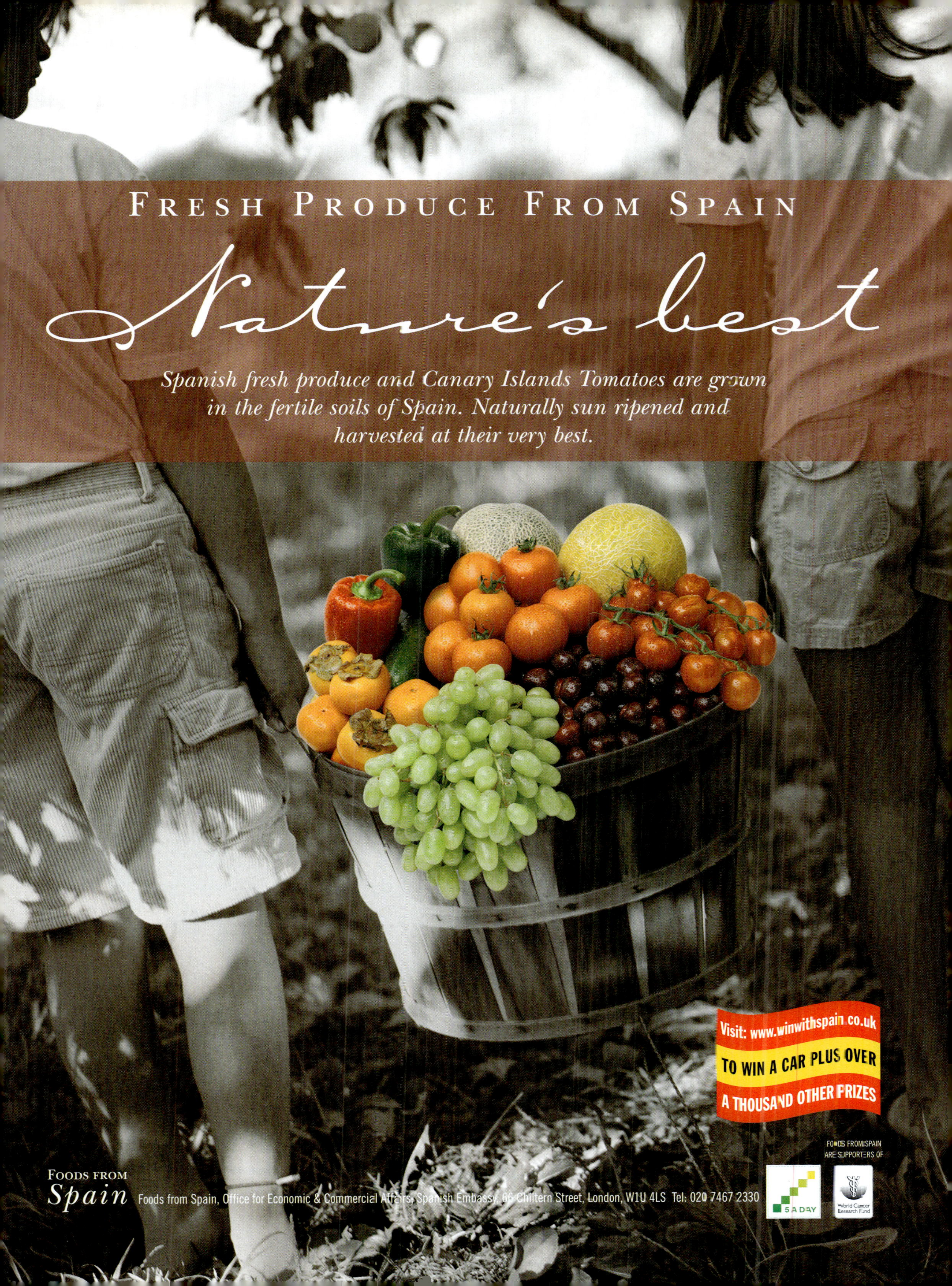

FRESH PRODUCE FROM SPAIN
Nature's best
Spanish fresh produce and Canary Islands Tomatoes are grown in the fertile soils of Spain. Naturally sun ripened and harvested at their very best.
Visit: www.winwithspain.co.uk
TO WIN A CAR PLUS OVER
A THOUSAND OTHER PRIZES
FOODS FROM SPAIN ARE SUPPORTERS OF
5 A DAY
World Cancer Research Fund
FOODS FROM Spain
Foods from Spain, Office for Economic & Commercial Affairs, Spanish Embassy, 66 Chiltern Street, London, W1U 4LS Tel: 020 7467 2330

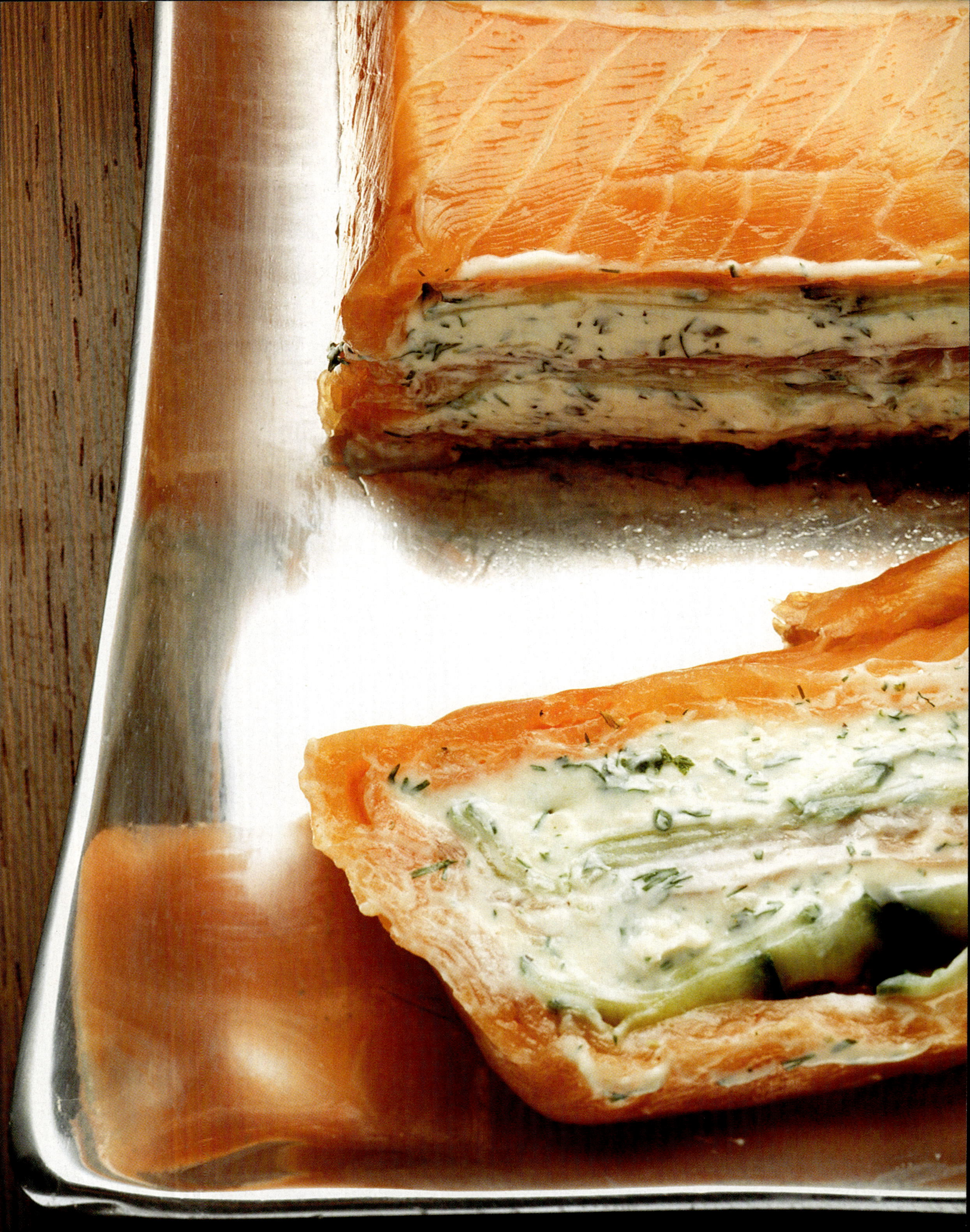

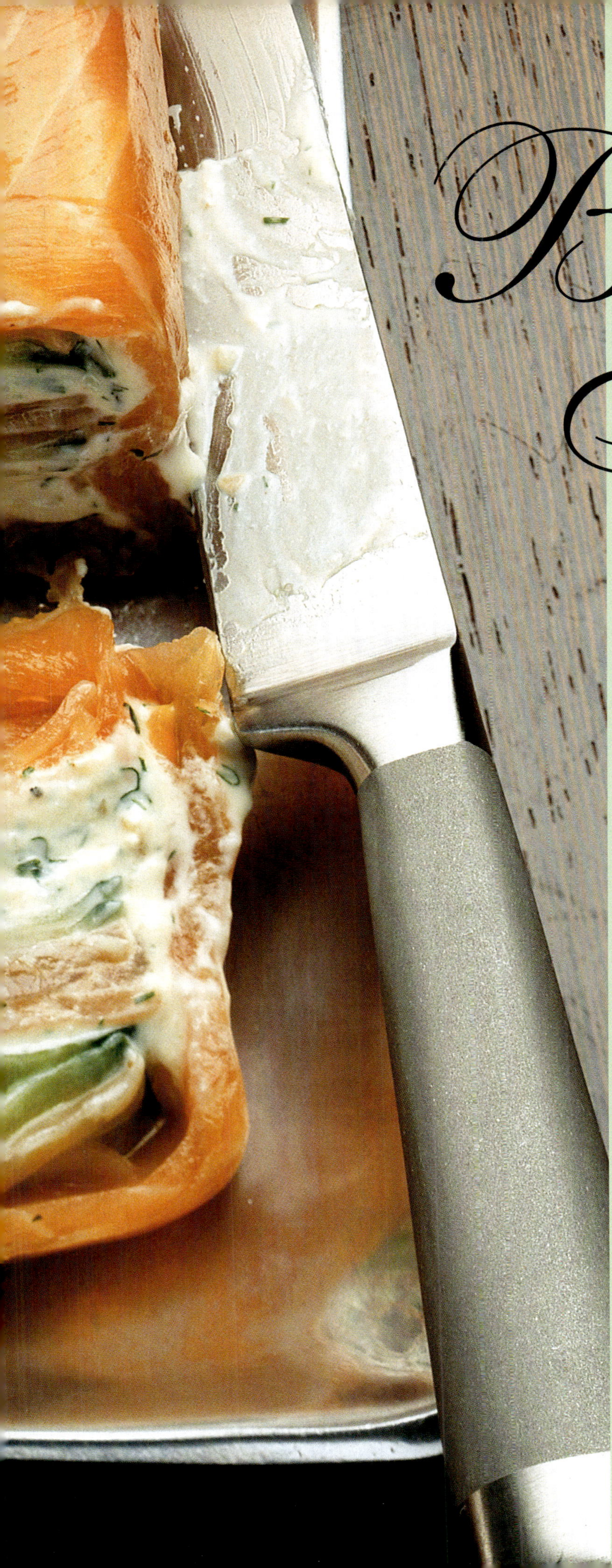

STUNNING YET SIMPLE

Best-ever Starters

Christmas lunch in your house may be a small affair for close family or entertaining on a much larger scale but, either way, you'll want to kick off the meal with a memorable starter. Here are some easy ideas when you're short of time yet the results are stunning. We've taken traditional **smoked salmon** and come up with some inspired ways to serve it. Then there's creamy Parsnip **Soup**, melt-in-your-mouth Lime and Coriander **Crab Cakes**, and for **vegetarians**, fancy **Mushroom Baskets** that taste as good as they look. Plus there's lots more ideas – and all our recipe suggestions will complement seasonal main courses perfectly.

Smoked Salmon and Potato Blinis

Preparation time: 30min
Cooking time: 30min
Serves: 6

FOR THE POTATO BLINIS

* 225g (8oz) floury potatoes, such as King Edward's, boiled and mashed with a little milk
* 3tbsp milk
* 5tbsp self-raising flour, sieved
* 4 large eggs, separated
* 3tbsp soured cream
* A pinch of cayenne pepper
* Vegetable oil for frying

FOR THE PICKLED VEGETABLES

* 75ml (3fl oz) white wine vinegar
* 2tbsp caster sugar
* 225g (8oz) cucumber, halved, deseeded and cut into thin strips
* 75g (3oz) radishes, cut into thin strips
* 1 spring onion, cut into thin strips
* 1tsp mustard seeds
* 1tbsp chopped fresh dill

TO SERVE

* 300ml (½ pint) full-fat crème fraîche
* 275–350g (10–12oz) smoked salmon
* Fresh dill and lemon wedges to garnish

1 To make the blinis, place the mashed potato in a large bowl and beat in the milk, flour, egg yolks and cream. Season, also adding a pinch of cayenne pepper. In a separate bowl, whisk the egg whites until they just hold their shape and fold into the potato mixture.

2 Lightly oil a non-stick frying pan and place over a high heat for 2–3min. Add 1–2tbsp batter and help it to spread to a circle 9cm (3½in) wide. Lower the heat and cook for 1–2min or until bubbles appear. Flip the blini over and cook for about 1min. Remove and repeat with the remaining batter to make 6 blinis. Interleaf the blinis with greaseproof paper and keep warm.

3 To make the pickled vegetables, place the vinegar and sugar in a saucepan and bring to the boil. Bubble for 2min, then leave to cool. Stir the cucumber, radishes, spring onion, mustard seeds and dill into the vinegar.

4 Top each blini with some crème fraîche, smoked salmon and the pickled vegetables. Garnish with fresh dill and wedges of lemon.

To freeze ahead: Complete the recipe to the end of step 2. Cool, wrap in clingfilm and freeze.
To use: Place the blinis on a non-stick baking sheet, cover with foil and warm at 190°C (170°C fan) mark 5 for 8–10min. Complete the recipe.

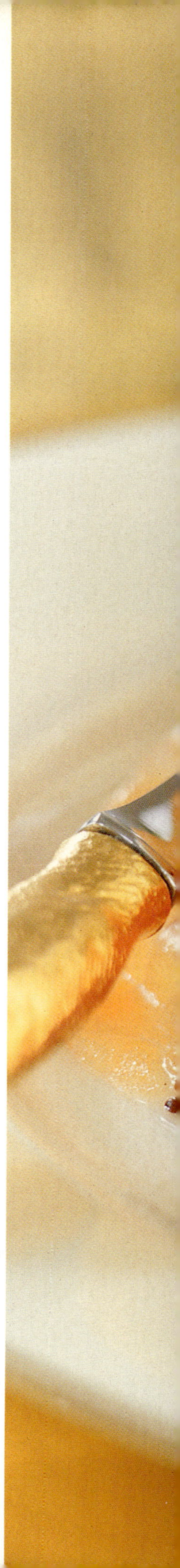

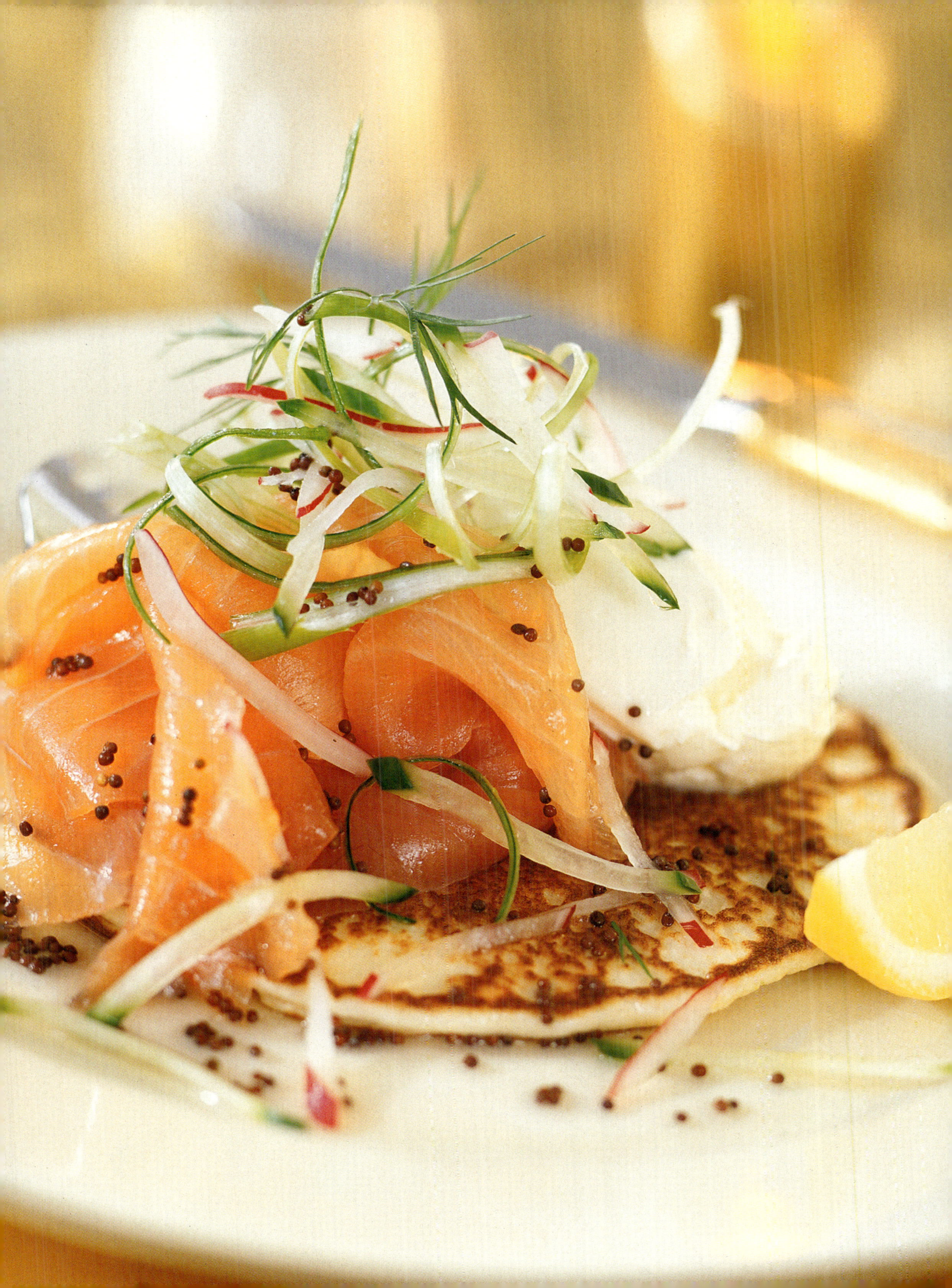

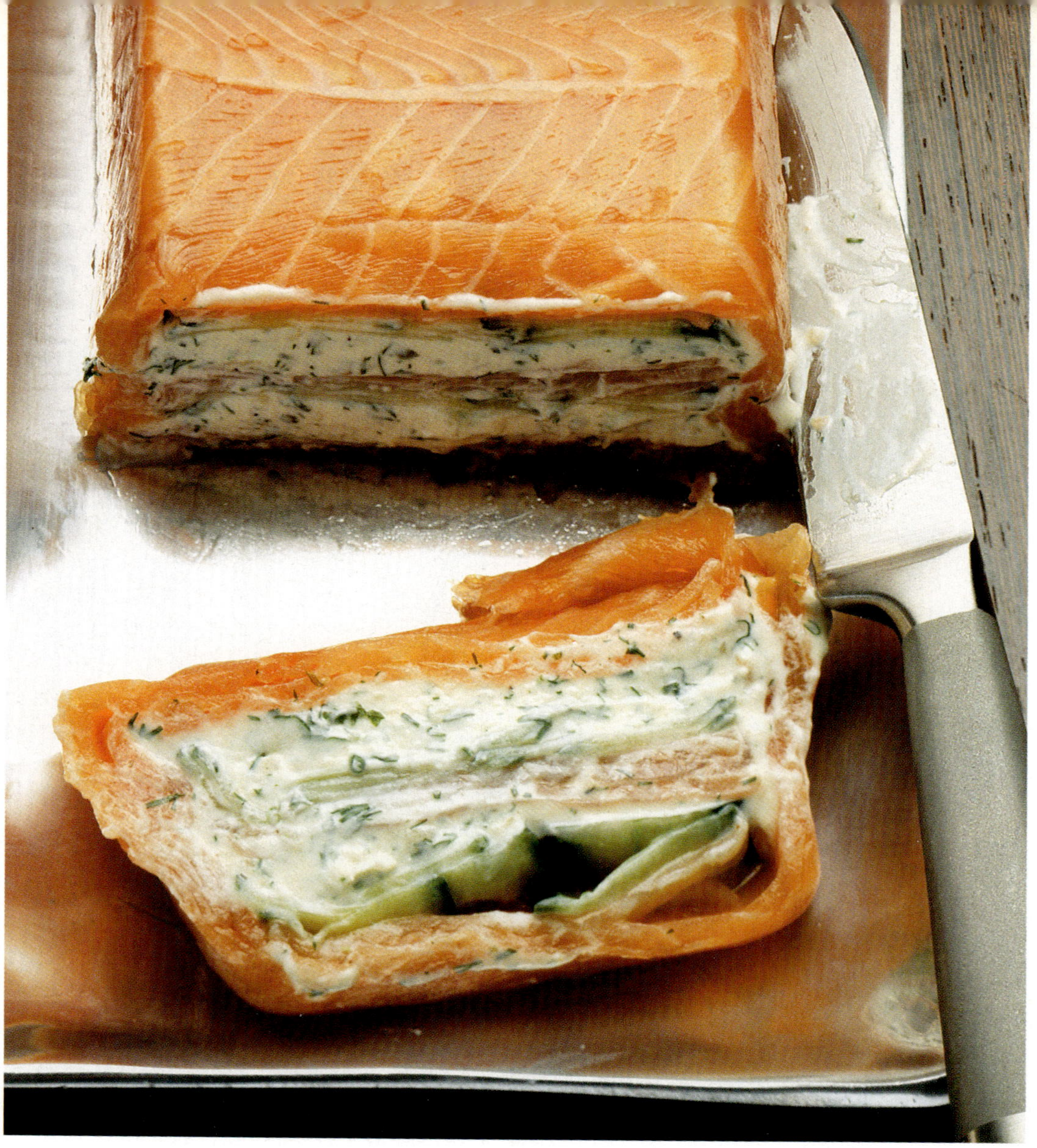

Smoked Salmon and Boursin Terrine

Hands-on time: 25min, plus 2hr chilling
Serves: 8

- 80g pack Boursin, garlic and herb variety
- 200ml tub crème fraîche
- 2tbsp freshly chopped dill
- 1tbsp horseradish
- 500g (1lb 2oz) oak-smoked salmon
- ½ cucumber, halved lengthways and seeds scooped out

1 Put the Boursin, crème fraîche, dill and horseradish into a bowl. Season and stir together until thoroughly mixed. Cover and chill.

2 Line a 900g (2lb) loaf tin with clingfilm, making sure there's enough to hang over the sides of the tin. Neatly line the base and sides of the tin with two layers of smoked salmon. Using a vegetable peeler, slice the cucumber lengthways into strips and arrange half on top of the salmon.

3 Spoon half the Boursin and dill mixture on top of the cucumber slices, smooth over using the back of the spoon, then top with two layers of smoked salmon and the remaining cucumber slices. Add the remaining cheese mixture and smooth over.

4 Top with a final two layers of smoked salmon to finish. Use the overhanging clingfilm to cover the terrine, weigh down and chill for at least 2hr. Unwrap and turn the terrine out onto a flat surface and carefully peel off the clingfilm. Cut into slices and serve.

Smoked Salmon and Scallop Parcels

Hands-on time: 40min
Cooking time: 6min
Serves: 6

FOR THE DRESSING

* 25g (1oz) coriander sprigs
* 1 small garlic clove, crushed
* 50ml (2fl oz) grapeseed oil
* 1tbsp lime juice
* A pinch of caster sugar

FOR THE PARCELS

* 6 large scallops or 12 small queen scallops with corals attached, about 225g (8oz) total weight
* 1 large ripe avocado
* 1 garlic clove, crushed
* 4 small spring onions, finely chopped
* 1 green chilli, deseeded and finely chopped
* 1tbsp grapeseed oil
* Zest and juice of 1 lime, plus extra to squeeze
* 6 large slices of smoked salmon, about 300g (11oz) total weight and 23cm (9in) in length
* Rocket leaves to garnish

1 To make the coriander dressing, place all the ingredients in a blender and process until smooth. Set aside.

2 To make the parcels, remove any tough membrane from the scallops and season. Place in a steamer and cook for about 5min or until the flesh is just white. Alternatively, put the scallops on a heatproof plate, cover with another plate and steam over a pan of simmering water for about 3min on each side. Drain and set on kitchen paper to cool.

3 Place the avocado, garlic, spring onions, chilli, oil, and lime zest and juice in a bowl. Mash the avocado with a fork, then mix together. Season.

4 Lay the salmon slices on a worksurface, place a large scallop or two small ones on each slice and spoon the avocado mixture on top. Roll the salmon around the filling.

5 To serve, place the parcels on serving plates and squeeze a little lime juice over each. Drizzle with the coriander dressing, garnish with salad leaves and sprinkle with freshly ground black pepper.

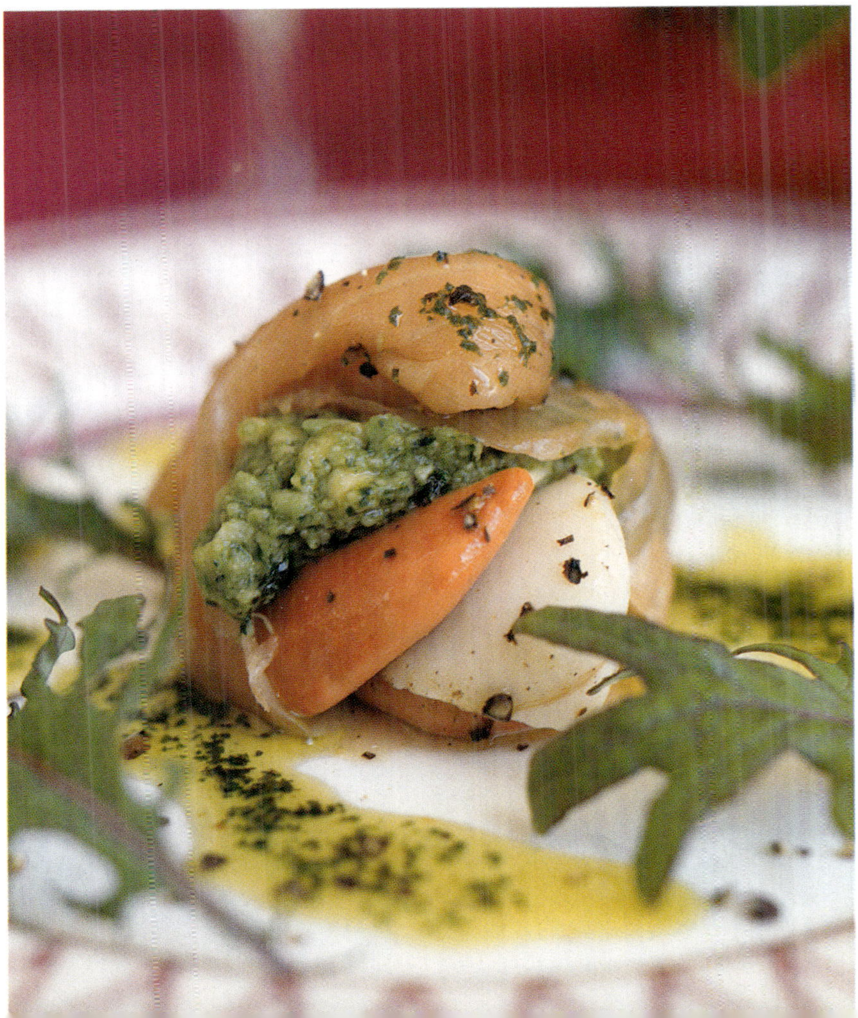

Parsnip Soup with Parmesan Crisps

Preparation time: 30min
Cooking time: 1hr
Makes: 2 litres (3½ pints)

- 40g (1½oz) butter
- 150g (5oz) onion, roughly chopped
- 225g (8oz) floury potatoes, such as King Edward's, peeled and chopped
- 400g (14oz) parsnips, peeled and chopped
- 4tsp paprika, plus extra to dust
- 1.1 litres (2 pints) vegetable stock
- 450ml (¾ pint) milk
- 4tbsp double cream
- 65g (2½oz) sliced chorizo sausage, cut into fine strips

FOR THE PARMESAN CRISPS

- 1 large parsnip, about 75g (3oz), peeled
- Vegetable oil for frying
- 3tbsp grated Parmesan cheese

1 Melt the butter in a large, heavy-based pan. Add the onion and cook over a gentle heat for 5min or until soft. Add the potatoes, parsnips and paprika, mix well and cook gently, stirring occasionally, for about 15min or until the vegetables begin to soften.

2 Add the stock, milk, and cream. Season. Bring to the boil and simmer for 25min or until the vegetables are very soft. Add 50g (2oz) of the chorizo.

3 Allow the soup to cool a little, then place in a blender or food processor and whiz until smooth. The soup can be thinned with additional stock or milk, if wished. Season to taste and return to the pan.

4 To prepare the Parmesan Crisps, using a vegetable peeler (the wide swivel ones are best for this), peel off long strips of parsnip until there is nothing left to peel. The strips should be as wide as possible.

5 In a large pan or deep-sided frying pan, pour in the oil to a depth of 2.5cm (1in) and heat to a moderate temperature. Shallow-fry the parsnip strips in batches until they're light golden and crisp. Drain on kitchen paper and sprinkle lightly with salt. Arrange the strips in six little piles on a baking sheet, then sprinkle with half the Parmesan cheese and the remaining chorizo. Set aside.

6 Cook the Parmesan Crisps at 200°C (180°C fan) mark 6 for 3–5min or until the cheese begins to melt. (Don't let the crisps become too brown or they'll taste bitter.) Reheat the soup. Serve topped with the Parmesan Crisps, sprinkled with the remaining Parmesan cheese and dusted with paprika.

To freeze ahead: Complete to the end of step 3, then cool, pack and freeze.
To use: Thaw the soup at cool room temperature overnight. Complete the recipe.

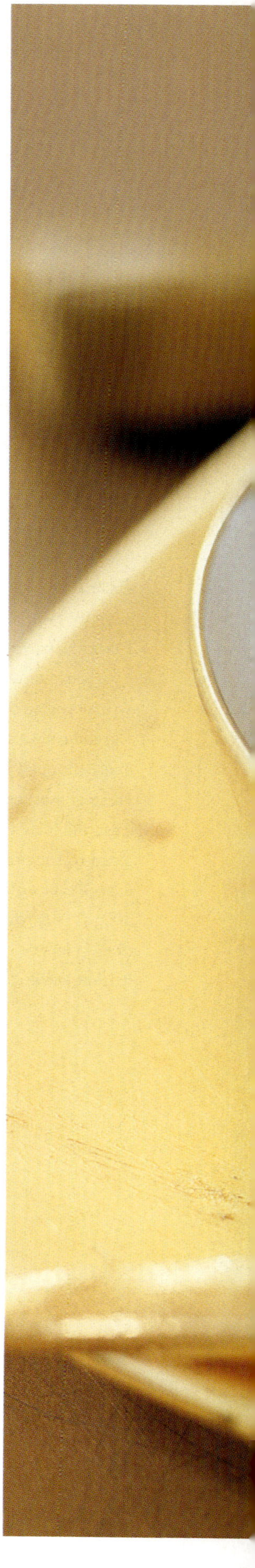

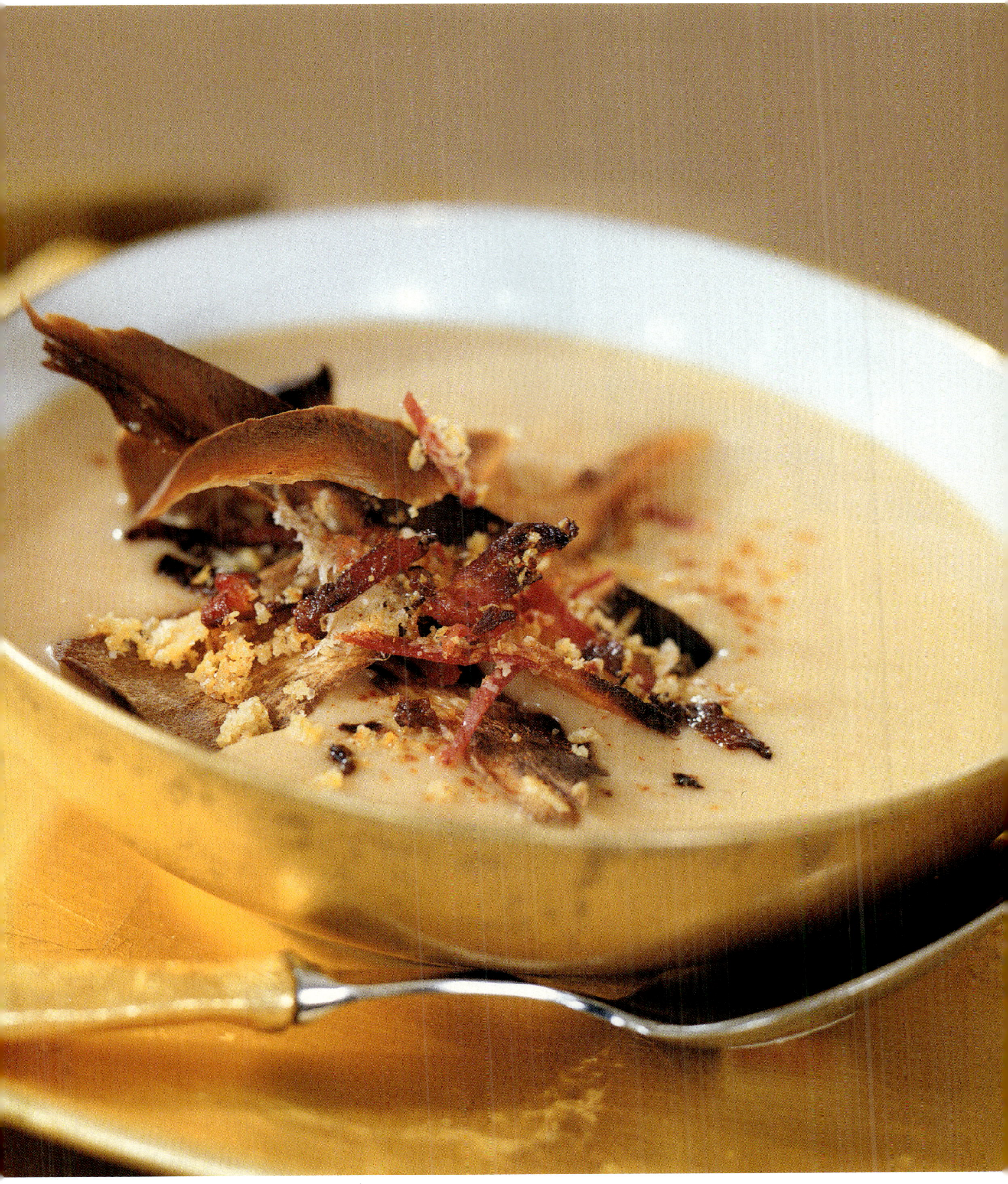

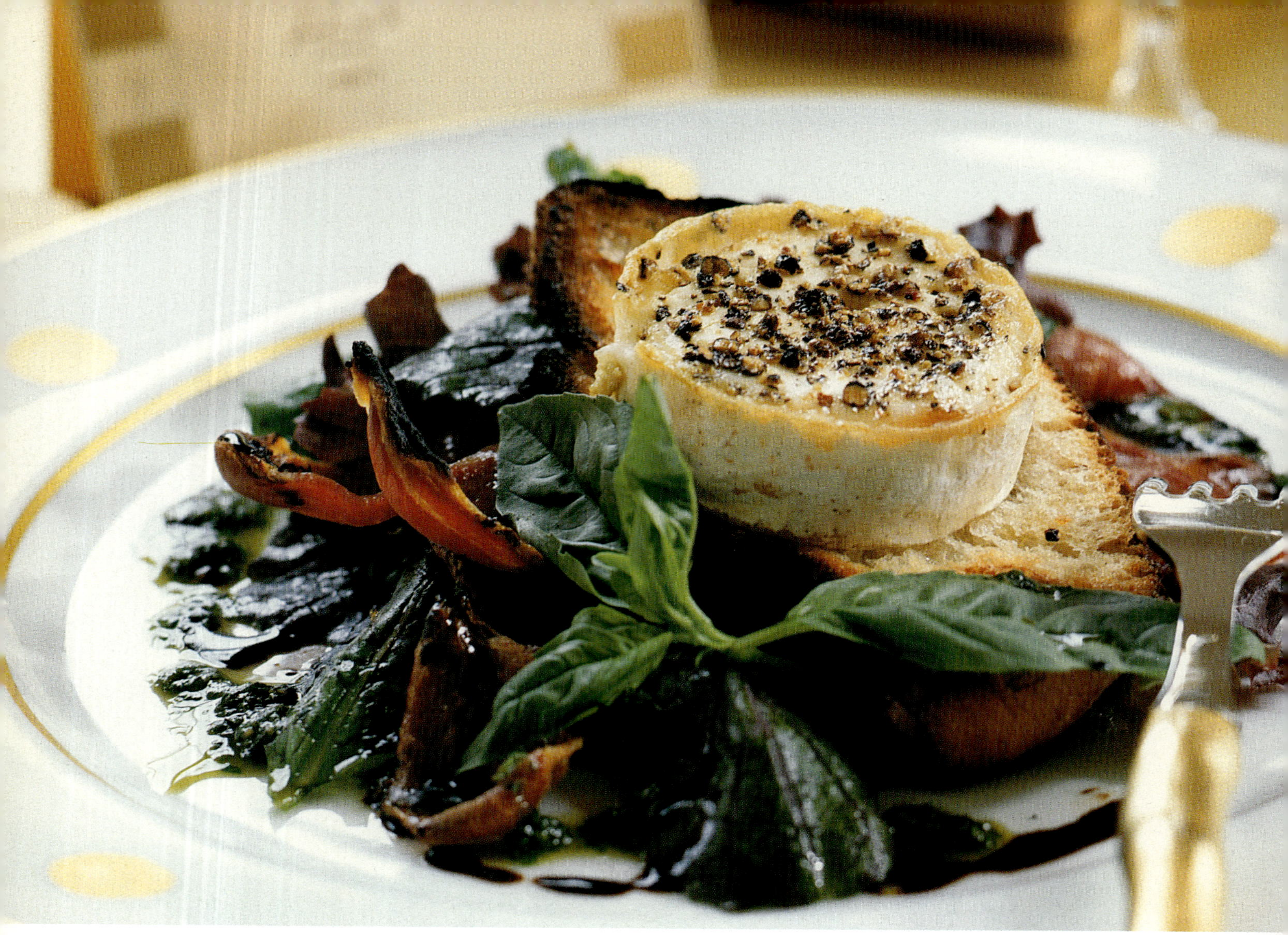

Peppercorn-crusted Goat's Cheese Salad

Hands-on time: 20min, plus 12hr marinating
Cooking time: 15min
Serves: 6

- 6 slices of hard goat's cheese
- 150ml (¼ pint) good quality olive oil
- 25g (1oz) fresh basil, leaves removed, stalks reserved
- 1tsp mixed peppercorns, crushed
- 175ml (6fl oz) balsamic vinegar
- 6 slices Parma ham, 140g (4½oz), cut in half
- 1tbsp soft brown sugar
- 6 slices ciabatta, cut at an angle
- 1 small garlic clove, crushed
- Lemon juice (optional)
- 125g (4oz) rocket or watercress sprigs
- Basil sprigs to garnish

1 Place the cheese in a bowl, pour the olive oil over and add the basil stalks. Cover and leave in a cool place to marinate for 12hr. Remove the cheese from the oil and dust with the peppercorns. Strain and reserve oil.

2 To make the balsamic dressing, place the vinegar in a pan, bring to the boil and bubble for 4–5min or until syrupy. Set aside to cool.

3 Place the Parma ham on a non-stick baking sheet, sprinkle with sugar and grill until crisp. Set aside. Brush the ciabatta slices with a little reserved oil and toast on one side. Set aside.

4 To make the basil dressing, place the basil leaves, garlic and reserved oil in a food processor and whiz until smooth. Season and add lemon juice, if using, to taste. Set aside.

5 Place the cheese on the untoasted side of the ciabatta. Grill until just melting. Divide the rocket and ham between six plates, top with the ciabatta, drizzle with the dressings and garnish with the sprigs of basil.

Crispy Duck Salad

Hands-on time: 30min, plus cooling and overnight chilling
Cooking time: 1hr 25min
Serves: 8

* 6 duck legs, each about 200g (7oz)
* 1tsp peppercorns
* 2 fresh thyme sprigs
* 2 bayleaves
* 125g (4oz) kumquats
* 125g (4oz) pecan nuts
* 2 oranges
* 225g (8oz) cranberries
* 125g (4oz) caster sugar
* 4tbsp white wine vinegar
* 135ml (9tbsp) sunflower oil
* 3tbsp walnut oil
* Frisée leaves to serve

1 Place the duck legs in a large, flameproof casserole, cover with cold water and bring to the boil. Simmer for 10min, skim the surface of the liquid and add the peppercorns, thyme, bay leaves and 2tsp salt. Cook at 180°C (160°C fan) mark 4 for 45min–1hr or until tender. Cool quickly and chill overnight.

2 Cut the kumquats into quarters. Place the pecan nuts on a baking sheet and toast lightly under a preheated grill.

3 Finely grate the zest and squeeze the juice from the oranges. Place the orange zest in a frying pan with 200ml (7fl oz) orange juice, along with the cranberries and sugar. Bring to the boil and simmer gently for 5min or until the cranberries are tender. Drain the cranberries, reserving the juice, and set aside the berries. Bring the juice to the boil and bubble until syrupy, then add the reserved cranberries back in.

4 In a small bowl, whisk in the vinegar followed by the oils and season. Add the kumquats to the cranberry mixture with the dressing and pecans. Set aside. Skim the fat from the surface of the jellied duck liquor and set aside. Cut the duck into thick shreds, leaving the skin on.

5 Just before serving, heat 1tbsp reserved duck fat in a large, non-stick frying pan and fry half the duck for about 5min or until very crisp and brown (the duck fat may splatter, so keep a lid handy). Set aside in a warm place. Repeat with the remaining duck. To serve, carefully toss the duck with the cranberry mixture and serve with salad leaves.

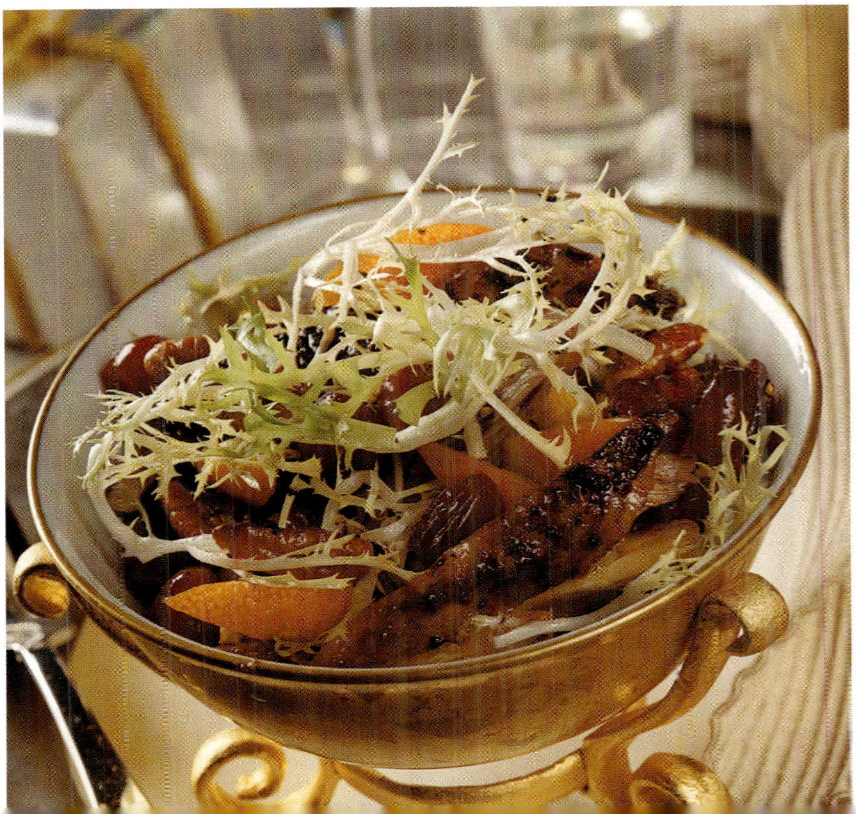

Lime and Coriander Crab Cakes

Hands-on time: 30min, plus 1½hr chilling
Cooking time: 15min
Serves: 4

FOR THE MAYONNAISE
* 2tbsp sweet chilli sauce
* 1tbsp chopped fresh coriander
* Zest and juice of 1 lime
* 5tbsp mayonnaise

FOR THE CRAB CAKES
* 1tbsp sunflower oil
* 3 spring onions, finely sliced
* 2 garlic cloves, crushed
* 1 red chilli, deseeded and chopped
* 350g (12oz) crabmeat
* 2tsp tomato ketchup
* 4tbsp mayonnaise
* 1tsp Worcestershire sauce
* 50g (2oz) fresh white breadcrumbs

FOR THE COATING
* 50g (2oz) seasoned flour
* 1 large egg, beaten
* 125 (4oz) fresh white breadcrumbs
* Vegetable oil for frying
* Spring onion curls, crushed
* Sliced red chilli to garnish

1 To make the chilli mayonnaise, combine the first four ingredients in a bowl. Season, cover and chill. Set aside. This can be made a day in advance.

2 To make the crab cakes, heat the oil in a pan, add the spring onions and cook, stirring, for 3min. Remove from the heat, stir in the garlic and chilli, transfer to a large bowl and cool. Add the remaining crab cake ingredients and stir until well combined. Season.

3 Using your hands, shape the mixture into 12 cakes, and place on a baking sheet. Cover and chill for a least 1hr.

4 To make the coating, dip the cakes into the seasoned flour, then the beaten egg and breadcrumbs. Return to the baking sheet and chill for 30min.

5 Heat 2.5cm (1in) oil in a pan. Fry the cakes in batches for 2–3min on each side or until golden. Remove the cakes from the pan and drain on kitchen paper. Season, garnish and serve with the chilli mayonnaise.

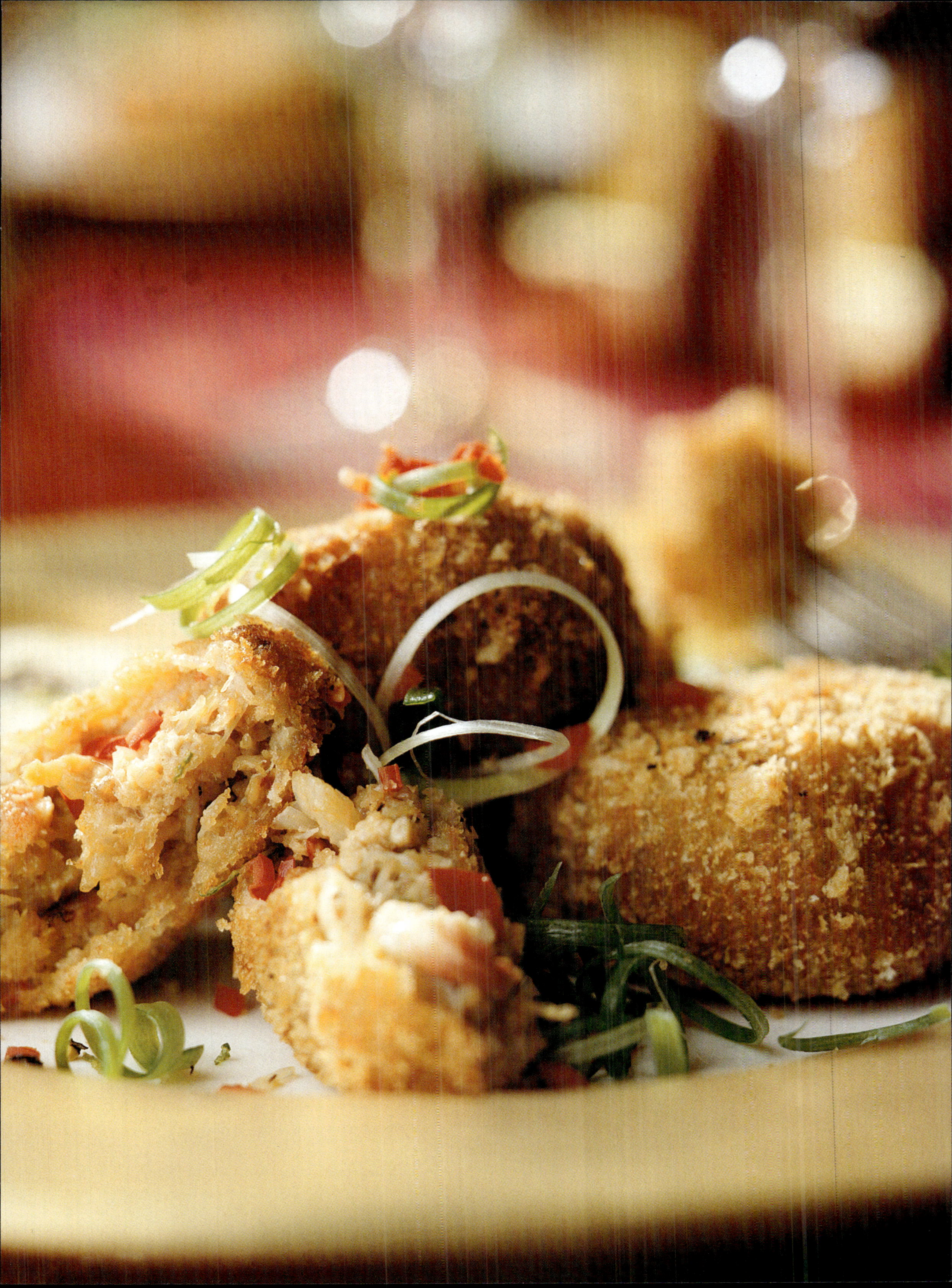

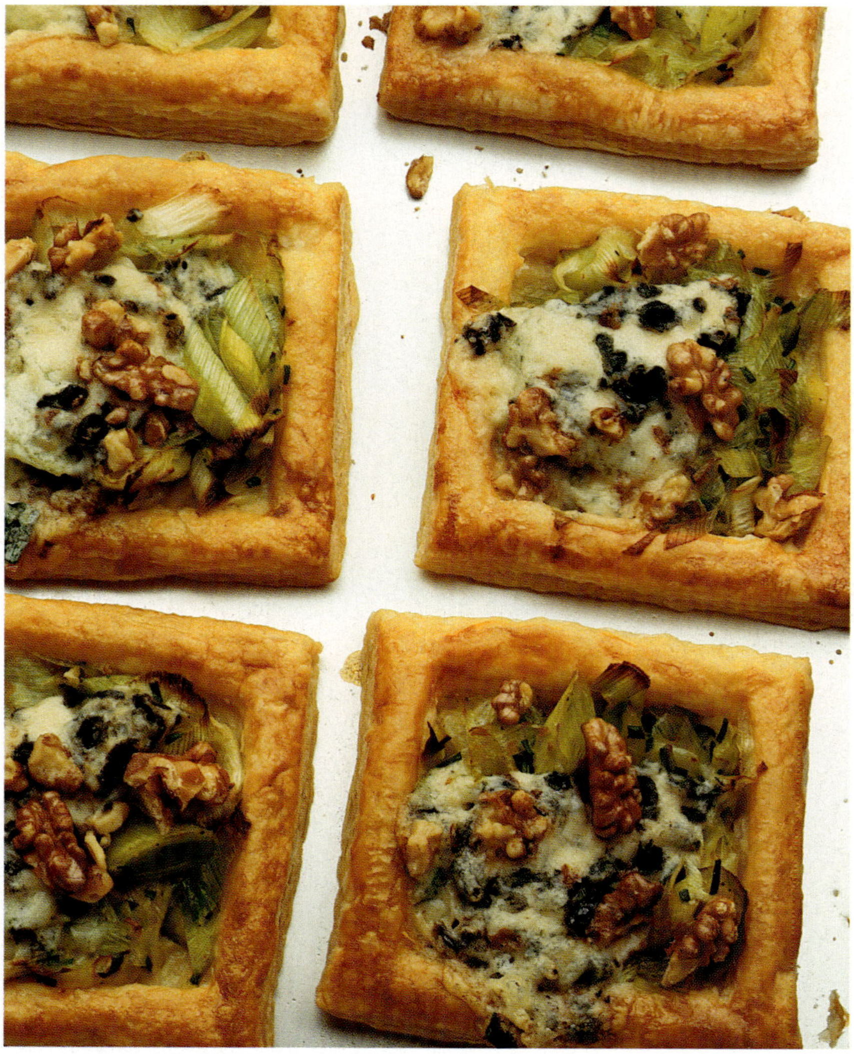

Roquefort, Leek and Walnut Tarts

Hands-on time: 25min
Cooking time: 30–35min
Serves: 6
Vegetarian

* 375g pack fresh ready-rolled puff pastry
* 2 medium eggs
* 40g (1½oz) butter
* 400g (14oz) trimmed leeks, thinly sliced
* 2tbsp chopped chives
* 100g (3½oz) Roquefort cheese, sliced into 6 triangles
* 75g (3oz) walnuts, chopped

1 Preheat the oven to 200°C (180°C fan) mark 6. Unroll the pastry and, leaving it on its plastic wrap, cut in half lengthways, then cut each half into three squares. Using the tip of a sharp knife, score a smaller square 1cm (½in) in from the edge of each to make a frame.

2 Put the squares on a greased baking tray. Beat one egg lightly and brush over each pastry case. Chill the pastry cases for 10min. Bake for 10min or until well risen and lightly golden. Carefully lift off the top layers of each inner square and discard, then use a fork to scoop out any uncooked pastry from each centre.

3 Melt the butter in a frying pan, add the leeks and cook for about 10min or until they're soft. Beat the remaining egg and add to the leeks with the chives. Season. Fill the pastry cases generously with the mixture.

4 Put a slice of cheese onto each tart and top with walnuts. Return the tarts to the oven and bake for 10–15min or until golden and heated through.

Mushroom Baskets

Hands-on time: 40min, plus 50min chilling
Cooking time: 50min
Serves: 6
Vegetarian

FOR THE PASTRY

* 250g (9oz) plain flour, plus extra to dust
* 150g (5oz) chilled butter, cubed
* 1 large egg

FOR THE FILLING

* 15g (½oz) dried mushrooms
* 50g (2oz) butter
* 225g (8oz) onion, finely chopped
* 450g (1lb) mixed mushrooms, sliced
* 1 garlic clove, crushed
* 300ml (½ pint) medium dry sherry
* 284ml carton double cream
* Thyme springs to garnish

1 To make the pastry, whiz the flour and butter in a food processor until the mixture resembles fine breadcrumbs. Add the egg and pulse until the mixture comes together. To make the pastry by hand, rub the butter into the flour until the mixture resembles breadcrumbs. Add the egg and stir until it just comes together. Knead lightly on a floured surface and shape into six balls. Wrap and chill for 30min.

2 On a floured worksurface, roll the pastry out and line six loose-bottomed tart cases 8.5cm (3¾in) across the base and 3cm (1¼in) high. Prick the bases and chill for 20min. Line with greaseproof paper and baking beans and bake at 200°C (180°C fan) mark 6 for 10min. Remove the paper and beans and bake for 5min or until cooked. The baskets can be frozen at this stage.

3 To make the filling, soak the dried mushrooms in 300ml (½ pint) boiling water for 10min. Heat the butter in a pan, add the onion and cook for 10min. Add the fresh mushrooms and garlic and cook for 5min. Remove from the pan and set aside. Put the dried mushrooms and their liquid in the pan and add the sherry. Bring to the boil, bubble for 10min, add the cream and cook for a further 5min or until syrupy.

4 To serve, warm the pastry at 180°C (160°C fan) mark 4 for 5min. Add the reserved mushrooms to the sauce, season and heat through. Pour into the cases and garnish.

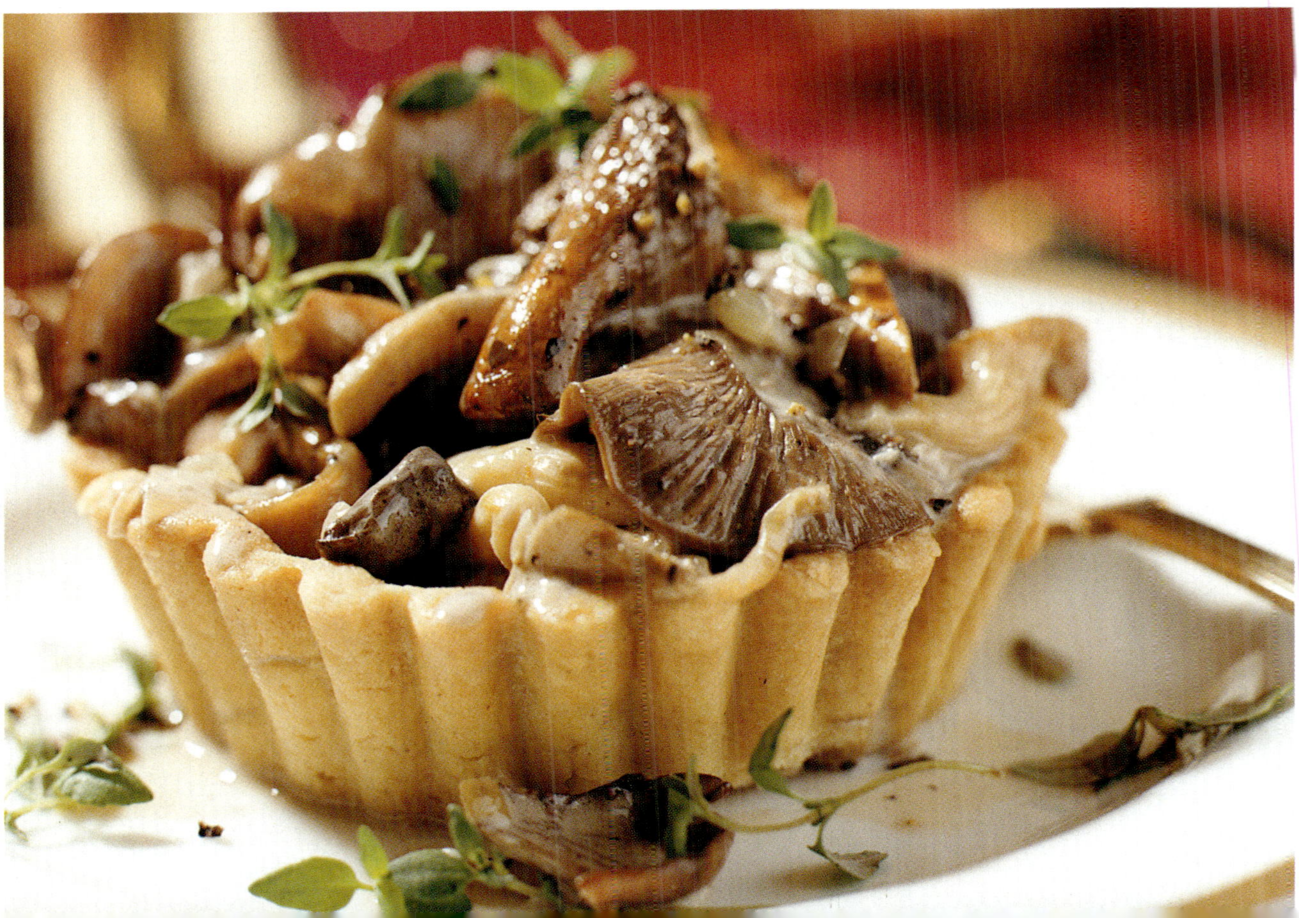

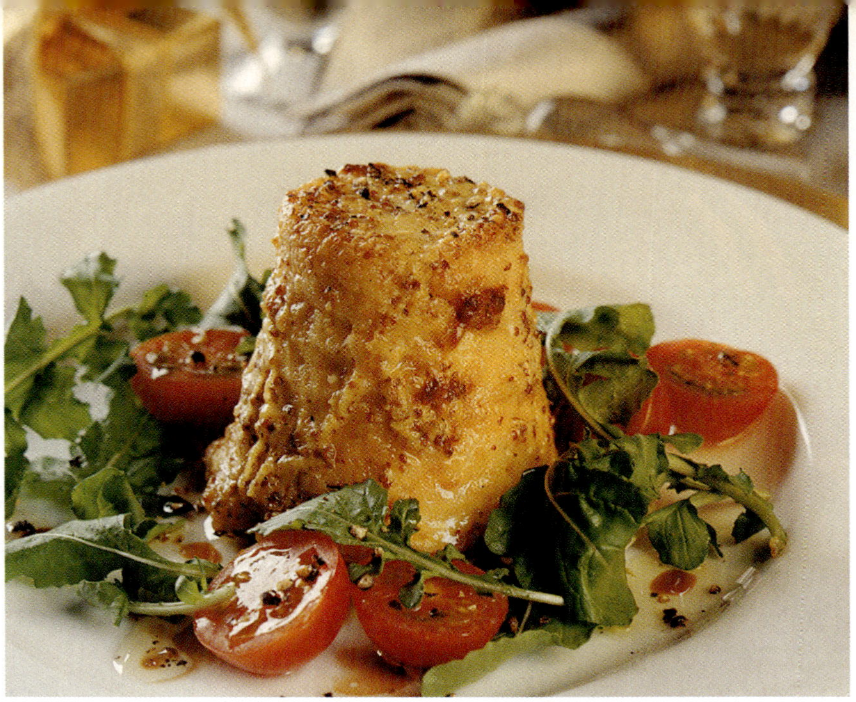

Twice-baked Cauliflower Cheese Souffles

Hands-on time: 20min
Cooking time: 1¼hr
Serves: 8
Vegetarian

* 75g (3oz) Cheddar cheese
* 75g (3oz) Emmenthal cheese
* 25g (1oz) ground almonds
* 50g (2oz) butter, plus extra for greasing
* 250g (9oz) cauliflower florets
* 150ml (¼ pint) milk
* 40g (1½oz) plain flour
* 3 large eggs, separated
* 284ml (10fl oz) carton double cream
* 1tbsp grainy mustard
* Rocket, leaves and cherry tomatoes to serve
* Olive oil and balsamic vinegar for drizzling
* Ramekins or dariole moulds

1 Finely grate the cheeses. Cook the almonds under a preheated grill, turning from time to time, until lightly toasted. Grease and baseline eight 150ml (¼ pint) ramekins or dariole moulds with greaseproof paper, then dust with toasted ground almonds.

2 Cook the cauliflower in salted, boiling water for 5–10min or until tender. Drain, plunge into iced water and drain again. Place in a food processor with the milk and whiz for 2–3min until smooth.

3 Melt the butter in a pan, add the flour and mix to a smooth paste. Blend in the cauliflower purée, stirring, and bring to the boil. Cool a little, then beat in the cheeses and egg yolks. Season. Whisk the whites to a soft peak and fold into the cauliflower mixture.

4 Fill the moulds with the cauliflower mixture and place in a roasting tin. Add enough hot water to come halfway up the side of the moulds. Cook at 180°C (160°C fan) mark 4 for 20–25min or until firm to the touch in the centre. Remove from the roasting tin and cool completely. Run a knife around the edge of the soufflés and carefully turn out onto a baking sheet.

5 Pour the cream into a wide pan, bring to the boil and bubble until syrupy and reduced by one-third. Add the mustard and season.

6 Spoon a little cream over the soufflés and bake at 200°C (180°C fan) mark 6 for 15–20min or until golden. Serve immediately with rocket leaves and cherry tomatoes. Garnish with freshly ground black pepper and drizzle with olive oil and balsamic vinegar.

To freeze ahead: Complete the recipe to the end of step 5, then wrap separately and freeze. **To use:** Complete the recipe, cooking the soufflés from frozen at 200 °C (180°C fan) for 25–30min or until golden.

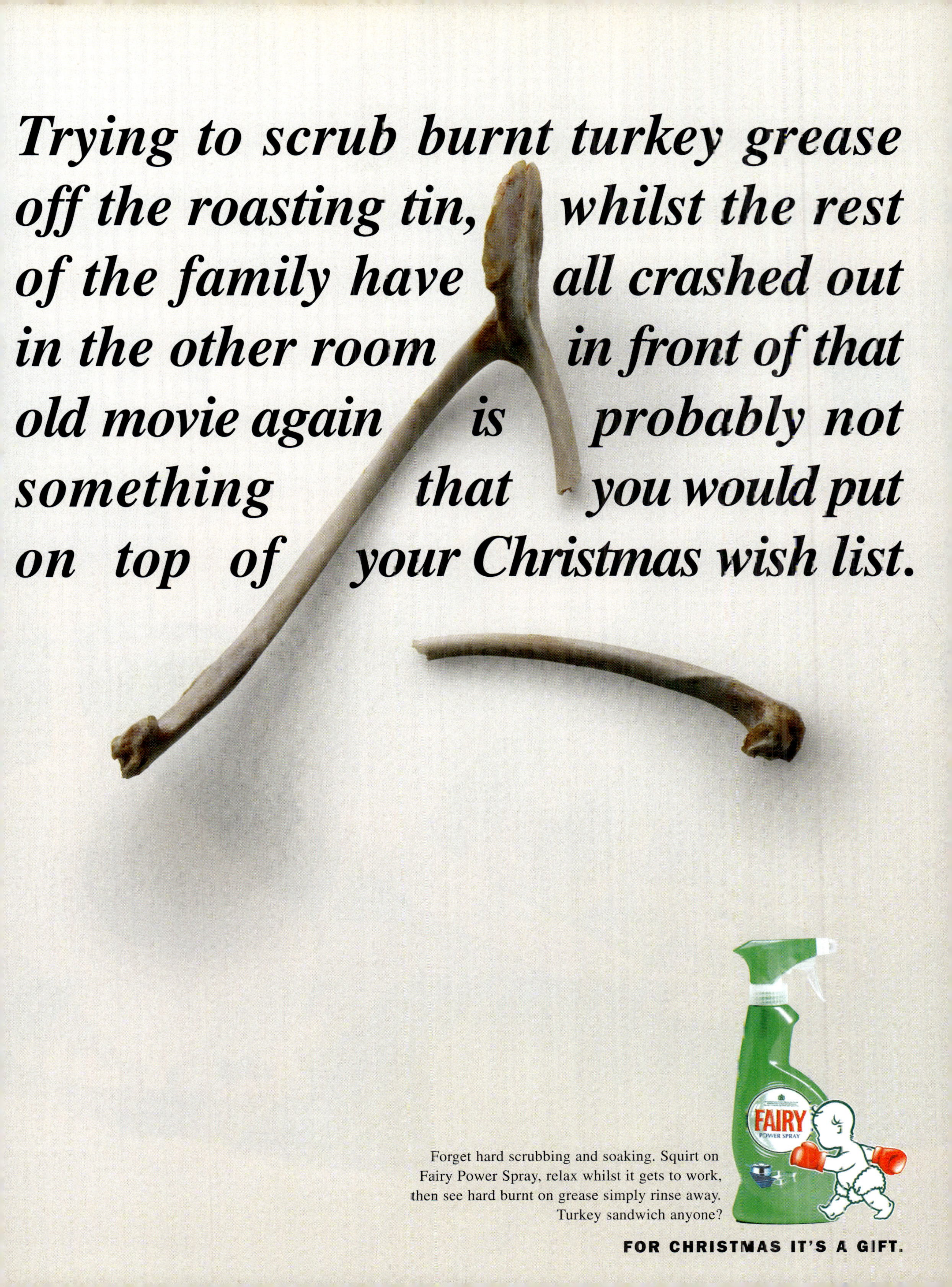
Trying to scrub burnt turkey grease off the roasting tin, whilst the rest of the family have all crashed out in the other room in front of that old movie again is probably not something that you would put on top of your Christmas wish list.
FAIRY
POWER SPRAY
Forget hard scrubbing and soaking. Squirt on Fairy Power Spray, relax whilst it gets to work, then see hard burnt on grease simply rinse away. Turkey sandwich anyone?
FOR CHRISTMAS IT'S A GIFT.

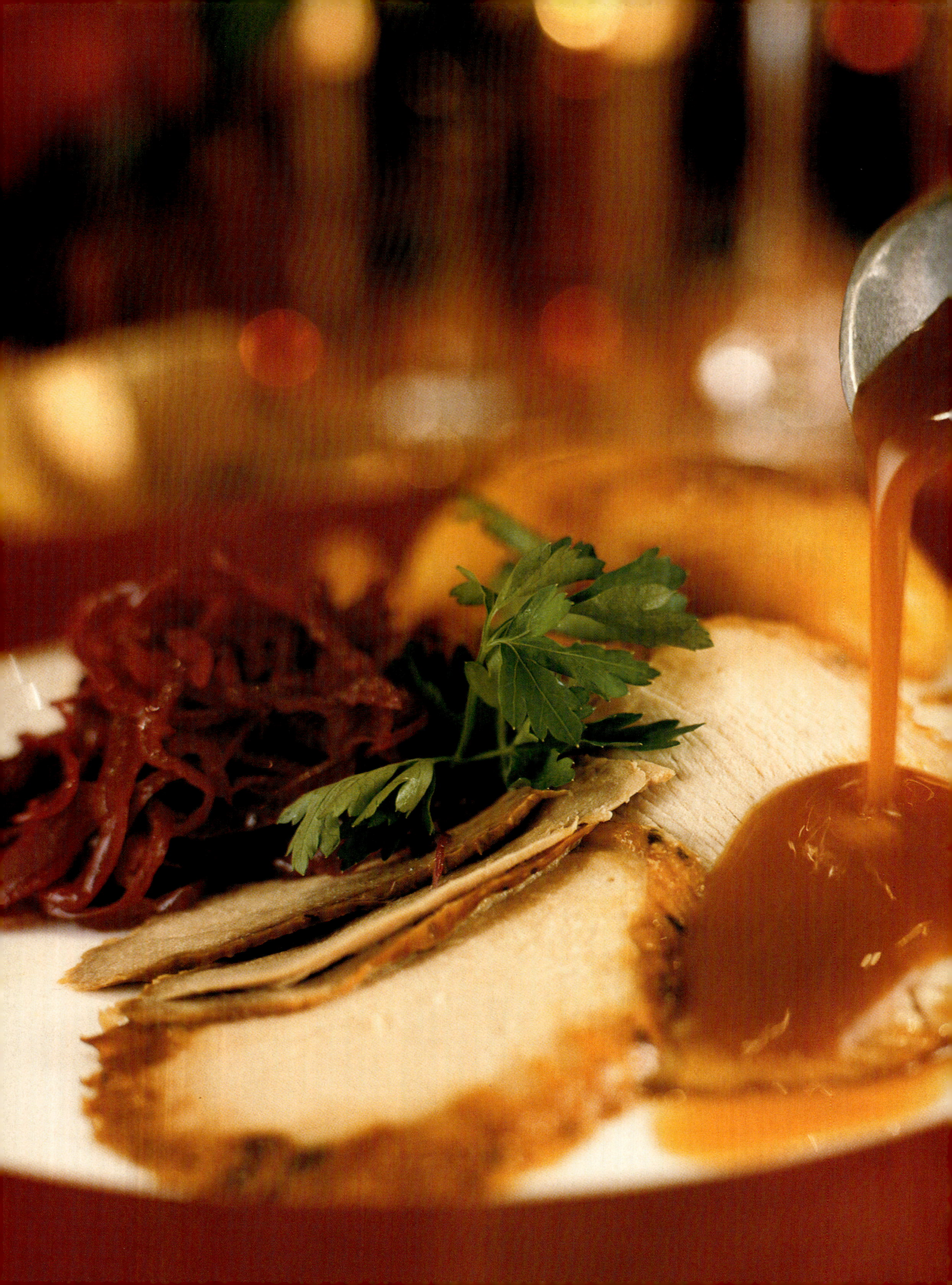

EVERYTHING YOU NEED TO KNOW ABOUT

Christmas Lunch

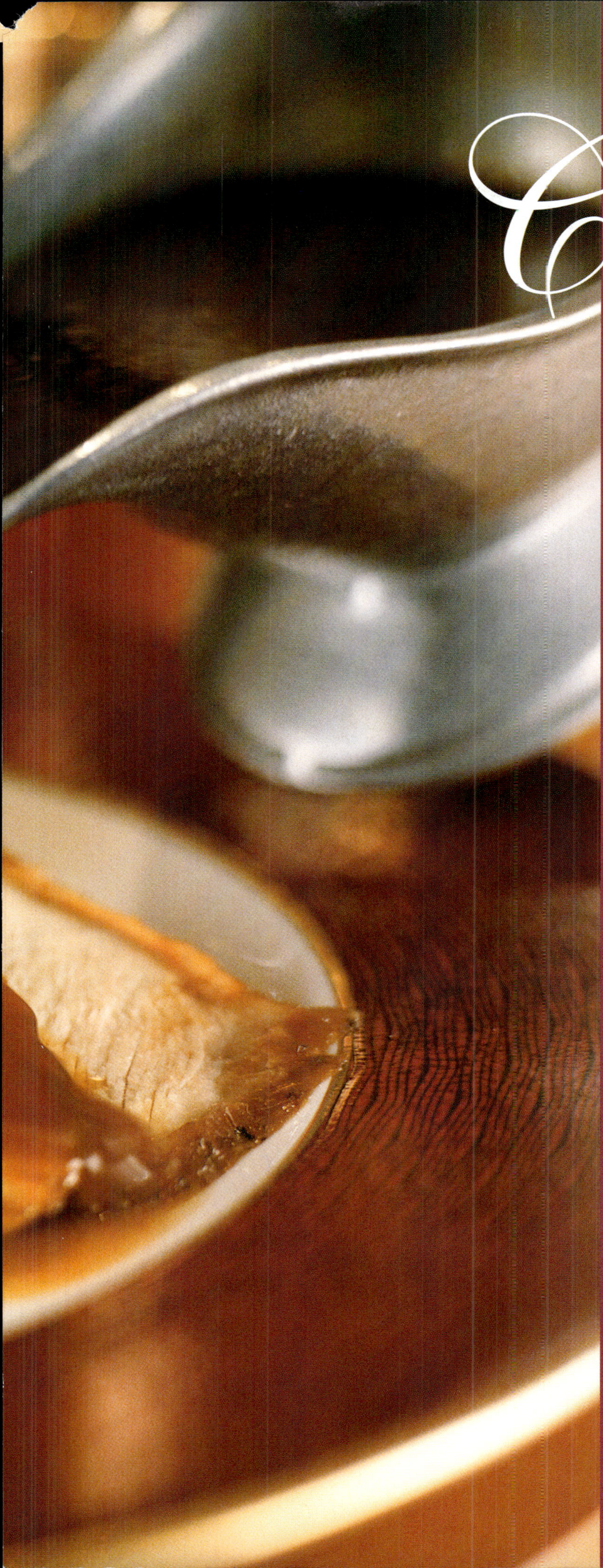

How can you guarantee a gorgeous Christmas lunch that everyone will love? For those of you who like to do things the traditional way, you can't go wrong with any of our delicious **turkey** recipes. If you fancy ringing the changes, why not try a **roast with a difference**, such as **goose, guinea fowl** or **gammon**? We haven't forgotten all the trimmings, either. You'll find an excellent selection of **sauces, relishes** and **gravies**, plus a mouthwatering array of seasonal **vegetables** and suggestions on how to serve up the crispiest **roast potatoes** around – which all adds up to your best Christmas lunch ever.

Parsley, Garlic, Sage and Thyme Turkey

Hands-on time: 40min
Cooking time: 3hr 45min
Serves: 16

FOR THE STUFFING

* 2tbsp olive oil
* 1 large onion, finely chopped
* 2 garlic cloves, crushed
* 75g (3oz) fresh white breadcrumbs
* 50g (2oz) pistachios, chopped
* Zest of 1 lemon
* 2tbsp each of freshly chopped flat-leafed parsley and sage
* 1 medium egg, lightly beaten
* Juice of ½ lemon

FOR THE TURKEY

* 6.3kg (14lb) turkey
* 2tsp sea salt
* 3tbsp chicken seasoning mix
* 2 small red onions, halved
* 1 garlic clove
* 1 lemon, halved
* 6 thyme sprigs
* 4 sage sprigs
* 4 sprigs of flat-leafed parsley
* A trussing needle and 2m fine string

FOR COOKING THE TURKEY

* 250g pack of butter
* 60cm (24in) square of muslin
* 12 sage leaves
* 10 sprigs of thyme
* 2 lemons, cut into wedges
* 4 small red onions, cut into wedges
* 4 garlic cloves

1 To make the stuffing (ideally the day before to enhance the flavour), heat the olive oil in a pan and fry the onion and garlic gently for 5min to soften but not brown, then cool. Put the breadcrumbs, pistachios, lemon zest, parsley, sage and egg into a bowl, then pour the lemon juice over. Add the onion mixture, then season. Stir to bind together, then cool.

2 Take the turkey (to save time, prepare the day before) and stand it upright on a board with the parson's nose facing upwards. Sprinkle the inside cavity with the sea salt, some coarse ground black pepper and 1tbsp of the chicken seasoning, then pack the onion, garlic, lemon, thyme, sage and parsley into the cavity.

3 Sit the turkey with the parson's nose facing away from you. Lift up the loose skin at the neck end with one hand and, using the other, fill the cavity with stuffing (for safety, it's essential the stuffing is cool). Turn the turkey onto its breast, lift the neck flap up and over the stuffing to cover, and rest the wing tips across it to secure.

4 Use the trussing needle and string to oversew the neck flap to the turkey to enclose the stuffing. Push the needle into one wing, then through to the other. Pull tight. Tuck in the parson's nose and secure with a skewer. Bring the string up and under the leg, and wrap tightly around the loop of the skewer. Tie the legs together, securing with a double knot. Weigh to calculate the cooking time (see Turkey Planner).

5 Melt the butter in a pan and pour into a roasting tin. Cool slightly before immersing the muslin, then stretch it out, with the edges overhanging the tin. Put the turkey in the middle, sprinkle with the remaining chicken seasoning, then season with ground black pepper. Scatter the sage and thyme across the turkey and arrange the lemon, onion and garlic around. Wrap the turkey in the muslin and turn it over so it's sitting breastside down in the tin. (If preparing ahead, cover the muslin-wrapped turkey with foil or clingfilm. Store in the bottom of the fridge. Remove from the fridge one hour before cooking.)

6 Roast in a preheated oven at 200°C (180°C fan) mark 6 for 3hr 40min (see the Turkey Planner). After 1hr 50min, turn the turkey over so that it's breastside up and continue roasting for a further 1hr 50min, or until the juices run clear when a knife is inserted into the thigh. Remove from the tin. Unwrap, put the turkey onto a serving dish, cover with foil and rest for 30min before carving.

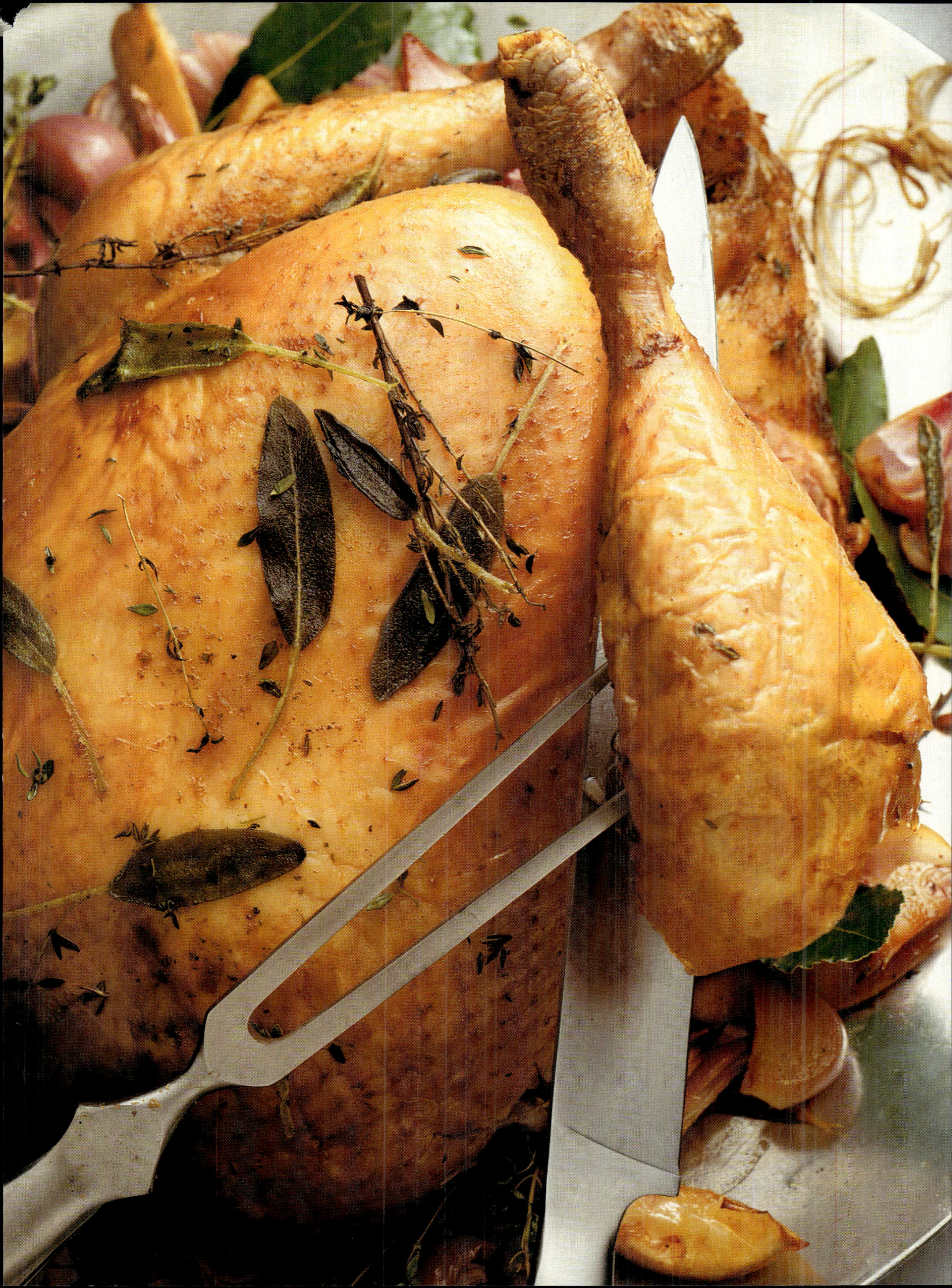

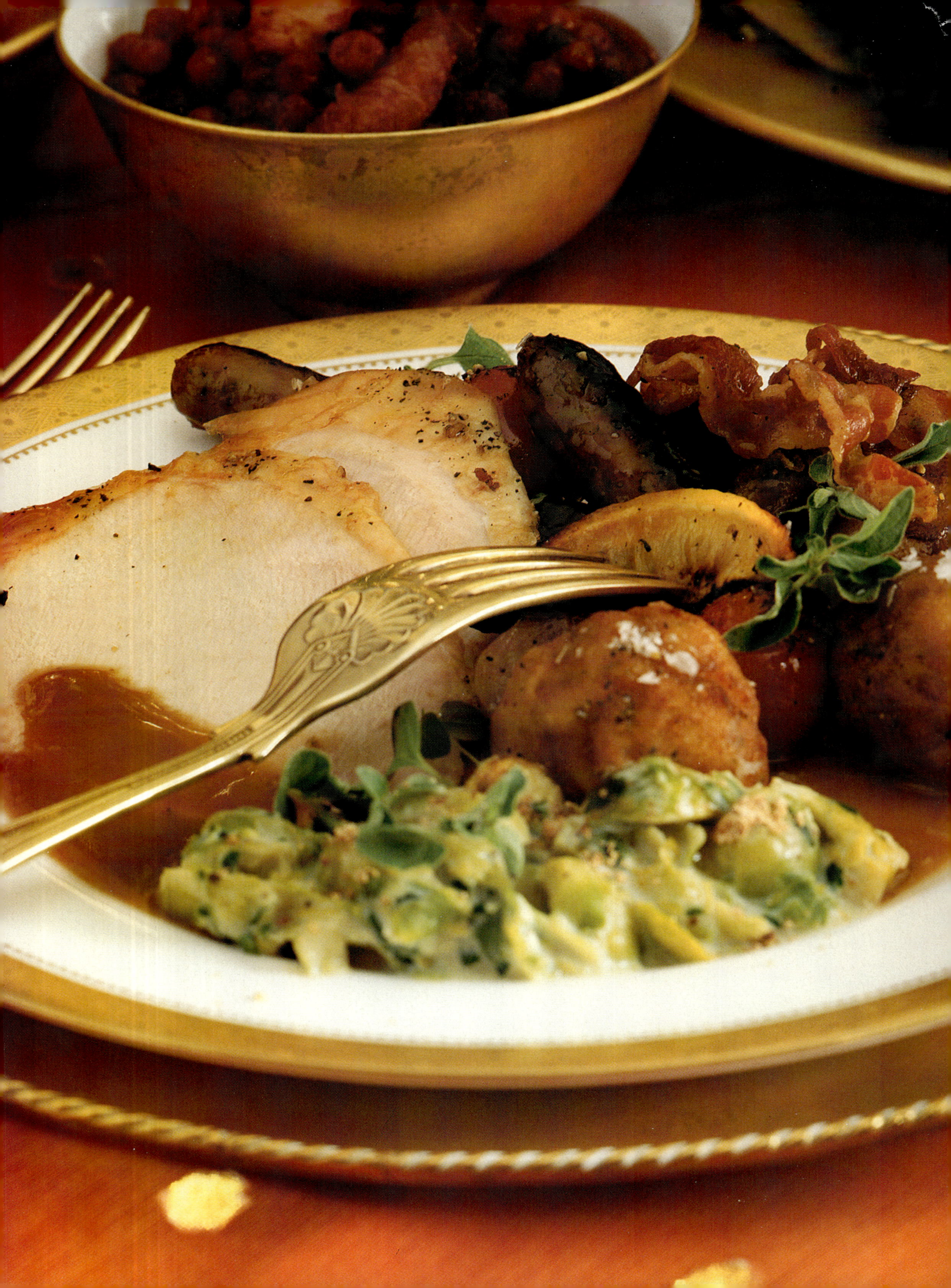

Lemon and Herb-roasted Turkey

Hands-on time: 20min
Cooking time: about 3hr, plus at least 30min resting
Serves: 8-10

* 4.5kg (10lb) turkey
* 1 large bunch fresh thyme
* 1 large bunch fresh rosemary
* 3 lemons, preferably unwaxed, cut into chunks
* 1 large Spanish onion, about 450g (1lb), cut into chunks
* 450g (1lb) prepared stuffing of your choice (see Stuffings)
* 125g (4oz) butter, softened
* 375g (13oz) pancetta or thinly sliced streaky bacon
* 150ml (¼ pint) white wine
* Fresh thyme and rosemary sprigs to garnish

FOR THE SAUSAGES WITH PLUM SAUCE

* 900g (2lb) sausages
* 250g pack of vacuum-packed chestnuts
* 4tbsp plum sauce

1 To make the carving easier, first remove the wishbone from the turkey. Loosen the skin at the neck end, then ease your fingers up between the skin and the breast and, using a small, sharp knife, remove the wishbone. Remove the giblets. Season the inside of the turkey, then stuff with thyme and rosemary sprigs and a few pieces of lemon and onion. Spoon the cold prepared stuffing into the neck end only, neaten the shape, tuck the skin under and secure with metal skewers or cocktail sticks. Weigh the turkey to calculate the cooking time (see Turkey Planner). To prepare ahead, cover and chill for up to 24hr; take the turkey out of the fridge 1hr before cooking.

2 Place the turkey in a large roasting tin, spread with the butter and arrange the slices of pancetta or bacon on the breast. Place the remaining lemon and onion chunks around the turkey and add the wine to the tin (this will keep the turkey succulent). Cover with a loose tent of foil. Roast at 190°C (170°C fan) mark 5 for about 3hr (see the Turkey Planner), basting from time to time. If the butcher has tied the legs together tightly, loosen after the first hour so they cook through more evenly. Remove the foil 45min before the end of the cooking time, lift off the pancetta and set aside.

3 Return the turkey to the oven to continue cooking. When it is cooked (the juices should run clear when a skewer is inserted deep into the thigh), tip up the turkey so the juices run into the tin, then place the turkey on a carving board. Place the pancetta back on the breast, cover the turkey with foil and set aside to rest for 30min.

4 To cook the sausages, place in a roasting tin and cook in the oven for 1¼hr below the turkey. After this time, stir in the chestnuts and plum sauce and return to the oven to cook for a further 15min on the top shelf.

5 Garnish the turkey with the thyme and rosemary sprigs and serve with roasted lemons, onions, fresh herbs, stuffing and sausages. You could also serve with grilled tomatoes drizzled first with balsamic vinegar and olive oil.

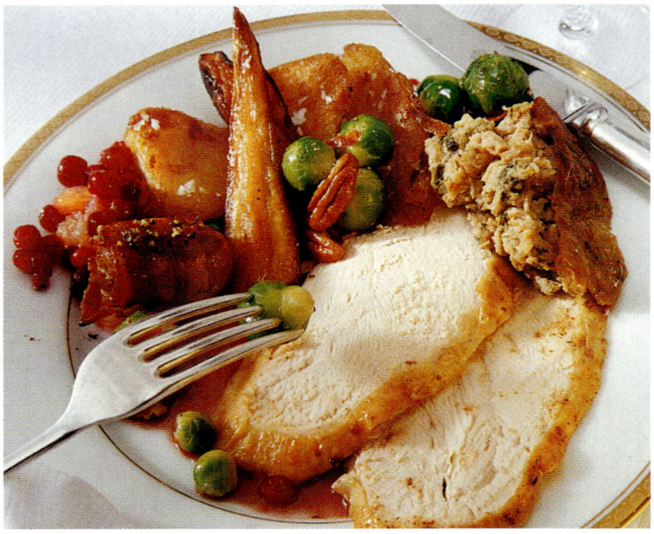

Spiced Roast Turkey

Hands-on time: 30min
Cooking time: 3hr
Serves: 8-10

* 4.5kg (10lb) turkey, with giblets
* Pork, Spinach and Apple Stuffing (see Stuffings)
* 2tsp Cajun spice mix
* 150g (5oz) salted butter, softened
* Holly sprig to decorate

1 Loosen the skin at the neck end of the turkey, then ease your fingers up between the skin and the breast and, using a small, sharp knife, remove the wishbone. Remove the giblets and reserve these to make the stock for the Turkey Gravy (see Sauces).

2 Season the inside of the turkey, then spoon the cold stuffing into the neck end only. Neaten, tuck the skin under and secure with skewers or cocktail sticks. (To prepare ahead, stuff the turkey 24hr earlier and remove from the fridge 1hr before cooking.) Weigh the turkey to calculate the cooking time (see Turkey Planner).

3 Put the turkey in a large roasting tin, mix the spice with the butter, smear over the turkey and season. Cover with a tent of foil. Roast at 190°C (170°C fan) mark 5 for about 3hr (see the Turkey Planner), basting from time to time. If the legs have been tied together tightly, loosen after the first hour so they cook through more evenly. Remove the foil covering 45min before the end of the cooking time.

4 When the turkey is cooked (the juices should run clear when a skewer is inserted deep into the thigh), tip up the turkey so the juices run into the tin, then serve on a platter together with Rosemary-roasted Bacon Rolls and Chipolatas (see Side Dishes). Decorate with a holly sprig.

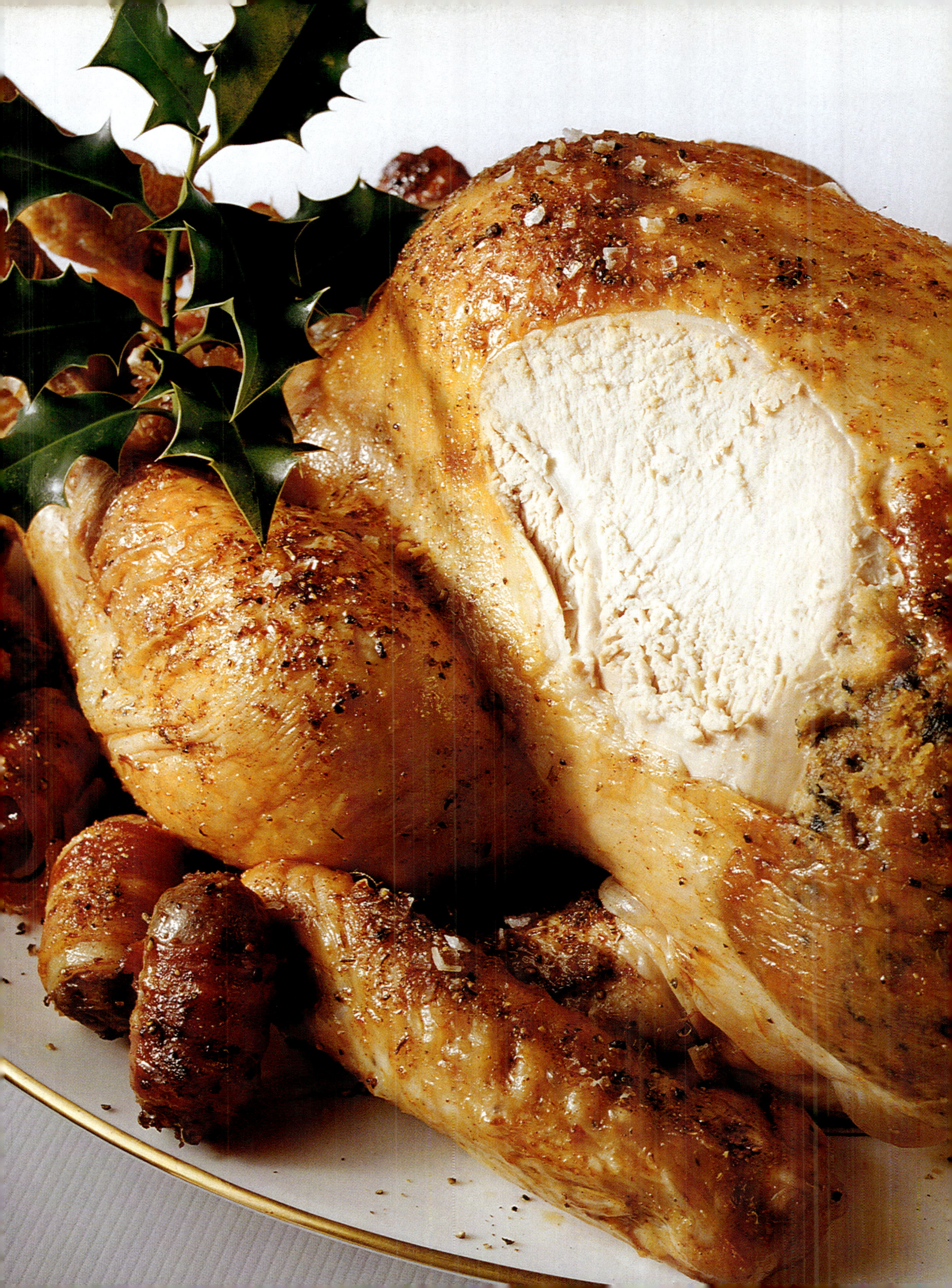

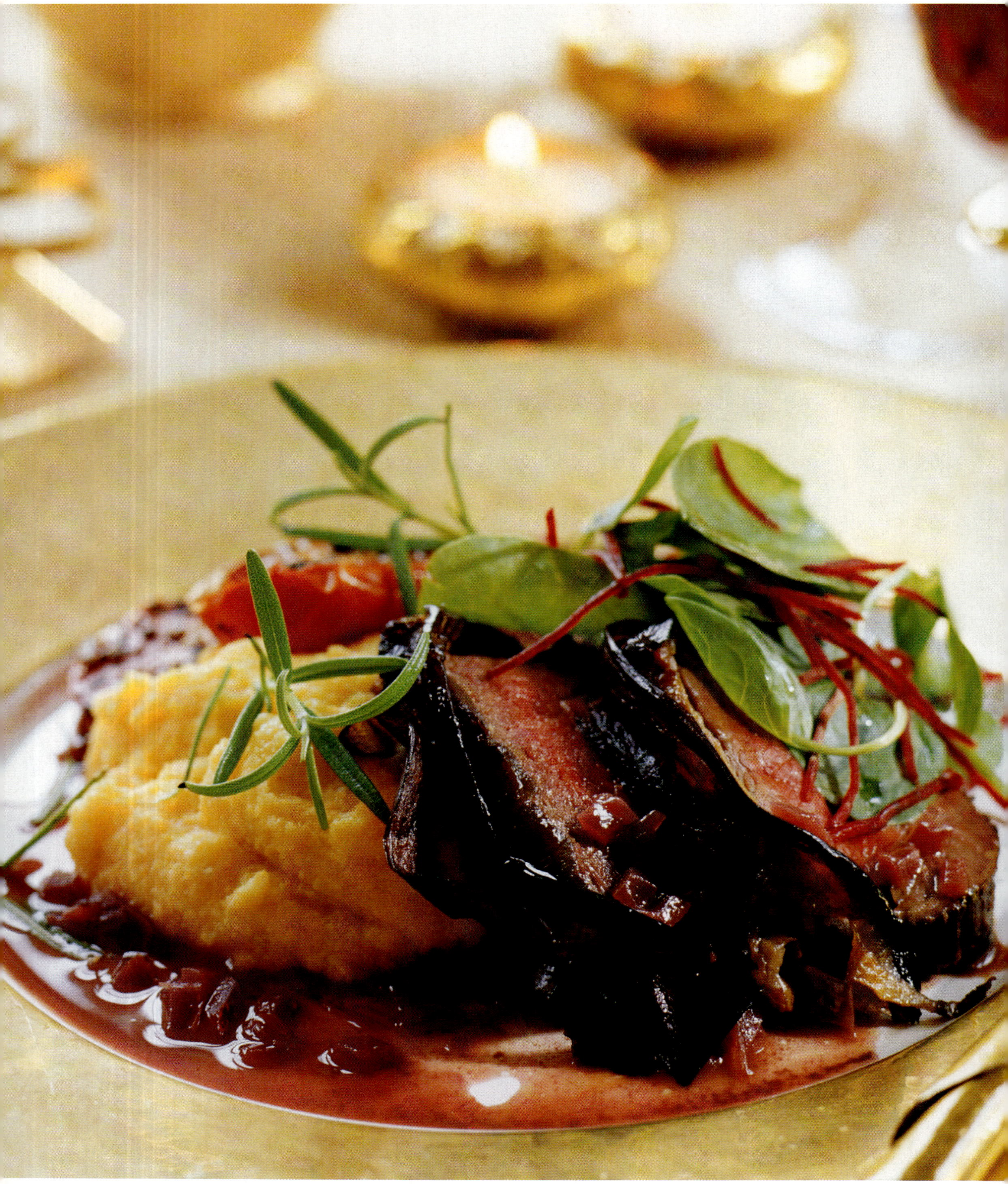

Fillet of Beef with Roquefort Butter Sauce

Hands-on time: 30min
Cooking time: About 1hr 10min
Serves: 6

* 125g (4oz) Roquefort cheese, crumbled
* 125g (4oz) unsalted butter, softened
* 900g (2lb) fillet beef
* 7tbsp vegetable oil
* 2 garlic cloves, crushed
* 2 large aubergines, 400g (14oz) each, cut lengthways into 1cm (½in) slices
* 150g (5oz) onion, finely chopped
* 150ml (¼ pint) medium-dry sherry
* 750ml (1¼ pints) fresh meat stock
* Lemon juice to taste
* Rosemary sprigs, baby spinach and beetroot shavings to garnish

For the polenta

* 900ml (1½ pints) milk
* 125g (4oz) polenta
* 4tbsp olive oil
* 75g (3oz) finely grated Parmesan cheese

1 Gently stir the cheese into the butter (don't overbeat or it will turn grey). Cover and chill. Season the beef. Heat 1tbsp oil in a frying pan for 1–2min, then brown beef for 1–2min on each side. Set aside to cool.

2 Rub the beef with the garlic. Brush each side of the aubergine slices with oil and fry in a non-stick frying pan for 4–5min on each side or until golden, then cool. Wrap the aubergine around the beef and tie at intervals with string. Season and set aside.

3 Heat 2tbsp oil in the frying pan, add the onion and cook for 10min or until golden. Add the sherry, bring to the boil and bubble to reduce by half. Add the stock, bring to the boil again and bubble for 10–15min or until reduced by half. Set aside.

4 Roast the beef at 220°C (200°C fan) mark 7 for 30min for rare, 35min for medium rare and 40min for well done. Cover and set aside in a warm place for 10min.

5 To make the polenta, pour the milk into a large pan, add a pinch of salt and bring to the boil. Remove from the heat and add the polenta in a slow, steady stream, stirring constantly. Return the mixture to a low heat and simmer, stirring, for 5min. Remove from the heat and stir in the olive oil and finely grated Parmesan cheese. Season and set aside.

6 To finish, reheat the sherry stock mixture, whisking in the reserved Roquefort butter a little at a time. Add the lemon juice. Remove the string from the beef and thickly slice. Stir any leftover pan juices into the sauce. Garnish and serve with the polenta and Roquefort Butter Sauce.

Goose with Roasted Apples and Onions

Hands-on time: 30min
Cooking time: 4hr 15min
Serves: 8

FOR THE STOCK

* Giblets removed from the goose
* 1 carrot, chopped
* 1 celery stalk, chopped
* 1 onion, quartered
* 1 bouquet garni (made from 1 bayleaf, 1 thyme sprig and 1 parsley sprig)
* 6 black peppercorns

FOR THE GOOSE

* 5kg (11lb) oven-ready goose
* 6 small red onions
* 7 small red eating apples
* A small bunch sage
* A small bunch rosemary
* 1 bayleaf
* Sea salt

FOR THE GRAVY

* 30g packet Madeira Wine Gravy Mix
* 300ml (½ pint) red wine
* 200ml (⅓ pint) giblet stock
* A bunch of watercress to serve

1 To make the stock, put the giblets into a pan, add the remaining ingredients and pour over 1.1 litres (2 pints) cold water. Cover and bring slowly to the boil, then simmer for 1hr. Strain and reserve the liquid.

2 Wash the goose and pat dry with kitchen paper, then season the bird inside and out. Cut one of the onions and two of the apples into quarters and put into the cavity of the goose with half the sage, half the rosemary and the bayleaf. Tie the legs together with string and push a long skewer through the wings to tuck them close to the body. Put the goose breastside up onto a rack in a large roasting tin. Use a metal skewer to prick the breast all over to help release the fat during cooking. Season generously with sea salt and freshly ground black pepper. Put the rest of the onions around the goose. Cover the goose and tin with foil, then chill until required.

3 When you're ready to cook, preheat the oven to 230°C (210°C fan) mark 8. Calculate the cooking time and cook for 15min per 450g (1lb) plus 15min – this works out to be 3hr for a 5kg (11lb) goose. Roast for 30min.

4 Reduce the oven temperature to 190°C (170°C fan) mark 5. Use a baster to remove the fat from the base of the tin – a sturdy, stainless-steel type where you squeeze the bulbous rubber end to suck up the excess fat is best. Drizzle some fat over the goose to keep the flesh moist, then chill the rest in a jar. (The goose fat can be used at a later date to make the most delicious crisp roast potatoes.) Roast the goose for a further 1hr, then remove and reserve the excess fat again from the base of the tin and chill it.

5 Cook the bird for a further 30min, then remove the foil. Extract, reserve and chill the fat again, then add the remaining apples to the tin. Sprinkle the goose with the remaining sage and rosemary sprigs, then return it to the oven and roast for a further 1hr. To test whether the goose is cooked, pierce the thigh with a skewer – it's ready when the juices run clear. Put the cooked bird onto a warm platter, cover tightly with foil and leave to rest for 30min. Remove the apples and onions, cover and keep warm.

6 To make the gravy, pour out and reserve all but 1tbsp of the fat from the tin, then sprinkle in the gravy mix and whisk in the wine. Put the tin directly onto the hob and bubble the gravy for 5min to reduce it slightly. Stir regularly, scraping up the goodness from the base of the tin, then whisk in the stock and bring to the boil.

7 Take one roast apple and onion and add them to the gravy, pressing them down with the back of a wooden spoon. Simmer the gravy for 10min, then strain it through a metal sieve into a clean pan, squeezing the onion and apple with the spoon to extract as much flavour as possible. Cut the remaining apples and onions into wedges and serve with the goose. Garnish with watercress.

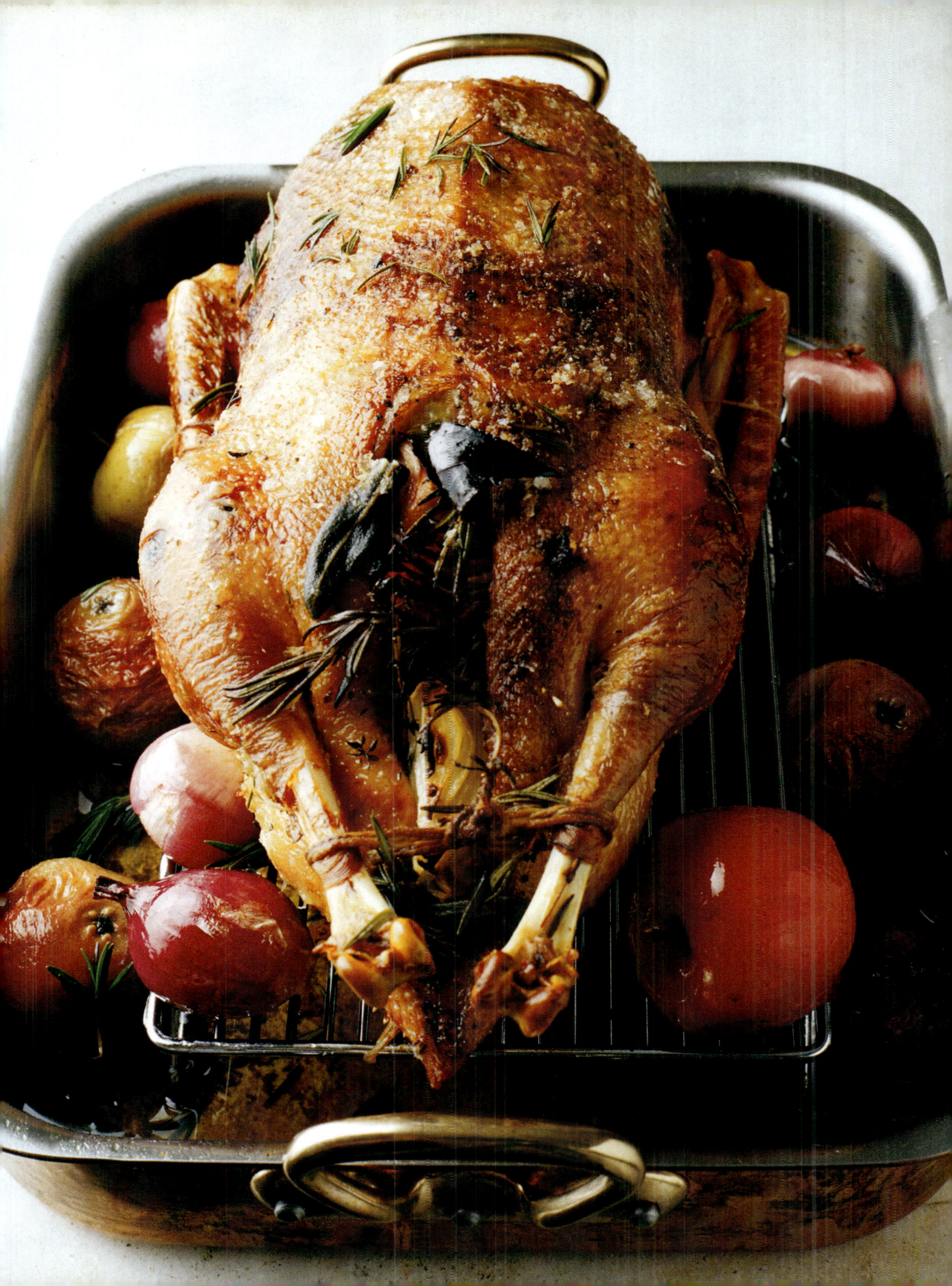

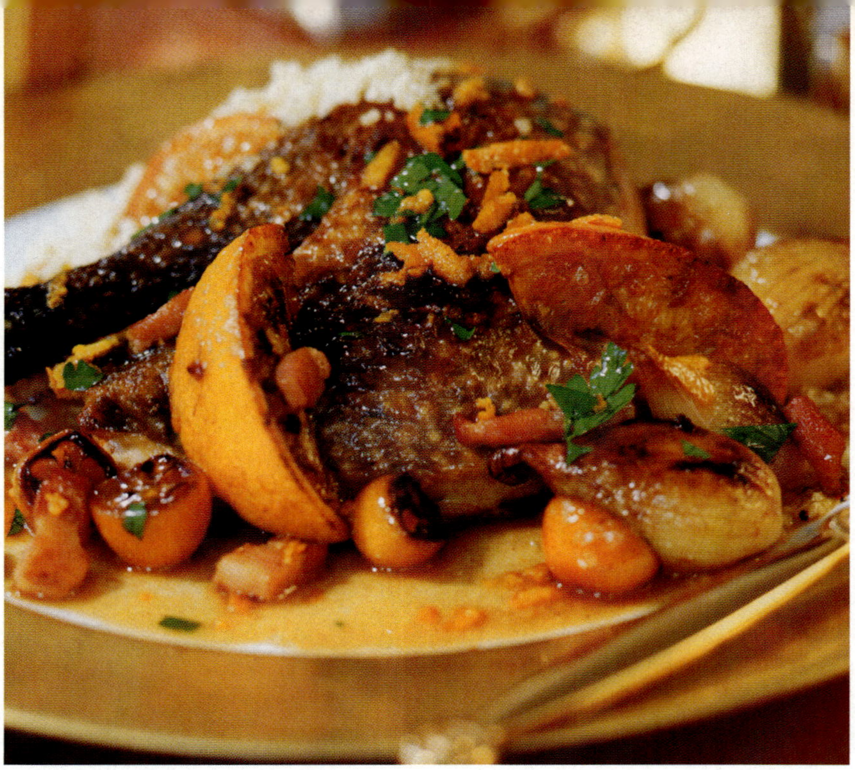

Guinea Fowl with Madeira

Hands-on time: 30min
Cooking time: 1½hr
Serves: 6

* 1tbsp oil
* 25g (1oz) butter
* 6–8 guinea fowl joints or corn-fed chicken joints, 2kg (4½lb) total weight
* 225g (8oz) shallots or button onions, peeled and with the root end trimmed
* 225g (8oz) streaky bacon, cut into thin strips or lardons
* 4 tangerines, halved, and the juice squeezed from 1
* 50g (2oz) kumquats, halved
* 2.5cm (1in) piece fresh root ginger, peeled and coarsely grated
* 2 garlic cloves, crushed
* 2tbsp plain flour
* 300ml (½ pint) Madeira
* 600ml (1 pint) fresh chicken stock
* 1 cinnamon stick
* 3tbsp redcurrant jelly
* 200g (7oz) vacuum-packed chestnuts (optional)
* Chopped flat-leafed parsley to garnish
* Couscous to serve

1 Heat the oil and butter in a deep flameproof casserole. Add the guinea fowl or chicken joints in batches and cook until brown on the skin side before turning and browning on the other side. (If you don't have a large enough casserole, brown the bird with the other ingredients in a large frying pan and continue the recipe using a large roasting tin covered with foil.) Remove the joints with a slotted spoon and set aside.

2 Add the shallots or button onions, bacon strips or lardons, tangerines and kumquats to the pan and cook, stirring, until brown. Stir in the ginger and garlic and cook for 1min. Stir in the flour, Madeira and chicken stock. Return the guinea fowl joints to the casserole, then add the cinnamon stick, tangerine juice and redcurrant jelly.

3 Bring to the boil, then cover, put in the oven and cook at 170°C (150°C fan) mark 3 for 50–60min or until tender. (The cooking time depends on the thickness of the joints rather than their weight, so return to the oven and cook for longer if necessary.)

4 Discard the cinnamon stick. Lift the guinea fowl out of the sauce and put on a serving dish. Cover with foil and keep warm. In a pan, bring the sauce to the boil, add the chestnuts, if using, and bubble for 10min or until the sauce has reduced by half. Pour the sauce over the guinea fowl and garnish with the parsley. If wished, serve with couscous.

To freeze: Complete the recipe. Cool, then pack and freeze.
To use: Thaw at cool room temperature overnight, then place the guinea fowl and sauce in a flameproof casserole, add 2tbsp water and bring to the boil. Place in the oven and reheat at 180°C (160°C fan) mark 4 for 30–40min or until hot to the centre.

Roast Pork with Apple and Saffron Chutney

Hands-on time: 20min, plus cooling
Cooking time: 1¾hr, plus 20min resting
Serves: 8

FOR THE CHUTNEY

* 30g (1¼oz) butter
* 75g (3oz) caster sugar
* 2 large Cox's Orange Pippin apples, peeled, cored and roughly diced
* 5tbsp cider vinegar
* A pinch of saffron, plus extra to garnish
* 100g (3½oz) dried cranberries
* 50g (2oz) sultanas
* 350g (12oz) pumpkin, peeled and diced
* ½ red chilli, deseeded and finely chopped

FOR THE PORK

* 2.3kg (5lb) loin pork (choose a thin, narrow joint), boned and skin finely scored
* Chopped flat-leafed parsley
* Root vegetable chips (such as parsnip) to serve

FOR THE CARAMELISED ONION SAUCE

* 40g (1½oz) butter
* 250g (9oz) onions, finely sliced
* 4tsp caster sugar
* 4tsp balsamic vinegar
* 200ml (7fl oz) white wine
* 450ml (¾ pint) fresh chicken or vegetable stock
* 20g (¾oz) softened butter
* 20g (¾oz) plain flour

1 To make the chutney, melt the butter and sugar in a heavy-based pan until golden. Add the remaining chutney ingredients and cook, stirring, over a medium heat until caramelised. Add 2tbsp water and simmer for 5–8min. Set aside to cool.

2 Slit the pork lengthways, almost through the muscle, and open out. Place two-thirds of the chutney down the middle and roll up. Tie the joint at intervals with string, but not too tightly. Reserve the leftover chutney.

3 Put the pork in a roasting tin, sprinkle the skin generously with salt, then cook at 200°C (180°C fan) mark 6 for 1¼hr. Add the reserved chutney to the tin for the last 10min of cooking time, then remove the pork from the oven, cover loosely and rest for 20min.

4 To make the caramelised onion sauce, melt the butter in a pan, add the onions and cook gently for 5–10min or until soft. Add the caster sugar and balsamic vinegar. Bring to the boil and bubble until almost all the liquid has evaporated and the onions are dark brown. Pour in the white wine and bring to the boil, then bubble to reduce by half. Add the fresh chicken or vegetable stock, bring to the boil and bubble for 5min. Season to taste.

5 To thicken the sauce, combine the softened butter and plain flour. Whisk the flour paste into the bubbling sauce, a little at a time. Cook for 3–4min. Remove the string, cut the pork into thick slices and garnish with the parsley and saffron. Serve with the Caramelised Onion Sauce and root vegetable chips.

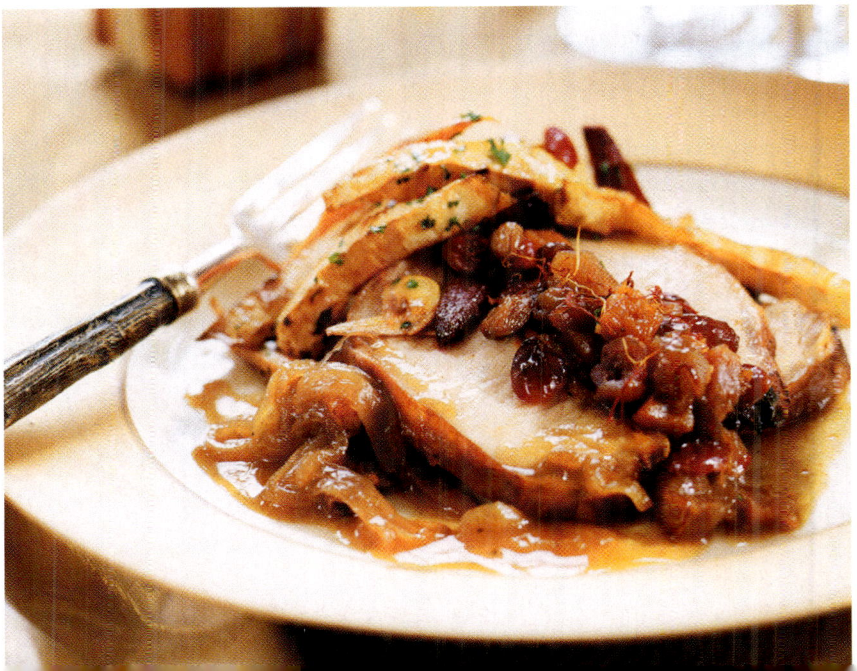

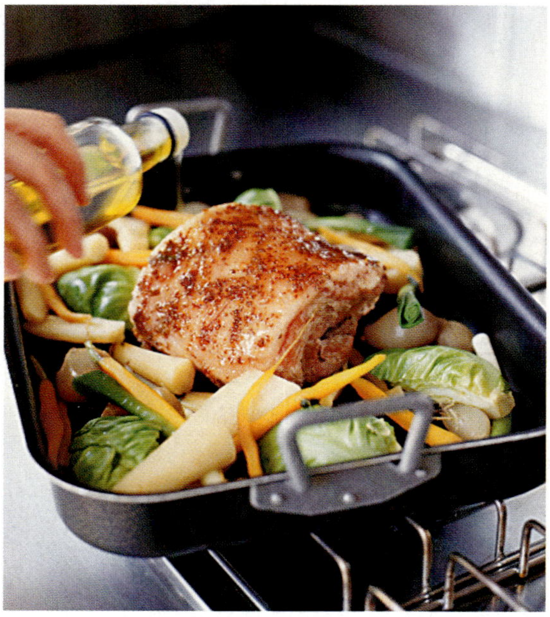

Glazed Roast Gammon

Hands-on time: 20min
Cooking time: 35–40min
Serves: 4

* 1kg (2¼lb) unsmoked gammon joint
* 6 whole allspice
* 6 peppercorns
* 2–3 sprigs each parsley and thyme
* 225g (8oz) each baby carrots and baby leeks
* 225g (8oz) baby parsnips, halved
* 225g (8oz) shallots, halved if large
* 2 small green cabbages, quartered, total weight around 450g (1lb)
* 3tbsp grainy mustard
* 3tbsp olive oil
* 3tbsp runny honey
* Fresh thyme sprigs to garnish

1 Put the gammon in a pressure cooker and add enough water to half fill the pan. Add the allspice, peppercorns and herbs, then cover and bring up to pressure. When hissing, set dial at number 2 or follow the instructions. Reduce the heat and cook for 25min. Run the cold tap in the sink and hold the pan under it to reduce the pressure quickly. Remove the lid, lift out the gammon, cover and put to one side.

2 Preheat the oven to 240°C (220°C fan) mark 9. Bring the stock back up to the boil, then add the baby carrots, leeks, parsnips, shallots and cabbage to the pan and blanch for 2min. Drain well.

3 Put the ham in a roasting tin with the vegetables. Mix together the mustard, 1tbsp olive oil and the honey, then drizzle over the ham. Pour the rest of the olive oil over the vegetables and season. Roast for 10–15min until golden and garnish with thyme to serve.

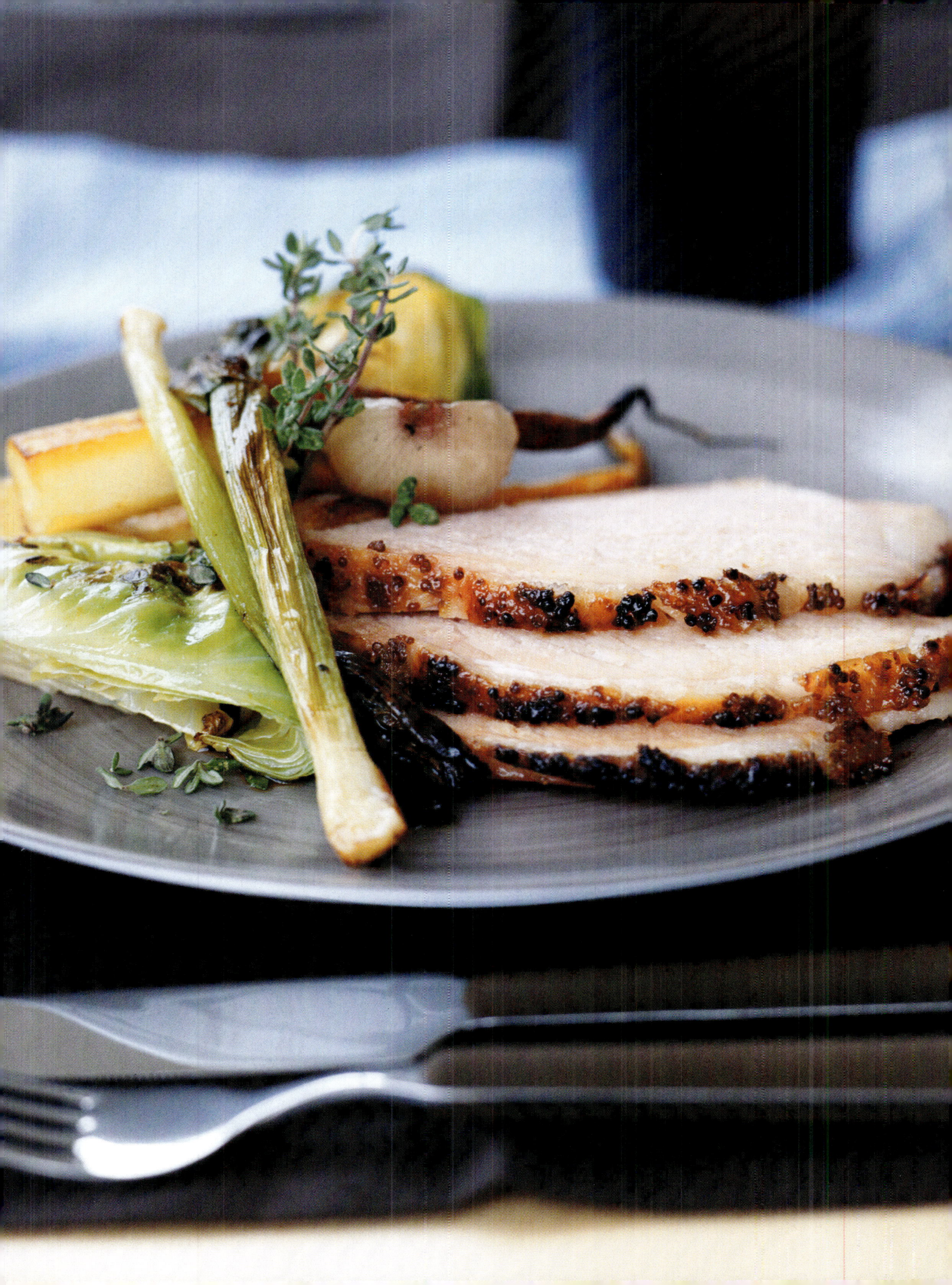

Spiced Cranberry and Orange Relish

Hands-on time: 15min, plus chilling
Cooking time: 1hr 5min
Serves: 8
Vegetarian

- 2tbsp olive oil
- 450g (1lb) red onions, thinly sliced
- Zest and juice of 1 large orange
- 1tsp coriander seeds, lightly crushed
- ½tsp ground cloves
- 1 bayleaf
- 150g (5oz) dark muscovado sugar
- 150ml (¼ pint) red wine
- 450g (1lb) cranberries

1 Heat the olive oil in a medium pan and gently cook the onions for 5min. Add the orange zest and juice, coriander seeds, ground cloves, bayleaf, sugar and red wine. Simmer gently for 40min, then discard the bayleaf.

2 Add the cranberries, bring back to the boil, then simmer for 20min. Cool. Cover and chill until ready to use.

Luxury Bread Sauce

Hands-on time: 10min
Cooking time: 15min
Serves: 8
Vegetarian

- 1 onion, peeled and quartered
- 4 cloves
- 1 bayleaf, plus another to garnish
- 450ml (¾ pint) milk
- 175g (6oz) fresh white breadcrumbs
- 50g (2oz) butter
- 200ml tub full-fat crème fraîche

1 Stud the onion with the cloves. Put into a medium pan with the bayleaf and add the milk. Gently heat on the lowest possible setting for 15min to let the flavours infuse.

2 Take the pan off the heat and discard the onion, cloves and bayleaf, then add the breadcrumbs and butter. Season. Stir in the crème fraîche, then cool. Cover and chill for up to two days. Garnish with a bayleaf to serve.

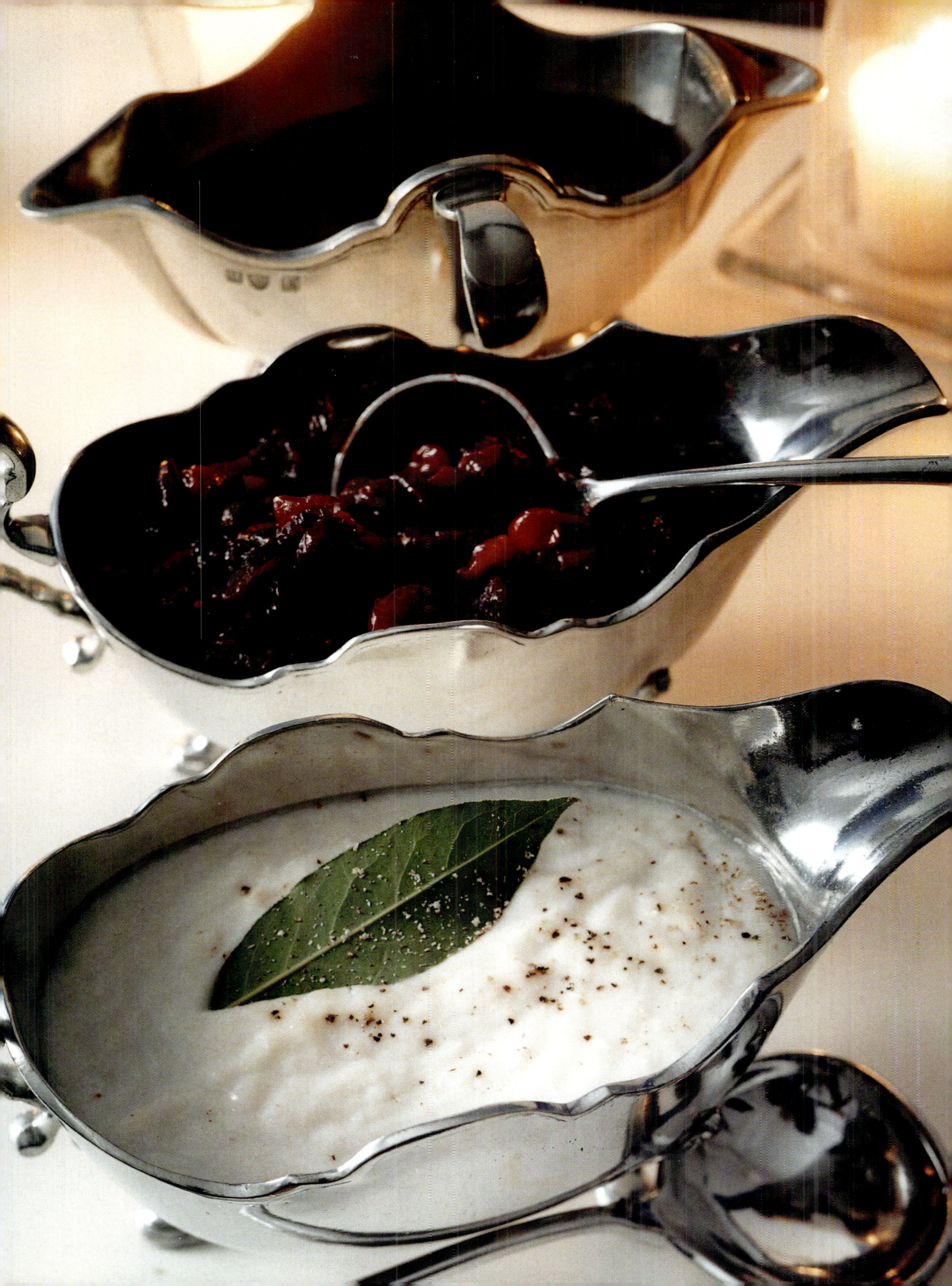

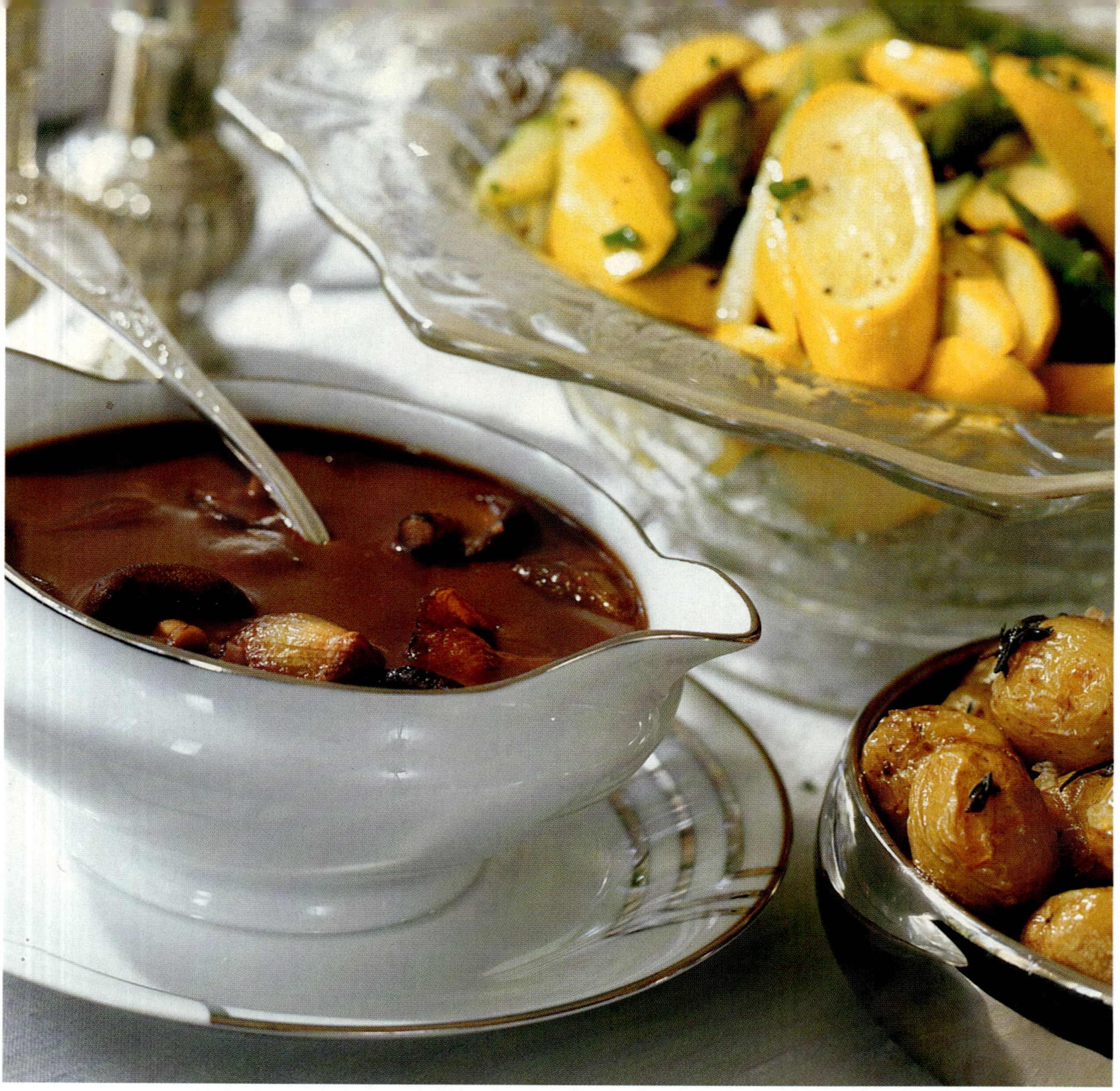

Shallot and Mushroom Sauce

Hands-on time: 15min
Cooking time: 1hr 10min
Serves: 6
Vegetarian

* 1tbsp olive oil
* 2 shallots, finely chopped and 350g (12oz) whole shallots, peeled
* 300ml (½ pint) red wine
* 225g (8oz) button mushrooms, quartered
* 1 celery stalk, cut in half
* 4 thyme sprigs
* 40g (1½oz) butter
* 1tsp caster sugar
* 15g (½oz) plain flour

1 Heat the olive oil in a medium pan and cook the chopped shallots until golden brown. Add the red wine, bring to the boil and bubble until reduced to about 2tbsp. Add the button mushrooms and cook for 3–4min. Add 600ml (1 pint) water, celery stalk and sprigs of thyme. Bring to the boil and simmer for 20min.

2 Meanwhile, heat 25g (1oz) butter in a frying pan, add the whole shallots and caster sugar. Cover and cook over a low heat for 20–25min.

3 Remove the thyme and celery from the sauce and pour over the shallots. Bring to the boil and bubble, uncovered, until reduced by half.

4 To thicken, combine the remaining butter, softened, and plain flour and whisk into the sauce. Simmer for 1–2min and season. Strain into a gravy boat and serve.

Cranberry Sauce

Hands-on time: 5min
Cooking time: 5min
Serves: 8
Vegetarian

- 350g (12oz) cranberries, fresh or frozen
- 125g (4oz) golden caster sugar
- Grated rind and juice of 1 orange
- 1–2tbsp port
- 8 juniper berries, crushed

1 Put all the ingredients in a medium pan, bring to the boil, then simmer until the cranberries pop and the sauce thickens. Cool, cover and chill until ready to use.

To freeze ahead: Complete the recipe, then cool, pack and freeze.
To use: Thaw at a cool room temperature for 2hr.

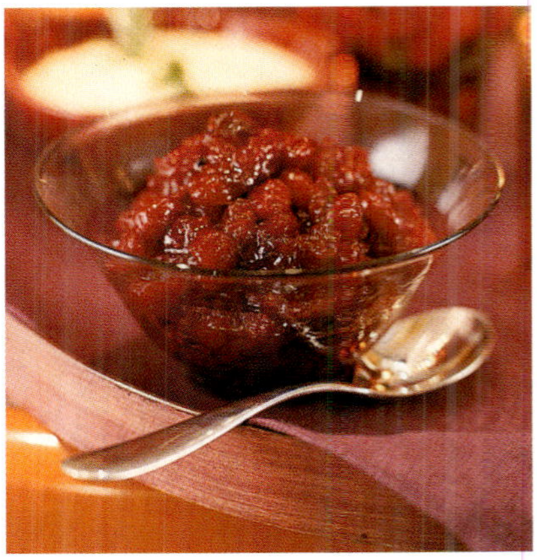

Cranberry, Orange and Port Sauce

Hands-on time: 10min
Cooking time: 20min
Serves: 8-10
Vegetarian

- 450g (1lb) cranberries
- Zest of 2 large oranges and flesh cut into segments
- 125g (4oz) caster sugar
- 150ml (¼ pint) port

1 Gently cook the cranberries and the orange zest in a heavy-based pan over a low heat for 5min or until the cranberry skins begin to split. Using a draining spoon, remove the cranberries from the pan and place in a bowl.

2 Add the caster sugar and port to the pan. When the sugar has dissolved, bring to the boil. Bubble until reduced by half and pour over the cranberries. Allow to cool, then add the orange segments. Cover and chill for up to four days.

To freeze ahead Complete the recipe, then cool, pack and freeze.
To use: Thaw overnight.

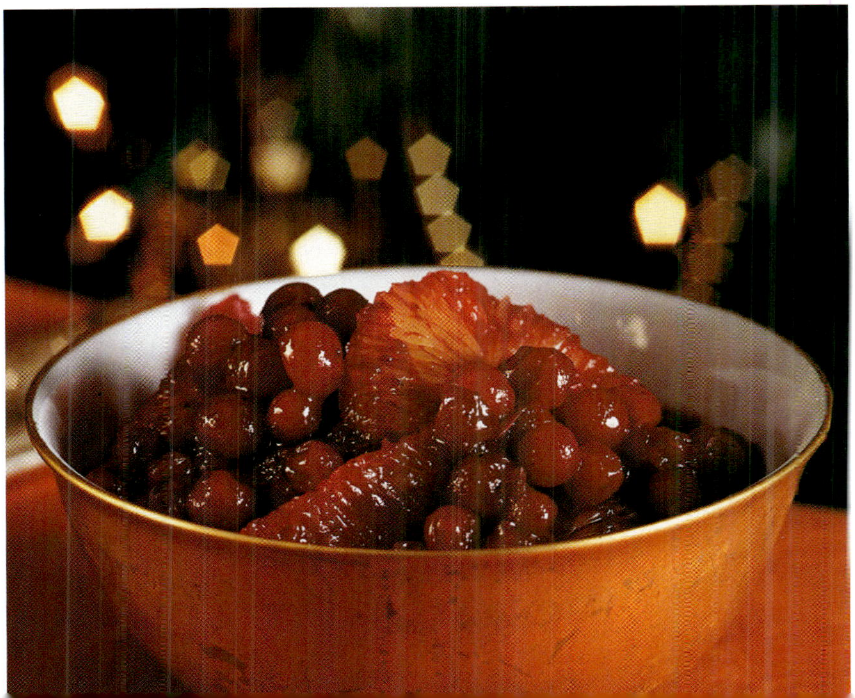

Turkey Gravy

Hands-on time: 5min
Cooking time: 2hr 20min
Serves: 8-10

* Turkey giblets
* Slices of onion, celery and leek
* Juices from the roast turkey
* 4tbsp plain flour
* 300ml (½ pint) red wine or port
* 1.1 litres (2 pints) turkey stock

1 To make the stock, place the giblets in a pan with 2.3 litres (4 pints) water and add the onion, celery and leek. Season, bring to the boil and simmer for 2hr. Strain, cool and chill until ready to use.

2 To make the gravy, strain the turkey juices from the roasting tin into a bowl and skim off any fat, reserving 3tbsp. Return the reserved fat to the tin and whisk in the flour to make a smooth paste. Cook over a moderate heat, whisking until the flour turns a russet brown.

3 Off the heat, add the red wine or port, stir until smooth, bring to the boil and bubble for 2–3min. Stir in the turkey juices and the stock, then bubble for 10–15min or until reduced by half. Skim off any fat and season. Strain into a gravy boat and serve.

Sherry Gravy

Hands-on time: 5min
Cooking time: 15min, if using ready-made turkey stock
Serves: 8-10

* Juices from the roast turkey
* Turkey giblets
* 3tbsp plain flour
* 200ml (7fl oz) dry sherry
* 1.1 litres (2 pints) turkey stock

1 Skim most of the fat from the turkey juices, leaving behind 2tbsp fat in the roasting tin. Add the giblets to the tin. Stir in the flour to make a paste, then put the tin over a moderate heat. Cook, stirring or gently whisking, for 2–3min until golden brown.

2 Add the dry sherry, bring to the boil and bubble for 1min. Add the stock, bring back to the boil and bubble for 5–10min until reduced by half and lightly thickened. Skim off any fat and season. Strain into a gravy boat and serve.

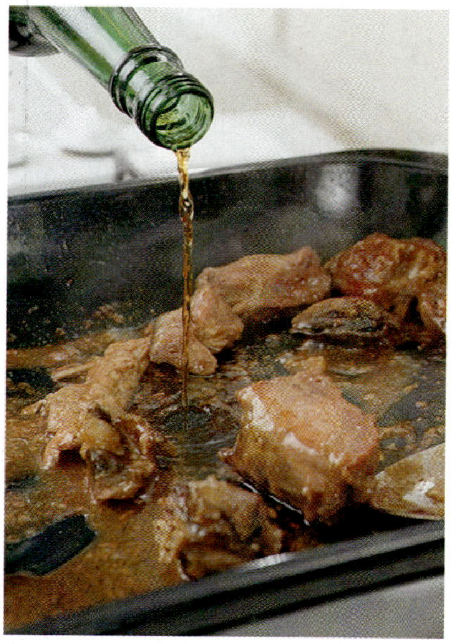

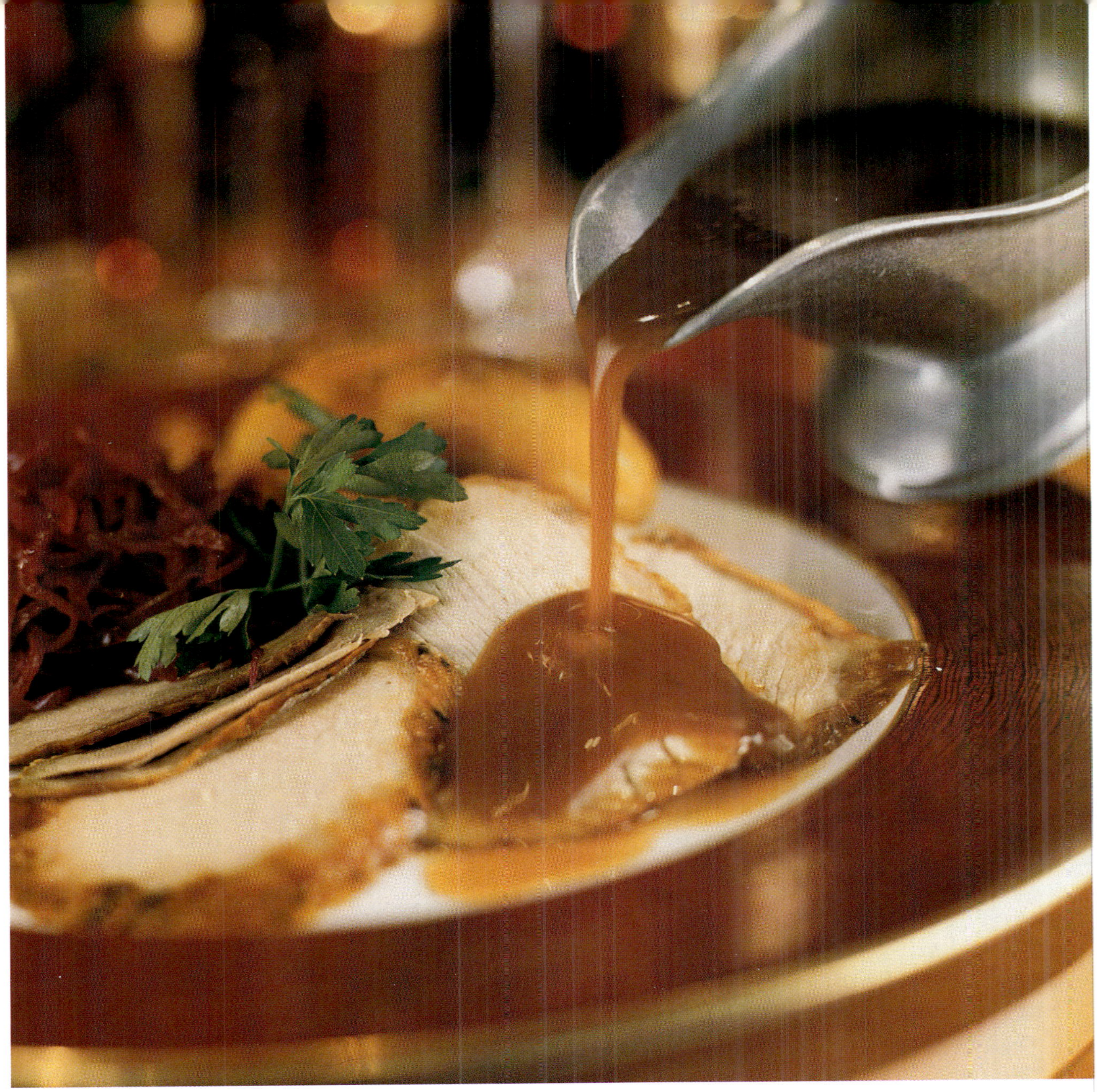

Rich Wine Gravy

Hands-on time: 5min
Cooking time: 40min
Serves: 8–10

* Turkey giblets
* 1 carrot, thickly sliced
* 1 onion, cut into wedges
* 1 stick celery, thickly sliced
* 8 black peppercorns
* 2 bayleaves
* Juices from the roast turkey
* 40g (1½oz) plain flour
* 150ml (¼ pint) white wine
* 2tbsp redcurrant jelly

1 Put the giblets, carrot, onion, celery, peppercorns and bayleaves in a large pan with 600ml (1 pint) cold water. Cover and bring to the boil. Simmer for 30min, skimming the surface from time to time, then discard the giblets and reserve the stock. The stock can be made the day before it is needed, then cooled and chilled before doing step 2 and 3.

2 Once the turkey has finished cooking (include quarters of lemon in the roasting tin for flavour), skim all the fat from the juices in the tin. In a bowl, mix 3tbsp of the juices to a smooth paste with the flour. Pour the stock into the tin with the wine and redcurrant jelly, scraping up all the goodness from the base of the pan.

3 Return the roasting tin to the heat, whisk in the flour mixture and bring to the boil. Simmer for 5–10min. Season. Strain into a gravy boat and serve.

Mushroom and Chestnut Wreath Stuffing

Hands-on time: 1hr
Cooking time: 1hr 5min
Serves: 16

FOR THE WREATH

* 50g (2oz) butter
* 1 onion, finely chopped
* 4tbsp chopped fresh sage
* 50g (2oz) walnut halves, toasted
* 125g (4oz) each ready-to-eat dried pears and apricots, roughly chopped
* 500g pack sausagemeat
* Oil to brush
* Plain flour to shape

FOR THE STUFFING

* 25g (1oz) butter
* 25g (1oz) dark muscovado sugar
* 2 onions, finely chopped
* 3tbsp balsamic vinegar
* 1 celery stalk, chopped
* 4tbsp chopped fresh oregano
* 75g pack dried cranberries
* 75g (3oz) fresh white breadcrumbs
* 125g (4oz) vacuum-packed chestnuts, chopped
* 350g (12oz) small chestnut mushrooms – around 16

TO FINISH

* 450g (1lb) chipolata sausages
* 12 rashers rindless streaky bacon, made into rolls
* 3 unwaxed oranges, cut into wedges
* Cocktail sticks
* 20 bayleaves, plus extra to garnish
* 2tbsp olive oil
* 4tbsp redcurrant jelly

1 To make the wreath, melt the butter in a pan and cook the onion until soft. Cool. Put the sage, walnuts, dried fruit and sausagemeat in a bowl with the onion, season and mix together.

2 Oil a round baking sheet or large, ovenproof glass dish. Dust your hands with flour and shape the stuffing on the baking sheet into a sausage, around 61cm (24in) long. Join the ends together to make a ring. Cover and chill.

3 To make the stuffing, melt the butter and sugar in a pan and cook the onions until soft. Add the vinegar and celery, bring to the boil and cook for 1min. Cool. Add the oregano, cranberries, breadcrumbs and chestnuts, season and mix well. Stuff the mushrooms with all the mixture.

4 Preheat the oven to 200°C (180°C fan) mark 6. Secure the chipolata sausages, bacon, mushrooms and orange to the sausage ring with cocktail sticks. Add the bayleaves, drizzle with oil and bake for 45min.

5 Melt the redcurrant jelly and brush over the wreath. Return to the oven for 10min or until cooked. Garnish.

To freeze ahead: Make the sausage ring, cover and freeze. Prepare the bacon rolls and freeze with the chipolatas. Make the stuffing and freeze. **To use:** Thaw for 2hr, stuff mushrooms, assemble wreath and follow the recipe from Step 4.

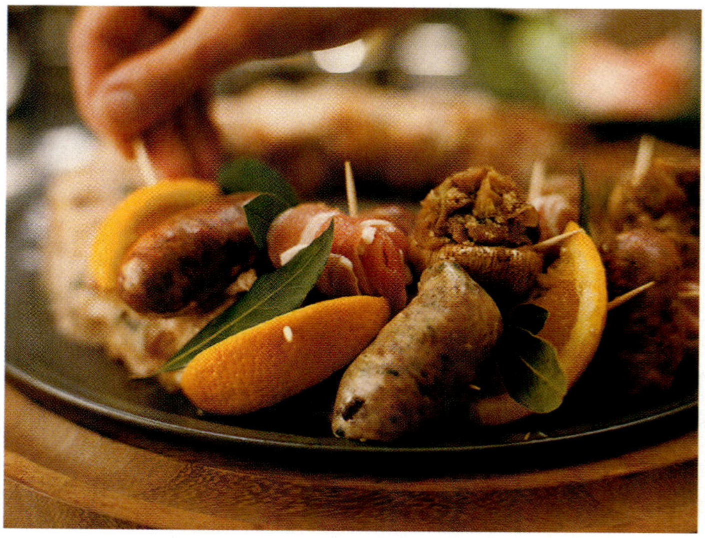

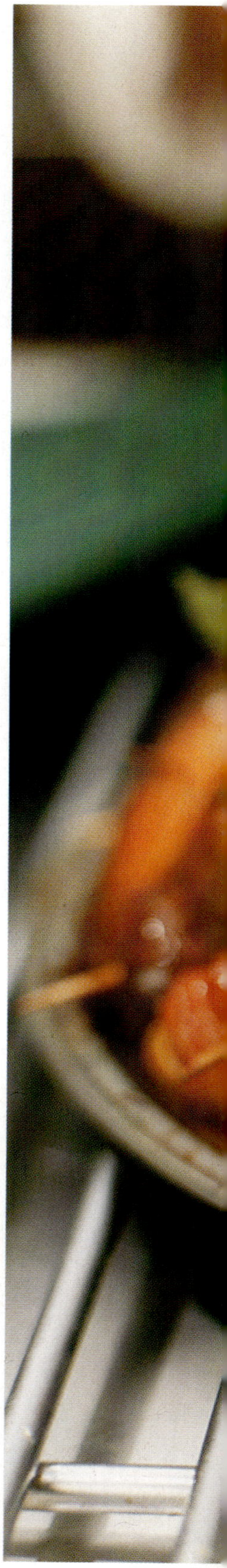

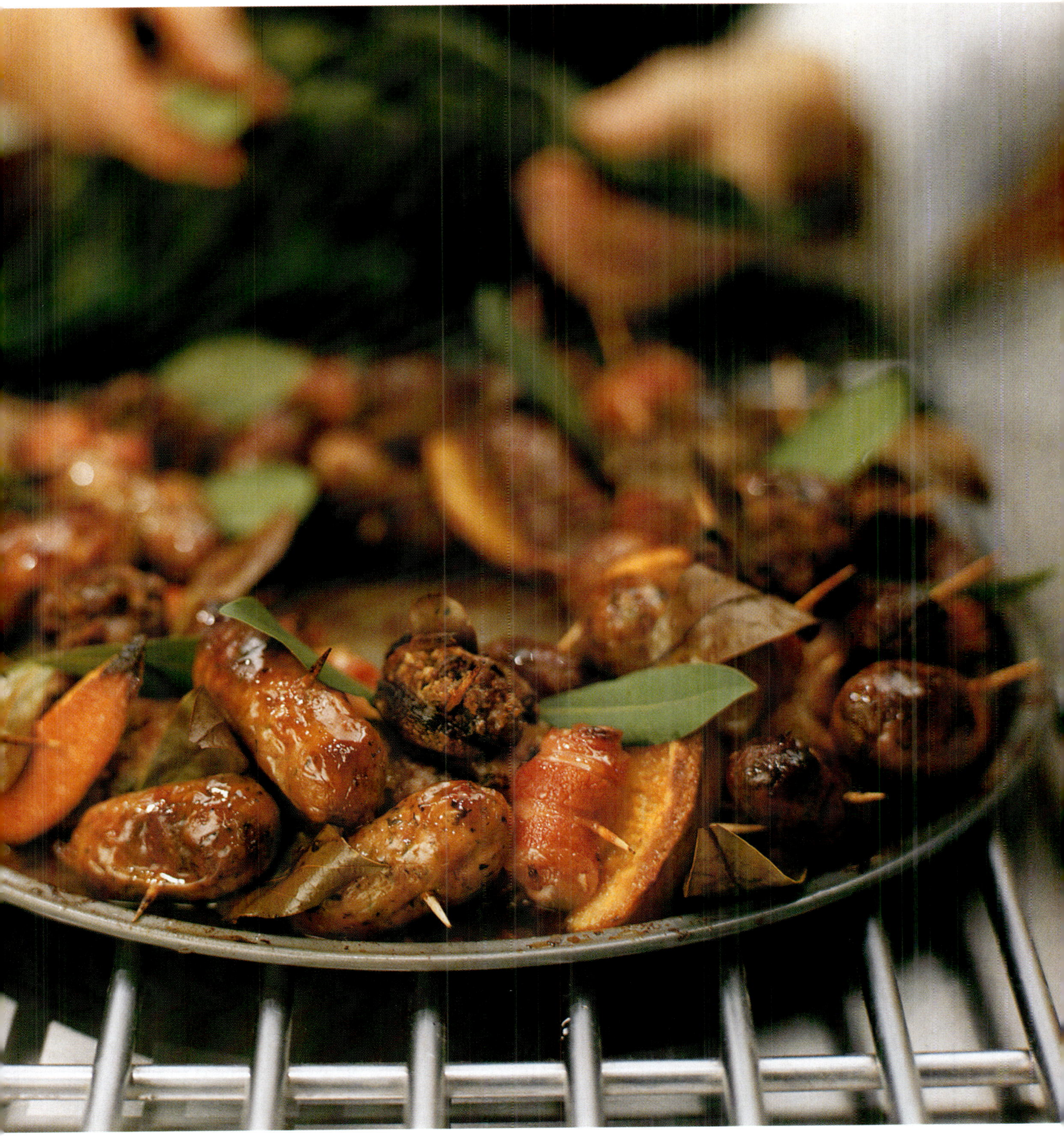

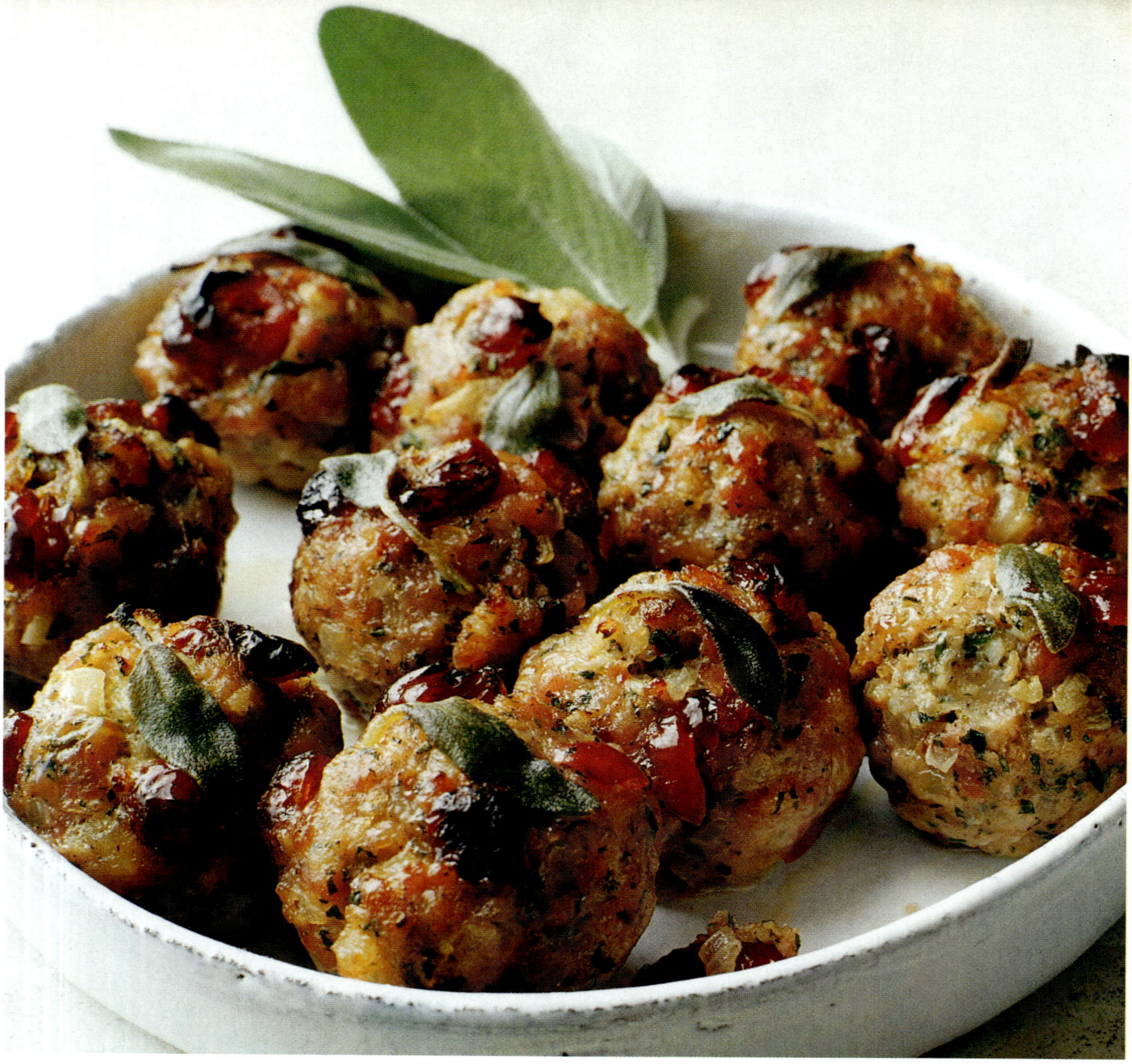

Cranberry and Lemon Stuffing Balls

Hands-on time: 35min
Cooking time: 20–25min (35–40min from frozen)
Makes: 18 balls

* 25g (1oz) butter
* 1 large onion, peeled and finely chopped
* 1 garlic clove, peeled and crushed
* 450g (1lb) best quality Lincolnshire sausages
* 4tbsp freshly chopped parsley
* 2tbsp freshly chopped sage, plus a few leaves to garnish
* Zest of 2 lemons
* 1tbsp brandy or Calvados (optional)
* 75g (3oz) dried cranberries

1 Melt the butter in a pan and sauté the onion for around 10min until soft but not coloured. Add the garlic and cook for a further 1min. Transfer to a bowl and cool.

2 Squeeze the meat from the sausages into the bowl with the cooled onion and garlic, discarding the sausage skins. Add the chopped parsley and sage, lemon zest, brandy (if using) and cranberries. Season, then mix well to combine – you may find it easiest to do this with clean hands.

3 Shape the mixture into 18 balls and put into mini paper muffin cases (to prevent it from sticking), then into mini muffin tins, if you like. Cover and freeze for up to one month.

4 Preheat the oven to 190°C (170°C fan) mark 5. Bake the stuffing balls from frozen for 35–40min until cooked and golden. Garnish with sage.

Orange, Sage and Thyme Stuffing

Hands-on time: 10min
Cooking time: 5min
Serves: 8
Vegetarian

* 2tbsp olive oil
* 1 large onion, finely chopped
* 2 garlic cloves, crushed
* 75g (3oz) fresh white breadcrumbs
* 50g (2oz) pine nuts, toasted and chopped
* Zest of 1 orange, plus 2–3tbsp juice
* 2tbsp each finely chopped fresh thyme and sage
* 1 medium egg yolk, beaten

1 Heat the olive oil in a frying pan and fry the onion and garlic gently for 5min to soften but not brown.

2 Put the breadcrumbs, pine nuts, orange zest and juice, herbs and egg yolk into a large bowl. Add the onion mixture, season and stir to bind, adding more orange juice if needed. Cool, bag and freeze for up to a month.

Couscous and Herb Stuffing

Hands-on time: 20min, plus 20min standing
Cooking time: 45min
Makes: about 450g (1lb)
Vegetarian

* 2tbsp olive oil
* 225g (8oz) onions, roughly chopped
* 1 garlic clove, crushed
* 100g (3½oz) couscous
* 1tsp paprika
* Zest of 1 lemon
* 1tbsp chopped fresh herbs
* 1 medium egg

1 Heat the olive oil and gently fry the chopped onion for 5min until soft but not coloured. Add the garlic and cook for 30sec.

2 Place the couscous in a heatproof bowl with freshly ground black pepper and 1tsp of salt. Pour boiling water over to cover the couscous by 5mm (¼in). Cover and leave in a warm place for 20min, then fluff up with a fork. Stir the onions and remaining ingredients into the couscous and season, then cool.

3 Use to stuff the turkey or butter a 450g (1lb) loaf tin, place the mixture in the tin and cover with foil. Cook at 200°C (180°C fan) mark 6 for 45min.

To freeze ahead: Complete the recipe, then pack and freeze.
To use: Thaw at cool room temperature overnight and use as wished.

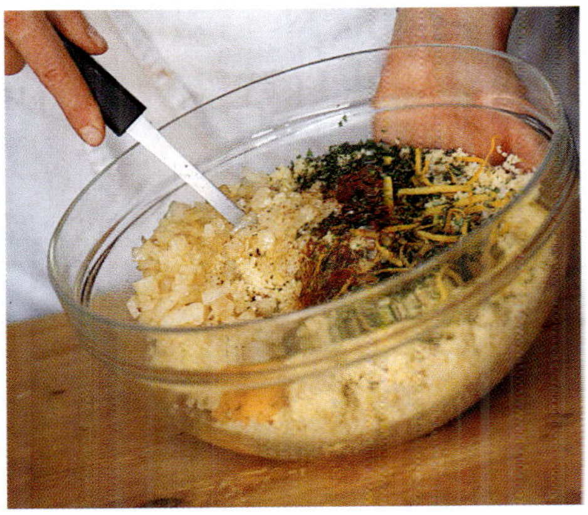

Rice and Apricot Stuffing

Hands-on time: 15min
Cooking time: about 1½hr
Makes: enough for a 4.5kg (10lb) turkey
Vegetarian

* 175g (6oz) mixed long-grain and wild rice, or basmati rice
* 150g (5oz) ready-to-eat dried apricots
* 50g (2oz) shelled, skinned pistachio nuts
* 200g (7oz) shallots or onions
* 3tbsp oil
* 4tbsp chopped flat-leafed parsley
* 1tbsp chopped fresh thyme
* 1 large egg, beaten

1 Cook the rice in a pan of boiling, salted water for 20min (12min for basmati). Drain and cool quickly. Cut the apricots into strips. Chop the nuts and shallots or onions.

2 Heat the oil and add the shallots or onions. Cook over a medium heat for 5–7min until soft. Add the apricots and fry for 1min. Place the rice in a bowl, add the onion mixture, nuts and herbs. Cool, then add the beaten egg. Mix well and season.

3 Use to stuff turkey or baseline a 900g (2lb) loaf tin with foil. Place the rice mixture in the tin, cover with foil and place in a roasting tin. Surround the loaf tin with hot water to come halfway up the sides. Cook at 190°C (170°C fan) mark 5 for 1¼–1½hr or until a skewer inserted in the centre feels hot.

To freeze ahead: Complete to the end of step 2 and freeze.
To use: Thaw at room temperature overnight, then cook as in step 3.

Pork, Spinach and Apple Stuffing

Hands-on time: 45min, plus cooling
Cooking time: 1hr 30min
Serves: 8-10

* 2tbsp olive oil
* 150g (5oz) onion, finely chopped
* 225g (8oz) fresh spinach, torn into pieces if the leaves are large
* 2 sharp apples, such as Granny Smith, peeled, cored and cut into chunks
* 450g (1lb) sausagemeat
* Coarsely grated rind of 1 lemon
* 1tbsp chopped thyme
* 100g (3½oz) fresh white breadcrumbs
* 2 large eggs, beaten

1 Heat the oil in a frying pan, add the onion for 10min or until soft. Increase the heat, add the spinach and cook until wilted.

2 Add the apples and cook for 2-3min, stirring, then cool. When cold, mix with the sausagemeat, lemon rind, thyme, breadcrumbs and beaten eggs, then season. The stuffing can be frozen at this stage or made up to two days in advance and kept in the fridge.

3 Cook the stuffing in the neck of the turkey or in a buttered 900g (2lb) loaf tin, covered with foil, at 180°C (160°C fan) mark 4 for 1½hr or until cooked to the centre.

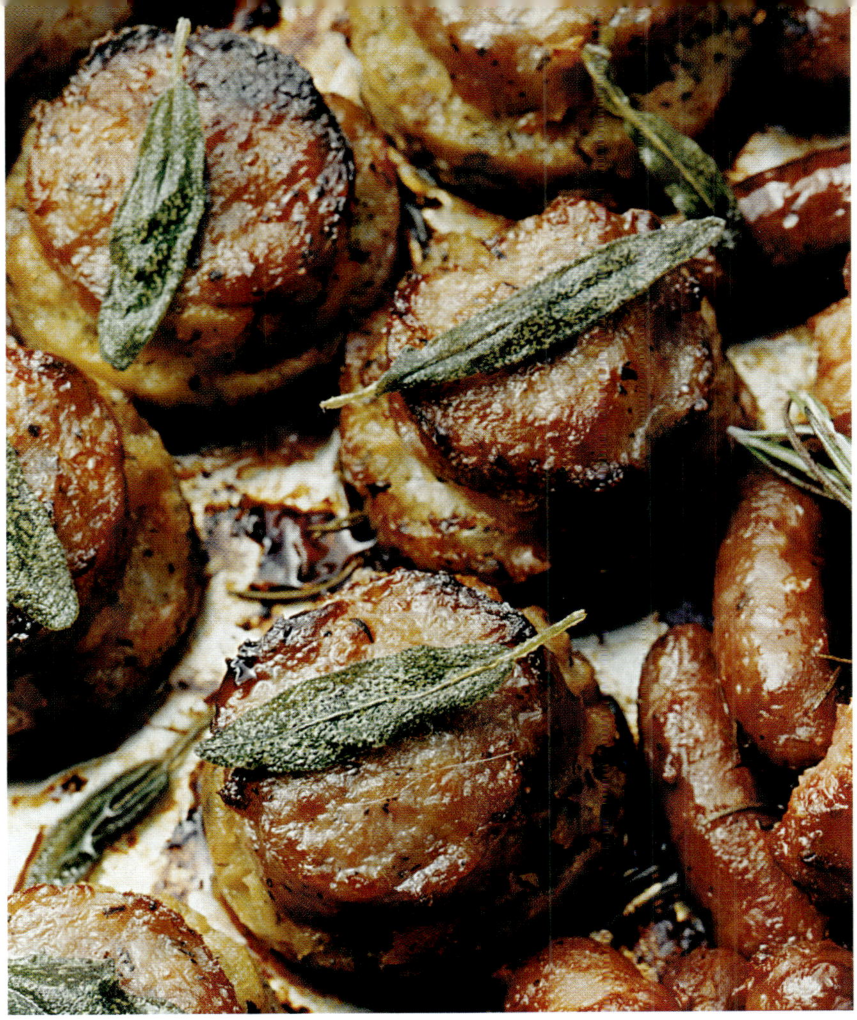

Sage, Onion and Sausage Timbales

Hands-on time: 15min, plus chilling
Cooking time: 30min
Serves: 8

* 2tbsp olive oil
* 1 large onion, finely chopped
* 2 garlic cloves, crushed
* 75g (3½oz) fresh white breadcrumbs
* 40g (1½oz) medium cornmeal or polenta
* 50g (2oz) hazelnuts, toasted and chopped
* Zest of 1 lemon and juice of ½
* 2tbsp each fresh flat-leafed parsley and sage, roughly chopped
* 1 medium egg, lightly beaten
* 400g (14oz) Lincolnshire sausages
* 8 sage leaves

1 Line a baking tray with baking parchment. Arrange eight 5cm (2in) greased plain ring cutters on top. Alternatively, make rings using 25.5x20.5cm (10x8in) strips of foil, folded five times (in half, then in half again, and so on, from the shortest side). Grease and shape each into a 5cm (2in) round and secure with a paper clip.

2 To make the stuffing, heat the oil in a pan and fry the onion and garlic gently for 10min to soften but not brown. Tip into a bowl to cool.

3 Put the breadcrumbs, cornmeal or polenta, hazelnuts, lemon zest, parsley, sage and egg into a large bowl and squeeze over the lemon juice. Add the cooled onion and garlic and season. Stir to bind together, then cool.

4 Spoon the stuffing into the base of each cutter or ring. Using a sharp knife, split open the sausages and squeeze the meat into a bowl. Stir to mix.

5 Divide the mixture among the eight cutters and smooth the tops with a palette knife. Cover and chill overnight or freeze for up to 1 month.

6 Preheat the oven to 200°C (180°C fan) mark 6. Top each stuffing timbale with a sage leaf and roast for 30min until cooked through and browned. Ease away cutters or foil rings to serve.

Mustard Roast Potatoes and Parsnips

Hands-on time: 25min
Cooking time: 1hr 25min
Serves: 8

* **1.4kg (3lb) small, even-sized potatoes, peeled**
* **800g (1lb 12oz) small parsnips, peeled**
* **50g (2oz) bought goose fat**
* **1–2tbsp black mustard seeds**
* **1tbsp sea salt**

1 Cut out small wedges from one side only of the potatoes and parsnips to help make them extra crispy. Put them into a pan of cold, salted water, bring to the boil and cook for 6min. Drain well.

2 Spread the potato and parsnip wedges out on a baking tray and leave to cool. Preheat the oven to 200°C (180°C fan) mark 6.

3 Heat the goose fat in a roasting tin for 4min until sizzling hot. Add the potatoes, toss in the fat and roast for 30min. Add the parsnips and sprinkle over the mustard seeds and sea salt. Roast for a further 45min, turning halfway, or until the vegetables are golden.

Crispy Roast Potatoes

Hands-on time: 20min
Cooking time: 1hr 20min
Serves: 8

* **1.4kg (3lb) medium, even-sized potatoes, peeled**
* **50g (2oz) bought goose fat**
* **2tsp sea salt**

1 Cut two or three small wedges from the top of each potato, then cut two or three wedges across to create a grid pattern to help make them extra crispy.

2 Put the potatoes into a pan of cold, salted water, bring to the boil and cook for 6min. Drain well. Spread the potatoes out onto a baking sheet.

3 Preheat the oven to 200°C (180°C fan) mark 6. Put the goose fat in a roasting tin and heat for 3–4min until sizzling. Add the potatoes and roast for 30min, then sprinkle over the sea salt. Roast for a further 40min, turning halfway through, or until golden.

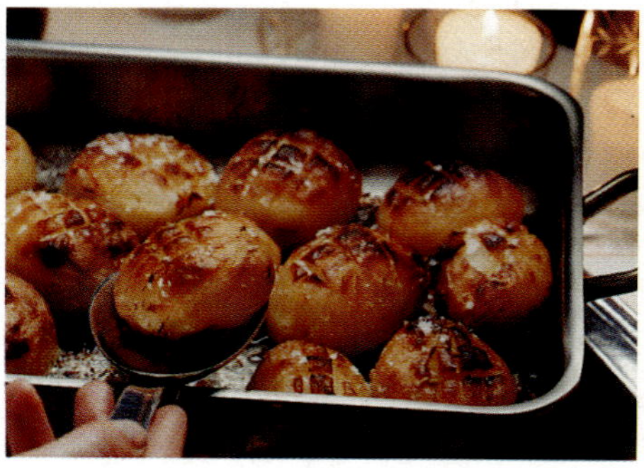

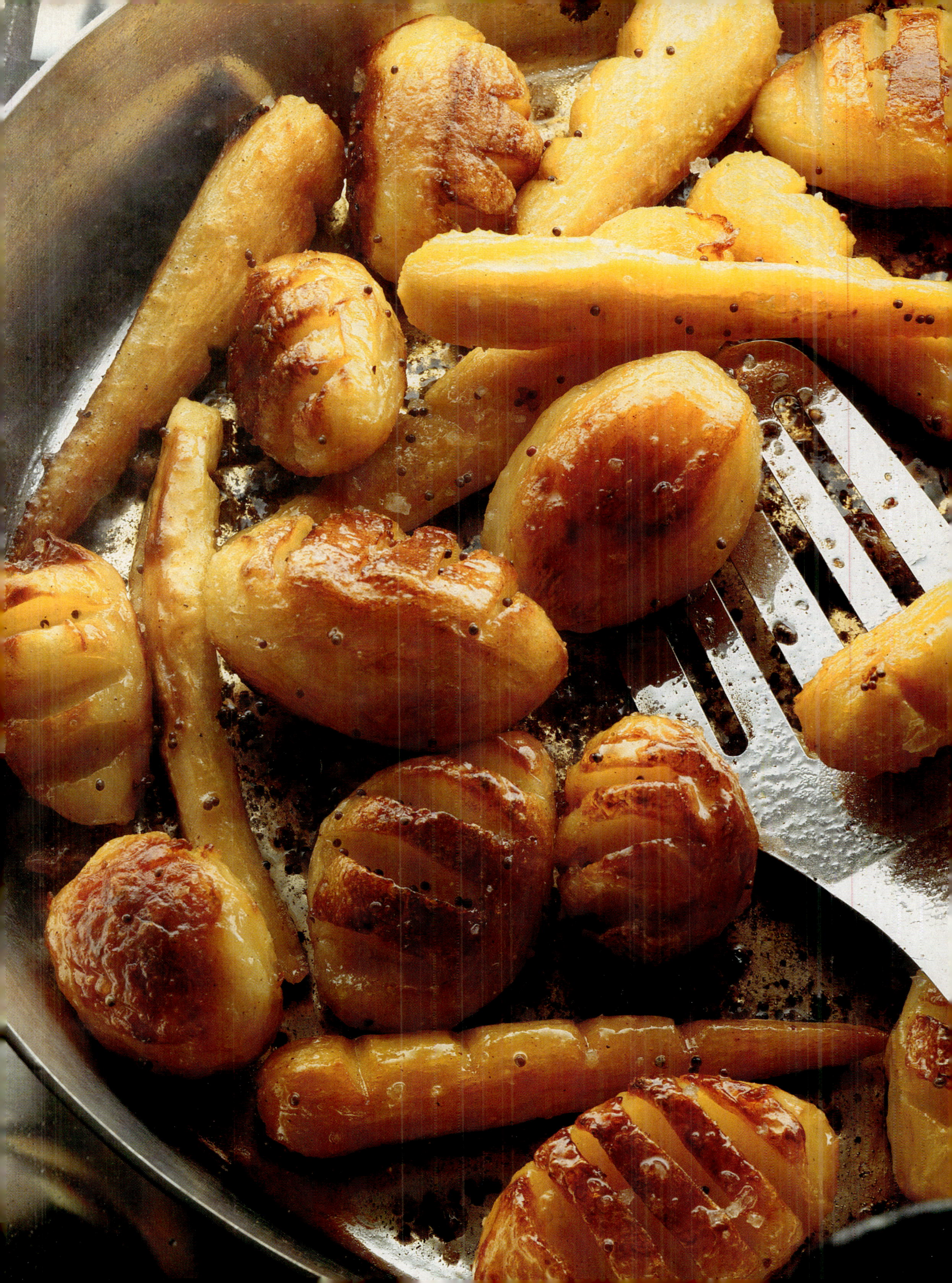

Roast Parsnips with Honey Glaze

Hands-on time: 15min
Cooking time: 1hr
Serves: 8–10
Vegetarian

* 2tbsp oil
* 700g (1½lb) each parsnips and sweet potatoes, peeled and cut into large chunks
* 4tbsp runny honey

1 Heat the oil in a roasting tin on the hob. Add the parsnips and sweet potatoes and shake the tin to coat them with the oil. Season. Roast at 200°C (180°C fan) mark 6 for 45min, turning the parsnips from time to time.

2 Mix in the runny honey and return to the oven for a further 10–15min or until the vegetables are glazed, sticky and a deep golden brown. Season to taste and turn into a serving dish immediately.

Caramelised Carrots

Hands-on time: 15min
Cooking time: 10–15min
Serves: 8
Vegetarian

* 700g (1½lb) baby carrots, thinly sliced lengthways
* 50g (2oz) butter
* 50g (2oz) light muscovado sugar
* 300ml (½ pint) vegetable stock
* 2tbsp balsamic vinegar
* 2tbsp freshly chopped flat-leafed parsley to serve

1 Put the baby carrots, butter, sugar and stock into a pan, season, then cover and bring to the boil. Reduce the heat and simmer for 5min.

2 Remove the lid, add the balsamic vinegar and cook for a further 5–10min or until the carrots are tender (the liquid should have evaporated enough to form a glaze). Sprinkle with the parsley to serve.

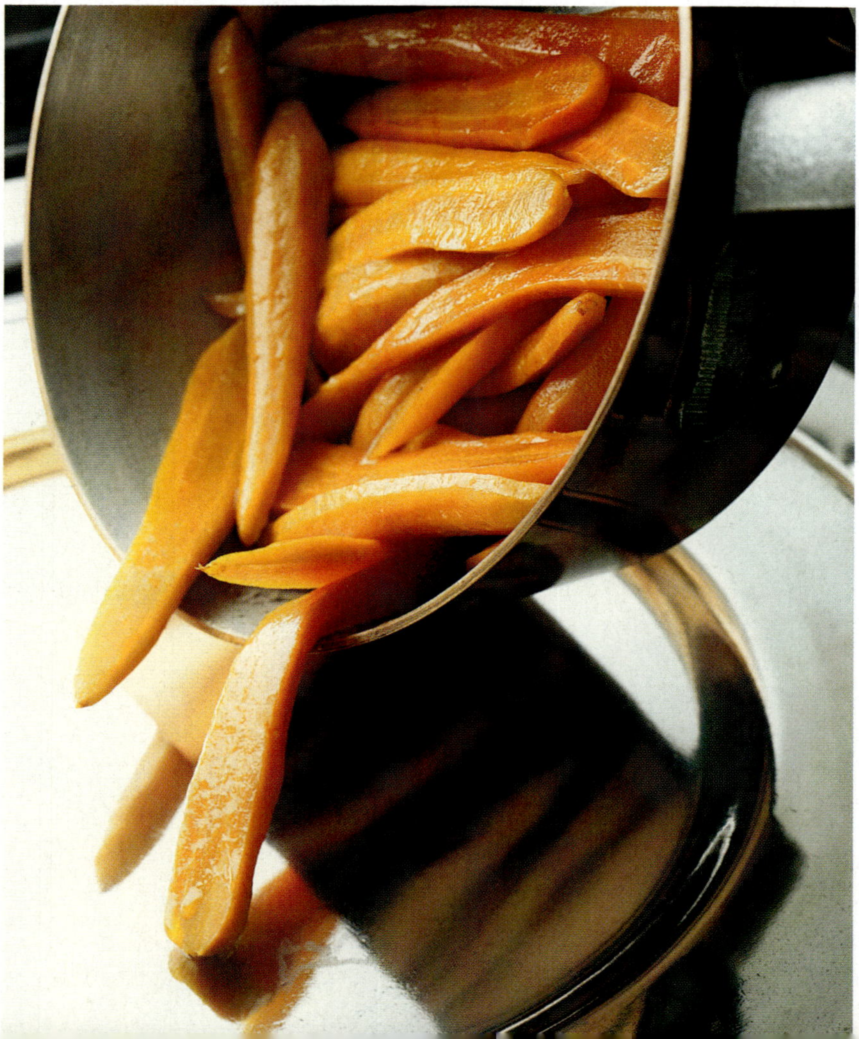

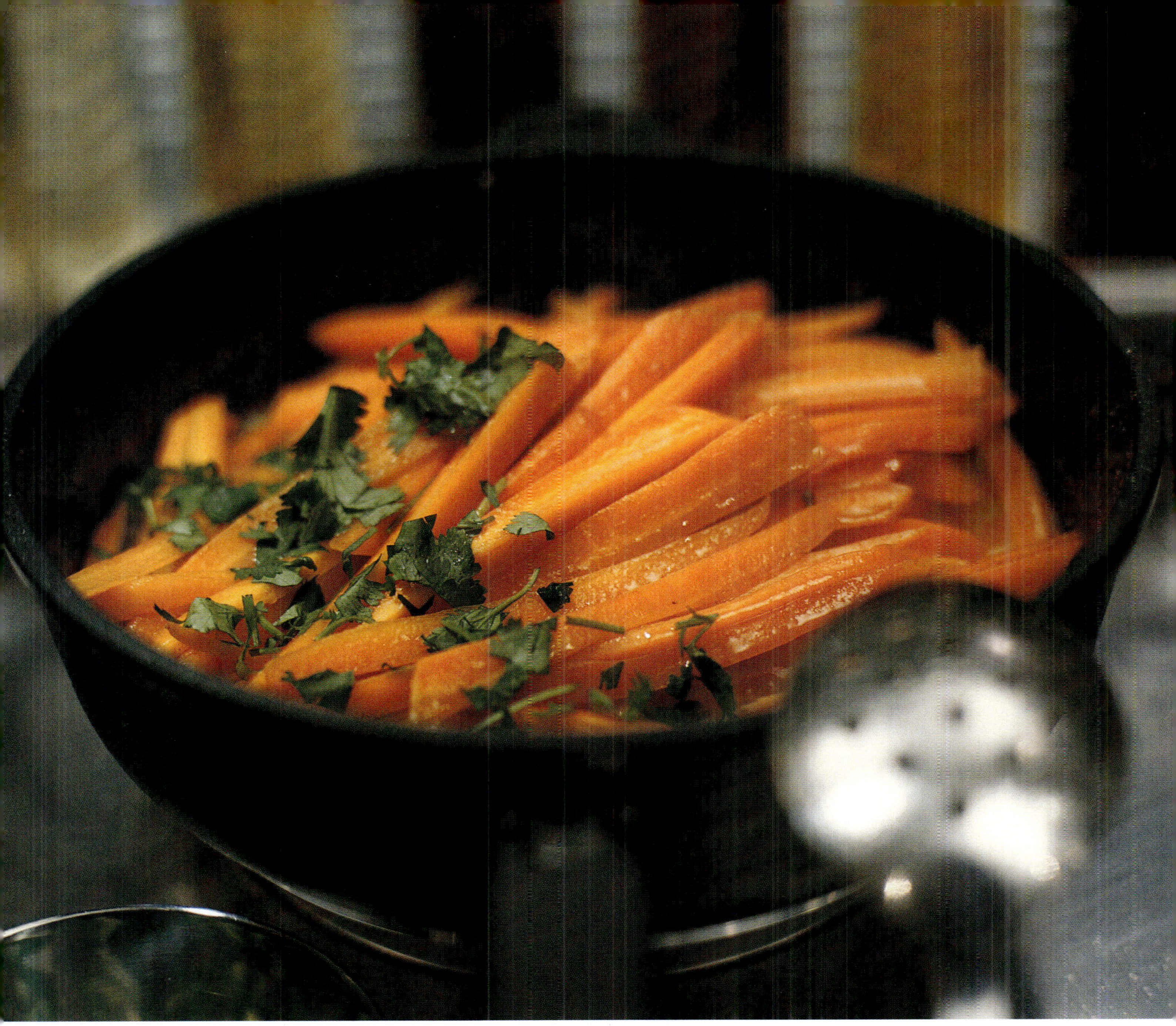

Lemon and Orange Carrots

Hands-on time: 5min;
Cooking time: 10–15min
Serves: 8
Vegetarian

- 900g (2lb) carrots, cut into long batons
- 150ml (¼ pint) orange juice
- Juice of 2 lemons
- 150ml (¼ pint) dry white wine
- 50g (2oz) butter
- 3tbsp light muscovado sugar
- 4tbsp fresh coriander, roughly chopped

1 Put the carrots, orange and lemon juice, white wine, butter and sugar in a pan. Cover and bring to the boil.

2 Remove the lid and cook until almost all the liquid evaporates – this should take about 10min. Sprinkle with the coriander to serve

Spicy Red Cabbage

Hands-on time: 30min
Cooking time: 1hr 10min
Serves: 8
Vegetarian

* 75g (3oz) butter
* 2 red onions, finely chopped
* 1 leek (about 175g/6oz), finely sliced
* 1 small red cabbage, about 1.1kg (2½lb), finely shredded
* 2 red apples, cored and sliced
* Juice of 1 lemon
* 2tbsp red wine vinegar
* 1tbsp light muscovado sugar
* 1 cinnamon stick, broken, 4 cloves and 2 star anise

1 Heat the butter in a large pan, add the onions and cook until soft. Add the leeks and cook for a further 5min.

2 Add the red cabbage, apples, lemon juice, vinegar, sugar and spices. Season. Cover and cook, stirring from time to time, over a low heat for 1hr or until the cabbage is just soft.

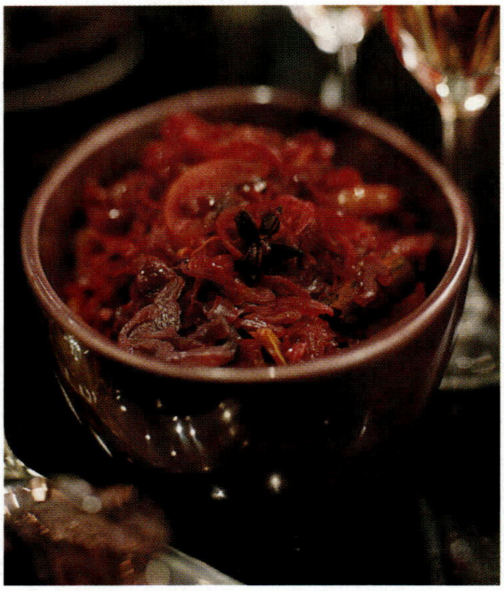

Creamy Brussels Sprouts

Hands-on time: 15min
Cooking time: 25min, plus 30min infusing
Serves: 8–10
Vegetarian

* 568ml (1 pint) milk
* 1 thick slice each onion and celery
* 6 peppercorns
* 1 small bayleaf
* 1.1kg (2½lb) Brussels sprouts, lightly trimmed
* 40g (1½oz) butter
* 40g (1½oz) plain flour
* ½ whole nutmeg, grated – about 1tsp
* 4tbsp single cream
* Oregano sprigs, flat-leafed parsley and grated nutmeg to garnish

1 Place the milk in a pan with the onion, celery, peppercorns and bayleaf. Bring to the boil, remove from the heat and leave to infuse for 20–30min.

2 Cook the sprouts in a pan of boiling salted water until just tender. Drain and plunge into a bowl of icy cold water. Drain again and dry well.

3 Strain and reserve the milk. Melt the butter in a heavy-based pan. Off the heat, add the flour and stir until smooth. Stir in the milk and mix until smooth. Return to the heat and bring to the boil, stirring. Simmer for 1–2min, add the nutmeg and season. Float the cream on top.

4 In a food processor, whiz the sprouts briefly until roughly chopped. Combine with the sauce. Place in a pan over a low heat and stir until hot. Garnish with oregano, parsley and nutmeg.

To freeze ahead: Complete to the end of step 4 but don't reheat. Pack and freeze.
To use: Thaw overnight at cool room temperature, then reheat as above.

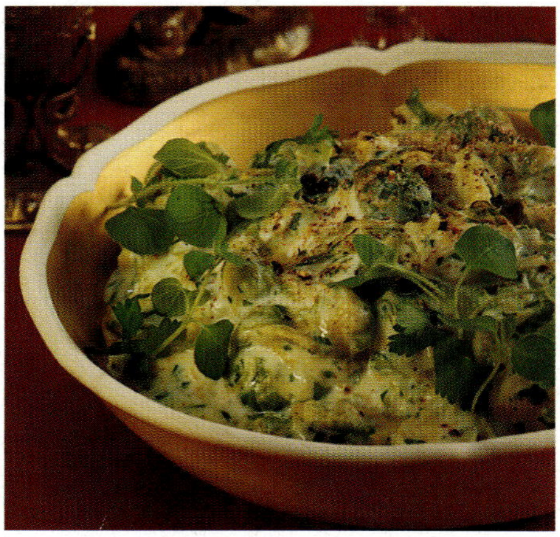

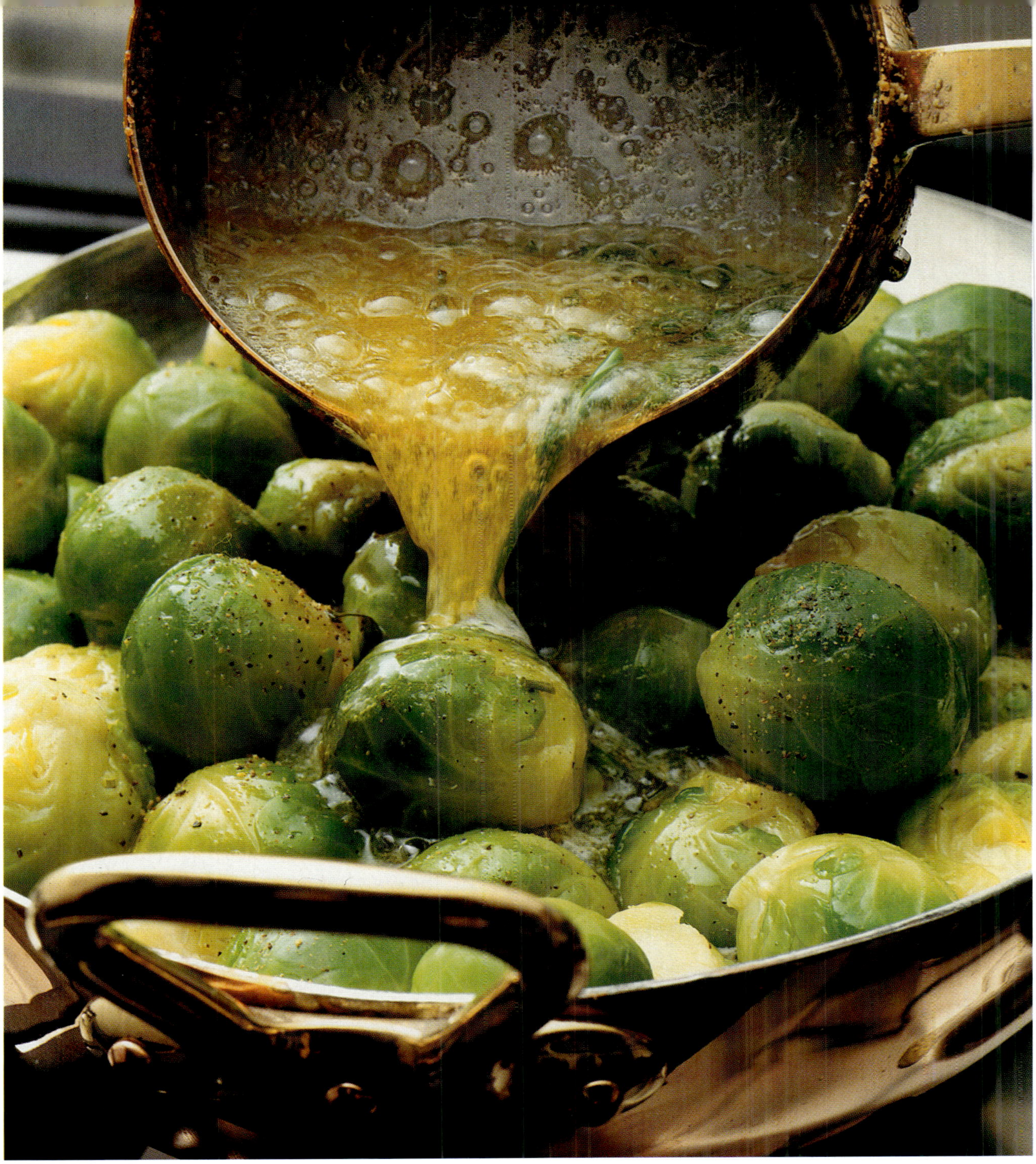

Herby Buttered Brussels Sprouts

Hands-on time: 10min, plus 10min standing
Cooking time: 8–10min
Serves: 8
Vegetarian

- 900g (2lb) Brussels sprouts, trimmed
- 125g (4oz) unsalted butter
- 4tbsp red wine vinegar
- 4tbsp each freshly chopped chives and tarragon

1 Bring a pan of salted water to the boil, add the Brussels sprouts and cook for 5min or until nearly tender. Drain the sprouts, plunge into cold water for 5min, then drain again thoroughly.

2 Melt the butter in a small pan and cook until brown. Add the red wine vinegar and cook for 2min. Stir in the herbs.

3 Heat a large frying pan and stir-fry the sprouts for 2–3min. Season. Pour the beurre noisette over, making sure the sprouts are evenly coated in butter and are thoroughly heated through.

Roast Potatoes with Rosemary and Garlic

Hands-on time: 20min
Cooking time: 1hr 10min
Serves: 8–10
Vegetarian

- 1.8kg (4lb) potatoes, peeled and cut into large chunks
- 3tbsp vegetable oil
- 75g (3oz) unsalted butter
- 6 rosemary sprigs
- 6 garlic cloves, unpeeled

1 Preheat the oven to 200°C (180°C fan) mark 6. Put the potatoes in a pan of cold, salted water, bring to the boil and cook for 5–10min or until the potatoes begin to soften. Drain and return to the pan, put over a low heat and shake the pan until the potatoes are dry and a little fluffy. Put to one side.

2 Heat the vegetable oil and butter in a roasting tin. Put the warm potatoes in the tin with the rosemary and garlic and toss to cover them evenly in the oil and butter mixture. Season. Cook the potatoes for 1hr or until the potatoes are brown and crisp, turning the potatoes over from time to time to ensure they're cooked evenly. Sprinkle with sea salt, if wished.

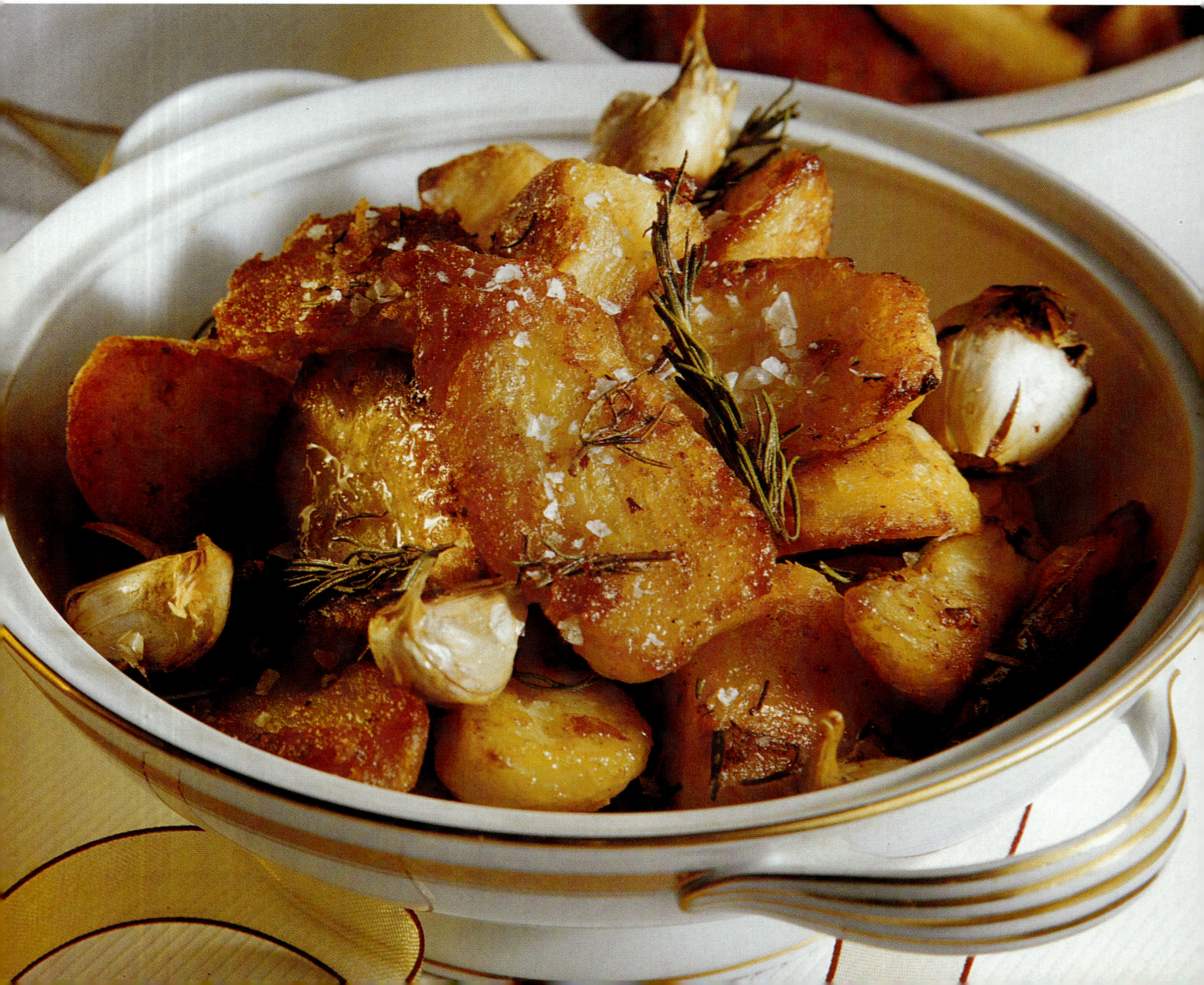

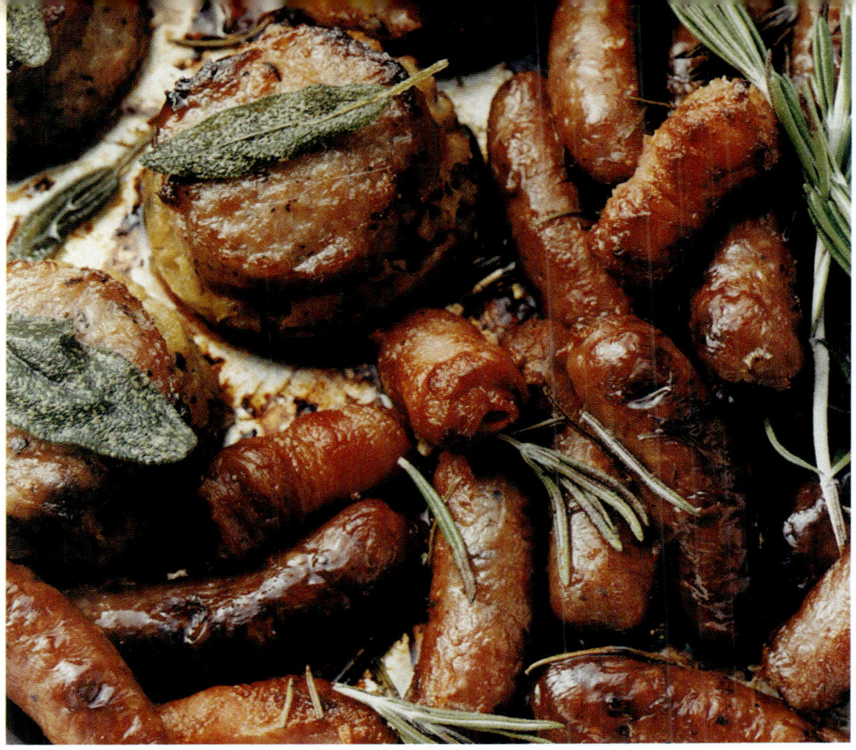

Rosemary-roasted Bacon Rolls and Chipolatas

Hands-on time: 15min
Cooking time: 30min
Serves: 8

* 10 maple-smoked, traditional-style, rindless streaky bacon rashers
* Sage, Onion and Sausage Timbales (see Stuffings)
* 10 chipolatas
* 4 fresh rosemary sprigs

1 Cut each bacon rasher in half. Use the back of a knife to stretch each rasher slightly, then roll up into bacon rolls. Put into a roasting tin with the Timbales.

2 Separate the chipolatas with scissors. Take each one, then twist twice in the centre and cut to make two mini chipolatas. Add to the roasting tin and scatter with the sprigs of rosemary.

3 Preheat the oven to 200°C (180°C fan) mark 6. Roast for 30min until cooked through and browned.

Roasted Sweet Potatoes with Sage

Hands-on time: 5–10min
Cooking time: 50min–1hr
Serves: 8
Vegetarian

* 5 sweet potatoes – around 1.1kg (2½lb)
* 2tbsp freshly chopped sage
* 2tsp yellow mustard seeds
* 3–4tbsp olive oil

1 Preheat the oven to 200°C (180°C fan) mark 6. Peel and cut the potatoes into wedges, then put into a large roasting tin. Add the sage, mustard seeds and olive oil. Season. Toss everything together to coat.

2 Roast the potatoes in the oven for 50min–1hr until golden and tender. Put in a large dish and serve.

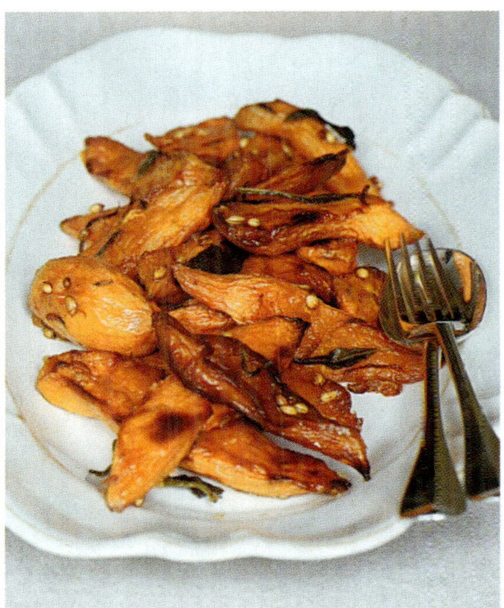

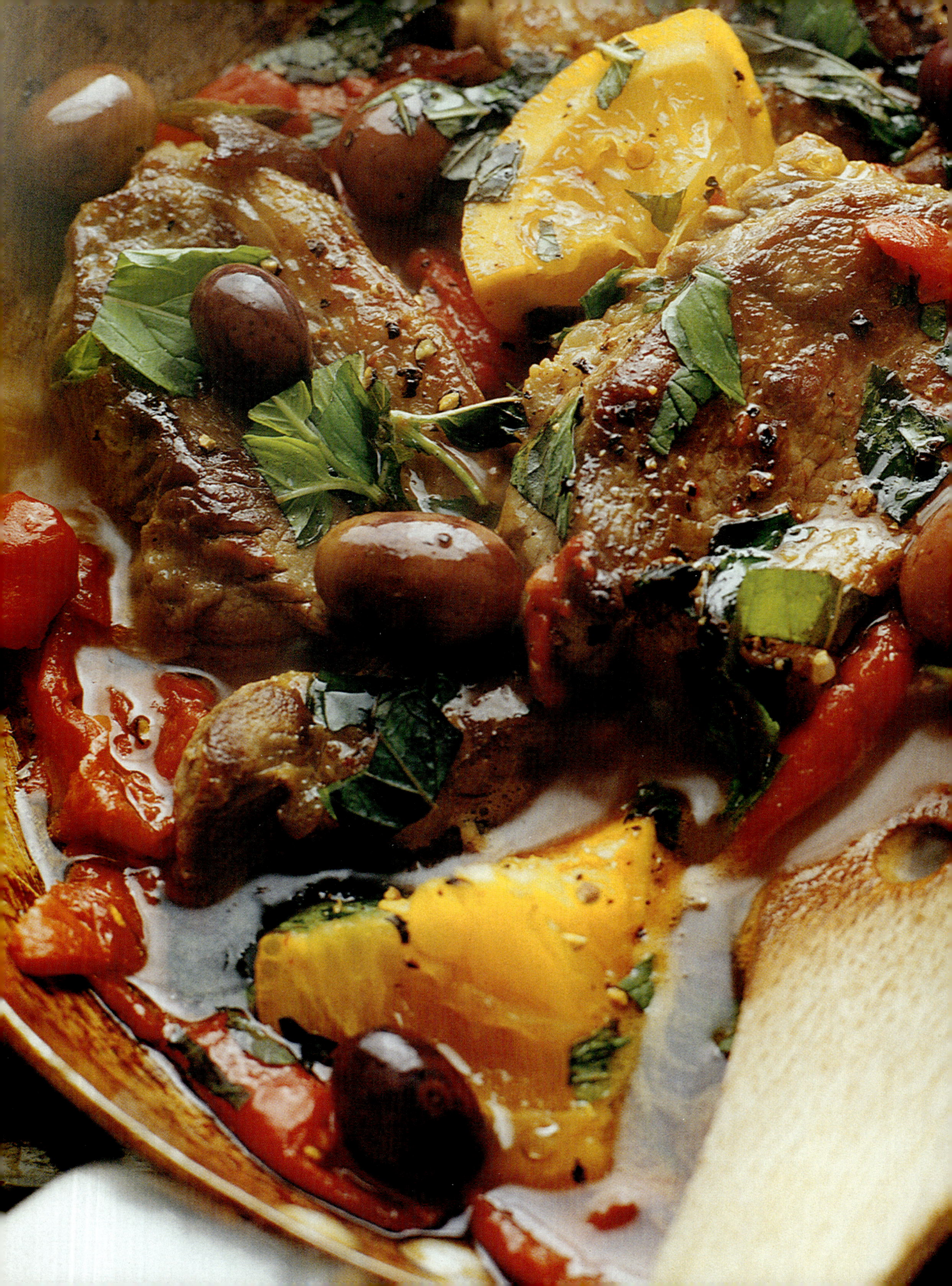

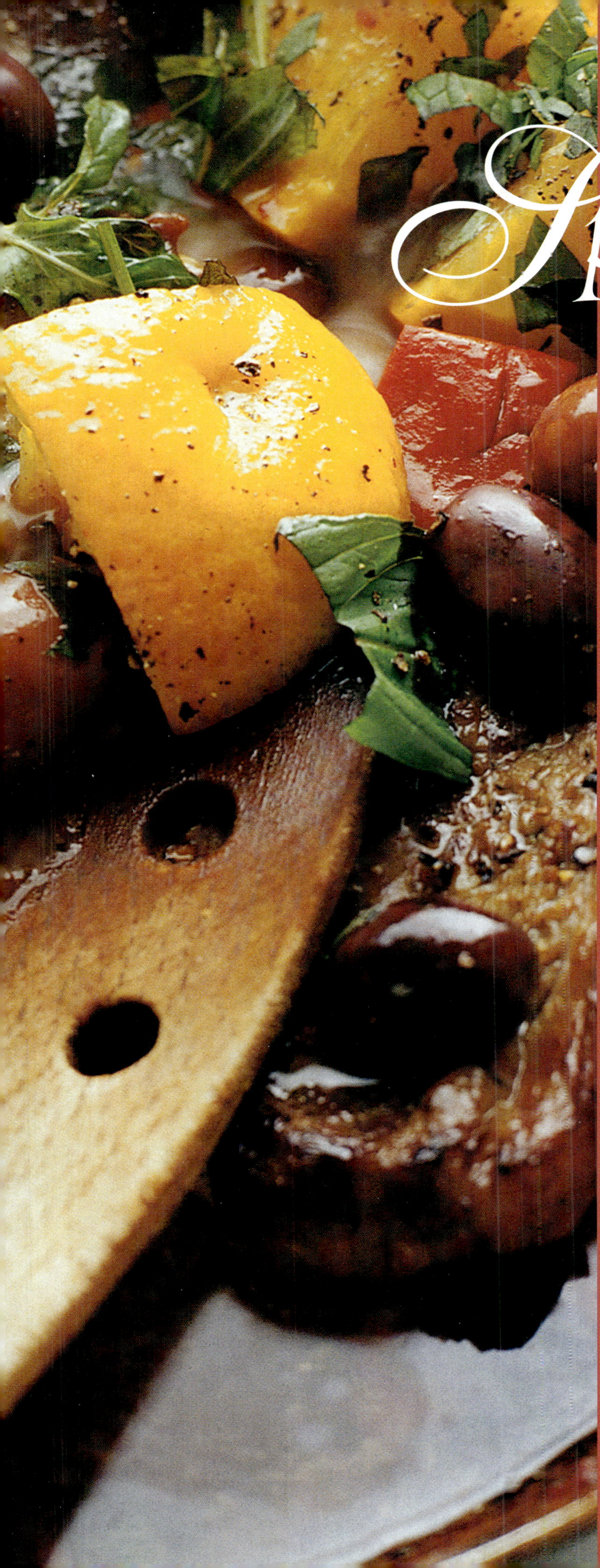

FOR FAMILY AND FRIENDS

Special Dishes

We spend so much time thinking about Christmas lunch, we often forget that the annual feast covers several other special meals. In our **Food For Friends** section, there is a selection of dishes that will really impress at this busy time of year. They can be prepared ahead of time and frozen, making your festivities truly stress-free. And you'll be spoilt for choice with the **vegetarian** options – the **White Nut Roast** is a new take on traditional nut roast, plus there are timbales, tarts, and tians for non-meat eaters to enjoy. Finally, our recipes for **leftovers** help you turn surplus turkey, vegetables and Christmas pudding into impressive, easy-to-make suppers.

Salmon and Fennel Rostí

Hands-on time: 20min, plus cooling
Cooking time: 1½hr
Serves: 4

- 700g (1½lb) medium-sized waxy potatoes, such as Desirée
- 75g (3oz) butter
- 300g (11oz) onions, sliced
- 350g (12oz) fennel, sliced
- 150ml (¼ pint) dry white wine
- 50ml (2fl oz) vermouth
- 25g (1oz) flour
- 450ml (¾ pint) fish stock
- 4tbsp double cream
- 2tbsp chopped fresh dill
- 4 x 150g (5oz) skinless salmon fillets

1 Bake the potatoes at 200°C (180°C fan) mark 6 for 30–40min or until just soft. Then cool, peel and coarsely grate. Melt 50g (2oz) butter and mix it with the potato. Season and put to one side.

2 Meanwhile, melt the remaining butter in a frying pan, then cook the onion and fennel for 10min or until just soft. Add the wine and vermouth, bring to the boil and bubble for 5min to reduce by half.

3 Sprinkle in the flour, stir until smooth, then add the stock and cream. Bring to the boil, stirring, then simmer for 2–3min. Add the dill, season and cool.

4 Put the salmon fillets in an ovenproof dish. Spoon the fennel mixture over them, then sprinkle the potato on top.

5 Cook at 200°C (180°C fan) mark 6 for 25–30min or until the topping is crisp and golden.

To freeze ahead: Complete the recipe to the end of step 4, then wrap and freeze.
To use: Thaw the rösti at cool room temperature overnight, then complete the recipe.

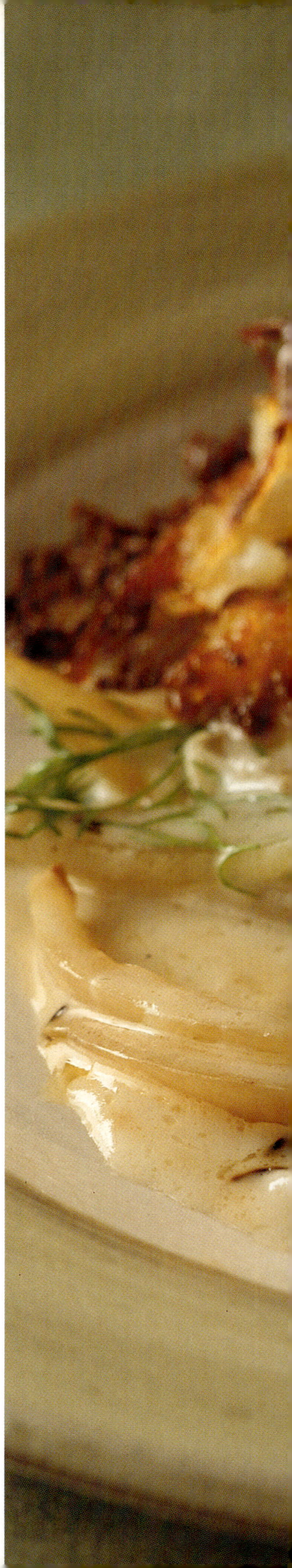

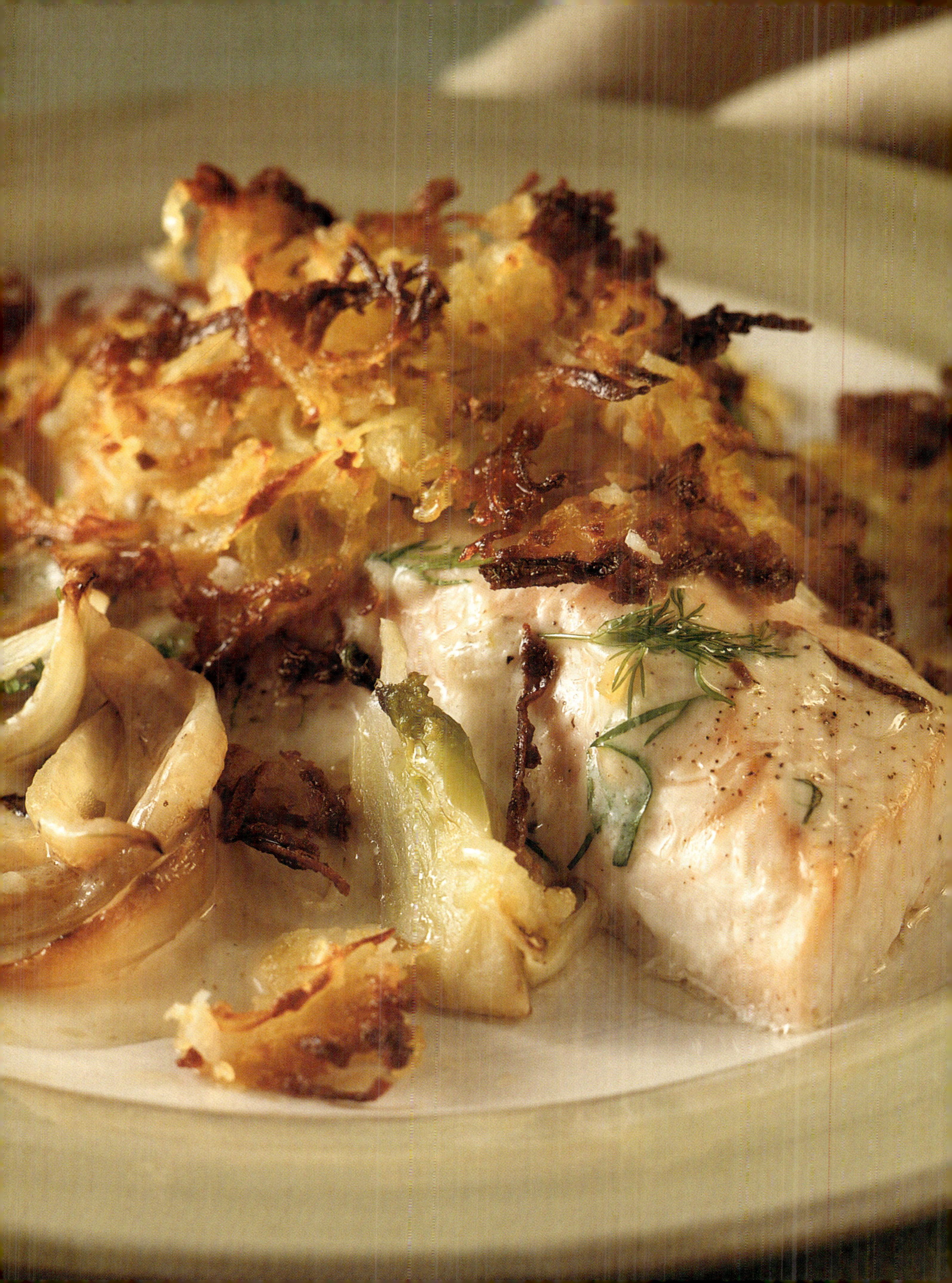

Provençale Fish Stew

Hands-on time: 20min
Cooking time: 1hr 5min
Serves: 6–8

* 3tbsp mixed chopped fresh herbs such as basil, parsley and coriander
* 50ml (2fl oz) olive oil
* 1 pack ready-made garlic bread, cut into rough chunks

FOR THE TOMATO SAUCE
* 2 x 400g cans chopped tomatoes
* 2tbsp olive oil
* Zest of ½ lemon
* ½tsp dried oregano
* 2 garlic cloves, peeled and crushed
* Sugar to taste

FOR THE FISH STEW
* 700g (1½lb) large potatoes, peeled and cut into small chunks
* 300ml (10fl oz) dry white wine
* 2tbsp Pernod (optional)
* 900ml (1½ pints) passata or homemade tomato sauce (see above)
* 2 x 284ml tubs fresh fish stock
* 3tbsp chopped fresh thyme
* 700g (1½lb) cod fillet, skinned and cut into 2.5cm (1in) cubes
* 2tbsp chopped fresh basil to serve

1 Whiz the herbs together in a food processor for about 10sec. Add the olive oil gradually until the mixture looks smooth. Transfer to a bowl, then season. Cover and chill until ready to use.

2 To make the croûtons, cut the bread into rough chunks, lay in a single layer on a baking sheet and season. Cook at 180°C (160°C fan) mark 4 for 15min or until crisp and golden, turning halfway through. Cool.

3 To make the tomato sauce, if you are not using the ready-made passata, put the chopped tomatoes with their juice in a pan with the olive oil, lemon zest and dried oregano. Bring to the boil, cover and simmer gently for 20min. Add the garlic cloves, season and add a little sugar to taste. Simmer, uncovered, for 10min or until the sauce has thickened slightly. It can be frozen at this point or kept in the fridge for a few days.

4 For the stew, put the potatoes in a large pan of salted water, bring to the boil and simmer for about 10min until just cooked. Drain and cool.

5 Put the wine and Pernod, if using, in a large pan and bring to the boil, then simmer for 10min to allow the alcohol to boil away. Add the passata or the homemade tomato sauce, then the fish stock, thyme and 300ml (10fl oz) water, season and bring to the boil, then simmer for 10min. Add the potatoes, reduce the heat a little and let them warm through for 5min. Just before serving, add the cod and cook for a further 5min or until white and firm. Stir very carefully so you don't break up the fish pieces. Season to taste.

6 Spoon the fish stew into bowls, top with the croûtons and drizzle liberally with the herb oil. Sprinkle with the chopped fresh basil to serve.

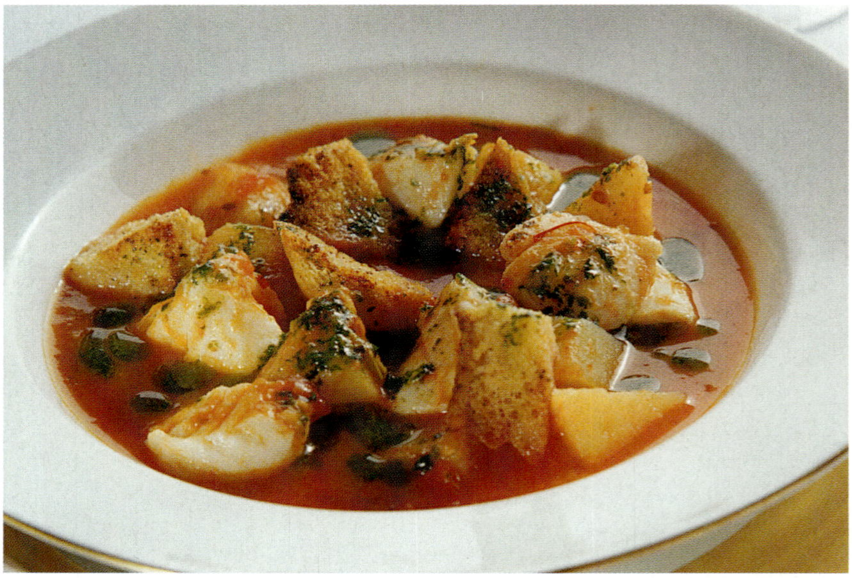

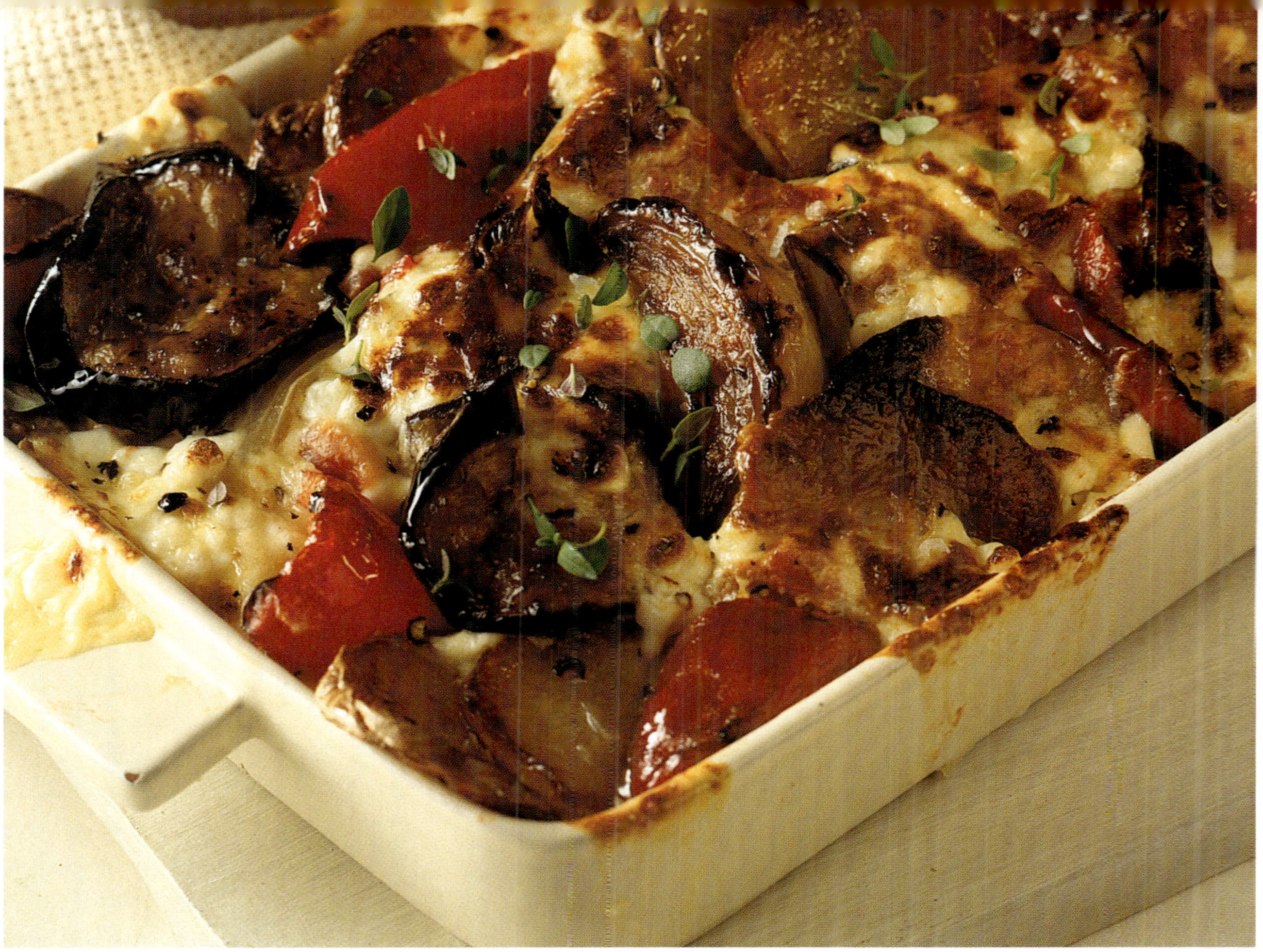

Roasted Vegetable Moussaka

Hands-on time: 45min
Cooking time: 1hr 45min
Serves: 4–6
Vegetarian

* 1 medium onion, cut into strips
* 2 fennel bulbs, cut into strips
* 2 red peppers, deseeded and roughly sliced
* 1 medium aubergine, sliced
* 350g (12oz) potato, peeled and sliced
* 5 whole garlic cloves
* 5tbsp olive oil
* 400g can chopped tomatoes
* 4 whole pieces of sun-dried tomato, chopped
* 227g tub cottage cheese
* 3 large eggs
* 175g (6oz) Cheddar cheese, grated
* 3tbsp natural yogurt
* Thyme leaves to garnish

1 Put the vegetables and garlic in two roasting tins, drizzle with the olive oil and season. Cook at 220°C (200°C fan) mark 7 for 1hr, tossing occasionally and swapping the tins around so the vegetables cook evenly and turn golden and soft.

2 Add the canned tomatoes and the sun-dried tomato to the vegetables then mix well to combine. Return the vegetables to the oven to cook for a further 10–15min.

3 In a bowl, beat together the cottage cheese, eggs, Cheddar cheese and yogurt, season. Spoon the vegetable mixture into a shallow 2–2.3 litre (3½–4 pint) ovenproof dish, then spread the cheese mixture over the top.

4 Cook at 200°C (180°C fan) mark 6 for 20–30min or until the moussaka is golden and bubbling. Garnish with thyme leaves to serve

To freeze ahead: Complete the recipe to the end of step 3, cooling the vegetable mixture before spooning the cheese mixture on top. Wrap and freeze.
To use: Thaw the moussaka overnight at cool room temperature, then complete the recipe. Cover the moussaka with foil after 20min if the top starts to turn too brown, then continue to cook for a further 20min until it's hot to the centre.

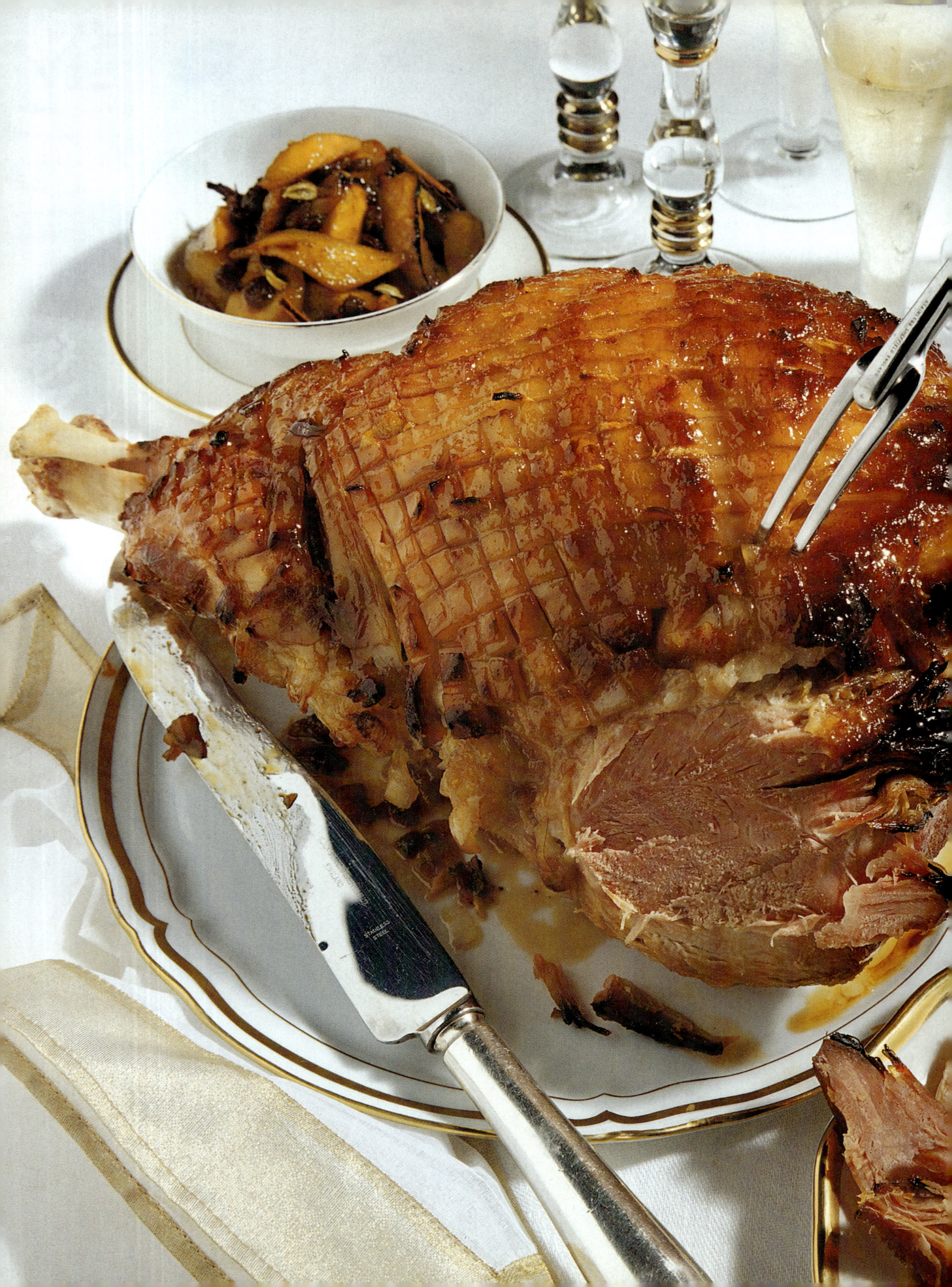

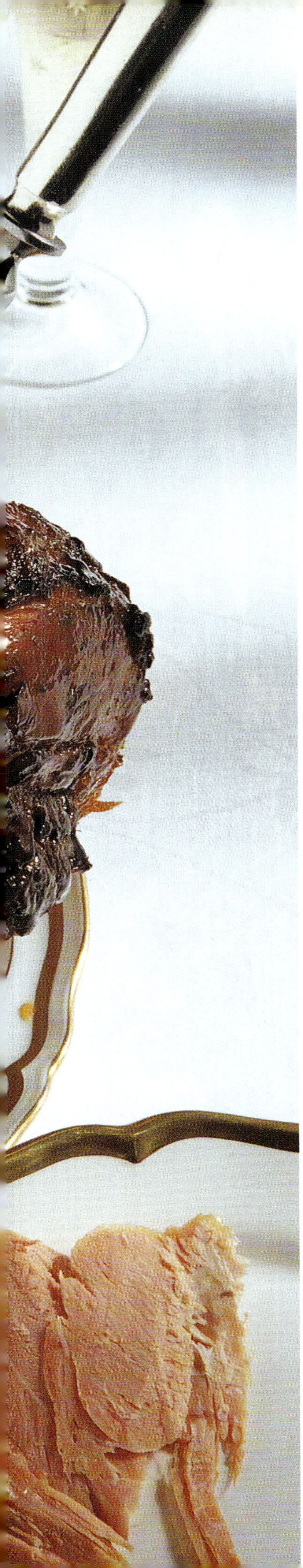

Ginger and Honey-glazed Ham

Hands-on time: 1hr
Cooking time: 5¾hr
Serves: 8–10

- 4.5kg–6.8kg (10–15lb) unsmoked gammon on the bone
- 2 shallots, peeled and halved
- 6 cloves
- 3 bayleaves
- 2 celery sticks, cut into 5cm (2in) pieces
- 2tbsp English mustard
- 5cm (2in) cube fresh ginger, peeled and thinly sliced

FOR THE GLAZE

- 225g (8oz) dark brown sugar
- 2tbsp runny honey
- 8tbsp brandy or Madeira

FOR THE CHUTNEY

- 4 mangoes, peeled, sliced and chopped into 5cm (2in) chunks
- 1tsp mixed spice
- 4 cardamom pods, seeds removed and crushed
- ½tsp ground cinnamon
- 4tbsp raisins

1 Put the gammon in a pan. Add the shallots, cloves, bayleaves, celery and enough cold water to cover. Bring to the boil, cover and simmer gently for about 5hr. Remove any scum with a slotted spoon. Lift the ham out of the pan, discard the vegetables and herbs and cool.

2 Using a sharp knife, carefully cut away the ham's thick skin to leave an even layer of fat. Score a diamond pattern in the fat. Put the ham into a roasting tin. Smother evenly with the mustard and tuck the ginger into the scored fat.

3 To make the glaze, put the sugar, honey and brandy in a pan and heat until the sugar has melted. Brush over the ham.

4 In a bowl, mix together the chutney ingredients, add any remaining glaze, then spoon around the ham.

5 Cook the ham at 200°C (180°C fan) mark 6 for 30-40min, basting every 10min. Remove the ham from the roasting tin and put to one side. Stir the chutney and place under a grill for 5min to allow the mango to caramelise. Decant the chutney into a side dish for serving.

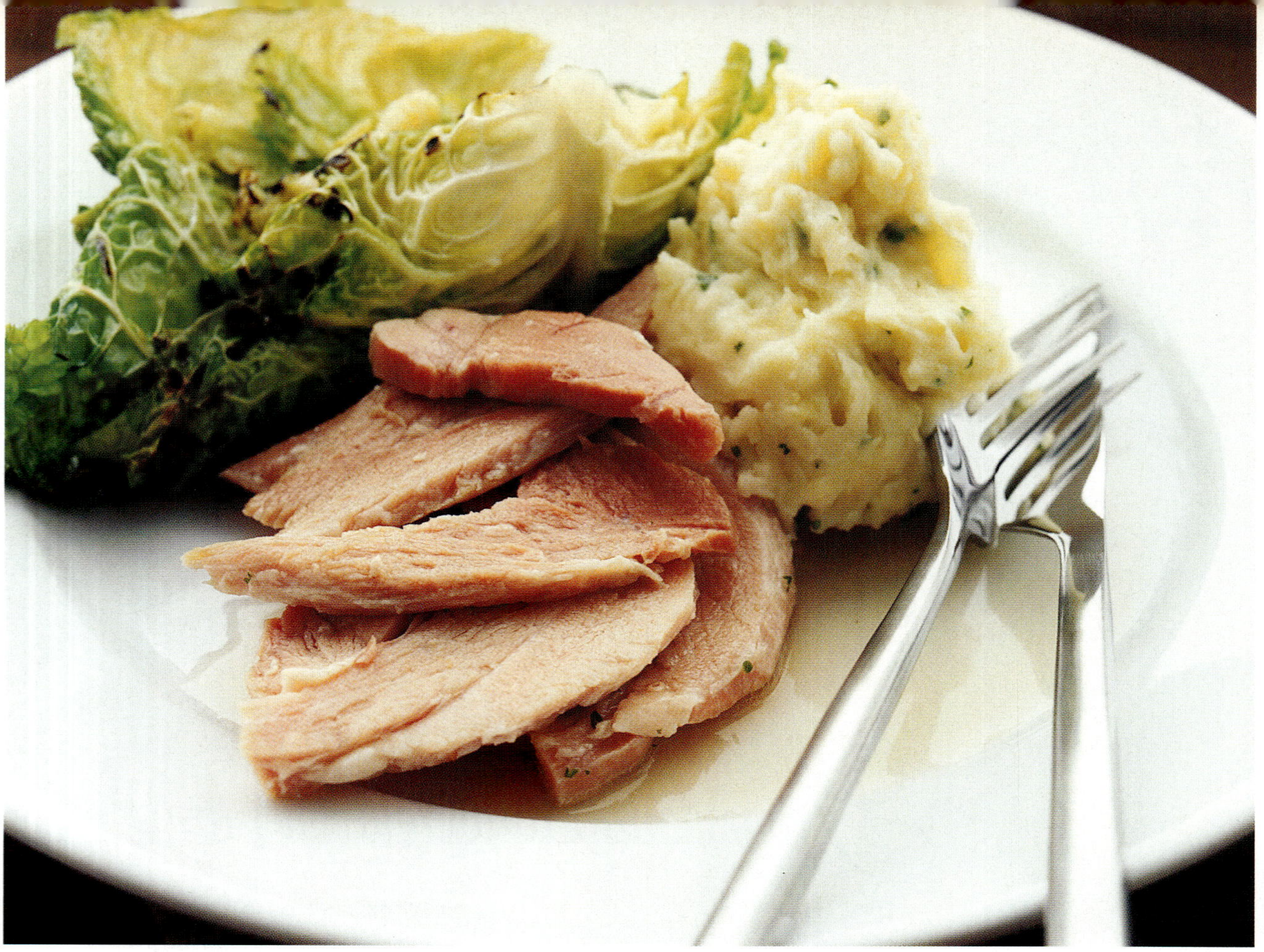

Gammon with Parsley Mash

Hands-on time: 20min
Cooking time: 1hr 50min, plus 15min resting
Serves: 4

- 1.4kg (3lb) gammon knuckle
- 1 onion, quartered
- 1 carrot, cut into chunks
- 1 stick celery, thickly sliced
- 1tsp black peppercorns
- 2 bayleaves
- 700g (1½lb) white potatoes, cut into large chunks
- 6–8tbsp milk
- 40g (1½oz) butter
- 1tbsp freshly chopped parsley
- 1 Savoy cabbage, cut into wedges

1 Put the gammon knuckle in a deep pan, add the onion, carrot, celery, peppercorns and bayleaves and cover with cold water. Bring very slowly to the boil – this should take 20–30min. Skim, then simmer very gently, covered with a lid, for 1½hr or until the meat is cooked through and tender. Allow the gammon to rest in the liquid in the pan for 15min.

2 Meanwhile, put the potatoes in a pan of cold, salted water, bring to the boil and simmer until they're soft to the centre – about 15min. Drain and put the potatoes back in the pan over a low heat to dry off. Take the pan off the heat and mash the potatoes.

3 Put the pan back on a low heat, push the potatoes to one side of the pan and add the milk and 25g (1oz) butter to warm through. Beat the milk and butter into the mashed potatoes until they're fluffy, adding more milk if necessary. Season and add the chopped parsley.

4 Bring a large pan of salted water to the boil, add the cabbage and return to the boil. Drain and dry on kitchen paper, then melt the remaining butter and brush over the cabbage. Heat a griddle or frying pan, add the cabbage and fry until beginning to brown – about 5min.

5 Lift the gammon from the cooking liquid, then remove the skin and slice. Serve with the mashed potatoes, cabbage and a little liquid from the pan.

Guinea Fowl with Prunes, Apples and Bacon

Hands-on time: 40min, plus 4hr marinating
Cooking time: 1hr 30min
Serves: 6

* 225g (8oz) onion, roughly chopped
* 125g (4oz) each carrot and celery, roughly chopped
* 6–8 guinea fowl joints or cornfed chicken joints, 2kg (4½lb) total weight
* 750ml (1¼ pints) red wine
* 1tsp black peppercorns, crushed
* 1tbsp chopped fresh thyme
* 2 bayleaves
* 175g (6oz) ready-to-eat dried prunes
* 3tbsp vegetable oil
* 3 garlic cloves, crushed
* 1tsp harissa paste
* 1tbsp tomato purée
* 2tbsp plain flour
* 300ml (½ pint) chicken stock
* 225g (8oz) streaky bacon, cut in strips
* 2 apples, cored and sliced
* Mashed potato to serve

1 Put the onion, carrot and celery in a large bowl with the guinea fowl, 600ml (1 pint) wine, peppercorns, thyme and bayleaves. Cover and marinate for at least 3–4hr. Place the remaining wine in another bowl with the prunes. Cover and soak for 3–4hr.

2 Drain the joints and pat dry (reserving the vegetables and wine). Heat 2tbsp oil in a large, flameproof casserole, add the joints in batches and cook, skin side down, over a medium heat so the skin browns, then turn over and brown the underside. Remove from the pan and put to one side. Add the marinated vegetables (reserving the marinade) and cook for 5min, stirring. Add the garlic, harissa and tomato purée and cook for 1min. Mix in the flour and cook for 1min.

3 Pour in the reserved wine marinade and stock and bring to the boil, stirring. Return the joints to the casserole (placing the legs at the bottom). Bring to the boil, then season. Cover and cook at 170°C (150°C fan) mark 3 for 40min.

4 Meanwhile, heat the remaining oil in a frying pan. Add the bacon and cook, stirring, for 5min or until golden brown. Remove from the pan and set aside. Add the apple and cook for 2–3min on each side or until golden. Put to one side with the bacon.

5 Remove the joints from the casserole and strain the sauce through a fine sieve. Return to the pan with the joints, then add the prunes and any juices, reserved bacon and apple. Heat through in the oven for a further 10min. If prepared ahead, bring to the boil and reheat at 180°C (160°C fan) mark 4 for 30–40min, plus 10min if frozen. Serve with mashed potato.

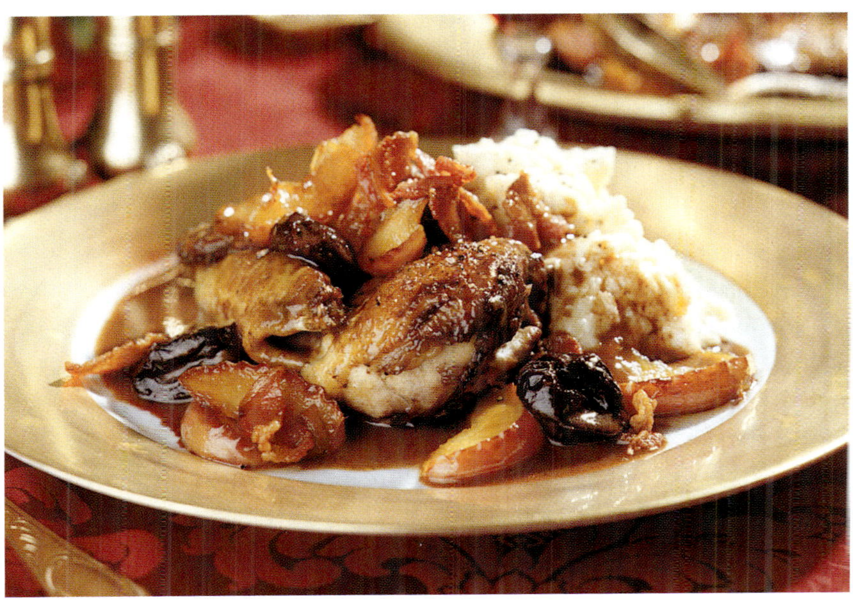

Marinated Duck with Prunes and Garlic

Hands-on time: 30min, plus overnight marinating and resting
Cooking time: 1hr 15min
Serves: 4

FOR THE MARINADE
* 1 carrot, finely chopped
* 2 shallots, finely chopped
* 1 sprig parsley
* 1 sprig thyme, plus extra to garnish
* 1 bayleaf
* 1tsp black peppercorns
* 250ml (9fl oz) prune juice
* 125ml (4fl oz) red wine
* 4tbsp brandy
* 4tbsp olive oil
* ½tsp salt

FOR THE DUCK
* 4 duck breasts
* 8 fat garlic cloves, unpeeled
* 8 ready-to-eat prunes
* 25g (1oz) butter
* 1tsp plain flour
* 4 wooden skewers

FOR THE RED CABBAGE
* 1tbsp olive oil
* 1 red onion, halved and sliced
* 2 garlic cloves, crushed
* 1 large red cabbage – approx 1kg (2lb 3½oz) – shredded
* 2tbsp light muscovado sugar
* 2tbsp red wine vinegar
* 8 juniper berries
* ¼tsp allspice
* 300ml (½ pint) vegetable stock
* 2 pears, cored and sliced

1 For the marinade, put all the ingredients (reserving half of the prune juice) into a dish large enough to hold the duck breasts in a single layer. Mix together, then add the duck. Cover and chill overnight, turning occasionally.

2 To make the red cabbage, heat the oil in a large pan, add the onion and fry for 5min to soften. Add the rest of the ingredients except the pears. Season with salt and freshly ground black pepper and bring to the boil. Reduce the heat, cover and simmer for 30min. Add the pears to the red cabbage and cook for a further 15min or until nearly all the liquid has evaporated and the cabbage is tender.

3 Boil the garlic for 10min, then drain, peel and set aside. Soak four small wooden skewers in warm water.

4 Remove the duck from the marinade and dry on kitchen paper. In a pan, bring the marinade to the boil, then reduce by half. Strain and keep warm. Push the prunes and garlic onto the skewers.

5 Melt the butter in a large frying pan and fry the duck, skin side down, for 8min or until golden. Turn and cook for 3–4min. Remove from the pan and put on a board to rest for 5–10min. Add the skewers to the pan and cook, turning regularly, until the garlic starts to colour. Remove and set aside.

6 Add the flour to the pan and cook, stirring, for 2–3sec. Add the marinade and the rest of the prune juice, bring to the boil and simmer, stirring, until the sauce thickens slightly and becomes glossy.

7 Arrange the duck breasts and prune skewers on individual plates and spoon over the sauce. Garnish with thyme sprigs and serve with the red cabbage and mashed potato.

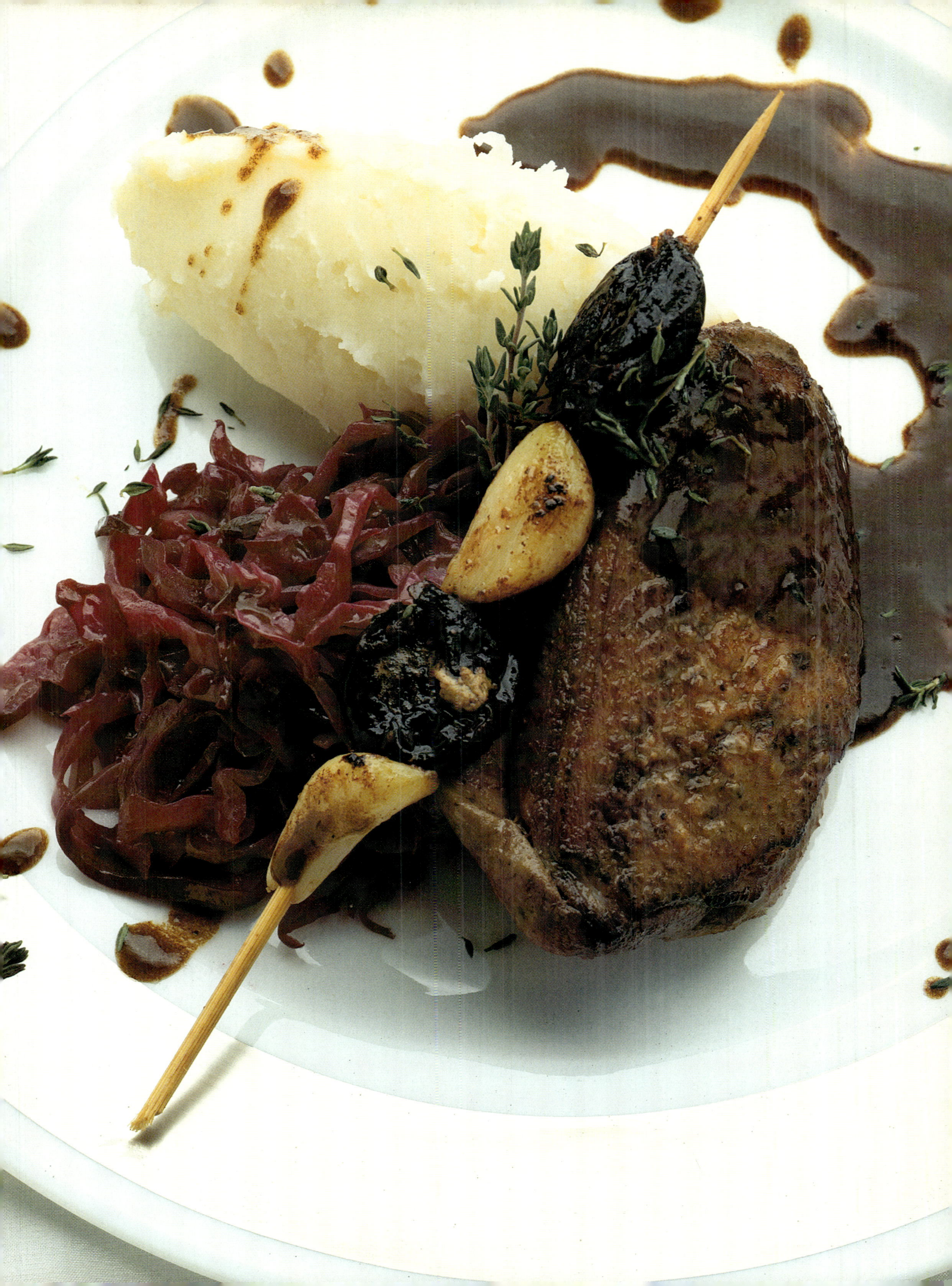

Lamb with Orange and Mint

Hands-on time: 10min
Cooking time: 20min
Serves: 4

* 4tbsp olive oil
* 4 lamb steaks – around 700g (1¼lb)
* 185g jar chargrilled sweet red peppers, drained and roughly chopped
* 50g (2oz) black olives
* 1 orange
* Juice of 1 lemon
* Small bunch of fresh mint, roughly chopped

1 Heat 2tbsp of olive oil in a large, non-stick frying pan. Brown the lamb in the hot oil, turning occasionally until the meat has formed a deep golden brown crust all over.

2 Reduce the heat and add the peppers and black olives. Chop up the orange, squeeze the juice directly into the pan and add the orange pieces for extra flavour. Add the lemon juice and the remaining olive oil.

3 Simmer for 5min, stirring to break down the peppers a little. Stir the mint into the pan. Season to taste and serve.

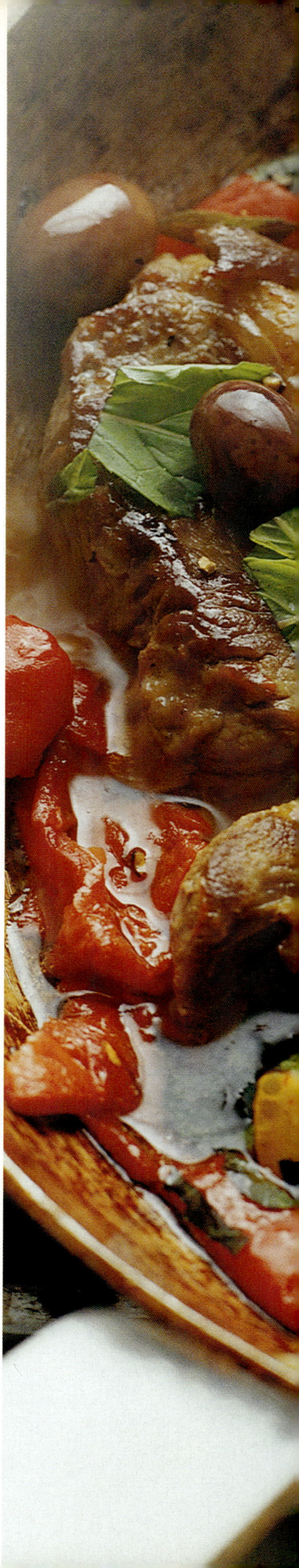

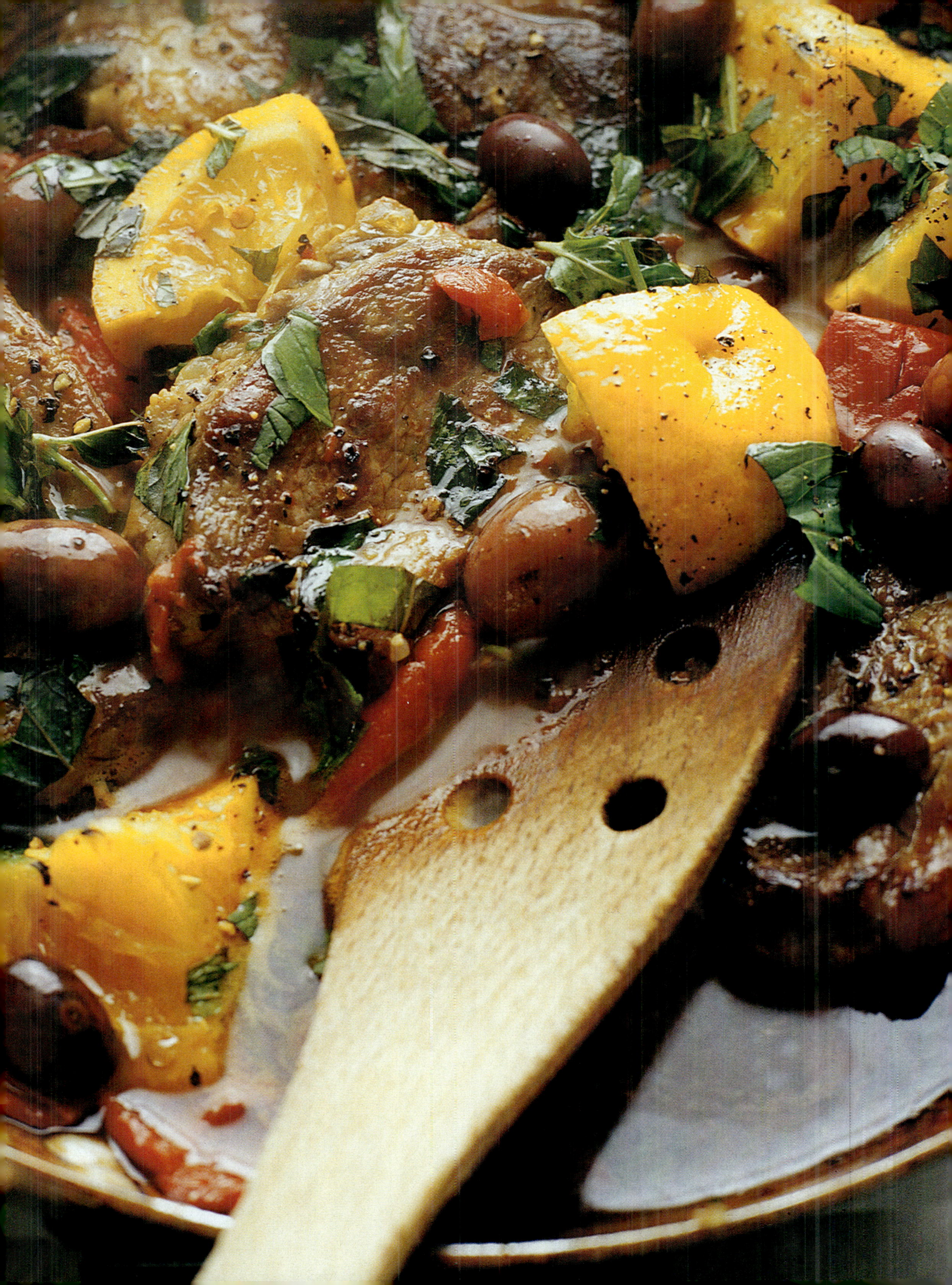

Winter Roasted Vegetable Tart

Hands-on time: for the marmalade, 10min, plus chilling; for the tart, 20min
Cooking time: for the marmalade, 1hr 5min; for the tart, 40min, plus 20min reheating
Serves: 3 (marmalade makes extra)
Vegetarian

FOR THE SAVOURY MARMALADE

* 2tbsp olive oil
* 500g (1lb 2oz) red onions, sliced
* Juice of 1 orange
* 1tbsp pickling spice
* 150g (5oz) dark muscovado sugar
* 150ml (¼ pint) ruby port
* 450g (1lb) fresh cranberries

FOR THE TART

* 250g ready-rolled shortcrust pastry, removed from fridge 5min before using
* 1 small red onion, cut into six wedges
* 1 raw baby beetroot, peeled and thickly sliced
* 1 baby aubergine, quartered
* 1 small red apple, quartered, cored and cut into chunky slices
* 1 garlic clove, crushed
* Juice of ½ lemon
* 1tsp freshly chopped thyme
* 1tbsp olive oil
* 125g (4oz) cranberry and red onion marmalade (see above)
* 25g (1oz) chestnut mushrooms, halved
* 50g (2oz) chestnuts, cooked and peeled
* 1tbsp redcurrant jelly, warmed

1 To make the savoury marmalade, heat the oil in a pan and gently fry the onions for 5min. Add the orange juice, spice, sugar and port and simmer gently for 40min. Add the cranberries and cook over a medium heat for 20min. Cool and chill until required – for up to two days.

2 To make the pastry case, first preheat the oven to 200°C (180°C fan) mark 6. Sit an 11.5x20.5cm (4½x8in) loose-bottomed tart tin on a baking sheet. Unroll the shortcrust pastry and use it to line the tin, trimming off any excess. Prick the base several times with a fork, then line with baking parchment and weigh down with pieces of leftover pastry or fill with baking beans. Bake the pastry case for 15min, then remove the weighted paper and cook for a further 5min until golden. Cool, remove from the tin, wrap in parchment and store in an airtight container for up to two days.

3 For the tart filling, put the onion, beetroot, aubergine, apple and garlic into a roasting tin. Squeeze over the lemon juice, scatter over the thyme and drizzle with olive oil, then roast for 20min. Put in a bowl, then cool, cover and chill for up to two days or until required.

4 Preheat the oven to 200°C (180°C fan) mark 6. To assemble the tart, put the cooked pastry case onto a baking sheet and spoon the marmalade over the base. Arrange the roasted vegetables and mushrooms on top. Chop the chestnuts and sprinkle over the tart, then season. Brush warmed redcurrant jelly over the vegetables to glaze. Cook for 20min and serve.

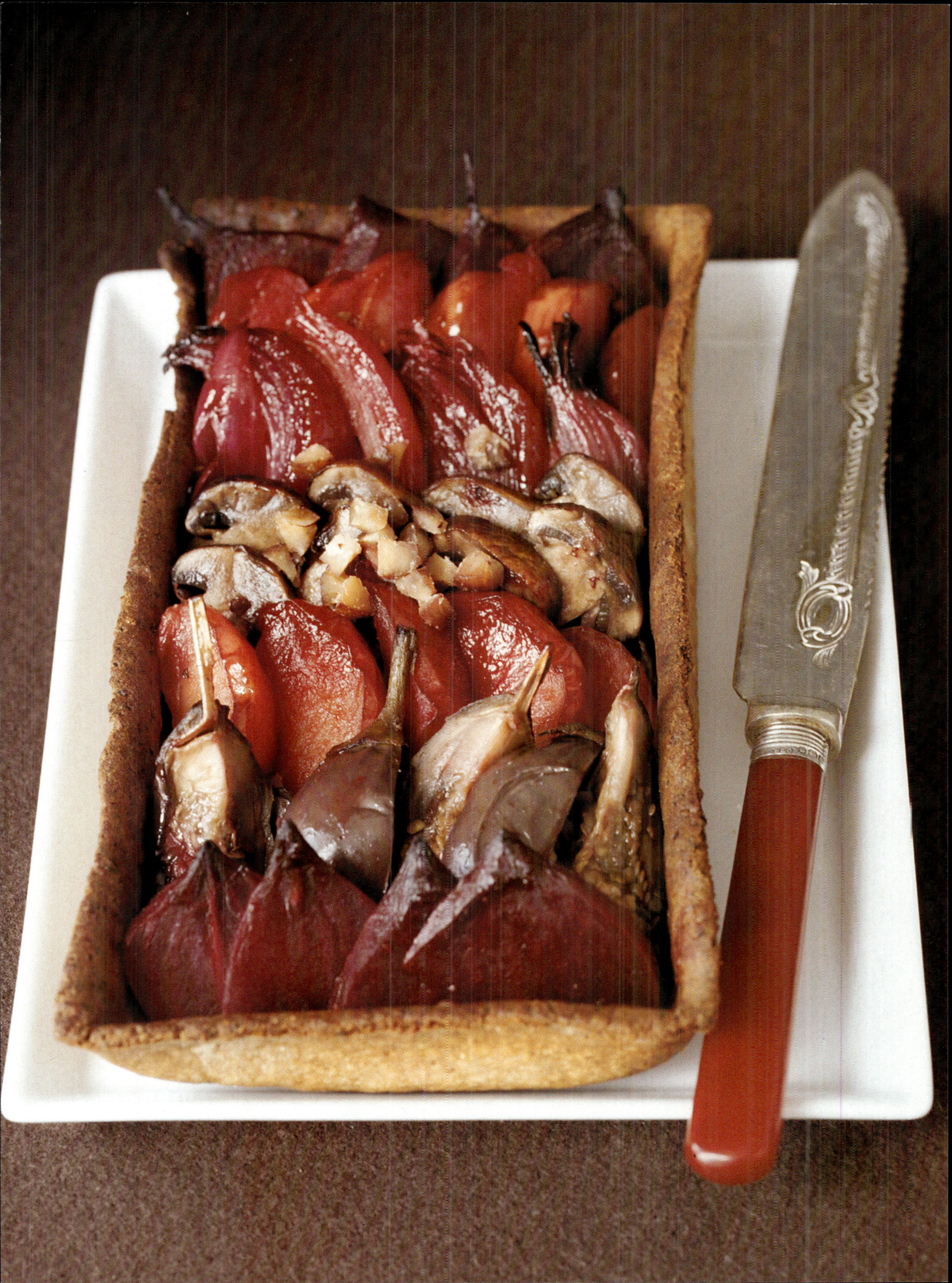

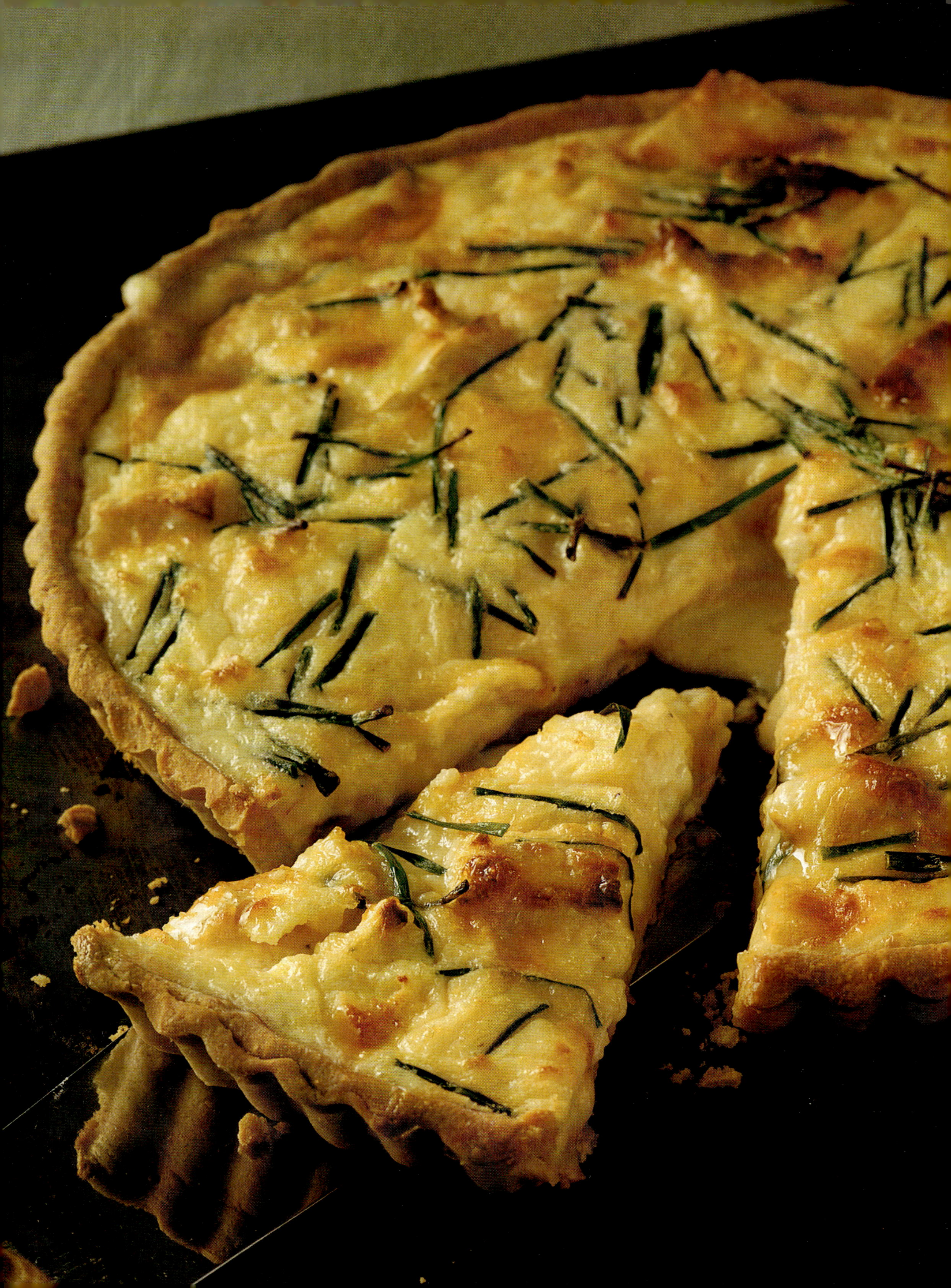

Cheese and Chive Tart

Hands-on time: 10min (20min if making pastry by hand), plus 30min chilling
Cooking time: 55min
Serves: 6–8
Vegetarian

FOR THE PASTRY

* 200g (7oz) plain flour
* 100g (3½oz) chilled butter, cubed
* A pinch of cayenne pepper
* 25g (1oz) Parmesan or Cheddar cheese, grated
* 2 large eggs

FOR THE FILLING

* 2 large eggs
* 125g (4oz) creamy goat's cheese
* 100ml (3½fl oz) crème fraîche
* 2tbsp chopped chives
* Ground nutmeg to taste
* 250g (9oz) goat's cheese with rind

1 Put the flour in a food processor with the butter and a pinch of salt and cayenne pepper. Whiz until the mixture resembles breadcrumbs. Add the grated hard cheese and one egg, then whiz or stir together until combined – you might need to add a little cold water. (If you're making the pastry by hand, rub together the flour and butter until the mixture resembles breadcrumbs, add the cheese and one egg, then stir until the mixture comes together.) Turn out the dough, wrap in clingfilm and chill for 20min.

2 Roll out the pastry on a lightly floured surface into a circle large enough to line a 23cm (9in) loose-bottomed tart tin, 2.5cm (1in) deep. Press the pastry into the tin, prick the base with a fork and line with greaseproof paper and baking beans. Cook at 200°C (180°C fan) mark 6 for 15min.

3 Remove the paper and beans and return the pastry case to the oven for 5–10min or until cooked in the centre. Lightly whisk one egg and brush over the inside of the pastry case. Return the pastry to the oven for 1min; reduce the temperature to 180°C (160°C fan) mark 4.

4 Mix two eggs with the creamy goat's cheese, crème fraîche and chives and season with pepper and a pinch of ground nutmeg. Crumble the rinded cheese into the egg mixture and pour the filling into the pastry case. Bake for 25–30min or until just set. Allow to cool for 15min, then turn the tart out of the tin. Serve warm.

To freeze: Complete the recipe, then cool, wrap and freeze.
To use: Reheat the tart from frozen at 200°C (180°C fan) mark 6 for 20min or until warm to the centre.

Potato and Celeriac Puffs

Hands-on time: 45min
Cooking time: 55min.
Allow extra time for the Shallot and Mushroom Sauce.
Serves: 6
Vegetarian

FOR THE CHUTNEY

* 700g (1½lb) tomatoes, peeled, deseeded and chopped
* 1 apple, peeled, cored and roughly chopped
* 50g (2oz) onion, finely chopped
* 1 garlic clove, crushed
* 125g (4oz) light, soft brown sugar
* 1tsp fresh ginger, finely chopped
* ½tsp turmeric
* 125g (4oz) sultanas
* 50ml (2fl oz) white wine vinegar

FOR THE POTATO BASE

* 350g (12oz) waxy potatoes, peeled and sliced
* 40–50g (1½–2oz) butter

FOR THE CELERIAC TOPPING

* 700g (1½lb) celeriac, peeled and cut into 2.5cm (1in) chunks
* 600ml (1 pint) vegetable stock
* 284ml carton double cream
* 2 garlic cloves, crushed
* 1 bayleaf
* A pinch of grated nutmeg
* 3 medium eggs, separated

TO SERVE

* Fresh chives to garnish
* Shallot and Mushroom Sauce (see Sauces)
* Blanched asparagus tips and yellow courgettes sprinkled with chopped herbs
* Roast potatoes with garlic and thyme

1 To make the chutney, mix in a pan the tomatoes, apple, onion, garlic, sugar, spices, sultanas and white wine vinegar. Bring to the boil and simmer for 30min or until reduced and thick. Cool, then use as required.

2 To make the potato base, place the sliced potatoes in a pan of cold, salted water and bring to the boil. Bubble for 1min, then drain. Heat half the butter in a non-stick frying pan and cook the potatoes in batches for 2–3min or until golden brown on both sides, adding more butter when necessary. Cool slightly and arrange in layers in the bottom of six 6.5cm (2½in) metal rings placed on a baking sheet, seasoning between each layer. (If you don't have ring moulds, make your own by folding extra-thick foil into strips and using to form rings. Fold over the ends to secure.) Set aside.

3 To make the celeriac topping, place the celeriac chunks in a pan and add the stock, cream, garlic, bayleaf and nutmeg. Season, bring to the boil and simmer for 15min. Drain and reserve the cooking liquid. Whiz the celeriac mixture with 2tbsp of the cooking liquid until smooth. Place the celeriac purée in a bowl and beat in the egg yolks. Whisk the egg whites until they form soft peaks and fold into the celeriac mixture.

4 Spoon the mixture on top of the potatoes, filling to the top of the rings. Cook at 200°C (180°C fan) mark 6 for 30min or until puffed and golden. Remove the rings from the puffs and place a spoonful of tomato and apple chutney on top. Garnish with chives and serve with the Shallot and Mushroom Sauce, blanched vegetables and roast potatoes.

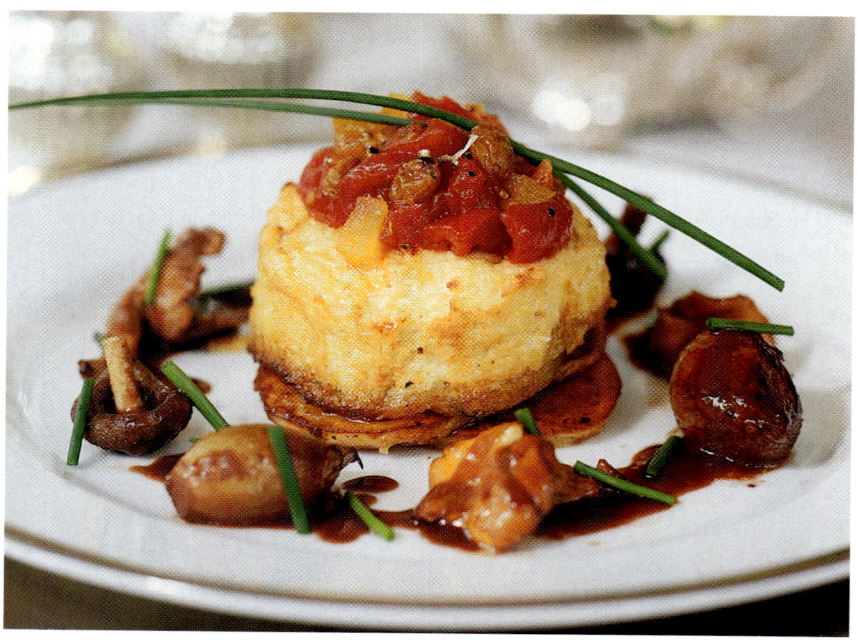

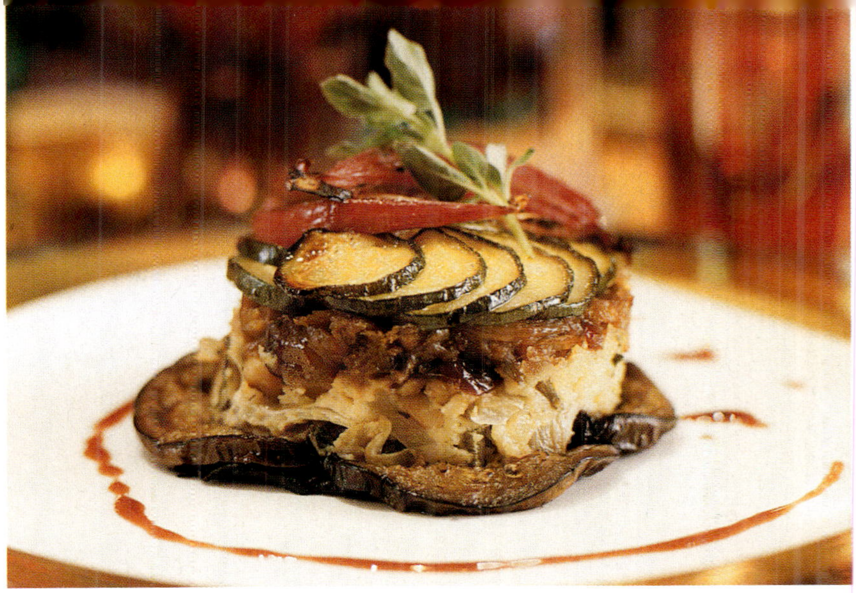

Mushroom and Aubergine Tian

Hands-on time: 50min
Cooking time: 58min. Allow extra time for the Mushroom and Chestnut Stuffing
Serves: 2
Vegetarian

FOR THE STUFFING

* 75g (3oz) butter
* 1 bunch spring onions, sliced
* 450g (1lb) fennel, roughly chopped
* 50g (2oz) pinenuts, toasted
* 150g (5oz) soft goat's cheese
* 4tbsp chopped fresh tarragon
* 125g (4oz) fresh breadcrumbs
* Zest and juice of 1 lemon
* 2 medium eggs, beaten

FOR THE TIAN

* 1 small aubergine, thinly sliced
* 1 courgette, thinly sliced
* ½ red onion, cut into thin wedges
* 3tbsp olive oil
* 2 portabella or large flat mushrooms
* 8tbsp Fennel and Pinenut Stuffing (see above)
* 8tbsp Mushroom and Chestnut Stuffing (see Stuffings)
* Oregano sprigs to garnish

FOR THE PORT WINE SAUCE

* 100ml (3½fl oz) port
* 150ml (¼ pint) vegetable stock
* 4tbsp redcurrant jelly
* 2 strips orange peel, finely sliced
* Juice of ½ lemon

1 First, to make the Fennel and Pinenut stuffing, heat the butter in a pan and cook the spring onions for 3min. Add the fennel and cook for 5min. Cool. Add the pinenuts, goat's cheese, tarragon, breadcrumbs, lemon zest and juice and eggs. Season mix well and set aside until required.

2 To make the tian, brush the aubergine and courgette slices and onion wedges with 2tbsp of olive oil. Heat a non-stick frying pan and fry the aubergine, courgette and onion in batches.

3 Preheat the oven to 200°C (180°C fan) mark 6. Lay half the fried aubergine slices overlapping on top of each mushroom. Divide the fennel stuffing equally between the two mushrooms. Season. Top with the mushroom stuffing and season. Arrange the courgette slices over the stuffing, overlapping them, then top with the onion wedges. Wrap a thick band of foil around each mushroom to keep the stuffing in place. Place in an ovenproof dish and drizzle the rest of the oil over the mushrooms. Bake for 40min.

4 Make the port wine sauce. Put the port, vegetable stock, redcurrant jelly, orange peel and lemon juice in a pan and bring to the boil. Simmer until syrupy.

5 Remove the foil from the mushrooms, then garnish each tian with the oregano sprigs and serve with the sauce drizzled round.

To freeze: Complete step 2, then freeze. Make the sauce and freeze.
To use: Thaw at room temperature for 4hr and continue from step 3.

White Nut Roast

Hands-on time: 20min, plus cooling and freezing
Cooking time: 50min–1hr 10min
Serves: 8
Vegetarian

* 40g (1½oz) butter
* 1 onion, finely chopped
* 1 garlic clove, crushed
* 225g (8oz) mixed white nuts, such as brazil, macadamia, pinenuts and whole almonds, ground down in a processor
* 125g (4oz) fresh white breadcrumbs
* Zest and juice of ½ lemon
* 75g (3oz) sage Derby cheese or Parmesan, grated
* 125g (4oz) canned peeled chestnuts, roughly chopped
* ½ x 390g can artichoke hearts, roughly chopped
* 1 medium egg, lightly beaten
* 2tsp each freshly chopped parsley, sage and thyme, plus extra sprigs

1 Melt the butter in a pan and cook the onion and garlic for 5min or until soft. Put into a large bowl and set aside to cool.

2 Add the ground nuts, breadcrumbs, lemon zest and juice, grated cheese, chestnuts and artichokes. Season generously and bind together with the beaten egg. Stir in the freshly chopped herbs.

3 Put the mixture onto a large buttered piece of foil and shape into a fat, tightly packed sausage. Scatter over the extra herb sprigs and wrap the sausage in the foil. Cool, cover and freeze until needed.

4 Cook the nut roast on an upturned Swiss roll tin at 200°C (180°C fan) mark 6 for 45min from frozen, then unwrap the foil slightly and cook for a further 15min until it is turning golden.

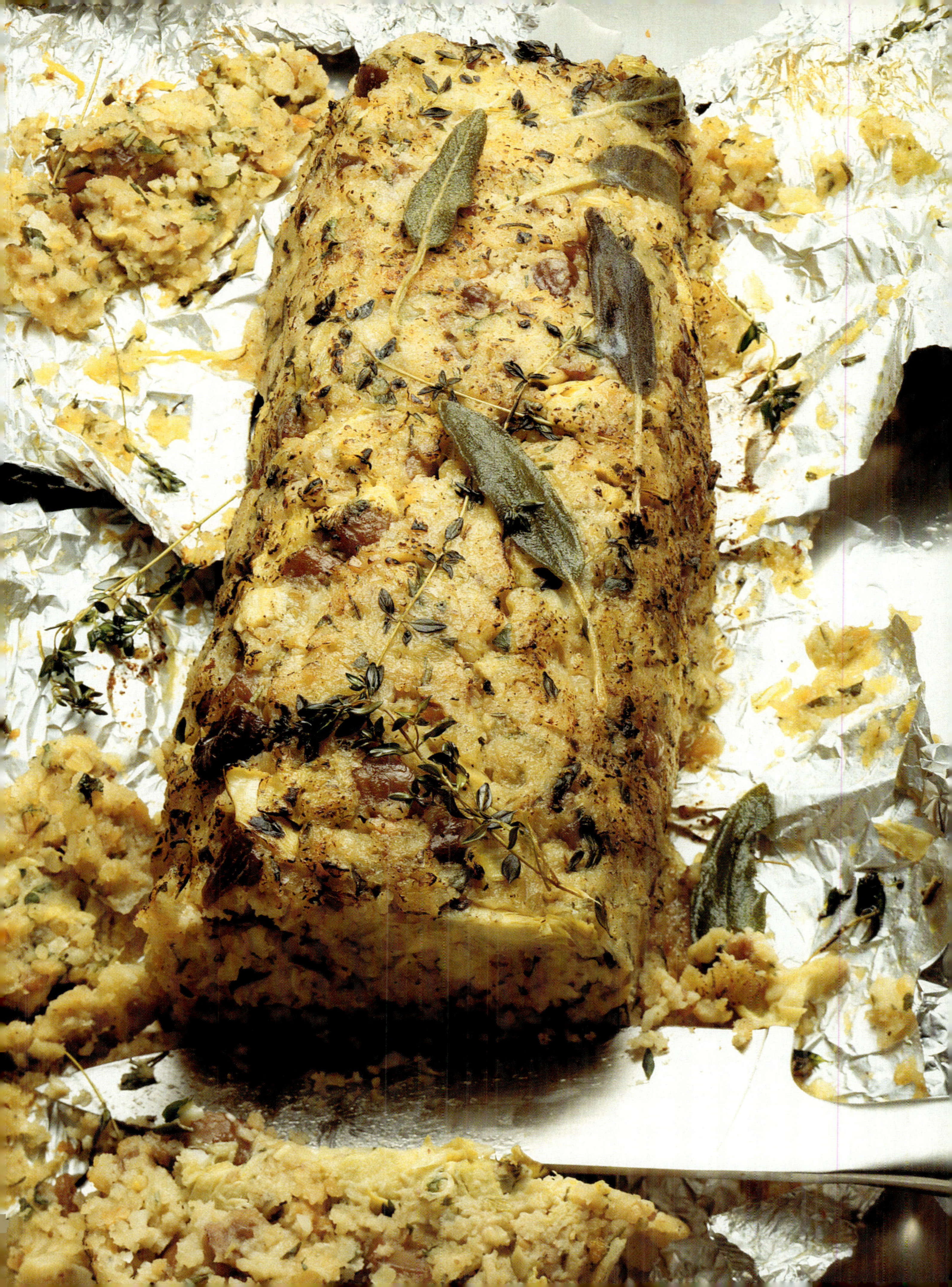

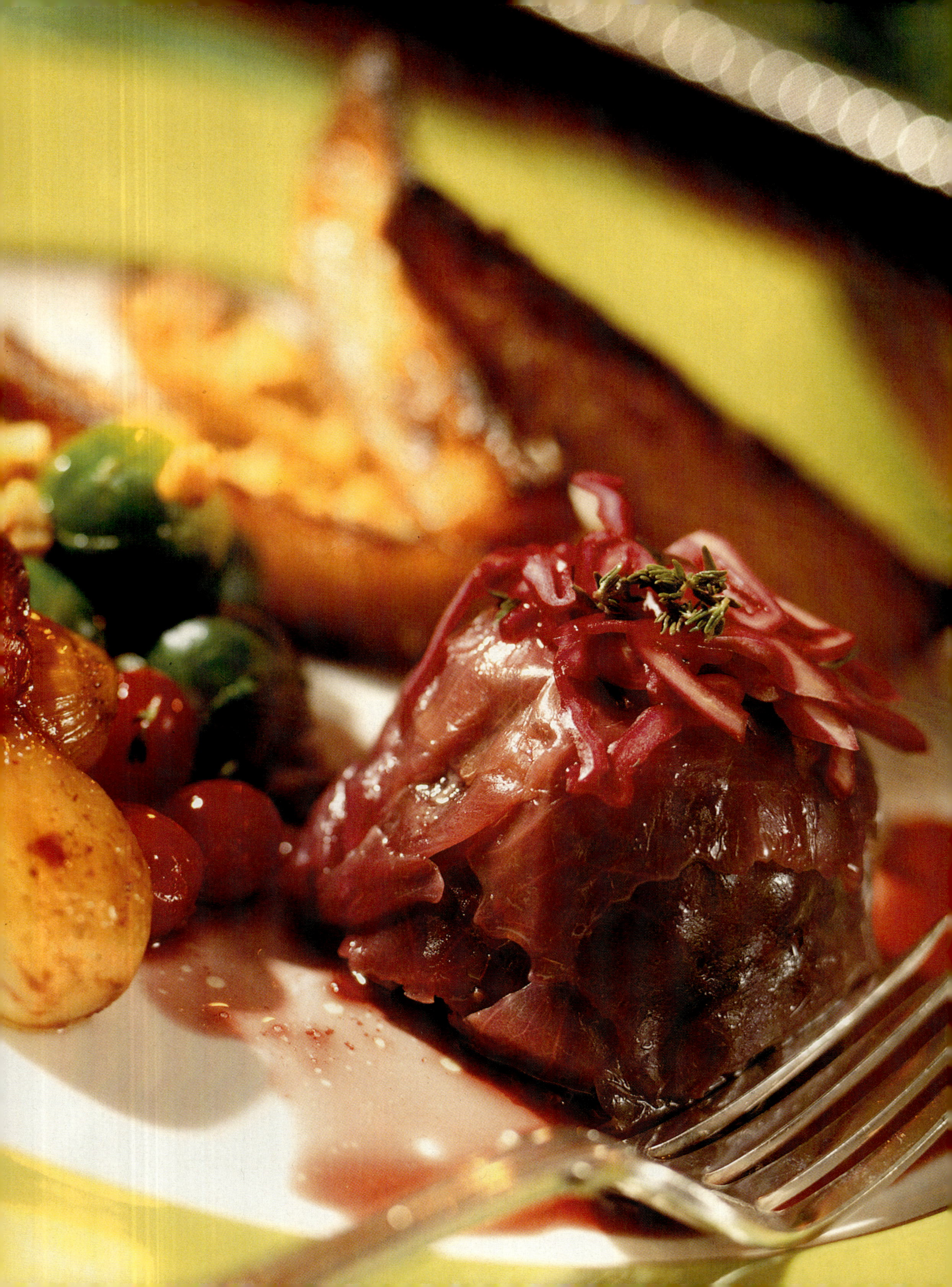

Red Cabbage Timbales with Mushroom Stuffing

Hands-on time: 1hr, plus cooling for 30min
Cooking time: 1hr
Serves: 6
Vegetarian

FOR THE STUFFING
* 50g (2oz) butter
* 200g (7oz) onions, finely chopped
* 450g (1lb) brown-cap mushrooms, roughly chopped
* 4tbsp chopped flat-leaf parsley
* 75g (3oz) toasted, salted cashew nuts, roughly chopped
* 125g (4oz) fresh breadcrumbs
* 2 large eggs, beaten

FOR THE TIMBALES
* 1 medium red cabbage, about 1.4kg (3lb)
* 375g (13oz) onions, finely chopped
* 40g (1½oz) butter
* 3tbsp balsamic vinegar

FOR THE RED WINE SAUCE
* 4tbsp caster sugar
* 4tbsp red wine vinegar
* 150ml (¼ pint) red wine
* 1tbsp lemon juice
* Small thyme sprigs to garnish (optional)

1 To make the stuffing, melt the butter in a pan, add the onions and cook until soft and golden. Add the mushrooms and fry over a brisk heat until the moisture has evaporated. Mix in the chopped parsley, cashew nuts and breadcrumbs. Leave to cool, then stir in the beaten eggs. Season and mix well. Cover and set aside.

2 To make the timbales, place the cabbage in a large pan of boiling water. Bring to the boil and simmer until the outside leaves have softened enough to be eased away. Lift the cabbage out of the pan and set aside, reserving the water. Remove the three outer leaves, boil them for a further 3–4min, then place in a bowl of cold water. Quarter the reserved whole cabbage and remove the core. Take 700g (1½lb) of the leaves; remove and discard any heavy central veins. Shred the leaves very finely, cover and set aside.

3 Line six 150ml (¼ pint) pudding moulds with microwave clingfilm. Drain the whole cabbage leaves and cut in half either side of the central vein. Discard the vein. Use the leaves to line the moulds. Fill with the stuffing mixture and cover with foil.

4 Place the moulds in a large roasting tin and pour in enough warm water to come halfway up their sides. Cook at 190°C (170°C fan) mark 5 for 30min or until just set to the centre. Meanwhile, melt the butter in a pan, add the onion and cook until soft. Mix in the reserved shredded cabbage, vinegar and 3tbsp of the reserved water. Season, then cook, stirring from time to time, for 15–20min or until beginning to soften.

5 To make the sauce, place the sugar and red wine vinegar in a small pan. Cook over a gentle heat until the sugar has dissolved, then bring to the boil and cook to a rich caramel. Pour in the wine and bubble until reduced by half. Add lemon juice to taste, and season. Cool.

6 To serve, turn out the timbales, spoon the shredded cabbage on top, drizzle over the red wine sauce and garnish with thyme sprigs, if using.

Leek, Mushroom and Artichoke Croûte

Hands-on time: 30min, plus cooling and chilling overnight
Cooking time: 30–35min
Serves: 8
Vegetarian

- 3tbsp olive oil
- 2 garlic cloves, crushed
- 125g (4oz) shiitake mushrooms, sliced
- 1tbsp balsamic vinegar
- 50g (2oz) whole cooked chestnuts, roughly chopped
- 1½tsp fresh young thyme sprigs
- 400g can artichoke hearts, drained and quartered
- 350g (12oz) leeks, washed and sliced
- 375g ready-rolled puff pastry
- Butter for greasing
- 1 egg, lightly beaten, to glaze
- Cranberry sauce and a little extra-virgin olive oil to serve

1 Heat 2tbsp of olive oil in a large pan and fry the garlic for 1min. Add the mushrooms and cook over a low heat for 3min to soften – cooking the mushrooms with the garlic before adding the other ingredients gives them depth of flavour. Add the balsamic vinegar, chestnuts, ½tsp of thyme leaves (stripped off the sprigs) and the artichokes, then cook for 1min. Cook the leeks separately: in a large clean pan, heat the remaining 1tbsp oil, add the leeks and cook for 4min to soften slightly. Turn into a bowl and cool for 5min.

2 Unroll the pastry and sprinkle the surface with the remaining thyme sprigs. Roll the leaves lightly into the pastry. Flip the pastry over so that the herbs are on the underside, then roll the pastry lightly to a 38x25.5cm (15x10in) rectangle. Using a sharp knife, cut the pastry in half vertically to create two long, thin rectangles.

3 Spoon half the mushroom mixture down the centre of each piece of pastry. Top with the leeks and season. Brush the pastry edges with water, then fold each side of the pastry up over the filling and seal. Cut both rolls in half and put onto a greased baking sheet. Cover and chill overnight.

4 Preheat the oven to 200°C (180°C fan) mark 6. Brush the pastry with egg to glaze. Cook for 20min until the pastry is golden. Slice each croûte into six and serve three slices per person, topped with a dollop of cranberry sauce and a light drizzle of olive oil.

To freeze: Complete the recipe to the end of step 3, then cover and freeze for up to one month.
To use: Cook the croûtes from frozen in a preheated oven at 200°C (180°C fan) mark 6 for 25min until the pastry is golden. Serve as above.

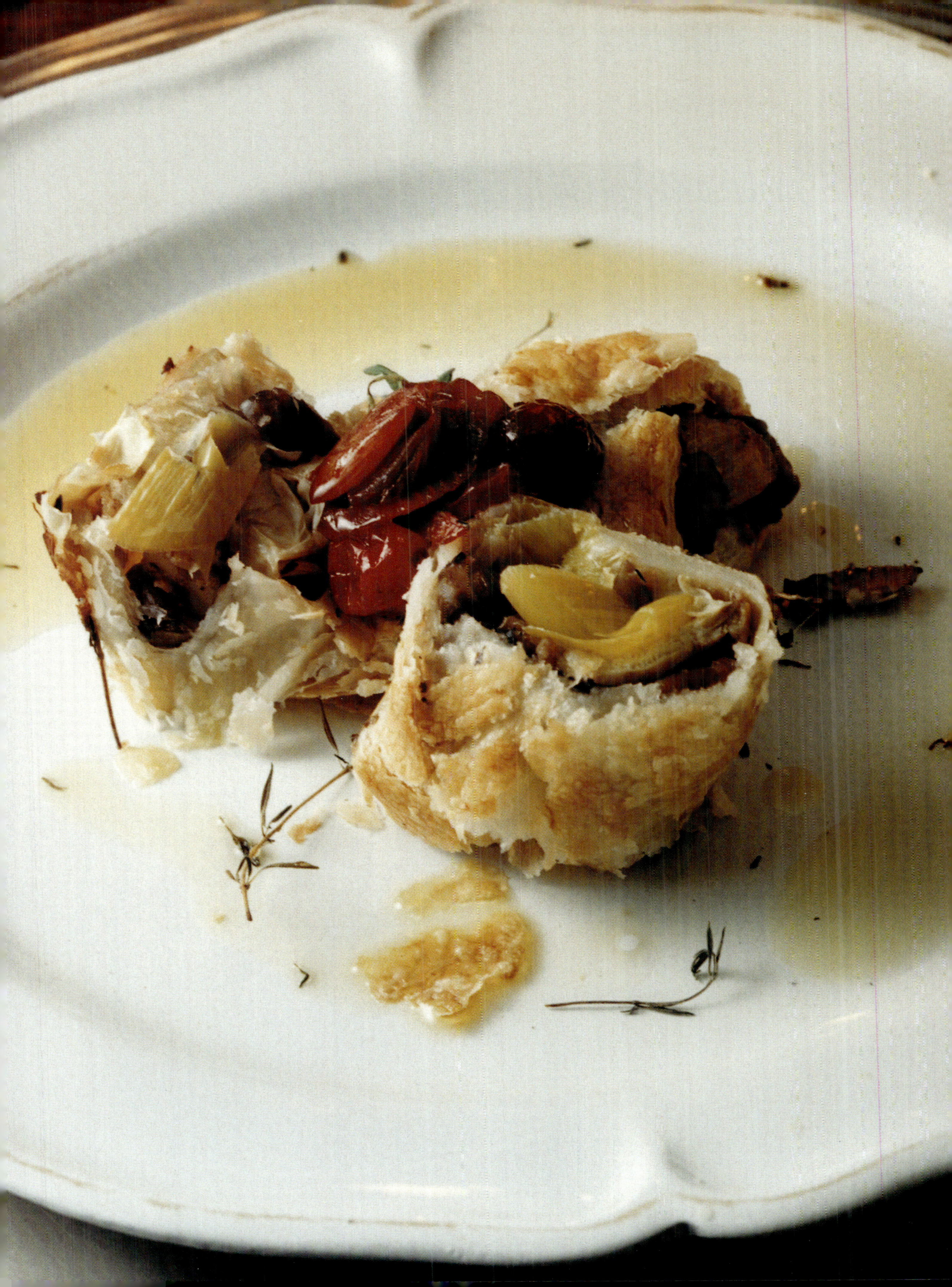

Bubble and Squeak

Hands-on time: 15min
Cooking time: 35min
Serves: 6

* 1tbsp oil
* 1 red onion, thinly sliced
* 4 rashers streaky bacon, cut into small pieces
* 550g (1½lb) mashed potato
* 300g (11oz) cooked Brussels sprouts, cut in half if large
* 25g (1oz) grated Parmesan cheese
* Butter for greasing, and a little extra, melted

1 Heat the oil in a large pan and cook the onion for 4–5min until soft. Add the bacon and cook for a further 3–4min until it begins to brown. Remove the pan from the heat and transfer the bacon and onions to a large bowl. Add the mashed potato and Brussels sprouts. Season. Add the Parmesan cheese, mix well and divide the mixture into six portions.

2 Using your hands, shape each portion into a small round cake, put onto a greased baking tray and brush with a little melted butter. Bake at 200°C (180°C fan) mark 6 for 25min until slightly golden.

Red Cabbage and Beetroot Salad

Hands-on time: 15min
Serves: 8
Vegetarian

FOR THE DRESSING
* 6tbsp extra-virgin olive oil
* 2tbsp sherry vinegar
* 3tbsp freshly chopped dill

* ½ red cabbage, finely sliced
* 500g (1lb 2oz) cooked beetroot (without vinegar), sliced into matchsticks or grated
* 8 cornichons (baby gherkins), sliced into rounds
* 2tbsp baby capers in vinegar, rinsed

1 To make the dressing, put the olive oil, vinegar and dill in a small bowl. Season, then add a splash of cold water to help emulsify the dressing. Whisk together thoroughly.

2 Put the cabbage, beetroot, cornichons and capers in a large bowl and mix. Pour the dressing over the salad and toss everything together well.

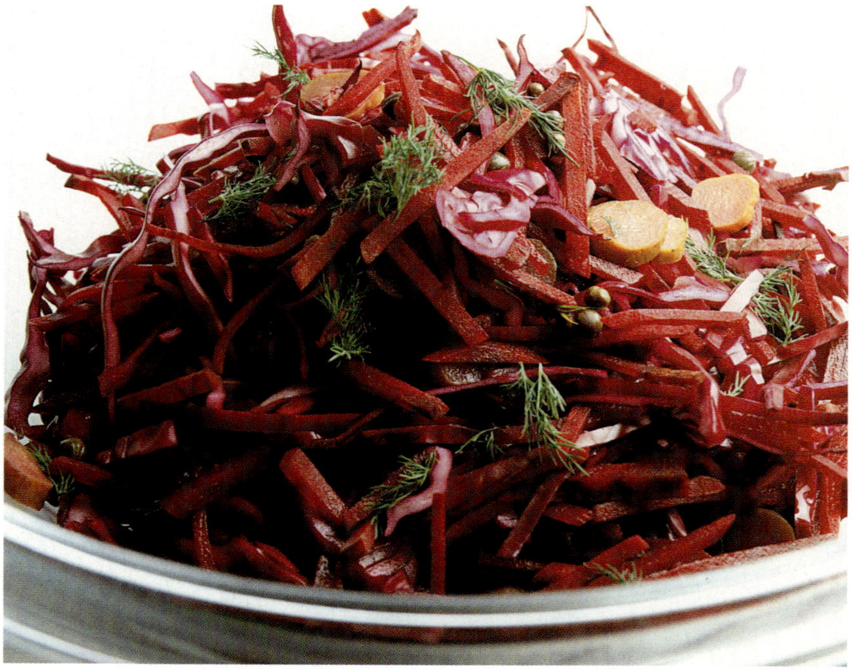

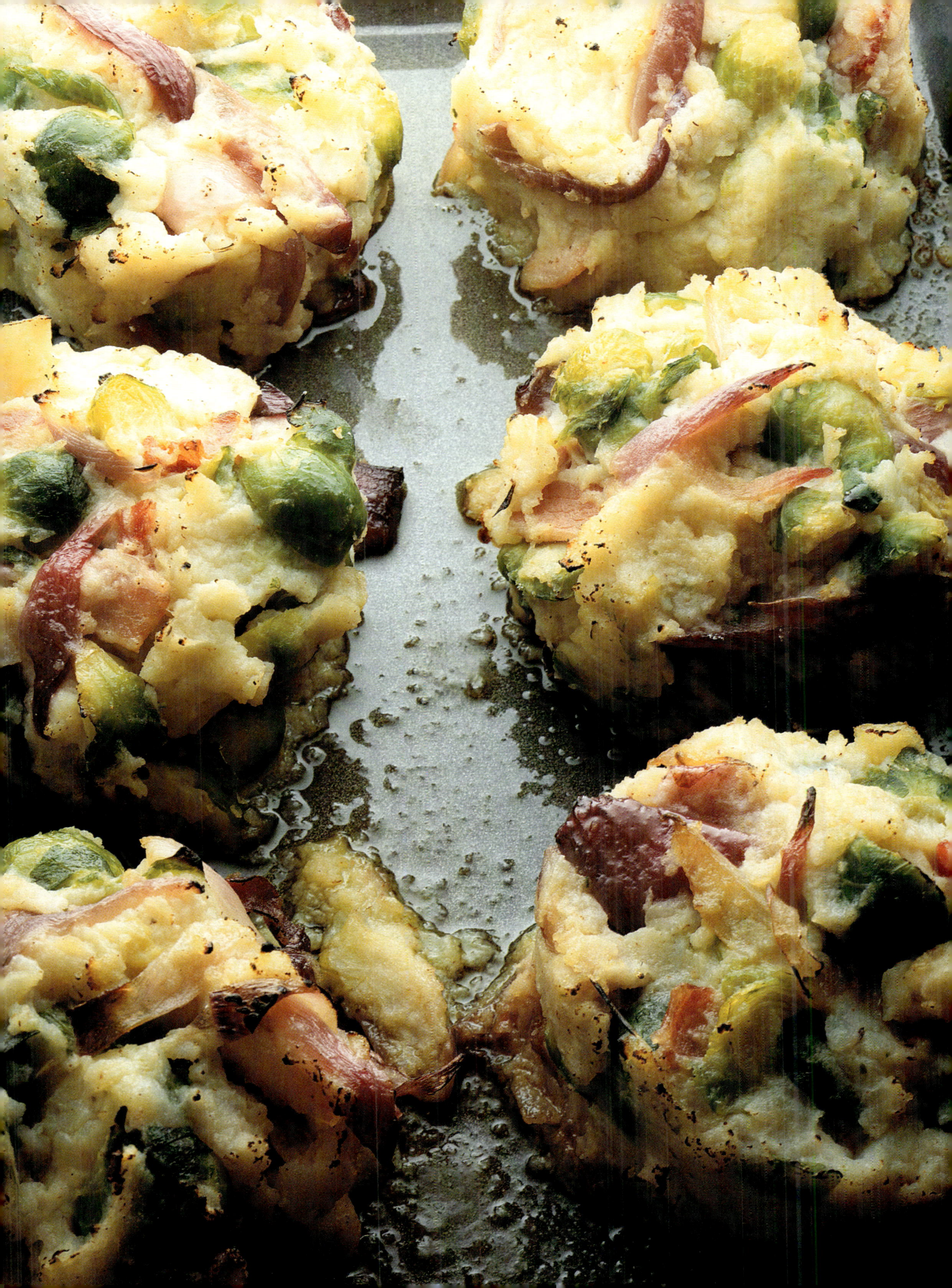

Salmon Rosti Pie

Hands-on time: 30min, plus 10min cooling
Cooking time: 1hr 40min
Serves: 8

- 1.5kg (3½lb) waxy potatoes, scrubbed
- 100g (3½oz) butter, melted, plus extra for greasing
- 900g (2lb) salmon fillet, skinned
- 200ml (7fl oz) dry white wine
- 2 x 250ml jars hollandaise sauce
- 2 x 250g bunches asparagus, cut into 7.5cm (3in) lengths, blanched
- Juice of ½ lemon
- 400g can artichoke hearts, drained and quartered
- 2tbsp roughly chopped fresh dill

1 Preheat the oven to 220°C (200°C fan) mark 7. Put the potatoes in a pan of cold, salted water. Cover, bring to the boil and cook for 5–8min. Drain the potatoes, tip them into a bowl, cool for 5–10min, then peel.

2 Slide each potato lengthways along a coarse grater to make long strands. Grease two baking trays (with a lip) and spoon the potato strands into 12 mounds onto each. Drizzle with the melted butter. Season. Bake for 50min or until golden brown.

3 Put the salmon in a large roasting tin with the white wine and 75ml (3fl oz) water. Season. Cover with foil and bake for 20min at the same temperature as the potatoes.

4 Lift the salmon out of the tin, reserving the juices – about 150ml (¼ pint) – and flake into a bowl. Mix the juices with the hollandaise sauce. Stir in the asparagus, lemon juice, artichoke hearts and dill. Season.

5 Put the salmon into the base of a 4 litre (7 pint) ovenproof dish. Pour the hollandaise mixture over and gently stir together. Turn the oven down to 200°C (180°C fan) mark 6. Arrange the rösti on top of the salmon and cook for 20–30min until heated through.

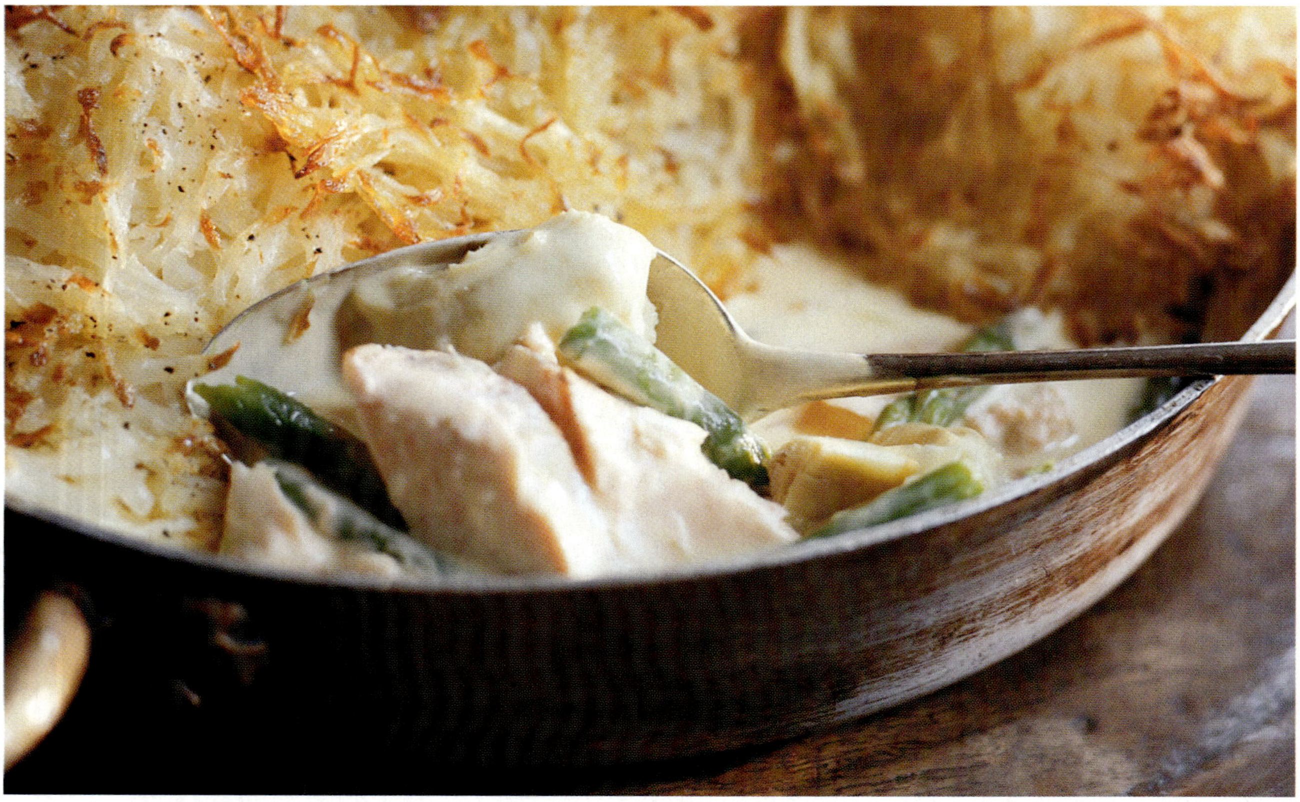

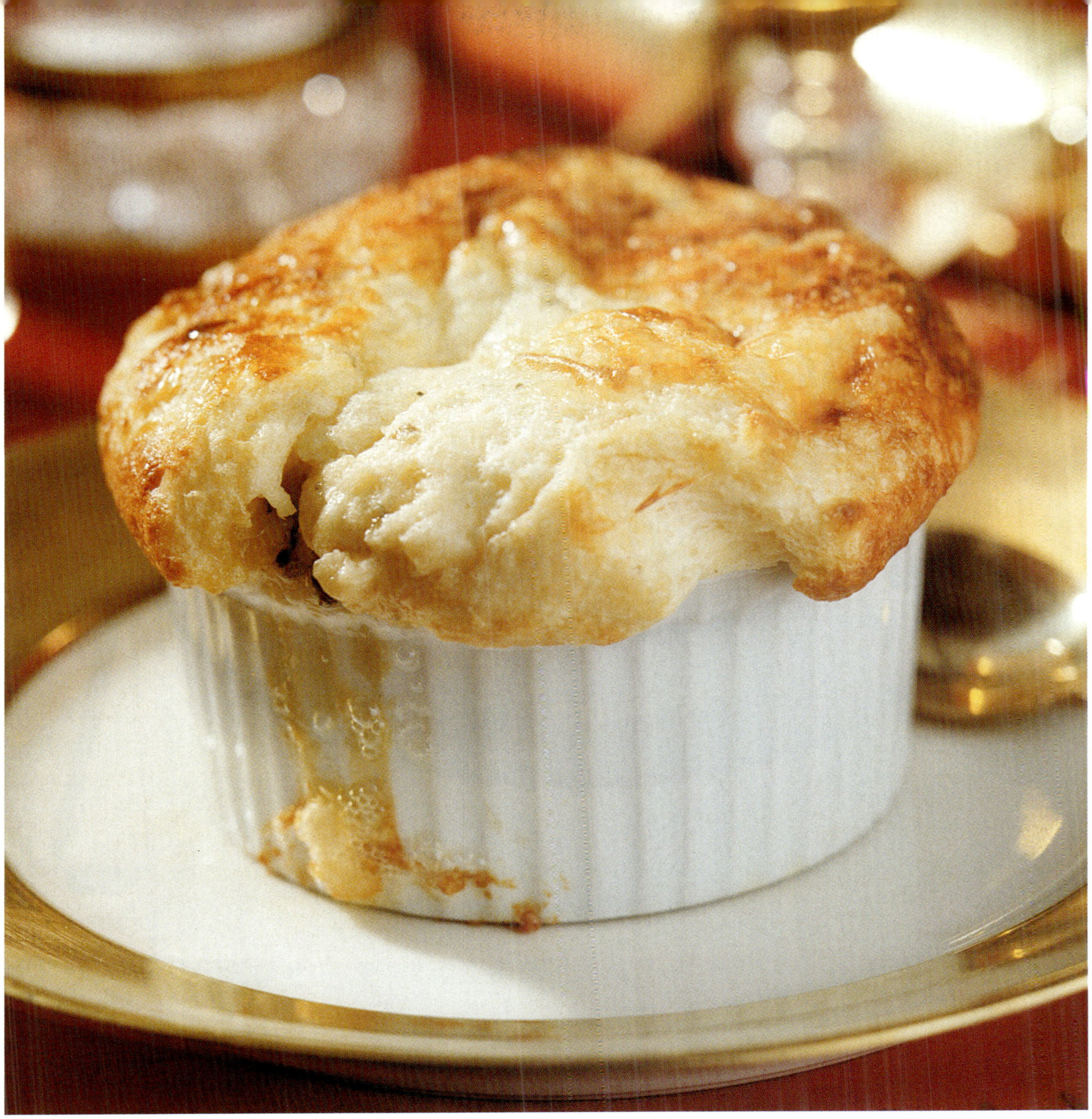

Blue Cheese and Parsnip Puffs

Hands-on time: 35min
Cooking time: 40min
Serves: 8

* 225g (8oz) parsnips, peeled and roughly chopped
* 50g (2oz) butter, plus extra for greasing
* 50g (2oz) flour
* 284ml carton milk
* 4 large eggs, separated
* 50g (2oz) Gruyère cheese, grated
* 75g (3oz) blue cheese, such as Stilton or dolcelatte, crumbled

1 Cook the parsnips in a large pan of boiling salted water until tender. Drain, dry well over a low heat then mash to a purée. Lightly butter eight 150ml (¼ pint) ramekin dishes and put on a baking sheet.

2 Melt the butter in a large pan, stir in the flour and mix into a smooth paste. Blend in the milk off the heat, then bring to the boil, stirring continuously. Cool a little, beat in the egg yolks, Gruyère and parsnip purée. Season. Whisk the egg whites to a soft peak, then, using a large metal spoon, fold into the parsnip mixture with the blue cheese (don't overstir).

3 Fill the ramekins almost to the top. Cook in the oven at 200°C (180°C fan) mark 6 for 15–20min or until puffed up and golden brown. Serve immediately.

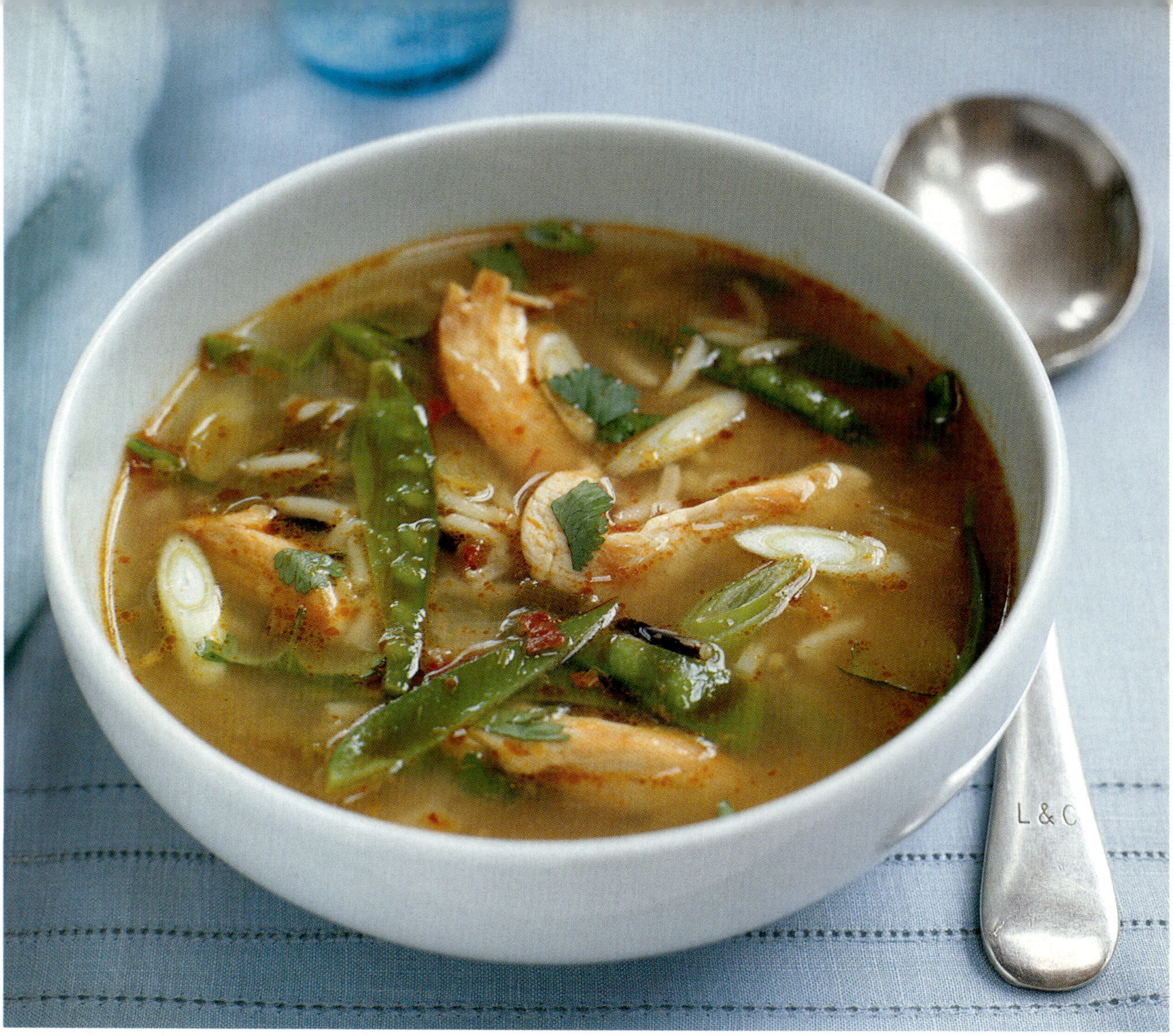

Hot and Sour Soup

Hands-on time: 20min
Cooking time: 30–35min
Serves: 4

- 1tbsp vegetable oil
- 2 turkey breasts, around 300g (11oz), or the same quantity of tofu, cut into strips
- 5cm (2in) piece fresh root ginger, grated
- 4 spring onions, finely sliced
- 1–2tbsp Thai red curry paste
- 75g (3oz) long-grain wild rice
- 1.1 litres (2 pints) hot weak chicken or vegetable stock or boiling water
- 200g (7oz) mangetout, sliced
- Juice of 1 lime
- 4tbsp roughly chopped coriander to sprinkle

1 Heat the vegetable oil in a deep pan. Add the turkey or tofu and cook over a medium heat for 5min until browned. Add the ginger and spring onions. Cook for a further 2–3min. Stir in the Thai red curry paste and cook for 1–2min to warm the spices.

2 Add the rice and stir to coat in the curry paste. Pour the hot stock or boiling water into the pan. Stir once, then bring to the boil. Turn the heat down and leave to simmer, covered, for 20min.

3 Add the mangetout and cook for a further 5min or until the rice is cooked. Just before serving, squeeze in the lime juice and stir to mix. Ladle into bowls and sprinkle with the coriander just before serving.

Cheesy Leek Soup

Hands-on time: 15min
Cooking time: 3hr 40min
Serves: 6

FOR THE STOCK

- Cooked carcass of a turkey
- Root vegetables, cut into slices
- 1tsp black peppercorns
- 2 bayleaves

FOR THE SOUP

- 50g (2oz) butter
- 225g (8oz) onions, finely chopped
- 700g (1½lb) trimmed leeks, roughly chopped
- 1tbsp flour
- 1.4 litres (2½ pints) turkey stock (see above)
- 142ml carton double cream
- 2tsp grainy mustard
- 225g (8oz) diced Gruyère or Stilton, plus extra shavings of Stilton to garnish
- Croûtons to serve

1 To make the stock, break the turkey carcass into pieces and place in a large pan with the root vegetables. Cover with cold water, bring slowly to the boil, skim and add the black peppercorns and bayleaves. Simmer, covered, for up to 3hr, then strain and cool quickly.

2 To make the soup, melt the butter in a large pan, add the onion and cook for 5min or until soft. Add the leeks and cook for 15min, stirring from time to time. Add the flour and mix until smooth, stirring continuously, then add the stock. Bring to the boil and simmer gently for 15min. Reduce the heat until the soup is bubbling gently, then stir in the cream and mustard. Add the cheese in batches, allowing it to melt between each addition. Season.

3 To make the soup garnish, chill a wedge of Stilton, then, using a swivel vegetable peeler, shave off thin slices. Store in a single layer on a baking sheet in the fridge until ready to use. Serve the soup in warmed bowls accompanied with croûtons and garnished with shavings of Stilton.

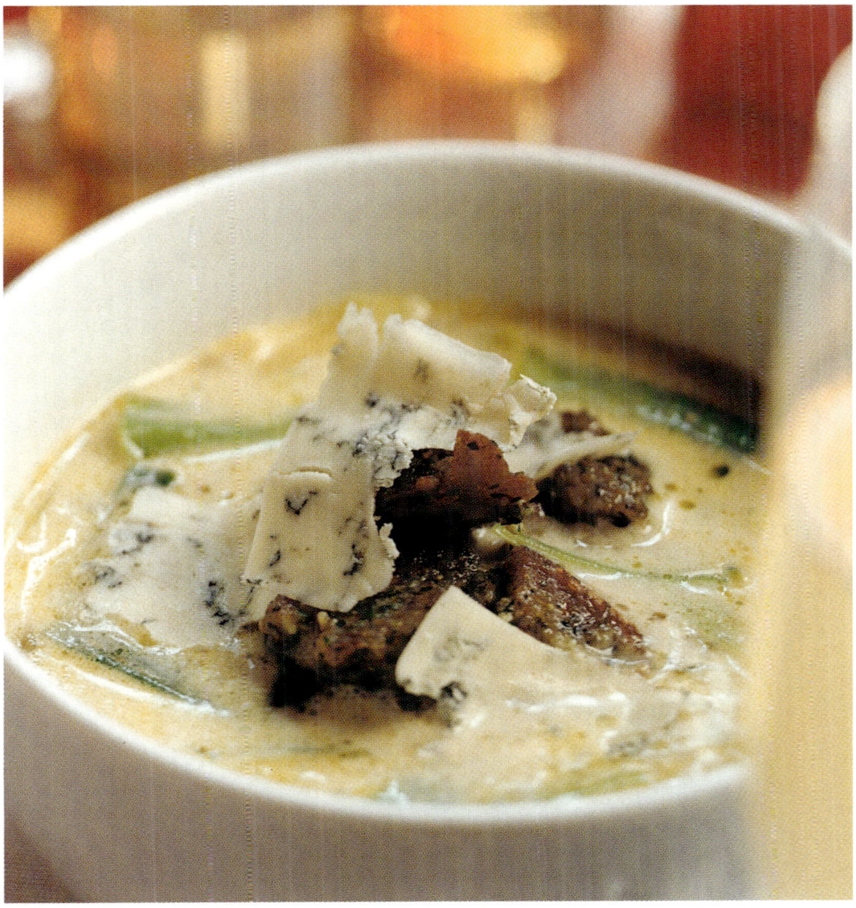

Turkey, Pepper and Haricot Casserole

Hands-on time: 20min, plus overnight soaking
Cooking time: 1hr 20min
Serves: 6

- 350g (12oz) dried haricot beans
- 2 small carrots, cut into chunks
- 2 large onions – 1 cut into quarters and 1 finely sliced
- 1 bouquet garni
- 1tbsp olive oil
- 2 medium red chillies, deseeded and chopped
- 2 garlic cloves, crushed
- 350g (12oz) lean turkey meat, cut into bite-size pieces
- 1 large red and 1 large orange pepper, deseeded and finely diced
- 2 courgettes, finely diced
- 400g can chopped tomatoes
- 1tbsp sun-dried tomato paste
- Large handful of fresh basil leaves

1 Soak the beans overnight in plenty of cold water. Drain, then put into a large casserole dish and cover with fresh water. Add the carrots, the onion quarters and the bouquet garni. Bring to the boil, cover, reduce the heat and simmer for 45min until the beans are tender. Drain, reserving the beans and 150ml (¼ pint) of the cooking liquid, then discard the vegetables.

2 Heat the oil in the casserole dish and cook the finely sliced onion for 5min. Add the chilli and garlic and cook for a further 1min until softened. Add the turkey and stir-fry for 5min, then add the peppers and courgettes. Season. Cover and cook for 5min, until the vegetables are slightly softened.

3 Add the tomatoes and tomato paste, cover and bring to the boil. Add the haricot beans and reserved cooking liquid. Season, cover and simmer for 15min. Stir in the basil leaves just before serving.

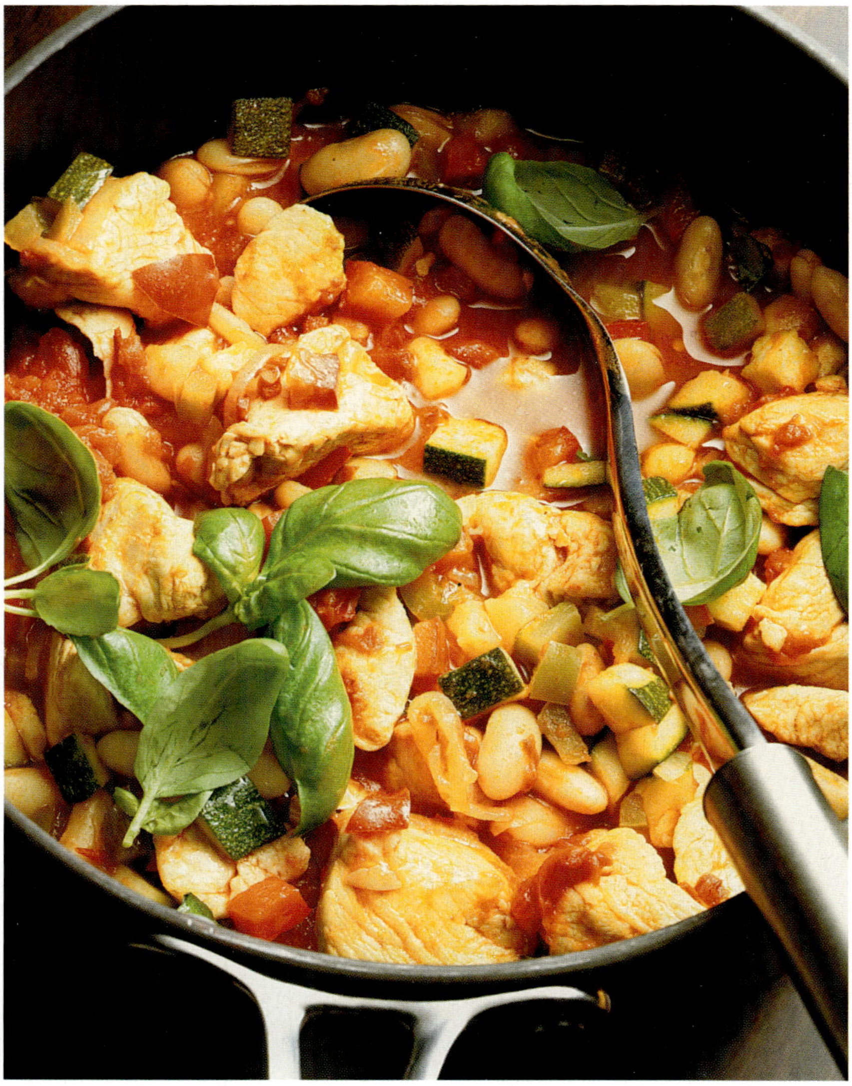

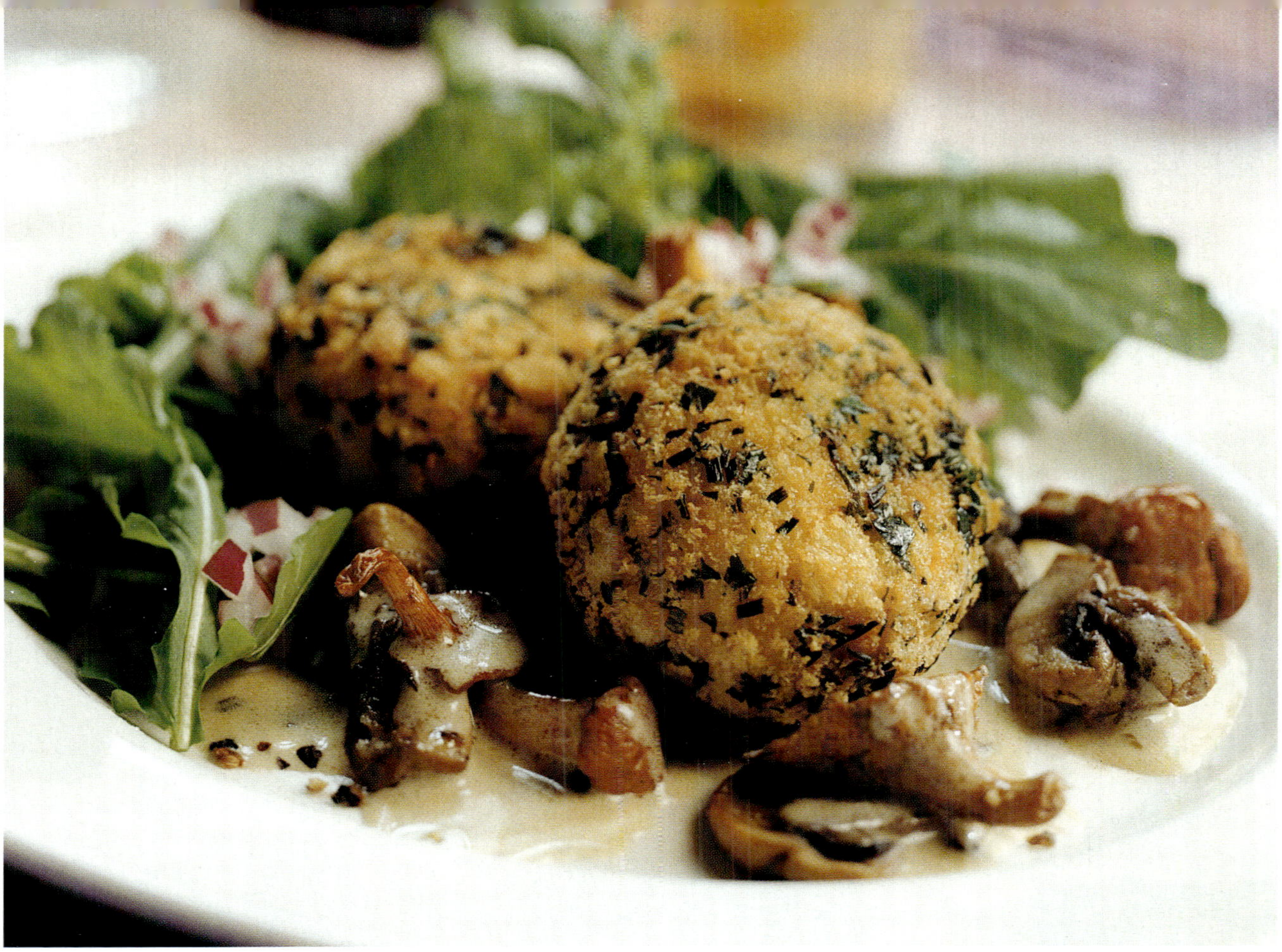

Turkey and Stilton Patties with Mushroom Sauce

Hands-on time: 1hr, plus 15min chilling
Cooking time: 30min
Serves: 6

- 125g (4oz) Stilton cheese
- 3tbsp chopped flat-leafed parsley
- 1tbsp chopped fresh thyme
- 125g (4oz) fresh breadcrumbs
- 700g (1½lb) cooked turkey meat
- 4 large eggs
- 2tsp ready-made English mustard
- 1 garlic clove, crushed
- Flour to dust

FOR THE MUSHROOM SAUCE

- 50g (2oz) butter
- 450g (1lb) wild or button mushrooms, finely sliced
- 300ml (½ pint) vermouth or white wine
- 500ml tub crème fraîche
- Vegetable oil
- Rocket leaves and finely chopped red onion to serve

1 Cut the Stilton cheese into 5mm cubes. Mix the chopped fresh herbs with the fresh breadcrumbs. Roughly cut the cooked turkey meat into pieces and place in a food processor with three eggs, the mustard and the garlic. Whiz until the mixture forms a fine paste. Season.

2 Divide the turkey mixture into 12 rounds. On a lightly floured surface, pat each round into a flat circle about 6.5cm (2½in) in diameter. Put a cube of cheese in the centre and gently bring the turkey mixture around to cover completely. Dust each patty with flour, brush with the remaining beaten egg and roll in the breadcrumb mixture. Chill, uncovered.

3 Melt the butter in a frying pan and cook the mushrooms for 5min over a high heat. Pour in the vermouth or white wine, bring to the boil and bubble until reduced by half. Add the crème fraîche, return to the boil and bubble for a further 10min or until the mixture is syrupy. Season.

4 To cook the patties, either shallow-fry for 3min on each side, then drain well on kitchen paper, or brush the crumbed surface lightly with oil and bake in the oven at 200°C (180°C fan) mark 6 for 20min or until crisp and brown. Serve with the mushroom sauce, rocket leaves and red onion.

Christmas Pudding Parfait

Hands-on time: 30min, plus 6hr freezing
Cooking time: 3–5min
Serves: 12

- Zest and juice of 1 orange
- 2tbsp brandy
- 125g (4oz) each sultanas and ready-to-eat prunes
- 1tsp ground mixed spice
- 568ml tub double cream
- 125g (4oz) dark muscovado sugar, plus 1tbsp extra
- 4 large eggs, separated
- Sprig of holly to decorate
- Icing sugar to dust

1 Line a 2.3 litre (4 pint) pudding basin with clingfilm. Put the zest and juice, brandy, sultanas, prunes and mixed spice in a pan. Heat gently for 3–5min until the liquid is absorbed, then purée in a food processor.

2 Whisk the cream in a bowl until just thickened. Put the sugar and the egg yolks in another bowl. Whisk for 5min until creamy and the sugar has dissolved. Fold in the cream.

3 Wash the whisks thoroughly. Put the egg whites in a clean, grease-free bowl and beat until soft peaks form. Beat in 1tbsp sugar. Stir a large spoonful of whites into the egg and cream mixture, then fold in the rest with a metal spoon. Add the puréed fruit and fold in. Pour the mixture into the lined bowl. Freeze for 6hr.

4 To serve, run the bottom of the bowl under a warm tap, turn out onto a serving plate and remove the clingfilm. Wrap the end of a holly sprig in clingfilm and insert into the top of the parfait to decorate. Dust with the icing sugar and cut into slices to serve.

Cheat's Festive Ice Cream

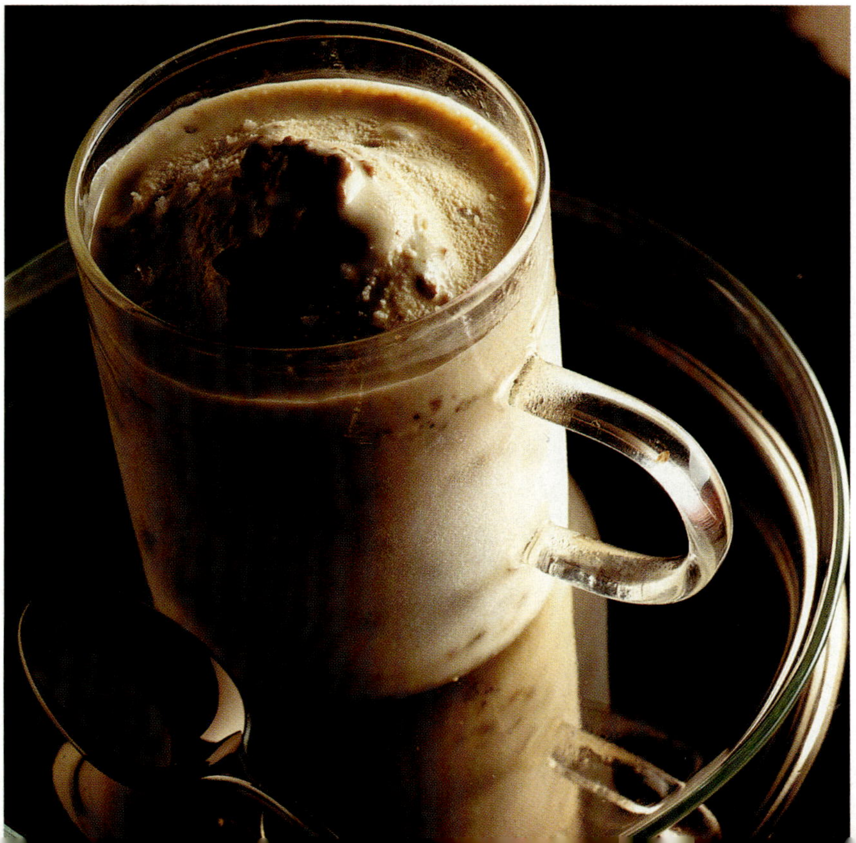

Hands-on time: 10 min
Serves: 4

- 500ml tub of vanilla ice cream
- 175g (6oz) cold Christmas pudding
- 1tbsp sweet sherry

1 Take the ice cream out of the freezer and leave to soften for 5min. Put the ice cream in a bowl, crush with a potato masher, then crumble in the cold Christmas pudding and mix well.

2 Stir in the sherry and spoon into four 150ml (5fl oz) freezerproof cups. Refreeze for 30min to set.

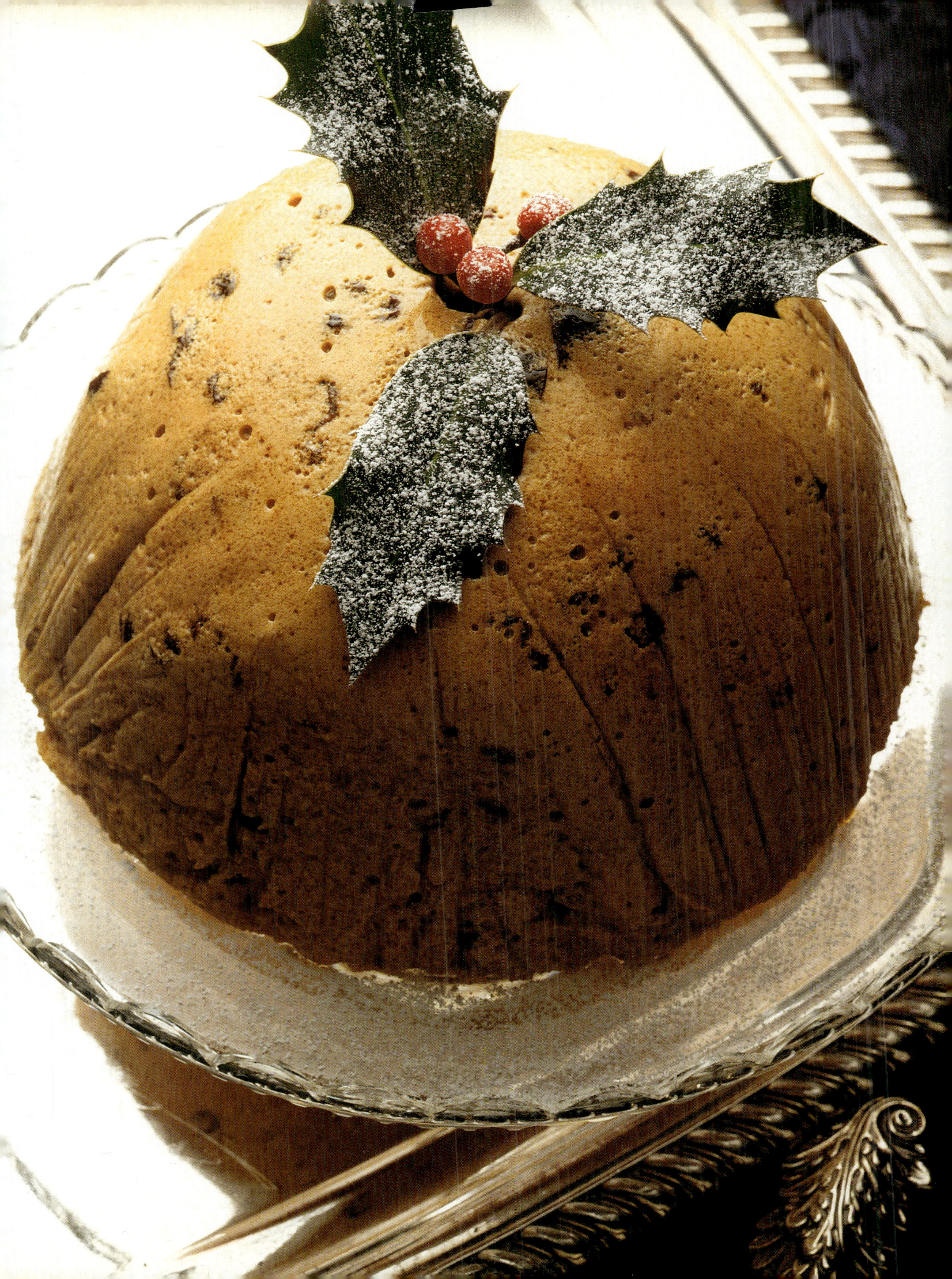

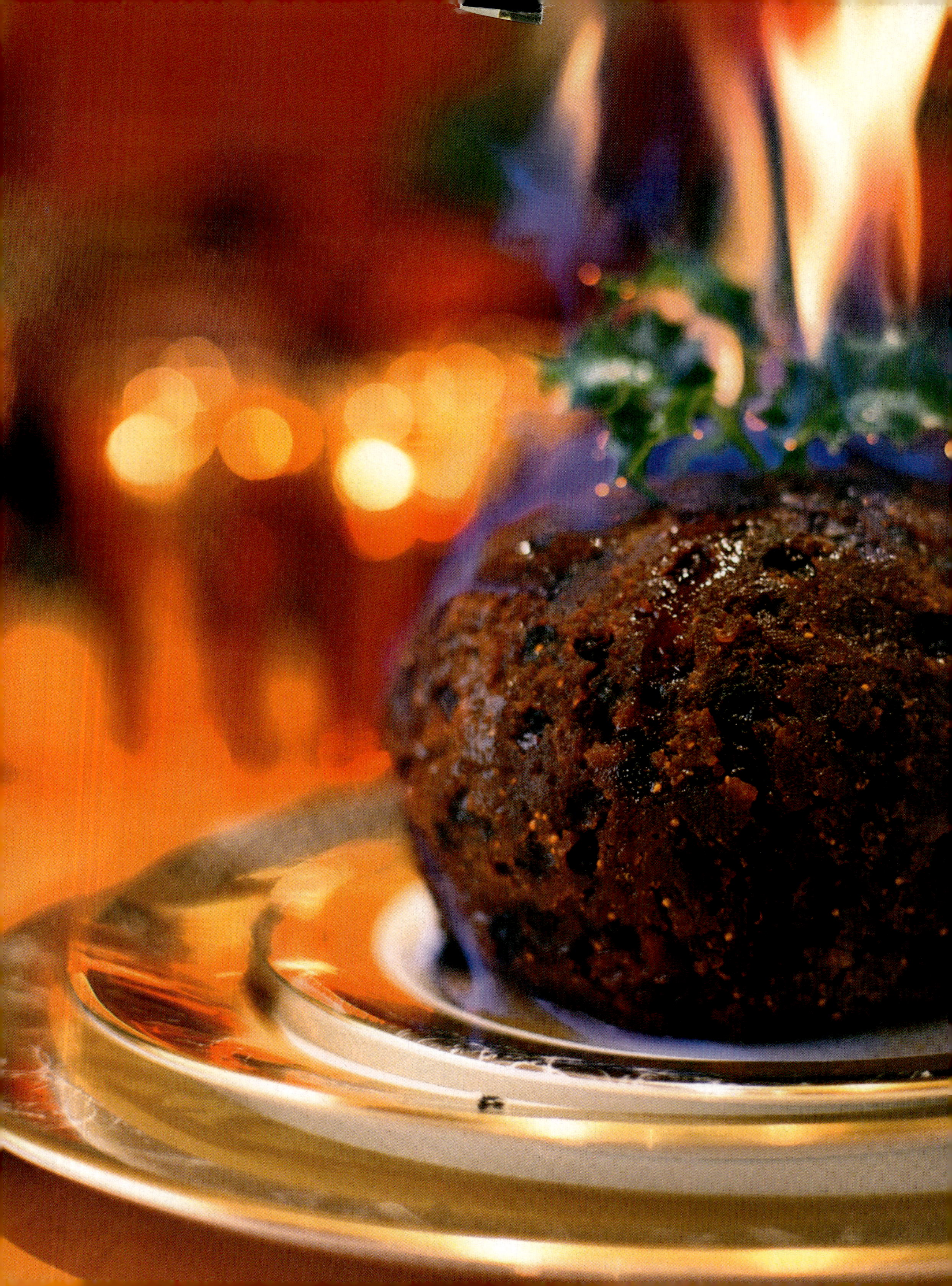

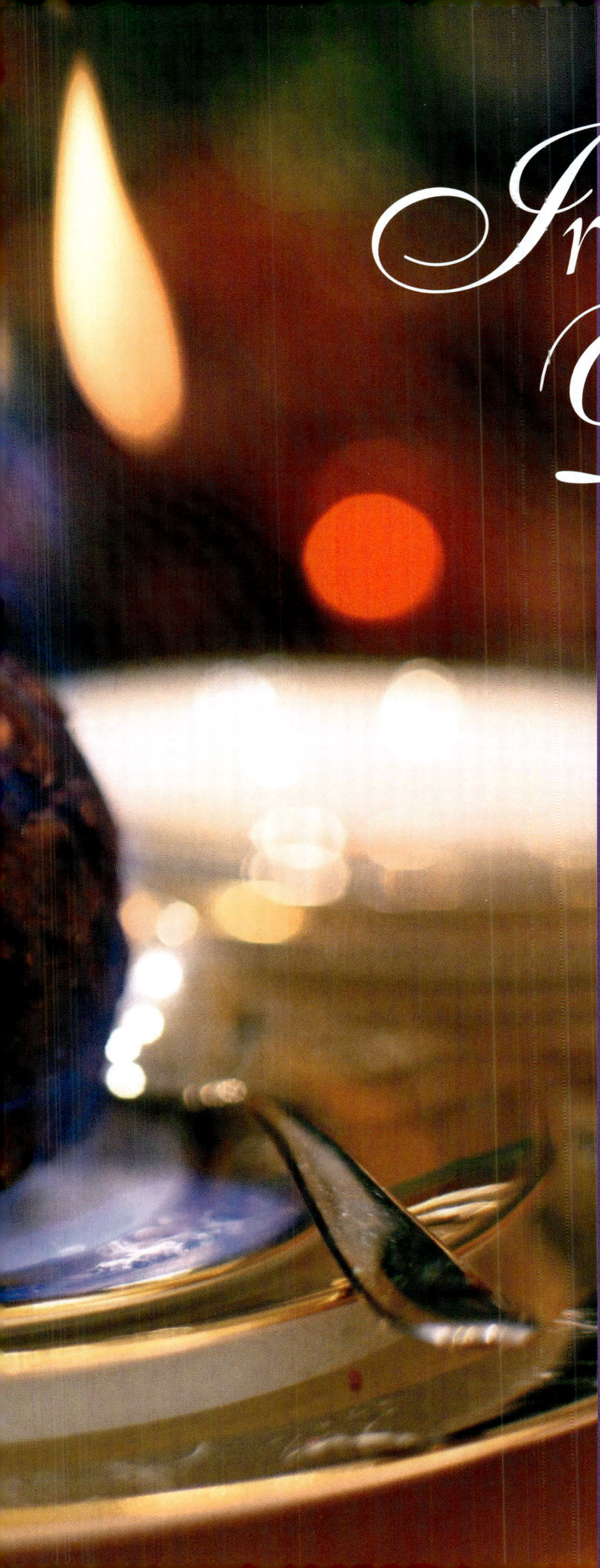

THE PERFECT FINISHING TOUCH

Irresistible Desserts

Traditions make Christmas special, whether they're handed down through generations or you start them yourself. Stir-up Sunday – the last Sunday before Advent – is the traditional day to make your own **Christmas pudding**, and we've given you three different recipes to choose from. **Desserts** come into their own during the festive season and ours are guaranteed to see everyone asking for seconds. From Mincemeat and Ricotta **Tart** and Pear and Cranberry **Strudel** to White Chocolate and Red Fruit **Trifle** and Champagne and Ginger **Jelly**, they all have the wow factor and are the perfect ending to a special meal.

Boozy Christmas Pudding

Hands-on time: 45min
Cooking time: 8–10hr
Makes: 2 x 900g (2lb) puddings that each serve 8–10
Vegetarian

- A little butter for greasing
- 225g (8oz) each currants and raisins
- 125g (4oz) sultanas
- 175g (6oz) ready-to-eat prunes, chopped
- 150g (5oz) shredded beef or vegetable suet
- 50g (2oz) flaked almonds
- Zest and juice of 1 large lemon, preferably unwaxed
- 1 medium carrot, around 75g (3oz), grated
- 175g (6oz) fresh white breadcrumbs, preferably farmhouse bread
- 50g (2oz) self-raising flour
- 175g (6oz) light brown muscovado sugar
- ½tsp each mixed spice and ground nutmeg
- 3 medium eggs, lightly beaten
- 50ml (2fl oz) each brandy and rum, plus 50ml (2fl oz) brandy, rum or Grand Marnier to serve
- 100ml (3½fl oz) sweet sherry
- 1tbsp Angostura bitters
- Sprig of holly to decorate

1 Grease two 1 litre (1¾ pint) pudding basins and line each with a 45.5cm (18in) square of muslin. Press against the basin sides and let the corners overhang the edges.

2 Put the currants, raisins, sultanas, prunes, suet, almonds, lemon zest and carrot into a very large bowl. Add the breadcrumbs, flour, sugar, mixed spice and ground nutmeg. Stir together well. Pour in the lemon juice, eggs, brandy, rum, sherry and Angostura bitters. Mix everything together until evenly combined (remember to make a wish as you stir).

3 Divide the mixture between the two basins and smooth the top. Gather the muslin up and over the puddings, then twist and secure with string. (The puddings can sit overnight in a cool, dry place before being cooked.)

4 To steam, put each basin in the top of a steamer filled with simmering water and steam for 8hr, topping up with boiling water as necessary. To boil, put the puddings on a trivet or an upturned, ovenproof saucer in a large pan. Add enough boiling water to come two-thirds of the way up the bowl. Cover with a tight-fitting lid and simmer for 6hr, topping up with water as necessary. Cool and wrap tightly with foil, then store in a cool, dry place for up to three months.

5 To serve, steam or boil each pudding for 2hr, topping up with water as necessary. Carefully lift the pudding out of the pan. Use scissors to cut off the string and release the muslin. Rest a slightly warmed serving plate on top of the pudding. Hold the basin and plate together and upturn the pudding. Lift off the pudding basin and carefully pull away the muslin. Push in the sterilised coins and decorate with holly.

6 Warm the brandy, rum or Grand Marnier in a small pan. Be careful not to boil furiously or it may burst into flames. Pour into a jug and carry to the table with the pudding. Ask someone to light a long taper and stand by. Pour your booze into a ladle, then onto the pudding. Wave the lit taper near to the pudding and stand well back. When the flames have died down, cut the pudding into wedges and serve with cream, vanilla custard or brandy butter.

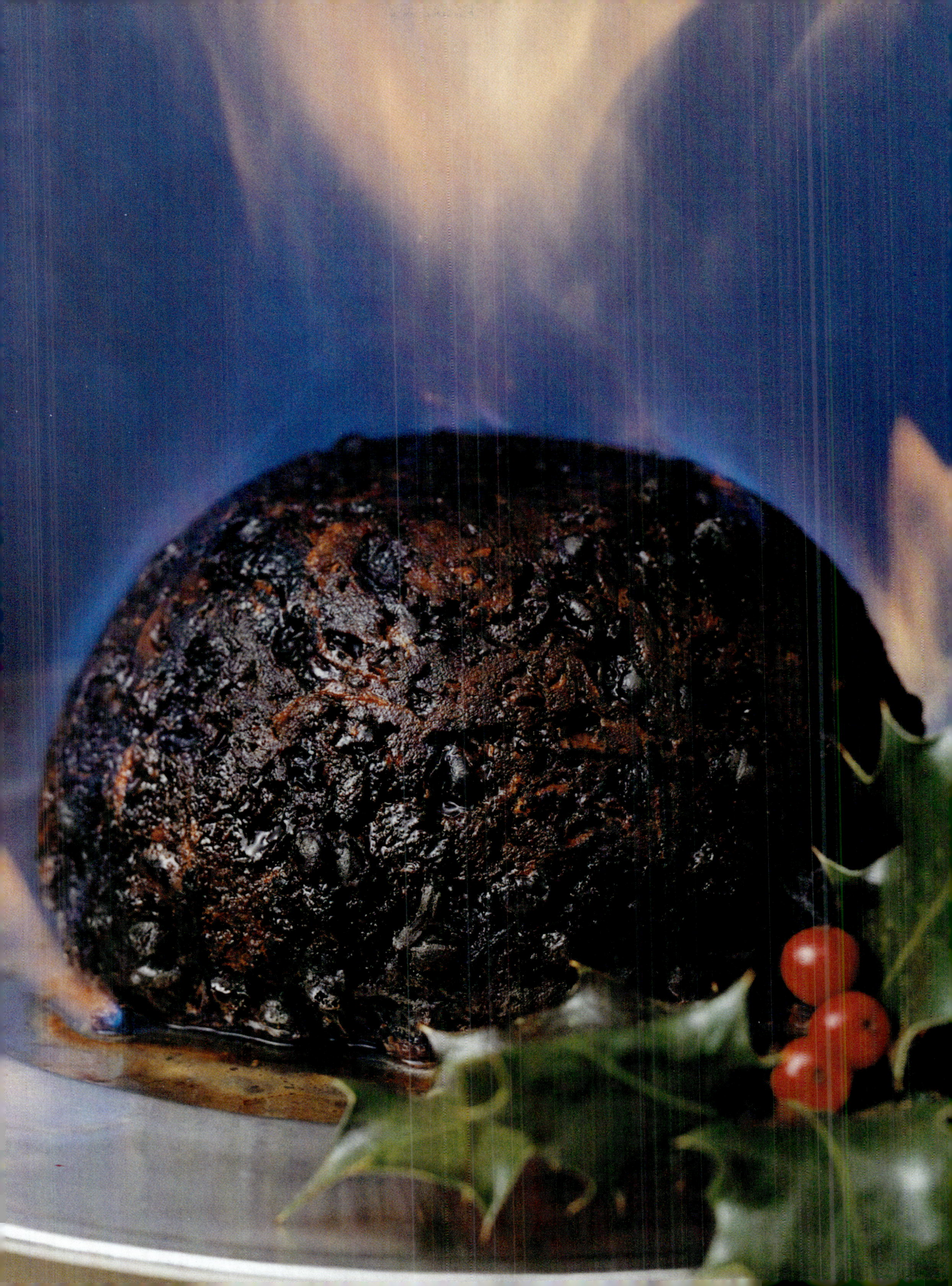

The Ultimate Christmas Pudding

Hands-on time: 45min, plus 30min standing
Cooking time: up to 6hr
Makes: 2 x 1 litre (1¾ pint) puddings that each serve 8, or 1 x 2 litre (3½ pint) pudding that serves 16
Vegetarian

* 500g bag luxury mixed dried fruit
* 125g (4oz) each dried, ready-to-eat figs, dates and pears, chopped
* 75g pack dried cranberries or dried sour cherries
* 1 sharp eating apple, cored and coarsely grated
* 227g can pineapple, drained and chopped
* 50g (2oz) whole blanched almonds, chopped
* 4tbsp maple syrup
* 4tbsp brandy
* 4tbsp sherry
* 125g (4oz) self-raising flour
* 1tsp ground nutmeg
* 1tsp ground ginger
* 1tsp ground cinnamon
* 1tsp mixed spice
* 50g (2oz) ground almonds
* 225g (8oz) shredded beef or vegetable suet
* 175g (6oz) fresh white breadcrumbs
* 125g (4oz) molasses sugar
* 4 large eggs, beaten
* 150ml (¼ pint) brown ale

1 Put all the dried, fresh and tinned fruit and nuts into a large mixing bowl, add the maple syrup, brandy and sherry and leave to stand for 30min.

2 Sift the flour, ½tsp salt and spices into a bowl, stir together and add the ground almonds, suet, breadcrumbs and sugar. In a separate bowl, beat the eggs and brown ale together. Add the egg mixture to the soaking fruit with the dry ingredients and stir to combine thoroughly.

3 Line the pudding moulds or basins with a single layer of muslin. Divide the mixture between the moulds, shape into a round, tie the muslin and secure the lid. Or spoon into the basins, tie up the muslin and cover with a double layer of pleated foil secured with string.

4 Place the puddings in a large pan or steamer half-filled with hot water. Cover and steam for 3–4hr for the small puddings or 5–6hr for a large pudding, keeping the water level topped up throughout. The pudding will keep in a cool, dry place for up to six months. To reheat, steam the small puddings for 1hr and the large pudding for around 2hr. Serve with cream, vanilla custard or brandy butter.

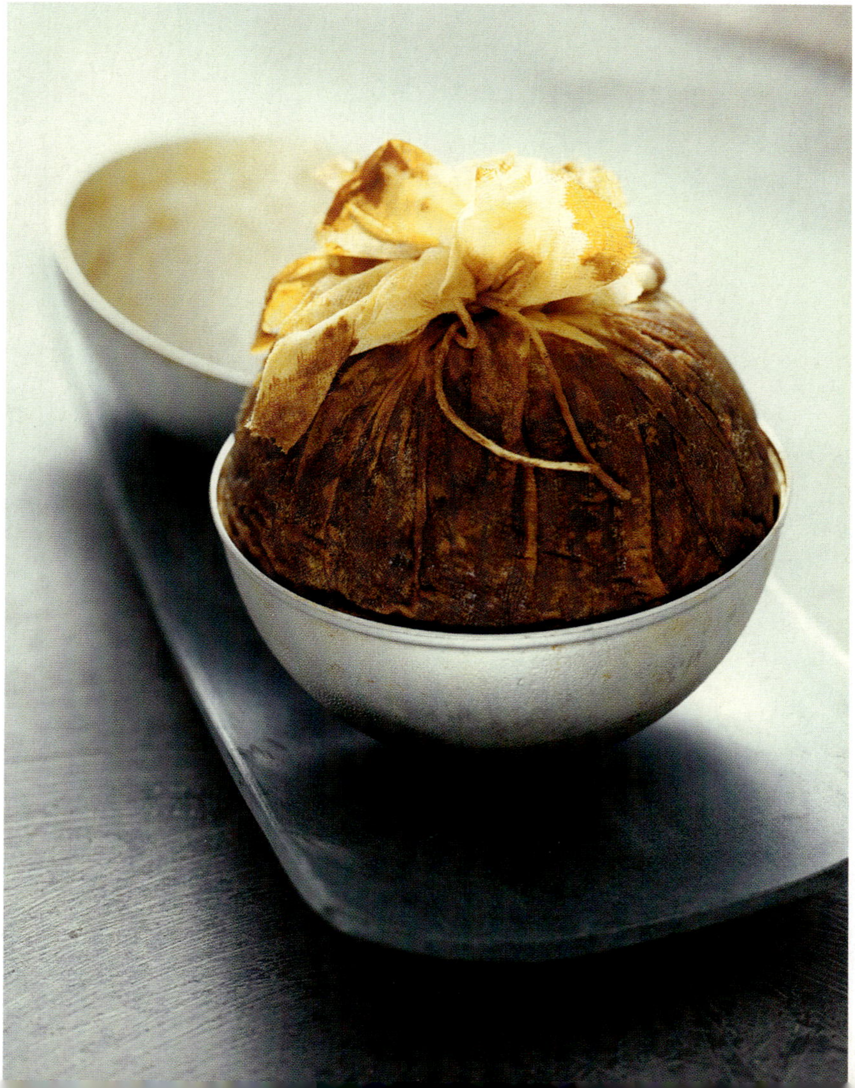

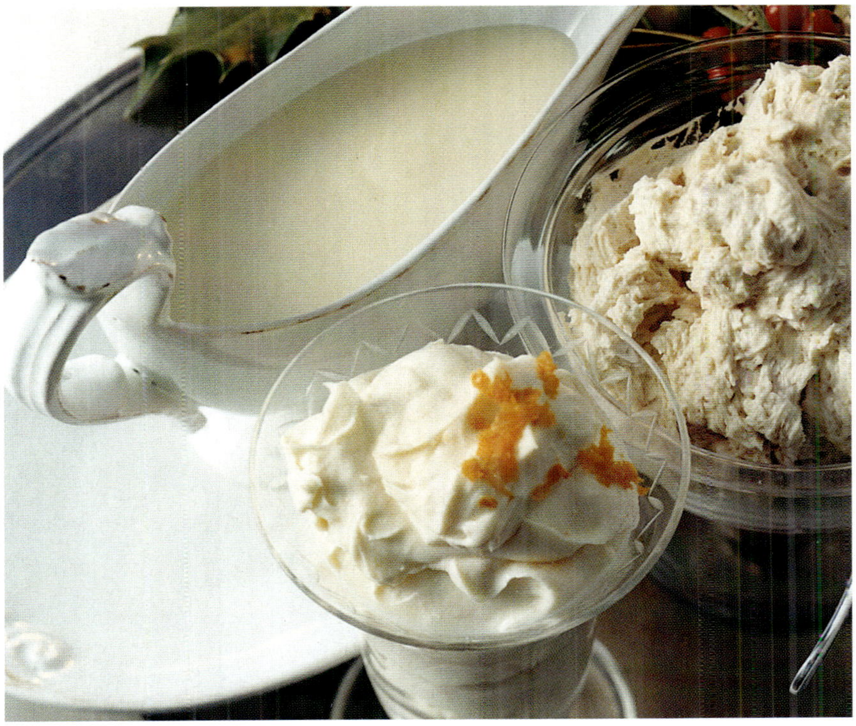

Brandy Butter

Hands-on time: 15min, plus 2-3hr chilling
Serves: 8–10

- 125g (4oz) unsalted butter
- 125g (4oz) light soft brown muscovado sugar, sieved
- 6tbsp brandy

1 Put the butter in a bowl and, using an electric whisk, beat until very soft. Gradually add the sugar to the butter, beating well between each addition, until very light and fluffy.

2 Beat in the brandy, spoonful by spoonful, then transfer to a bowl. Chill for at least 2–3hr before serving.

Fresh Vanilla Custard

Hands-on time: 20min, plus 5min cooling
Cooking time: 10min
Serves: 8

- 600ml (1 pint) full-fat milk
- 1 vanilla pod or 1tbsp vanilla extract
- 6 large egg yolks
- 2tbsp golden caster sugar
- 2tbsp cornflour

1 Pour the milk into a pan. Cut a slit down the length of the vanilla pod and scrape the seeds into the pan with the pod or pour in the vanilla extract. Bring to the boil. Turn off the heat immediately and leave to cool for 5min.

2 Put the egg yolks, caster sugar and cornflour in a bowl and whisk together. Remove the vanilla pod if using, and gradually whisk the warm milk into the egg mixture.

3 Rinse the pan and pour the custard back in. Heat gently, whisking continuously for 2–3min or until the mixture thickens (it should just coat the back of a wooden spoon in a thin layer). Serve immediately. If you don't wish to serve immediately, pour the custard into a jug, cover the surface with a round of wet greaseproof paper, then cover with clingfilm and chill. Reheat gently in a pan over a medium heat.

Last-minute Christmas Pudding

Hands-on time: 25min
Cooking time: 2hr
Serves: 12
Vegetarian

* Butter for greasing, plus 175g (6oz) butter, softened
* 3tbsp golden syrup, plus extra to drizzle
* 4 thin orange slices, plus the zest and juice of 1 orange and 1 lemon
* 175g (6oz) light muscovado sugar
* 3 medium eggs, beaten
* 75g (3oz) self-raising flour
* 75g (3oz) fresh breadcrumbs
* 75g (3oz) ready-to-eat prunes, roughly chopped
* 75g (3oz) ready-to-eat dates, roughly chopped

1 Generously grease the inside of a 1.2 litre (2 pint) pudding basin. Spoon the golden syrup into the base and cover with the thinly sliced orange.

2 Put the butter into a large bowl. Add the sugar and use an electric hand whisk to beat together until light and fluffy. Gradually beat the eggs into the butter and sugar mixture a little at a time.

3 Using a large metal spoon, fold in the flour, breadcrumbs, chopped fruit and the orange and lemon zest and juice. (Don't worry if the mixture looks a little bit curdled.) Spoon into the pudding basin and smooth the top.

4 Cut out two large 25.5 (10in) circles – one of greaseproof paper and one of foil. Lightly butter the greaseproof paper. Cover the top of the pudding with greaseproof paper, butter side down, then the foil. Secure with string and tie a piece of string over the top to act as a handle.

5 Put a small, heatproof plate upside down into the bottom of a pan. Put the pudding on top. Pour in boiling water to come halfway up the basin. Cover and steam at a medium heat for 2hr until cooked in the centre. Turn out onto a plate. Drizzle with the syrup and serve with cream or fresh custard. The pudding will keep for up to five days in the fridge.

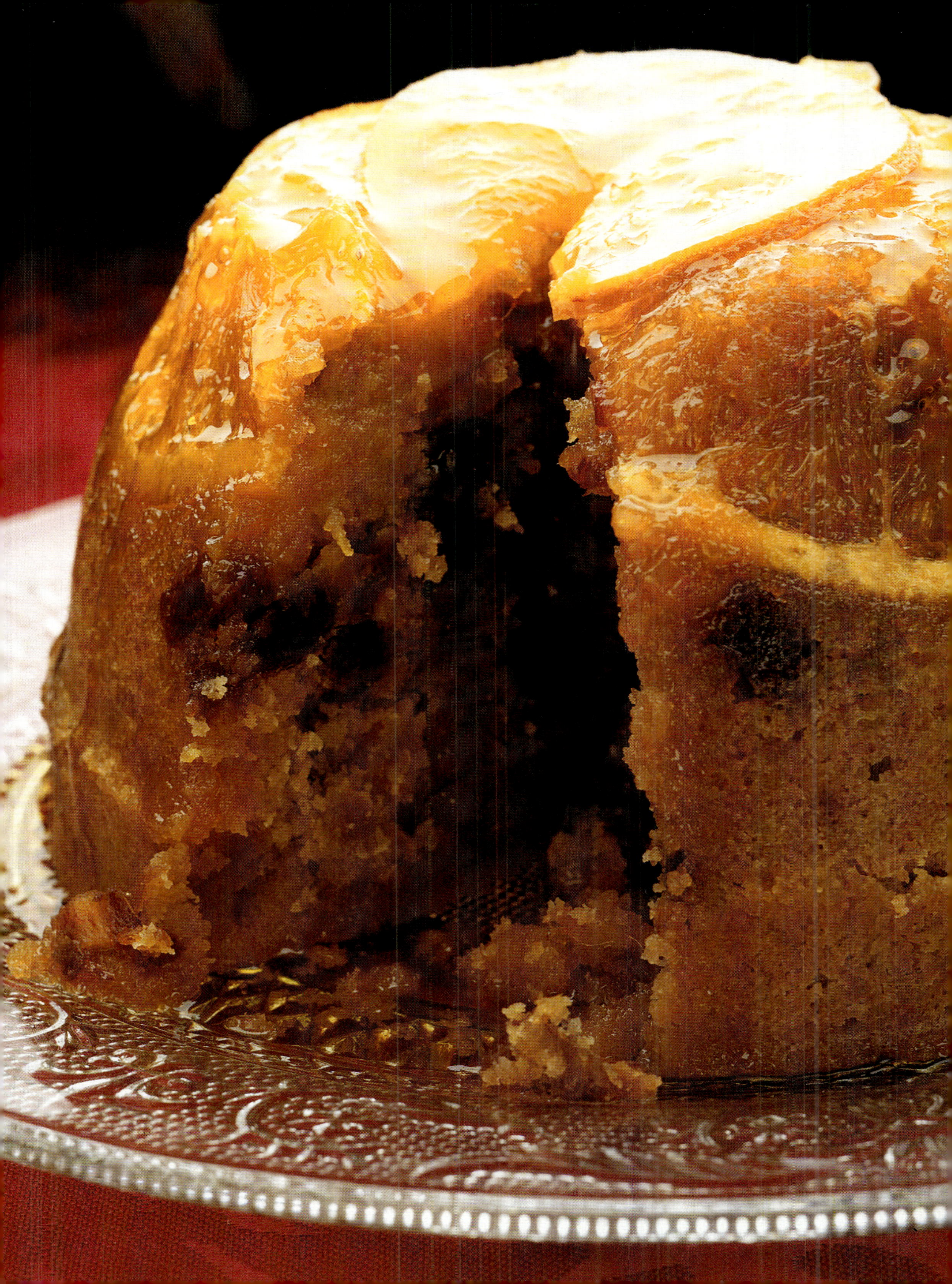

Chocolate and Cherry Gateau

Hands-on time: 1hr, plus 6hr marinating and 2hr chilling
Cooking time: 45min
Serves: 10–12

* 350g (12oz) cherries, plus optional extra cherries for decoration (if you can't find fresh cherries, use a 400g can of pitted cherries, drained)
* 3tbsp dark rum
* 50g (2oz) almonds
* 50g (2oz) plain flour
* 350g (12oz) plain chocolate, preferably with 70% cocoa solids, plus 75g (3oz) extra for the chocolate curls
* 3 large eggs, separated
* 125g (4oz) butter, softened, plus a bit extra for greasing
* 125g (4oz) caster sugar
* 450ml (¾ pint) double cream
* Cocoa powder to decorate
* Single cream to serve

1 Stone the cherries and place in a bowl with 2tbsp rum. Cover and leave to marinate for at least 6hr or overnight.

2 Spread the almonds on a baking sheet and cook under a preheated grill until golden brown. Leave to cool, then put in a food processor with the flour and whiz until finely ground.

3 Preheat the oven to 180°C (160°C fan) mark 4 and grease and baseline a 23cm (9in) diameter deep cake tin. Melt 125g (4oz) chocolate with 3tbsp water in a bowl over a pan of simmering water. Remove from the heat, add the remaining rum and the egg yolks and beat until smooth.

4 Beat the butter and sugar together in a bowl until light and fluffy. Stir in the chocolate mixture and fold in the flour and almonds. Whisk the egg whites until they form soft peaks, then fold into the chocolate mixture. Pour into the prepared tin and bake for 30–35min or until a skewer inserted into the cake comes out clean with a few crumbs on it. Leave to cool in the tin for 10min, then turn out onto a wire rack to cool completely.

5 Roughly chop the remaining chocolate. In a small pan bring the cream to the boil. Pour the hot cream over the chocolate, allow to stand for 5min, then stir until melted. Allow to cool, then, using an electric whisk, beat the mixture until thick and lighter in colour.

6 Clean the cake tin and return the cake to the tin. Spoon the cherries and any juice over the cake. Spread the chocolate cream on top of the cherries, smooth the surface, then cover and chill for at least 2hr.

7 To make the chocolate curls, melt the extra chocolate and spread a thin layer over a clean, smooth worksurface, marble slab or baking sheet. When it has just set, push a large knife across it at an angle of about 25° to make a curl. Melt the chocolate and repeat until you have enough curls.

8 To serve the cake, decorate with chocolate curls and dust heavily with cocoa powder. Serve in thin slices with cream and cherries, if wished.

To freeze ahead: Complete to the end of step 6, pack and freeze.
To use: Defrost overnight at cool room temperature. Complete the recipe.

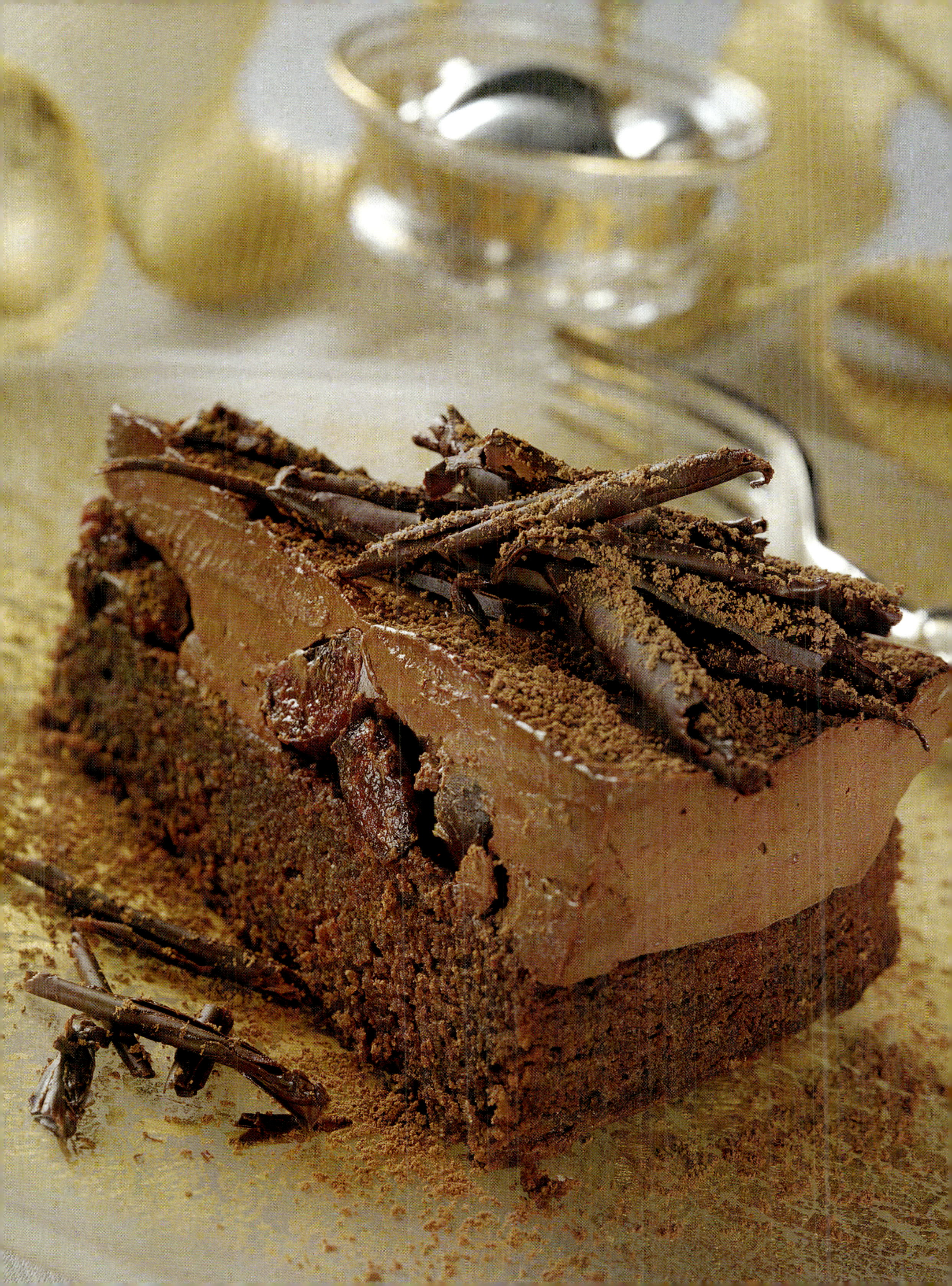

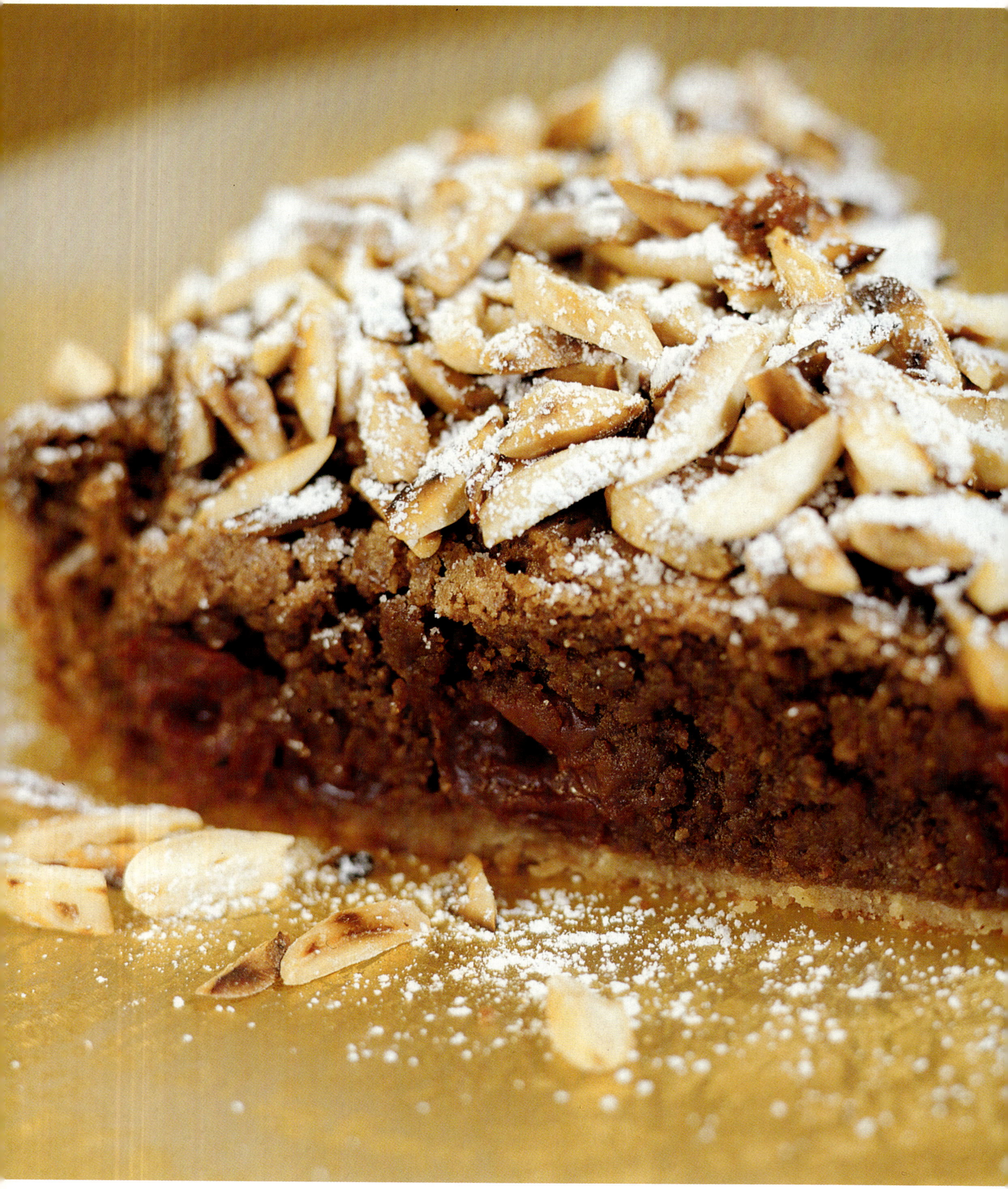

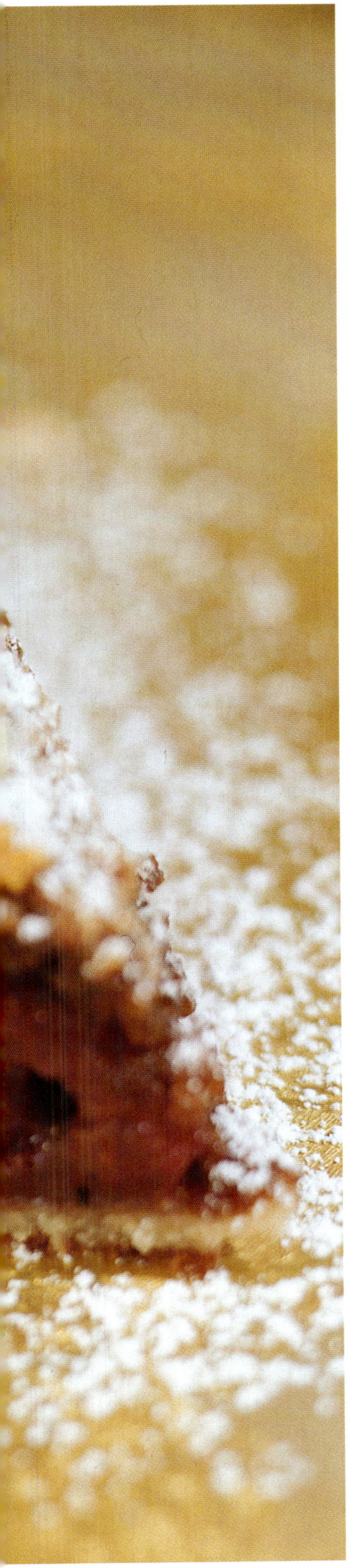

Chocolate Amaretti Tart

Hands-on time: 30min, plus 50min chilling
Cooking time: 1½hr, plus cooling
Serves: 8

- 400g (14oz) pitted morello cherries (bottled or canned), drained
- 3tbsp brandy, sloe gin or almond-flavoured liqueur

FOR THE PASTRY

- 150g (5oz) butter, softened
- 50g (2oz) icing sugar
- 1 small egg, beaten
- 225g (8oz) plain white flour, sieved, plus extra for dusting

FOR THE FILLING

- 100g (3½oz) plain chocolate
- 125g (4oz) butter, softened
- 125g (4oz) caster sugar
- 3 large eggs, beaten
- 125g (4oz) ground almonds
- 25g (1oz) self-raising flour
- 50g (2oz) amaretti biscuits, crushed
- 75g (3oz) slivered or flaked almonds
- Icing sugar to dust

1 Place the morello cherries in a bowl with the brandy, sloe gin or almond-flavoured liqueur and set aside for 30min to allow the flavours to develop. Meanwhile, make the pastry. Place the butter, icing sugar and egg in a food processor and whiz until almost smooth. Add the flour and whiz until the mixture just begins to form a dough. On a floured worksurface, lightly knead the pastry, then wrap and chill for 30min.

2 On a lightly floured worksurface, roll out the pastry and line a 24cm (9½in) fluted, loose-bottomed flan tin. Chill for 20min. Line with greaseproof paper and baking beans and cook at 200°C (180°C fan) mark 6 for 15min. Remove the paper and beans and return to the oven for a further 5min.

3 To make the filling, place the plain chocolate in a heatproof bowl over a pan of simmering water and stir until melted and smooth. Set aside to cool. In a bowl, beat together the butter and sugar until pale and fluffy. Gradually beat in the eggs alternately with the almonds and flour. Finally, fold in the cooled melted chocolate and amaretti biscuits.

4 Spoon about one-third of the mixture over the base of the pastry case. Spoon the morello cherries evenly over the surface, then top with the remaining filling mixture and spread out carefully to cover the cherries. Sprinkle the almonds over the top and bake at 150°C (130°C fan) mark 2 for about 1hr. The tart will have a thin crust on top but be quite soft underneath.

5 Cool in the tin for 10–15min before unmoulding and dusting with icing sugar. Serve warm.

To freeze ahead: Complete the recipe up to the end of step 4, then cool, wrap and freeze. **To use:** Thaw at cool room temperature overnight. Warm through as above and dust with icing sugar before serving.

Mincemeat and Ricotta Tart

Hands-on time: 45min, plus 1hr chilling and 30min cooling
Cooking time: 1hr 15min
Serves: 8

FOR THE PASTRY

* 175g (6oz) plain flour, plus extra to dust
* 125g (4oz) butter, cut into cubes
* 25g (1oz) ground almonds
* 25g (1oz) caster sugar
* 1 large egg yolk

FOR THE FILLING AND TOPPING

* 250g tub ricotta cheese
* 25g (1oz) icing sugar
* 2 large egg yolks
* 3tbsp double cream
* 700g (1½lb) good quality mincemeat
* Zest of 1 lemon
* 1tbsp brandy or lemon juice
* 25g (1oz) glacé cherries, sliced
* 2tbsp flaked almonds or pecan or walnut pieces
* Icing sugar to dust

1 To make the pastry, whiz the flour and butter in a food processor until the mixture resembles fine breadcrumbs. Add the ground almonds, caster sugar and egg yolk with 1tbsp cold water. Pulse until the mixture just comes together, then turn out onto a floured worksurface. Knead lightly, then wrap in clingfilm and chill for at least 30min.

2 Roll out the pastry on a lightly floured worksurface to a 15x38cm (6x15in) rectangle. Line a 10x33cm (4x13in) loose-based tin with the pastry, prick the bottom with a fork, then chill for 30min.

3 Line the pastry case with greaseproof paper and fill with baking beans. Bake at 190°C (170°C fan) mark 5 for 15min, then remove the paper and beans and cook for 10–15min until the pastry is cooked in the centre. Cool for 15min and reduce oven to 180°C (160°C fan) mark 4.

4 To make the filling, beat the ricotta cheese with the icing sugar, egg yolks and cream until combined. Spread over the base of the pastry and cook for 20–25min until lightly set.

5 Mix the mincemeat with the lemon zest and brandy or lemon juice, then spoon over the tart. Scatter the cherries and nuts on top and cook for 20min. Allow to cool a little, then dust with icing sugar to serve.

To freeze ahead: Complete up to Step 5, wrap and freeze for up to one month. **To use:** Thaw overnight, then warm in a moderate oven before serving.

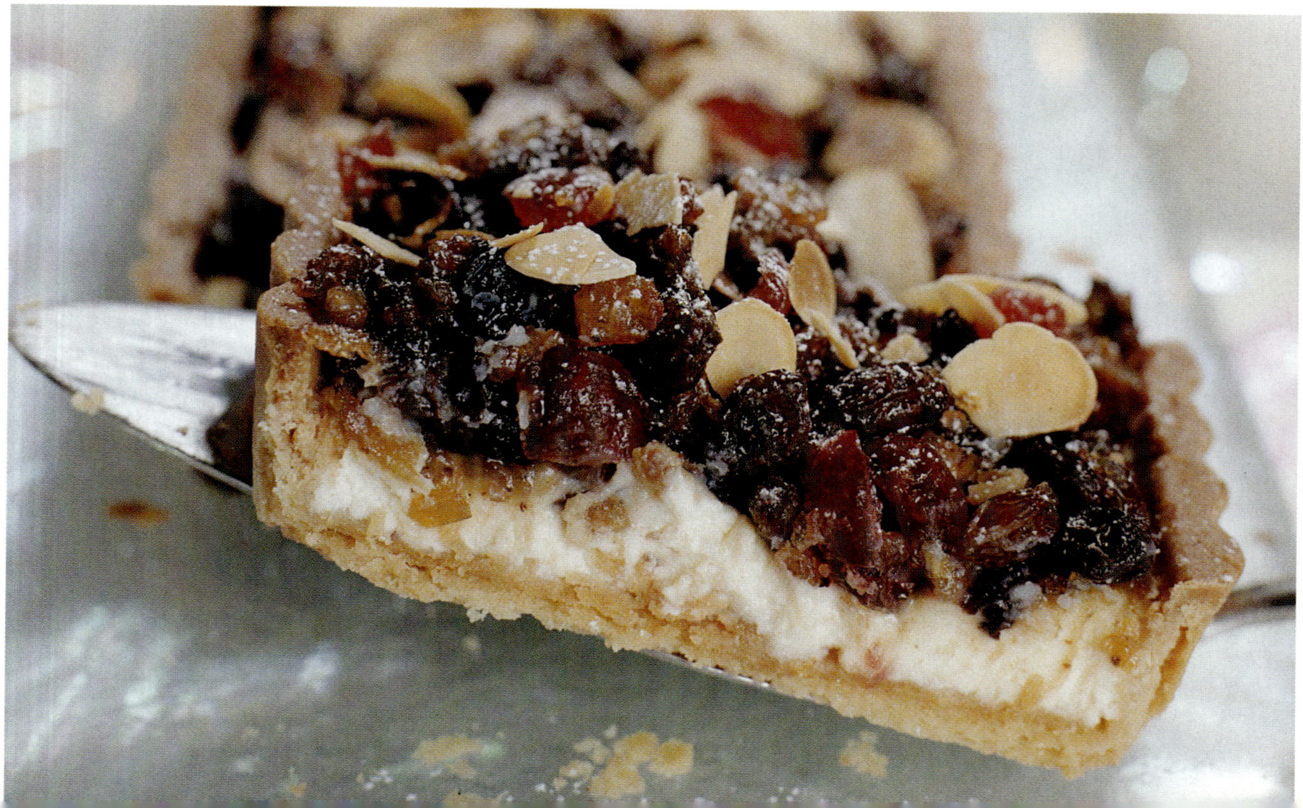

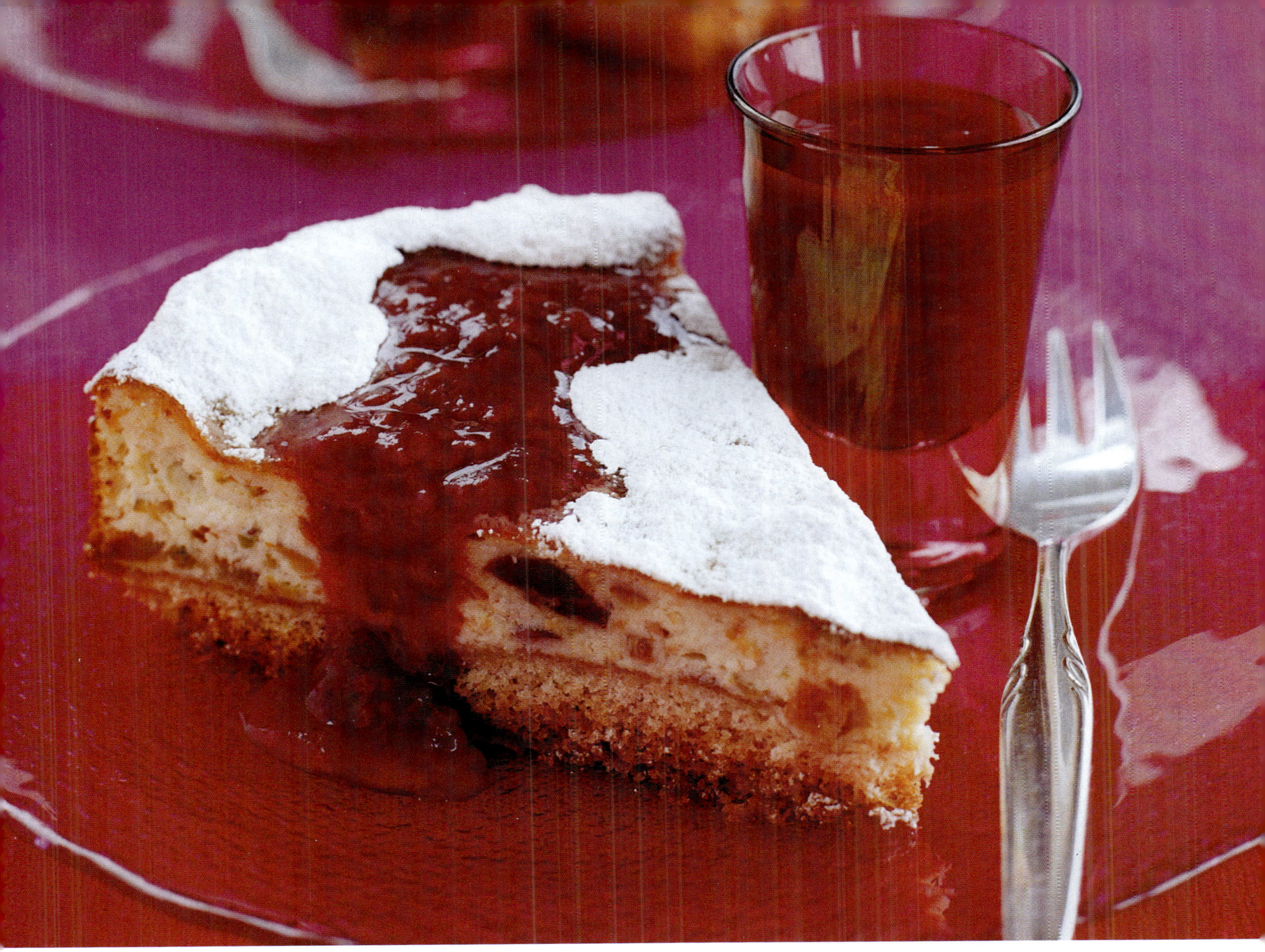

Jewelled Cheesecake

Hands-on time: 20min
Cooking time: 50–55min
Serves: 8

* I large sponge flan case
* 2tbsp orange-flavoured liqueur, such as Cointreau or Grand Marnier (optional)
* 500g (1lb 2oz) cream cheese
* 125g (4oz) golden caster sugar
* 3 medium eggs
* Zest of ½ orange
* 40g (1½oz) chopped mixed peel
* 50g (2oz) natural colour glacé cherries, thinly sliced
* 25g (1oz) pistachio nuts, chopped
* Golden icing sugar to dust
* Ready-made raspberry coulis

1 Preheat the oven to 180°C (160°C fan oven) mark 4. Grease and line a 23cm (9in) springform cake tin. Cut off the raised edge of the sponge flan case so that it fits snugly inside the tin. You can reserve the edges for a trifle or just eat them! If using, drizzle the liqueur over the sponge base.

2 Put the cheese in a large bowl. Add the sugar and beat together, then mix in the eggs. Add the orange zest, mixed peel, glacé cherries and nuts, mixing well. Spoon into the tin on top of the sponge and level the top. Bake for 50–55min until slightly risen and firm to the touch. Leave to cool in the tin.

3 Carefully remove the cheesecake from the tin. Put it on a plate, then dust thickly with golden icing sugar. Cut into slices and drizzle with coulis.

To freeze ahead: Leave the cheesecake in tin or transfer to a plate. Wrap in a double layer of foil and freeze for up to one month. **To use:** Thaw in the fridge for 12hr before serving. Complete the recipe. The cheesecake will keep for three days in the fridge.

Pear and Cranberry Strudel

Hands-on time: 20min
Cooking time: 40–45min
Serves: 8

* Zest and juice of 1 lemon
* 25g (1oz) golden caster sugar
* 1tbsp fresh white breadcrumbs
* 1tsp ground cinnamon
* 125g (4oz) fresh cranberries
* 550g (1¼lb) William or Comice pears, cored and sliced
* 50g (2oz) Brazil nuts, chopped and toasted
* 7 sheets ready-made filo pastry
* 75g (3oz) butter, melted
* Icing sugar to dust
* Double cream to serve

1 Preheat the oven to 190°C (170°C fan) mark 5. Mix the lemon zest with 1tbsp of the caster sugar, the breadcrumbs and the cinnamon and put to one side.

2 Put six cranberries on one side, then toss the rest with the pears, lemon juice and nuts. Mix in the breadcrumb mixture.

3 Lay a clean tea-towel on a board and put three sheets of filo pastry on it, each overlapping the other by 12.5cm (5in) to make a rectangle measuring 56x48cm (22x19in). Brush with the melted butter, then put three more sheets on top and brush again.

4 Spoon the pear mixture along the nearest, longest length and roll up. Trim the edges, then carefully lift onto a large, greased baking sheet so the seam is underneath.

5 Brush the remaining sheet of filo pastry with butter, fold in half and cut out six holly leaves. Arrange three each together on the log and brush with melted butter.

6 Sprinkle the strudel with the rest of the caster sugar and bake for about 40–45min, covering with foil if the top browns too quickly.

7 Arrange the reserved cranberries on the holly leaves and dust the strudel heavily with icing sugar. Serve at once with a dollop of thick cream.

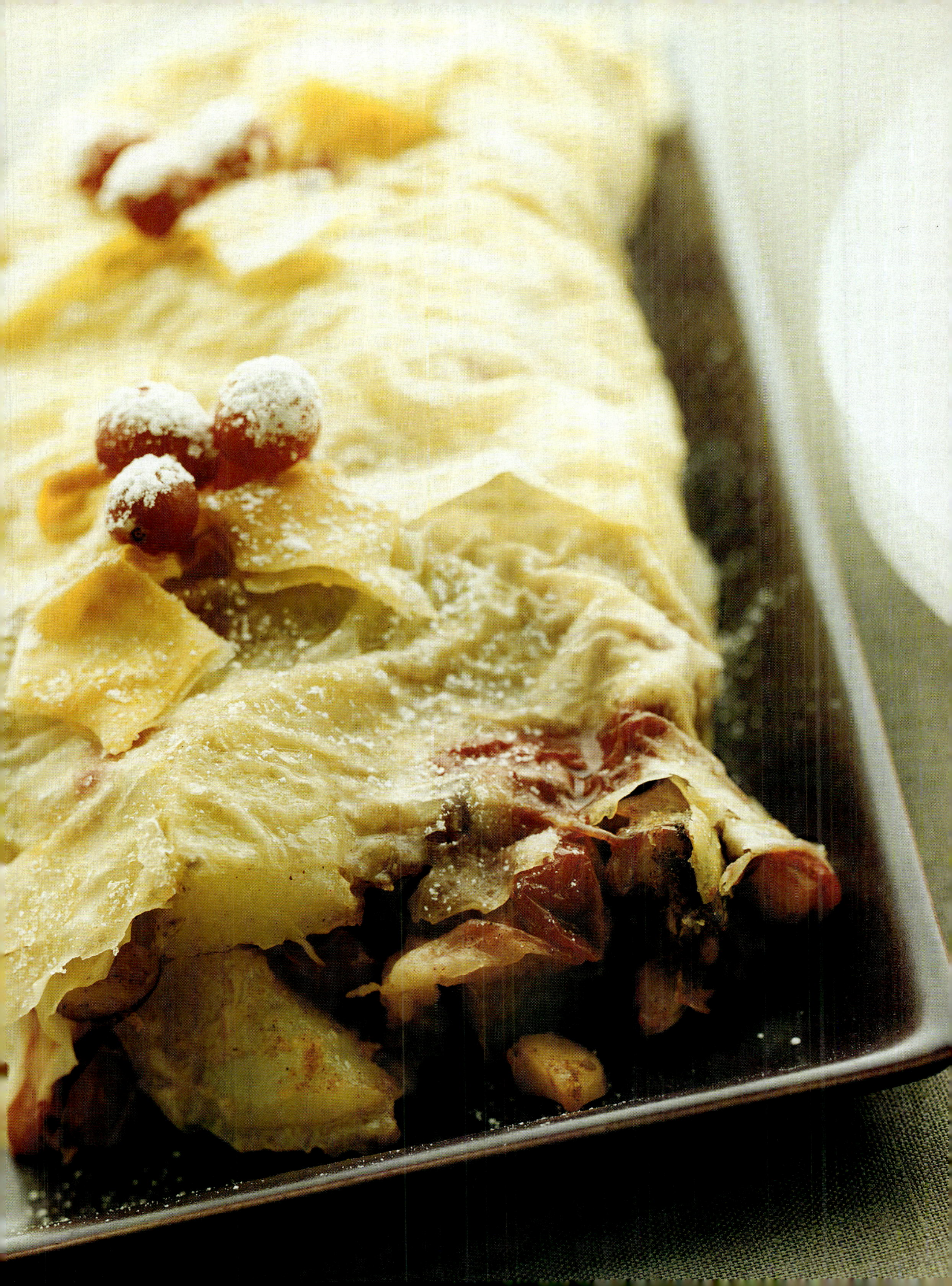

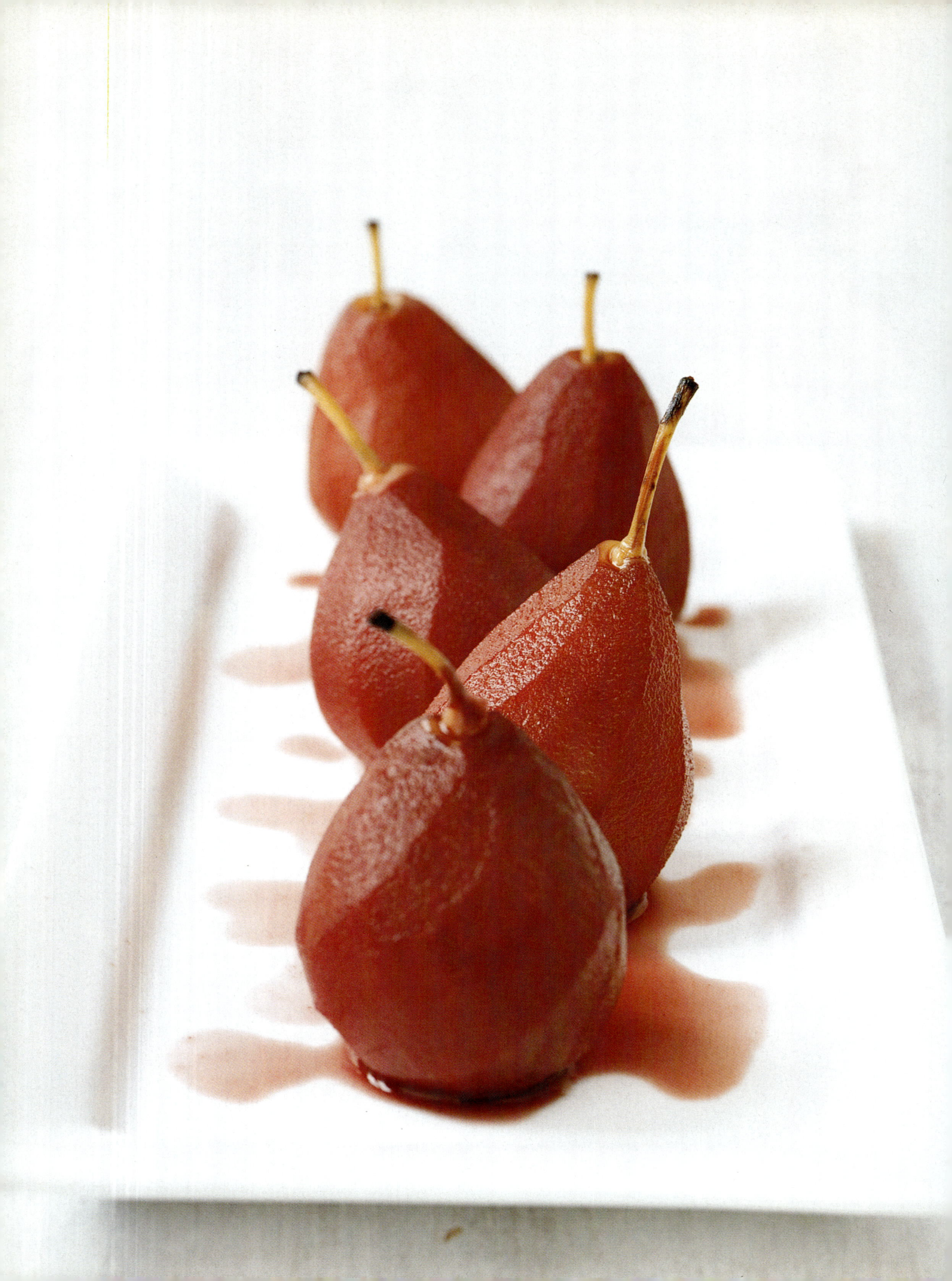

Spiced Pears in Mulled Wine Syrup

Hands-on time: 15min, plus overnight chilling
Cooking time: 35–45min
Serves: 6

* 6tbsp honey
* 6tbsp light muscovado sugar
* 300ml (½ pint) full-bodied and fruity red wine
* 1 cinnamon stick or large pinch of ground cinnamon
* Pared rind and juice of 1 large orange
* 6 small Comice or Conference pears, ripe but firm

1 In a medium pan, mix together the honey, sugar, wine, cinnamon, pared orange rind and juice. Gently heat together until the sugar dissolves, bring to the boil, then reduce to a simmer.

2 Meanwhile, peel the pears with a vegetable peeler, leaving the stalks intact to make them easier to handle. Cut a thin slice from the base of each pear so that it sits upright. Lower into the wine.

3 Add enough water just to cover the pears and set a heatproof plate on top to keep them immersed in the liquid. Poach the pears at a gentle simmer for 20–25min until tender when pierced with a knife.

4 Gently lift the cooked pears from the pan and lie them flat in a serving dish. Put the pan back on the hob, bring to the boil and bubble for about 15–20min until the syrup has reduced and is syrupy. Strain over the pears to colour them evenly, then cover with clingfilm and chill overnight (this allows the flavour and colour to intensify). Stand the pears upright in the syrup to serve.

To freeze ahead: Cool and freeze the cooked pears in the syrupy wine.
To use: Thaw the pears overnight in the fridge and serve chilled. To serve hot, return the pears and syrup to a pan and warm through gently on the hob for about 10min.

White Chocolate and Red Fruit Trifle

Hands-on time: 45min, plus 20min cooling and 2hr chilling
Cooking time: 15min
Serves: 8–10

- 3 x 500g bags frozen mixed berries
- 125g (4oz) caster sugar, plus 1tsp
- 250g (9oz) Italian biscotti or cantuccini biscuits
- 5tbsp dessert wine or fruit juice

FOR THE TOPPING

- 450ml (¾ pint) double cream
- 200g (7oz) good quality white chocolate, broken into pieces
- 500g carton fresh custard (remove from fridge 20min before using)
- 500ml carton crème fraîche

1 Put the berries in a large pan with 125g (4oz) caster sugar and heat gently for about 5min until the sugar has dissolved and the berries have thawed.

2 Drain the berry mixture through a sieve with a bowl underneath to catch the juices. Return the juices to the pan, bring to the boil, then simmer for around 10min or until reduced to about 150ml (¼ pint). Mix with the berries and leave to cool in the bowl.

3 Lay the biscotti in the bottom of a 3 litre (5¼ pint) trifle dish and spoon the dessert wine or fruit juice on top, followed by the cooled berries.

4 To make the topping, lightly whip the cream, then place half in the fridge and leave the remainder at room temperature. Put the chocolate in a bowl over a pan of gently simmering water, making sure the bowl doesn't touch the water, and stir until melted. Pour into a cold bowl, fold in the custard a little at a time, then fold in the room temperature cream. Doing it in this order stops the chocolate separating.

5 Cover the fruit evenly with the custard mixture. Beat the crème fraîche until smooth, fold in the reserved chilled whipped cream and extra sugar, then spoon it over the trifle. Chill for 2hr. (You can make this trifle a day ahead so the flavours have time to develop.) Remove from the fridge at least 20min before serving.

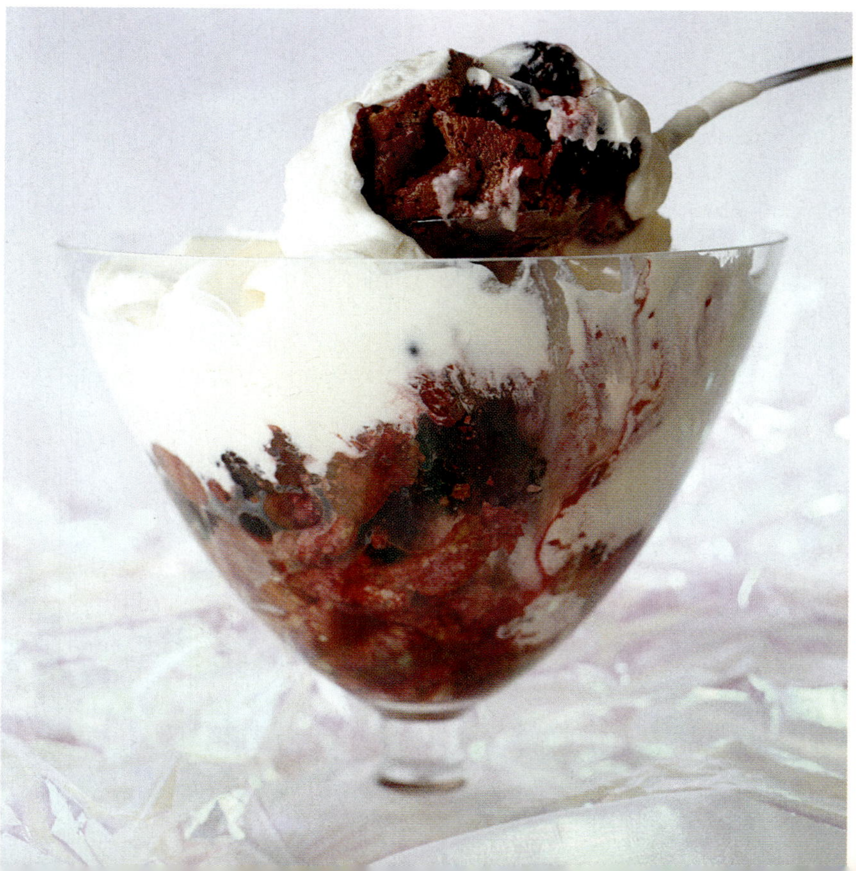

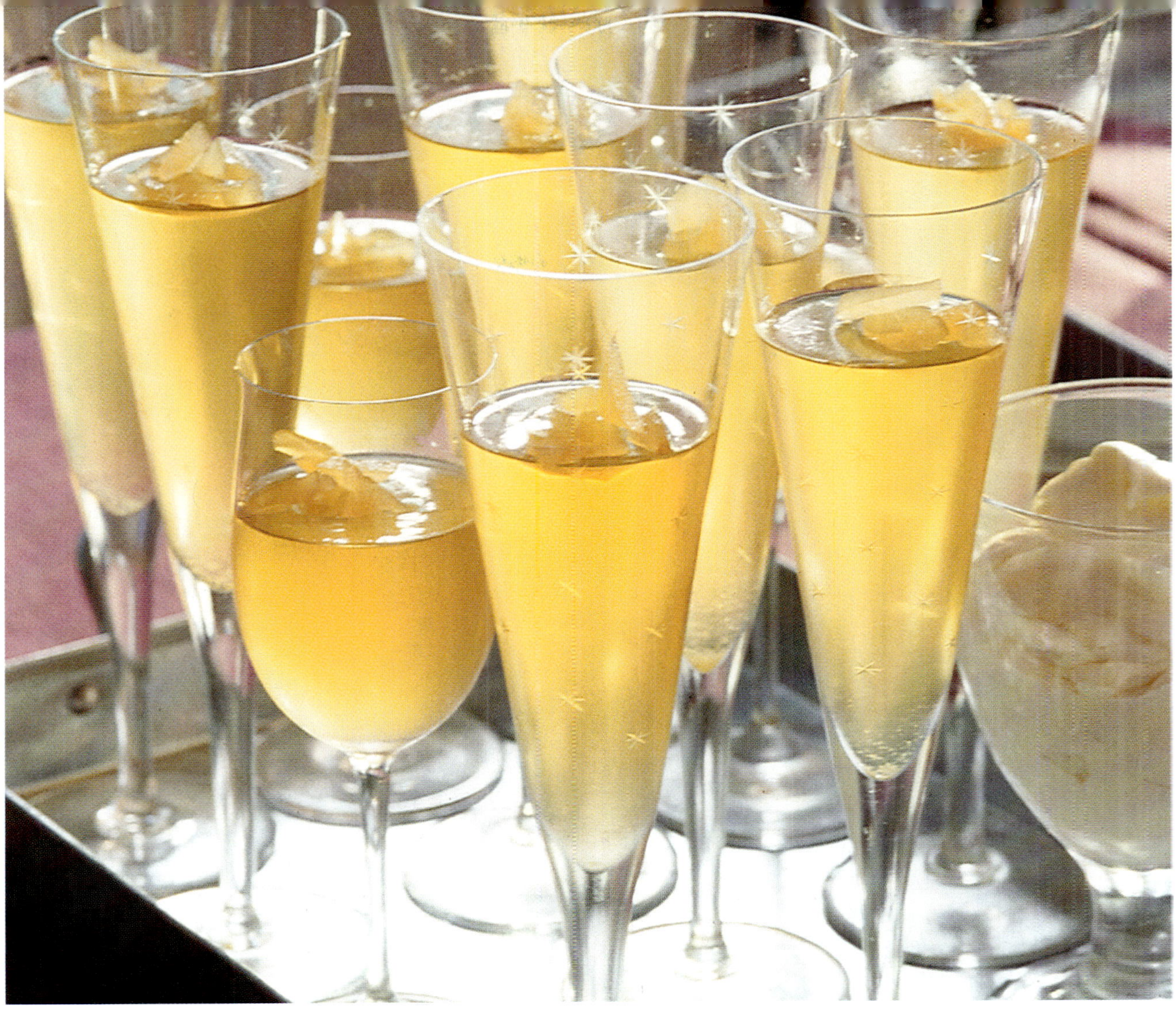

Champagne and Ginger Jelly

Hands-on time: 15min
Cooking time: 15min
Serves: 10

For the jelly

* 8 gelatine leaves – around 25g (1oz)
* 175g (6oz) golden caster sugar
* Pared rind of 2 unwaxed lemons (use a vegetable peeler to make long strips)
* 75cl bottle champagne or sparkling white wine
* 6–8tbsp ginger wine
* 4 pieces stem ginger, cut into slivers and drained of syrup (reserving 2tsp syrup for the Ginger Cream)

For the ginger cream

* 284ml carton double cream
* 3 pieces stem ginger
* 2tsp ginger syrup

1 Pour 600ml (1 pint) cold water into a bowl. Break up the gelatine and add to the water. Soak for 5min.

2 Put the sugar in a pan. Add the pared lemon and 400ml (14fl oz) cold water. Heat gently to dissolve the sugar, then simmer for 2–3min. Take off the heat and cool a little, then remove the pared lemon strips.

3 Lift the soaked gelatine out of the water and add it to the pan. Stir until it has melted. Stir in the champagne and ginger wine. Ladle the jelly into 10 wine glasses and chill until set.

4 To make the Ginger Cream, empty the double cream into a bowl and whip until soft peaks form. Chop the stem ginger and fold into the cream with the ginger syrup. Spoon into a serving dish and chill until ready to serve.

5 Just before serving, decorate the jelly with slivers of stem ginger. Serve with the Ginger Cream.

Cranberry Christmas Bombe

Hands-on time: 30min, plus 30min chilling and around 6hr freezing
Cooking time: 15min
Serves: 8–10

- **125g (4oz) granulated sugar**
- **300ml (½ pint) cranberry juice**
- **225g (8oz) each cranberries and raspberries, fresh or frozen (fresh cranberries will give a better colour)**
- **2 large egg whites**
- **75g (3oz) caster sugar**
- **Groundnut oil for greasing**
- **500ml tub good quality vanilla ice cream**

FOR THE SUGARED REDCURRANTS

- **A few sprigs of redcurrants**
- **1 large egg white, lightly beaten**
- **A little caster sugar**

1 If you don't have an ice cream maker, put a large enamelled roasting tin in the freezer before you start. Put the granulated sugar and cranberry juice in a pan and heat gently until the sugar has dissolved. Bring to the boil, then add the cranberries, cover and simmer for 15min or until very soft. Leave to cool.

2 Whiz the cranberry mixture and raspberries in a food processor until well broken down. Press through a nylon sieve into a bowl, then chill. Whisk the egg whites until soft peaks form, then add the caster sugar a spoonful at a time and continue whisking until stiff and glossy. Fold into the fruit purée.

3 Pour the cranberry sorbet mixture into an ice cream maker and churn until stiff. Alternatively, pour into the chilled roasting tin and freeze for 1hr or until it begins to solidify round the edges. Crush with a fork, mix together well, then put back in the freezer for another hour or until almost frozen.

4 Meanwhile, lightly grease a 1.4 litre (2½ pint) pudding basin with a little groundnut oil, then put a disc of foil in the bottom. Put the basin in the freezer for 30min.

5 Spoon the sorbet into the basin, reserving 3–4tbsp, creating a hollow in the centre for the ice cream. Put the sorbet in the freezer and leave the ice cream at room temperature for 10min, then spoon the ice cream into the centre of the sorbet and press down well. Spread the reserved sorbet on top to enclose the ice cream. Freeze for 4hr or until firm.

6 To make the Sugared Redcurrants, dip the sprigs in the beaten egg white, then in the sugar. Allow to harden on a baking sheet lined with greaseproof paper. To unmould the bombe, dip the basin in hot water for 10sec, then loosen the edges with a round-bladed knife, invert onto a plate, shake firmly and remove foil. Decorate with redcurrants, then use a warm knife to cut into wedges. The bombe will keep in the freezer for up to two weeks.

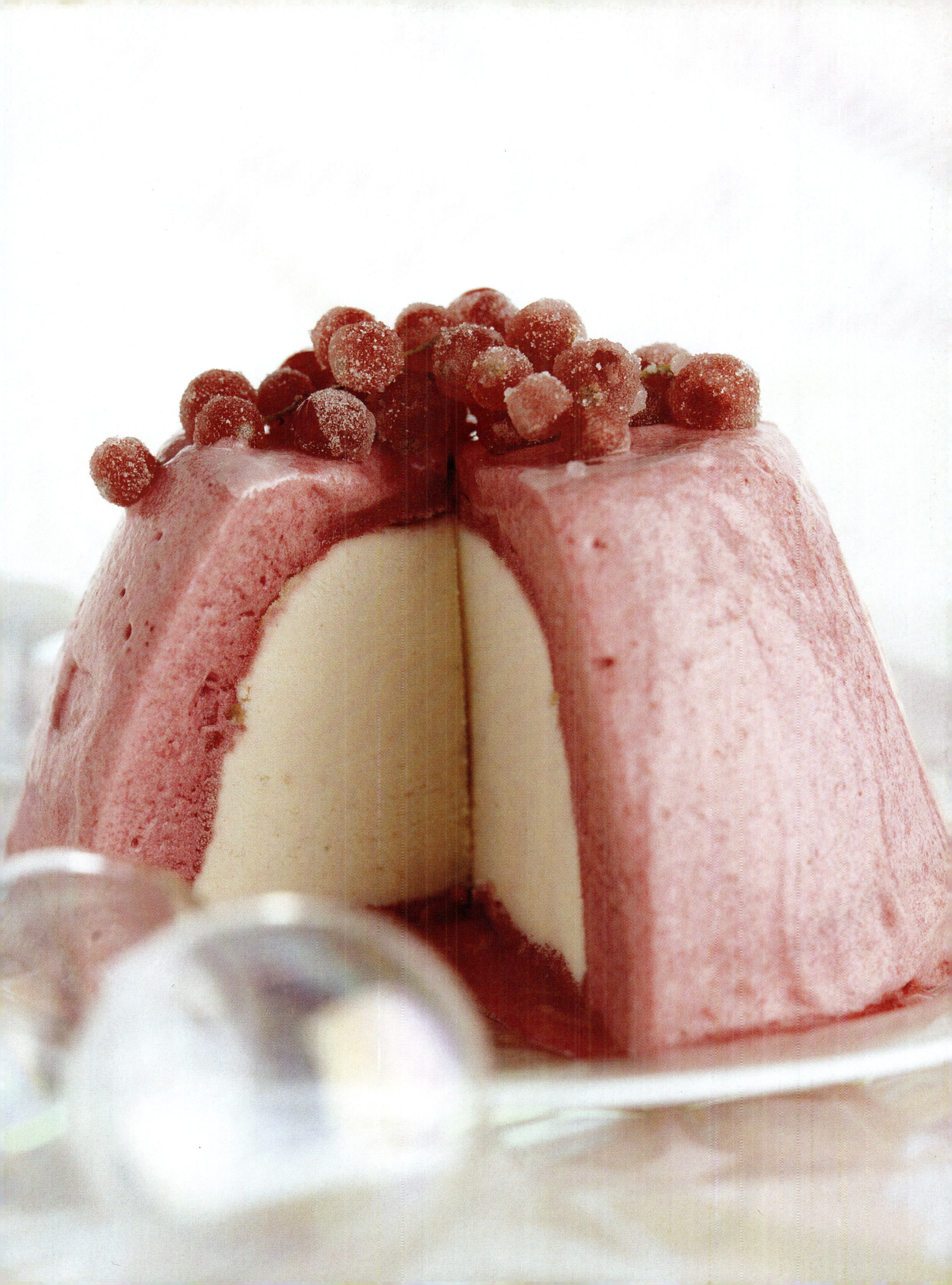

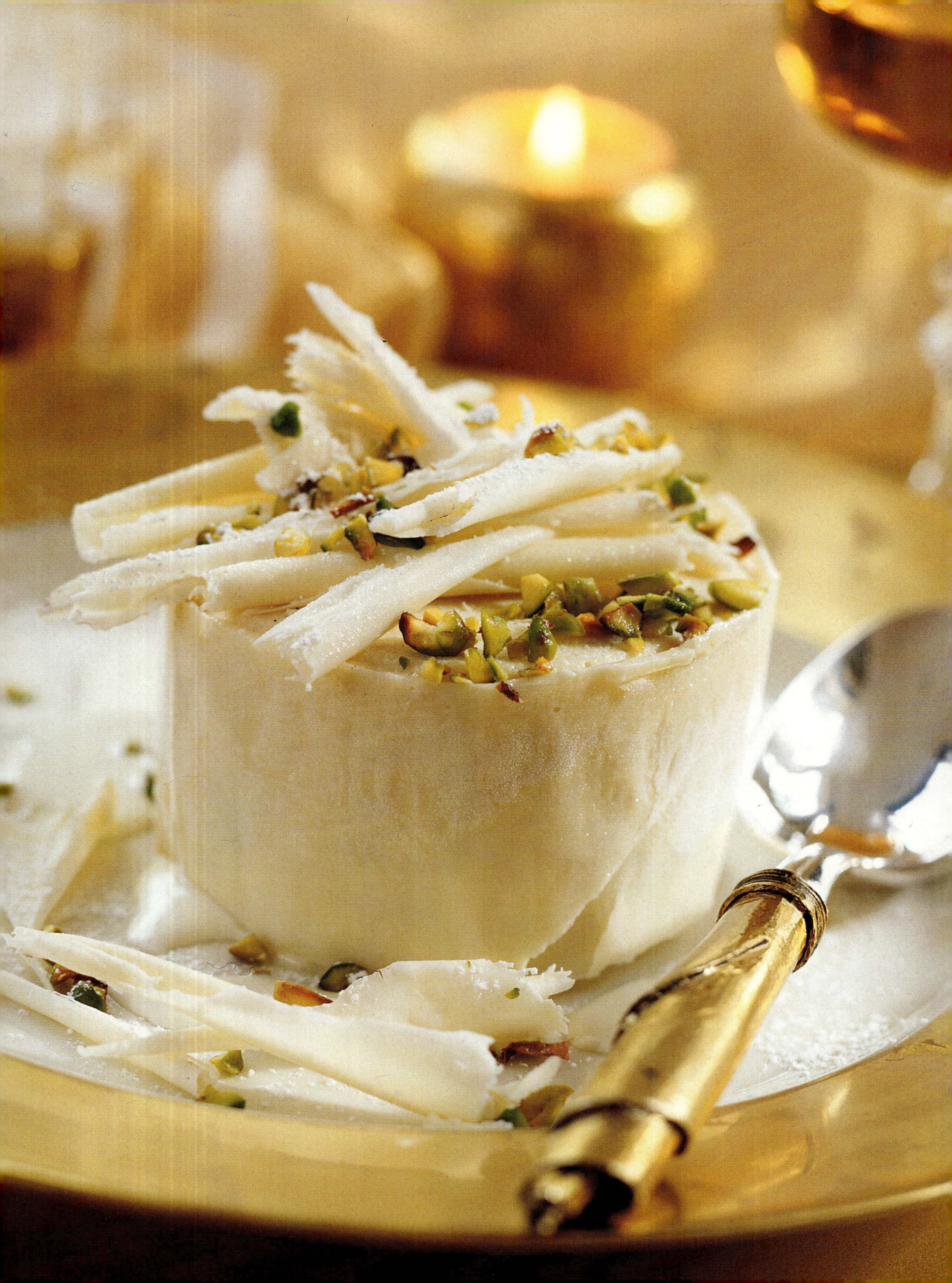

Iced Pistachio and Orange Parfait

Hands-on time: 1hr, plus at least 4½hr freezing
Serves: 6

- Flavourless oil, such as safflower, for greasing
- 75g (3oz) shelled, unsalted pistachio nuts, lightly toasted and finely chopped, plus extra to decorate
- 200ml (7fl oz) double cream
- 4 large egg whites
- 75g (3oz) icing sugar, sieved
- 2tbsp orange-flavoured liqueur, such as Grand Marnier
- 75g (3oz) white chocolate, plus 75g (3oz) for the chocolate curls (optional)

1 Lightly oil and baseline six 150ml (¼ pint) ramekins with greaseproof paper. Sprinkle base lightly with 1oz of the chopped pistachio nuts. Cut six strips of greaseproof paper, each measuring 5x25.5cm (2x10in). Lightly oil one side of the paper and sprinkle with 1oz nuts. Reserve the remaining nuts. With the nut side facing inwards, curl the paper around the insides of the ramekins.

2 Lightly whip the cream. Whisk the egg whites until stiff, then gradually whisk in the icing sugar. Fold in the reserved nuts, liqueur and cream. Don't overmix. Divide mixture between ramekins and freeze for 4hr or overnight.

3 Melt the chocolate in a bowl over a pan of simmering water. Cut six strips of non-stick baking parchment, each measuring 5x25.5cm (2x10in). Spread the chocolate thinly over each strip and leave to firm slightly. Unmould the parfaits and remove lining papers. Lift the chocolate-covered strips and wrap around the parfaits, chocolate side inside. Freeze until set (about 30min).

4 To make the white chocolate curls, melt the white chocolate in a bowl over a pan of simmering water. Spread out thinly on a marble slab or worksurface and leave to set until no longer sticky to the touch. Holding a large knife at a slight angle to the surface, push the blade across the chocolate, towards you, to shave off long, thin curls. Adjust the angle of the blade to obtain the best curls. Store in an airtight container for up to one week.

5 To serve the iced parfaits, peel away the parchment and decorate generously with pistachio nuts and chocolate curls.

To freeze ahead: Complete the recipe to the end of step 3. Pack the parfaits and freeze for up to four weeks. Complete step 4 up to one day in advance.
To use: Complete the recipe.

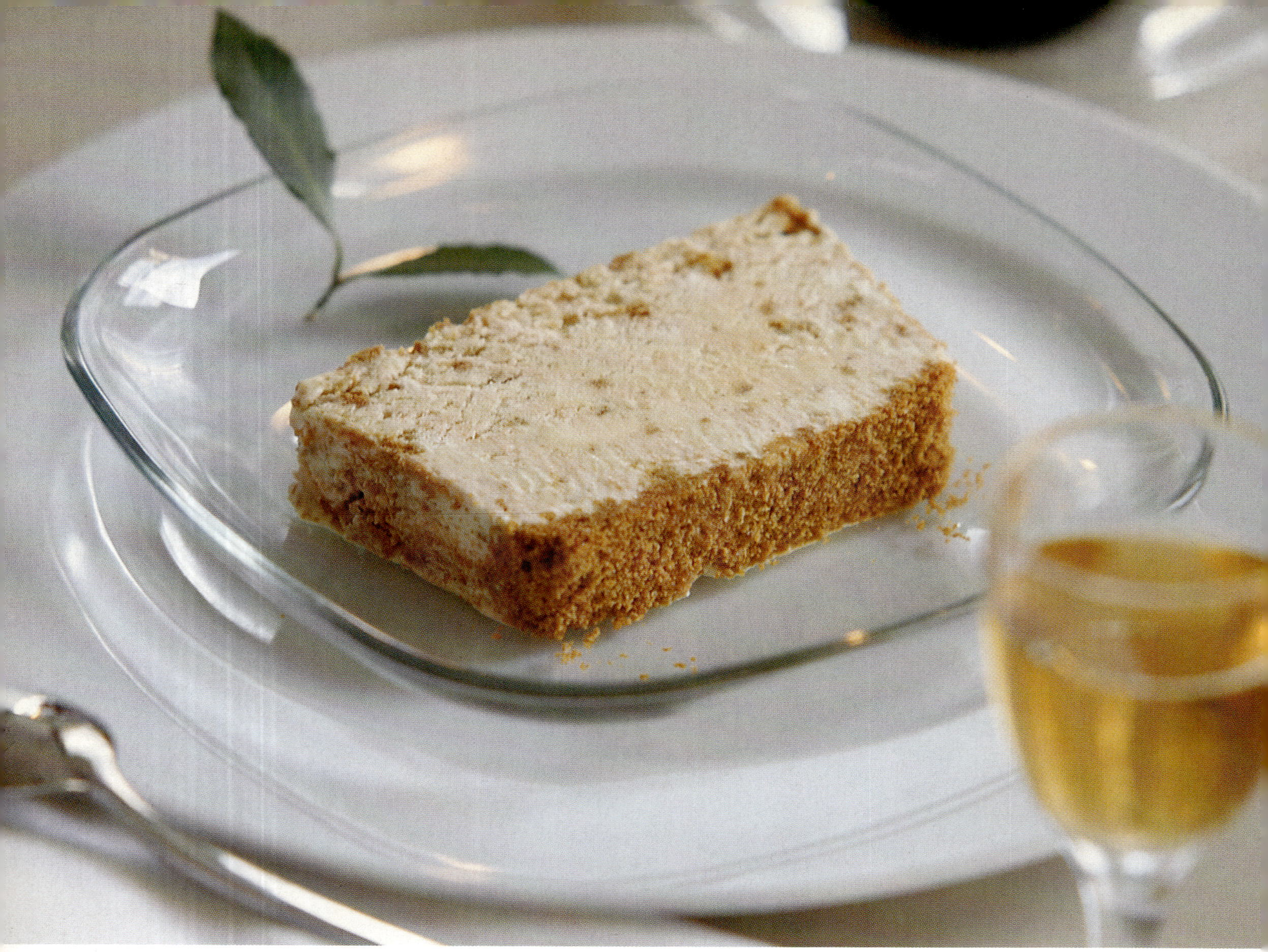

Ginger Parfait

Hands-on time: 20min
Freezing time: 6hr
Serves: 10

- 150g (5oz) ginger nut biscuits
- 15g (½oz) unsalted butter, melted
- 2 large eggs
- 175g (6oz) golden icing sugar
- 1 tbsp ground ginger
- 568ml carton double cream

1 Put the biscuits in a food processor and whiz for 10sec to make crumbs. Use most of the butter to grease a 900g (2lb) loaf tin. Line the tin with clingfilm, then brush the clingfilm with the rest of the melted butter.

2 Spoon about 3tbsp of the biscuit crumbs into the loaf tin and tip the tin around to give it an even coating of crumbs. Place in the freezer.

3 Put the eggs, icing sugar and ginger in a bowl and whisk together for 5–10min until the mixture is thick, moussey and leaves a ribbon-like trail.

4 Whisk the cream until soft peaks form, then fold into the egg mixture. Put 3tbsp biscuit crumbs to one side, then fold in the remainder. Pour the mixture into the prepared loaf tin and sprinkle with the remaining biscuit crumbs. Cover with clingfilm, then freeze for 6hr.

5 Dip the tin into hot water for 10sec, then unwrap and turn out onto a board. Cut into 2cm (¾in) slices and serve.

Mango Ice Cream Terrine

Hands-on time: 20–25min plus freezing
Serves: 8

* A little vegetable oil for greasing
* 2 small mangoes, peeled and chopped
* 2 medium eggs
* 125g (4oz) golden caster sugar
* 284ml carton double cream, whipped
* 1½tbsp Malibu
* 4 ratafia biscuits, roughly crushed

1 Lightly oil a 900g (2lb) loaf tin, then line with clingfilm, leaving enough to hang over the edges and smoothing any creases.

2 Whiz the mangoes in a food processor until smooth. Set aside. Put the eggs and sugar into a large bowl. Using an electric hand whisk, mix together until thick – this should take 5min.

3 Add the whipped cream to the mixture and fold together with a large metal spoon. Fold in three-quarters of the puréed mango and the Malibu. Spoon the remaining mango purée into the lined tin to cover the base, then pour in the ice cream mixture. Cover with the overhanging clingfilm and freeze overnight or for up to one month.

4 To serve, remove the ice cream from the freezer 5min before serving. Unwrap the clingfilm. Turn out onto a serving dish, cover with the biscuits, slice and serve.

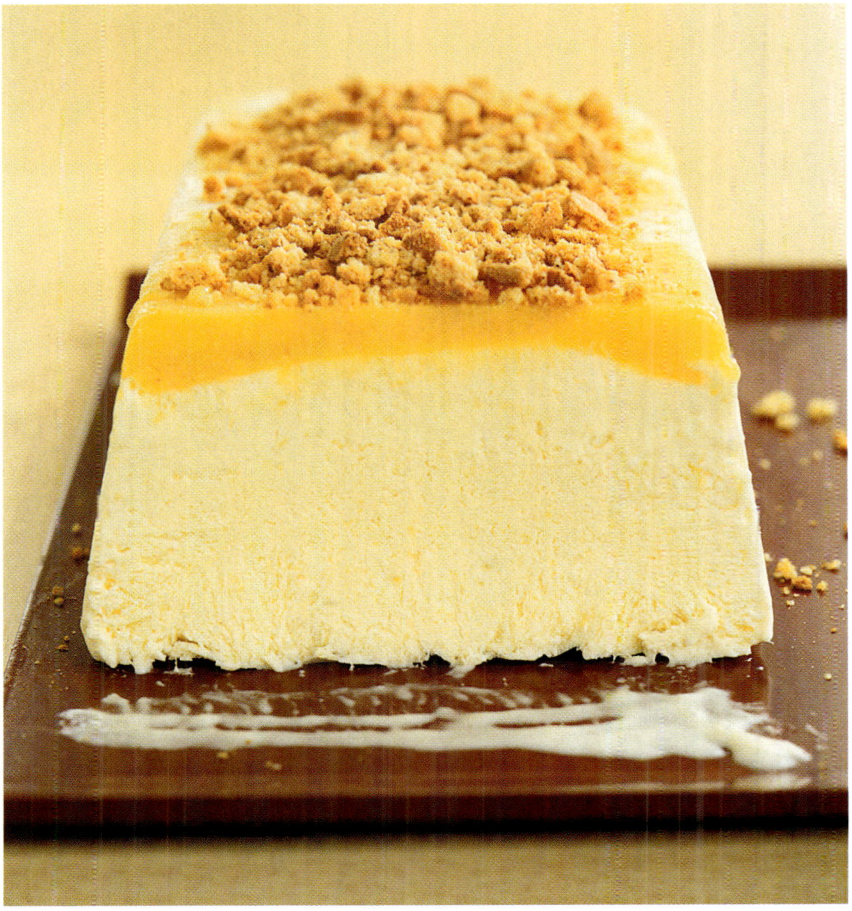

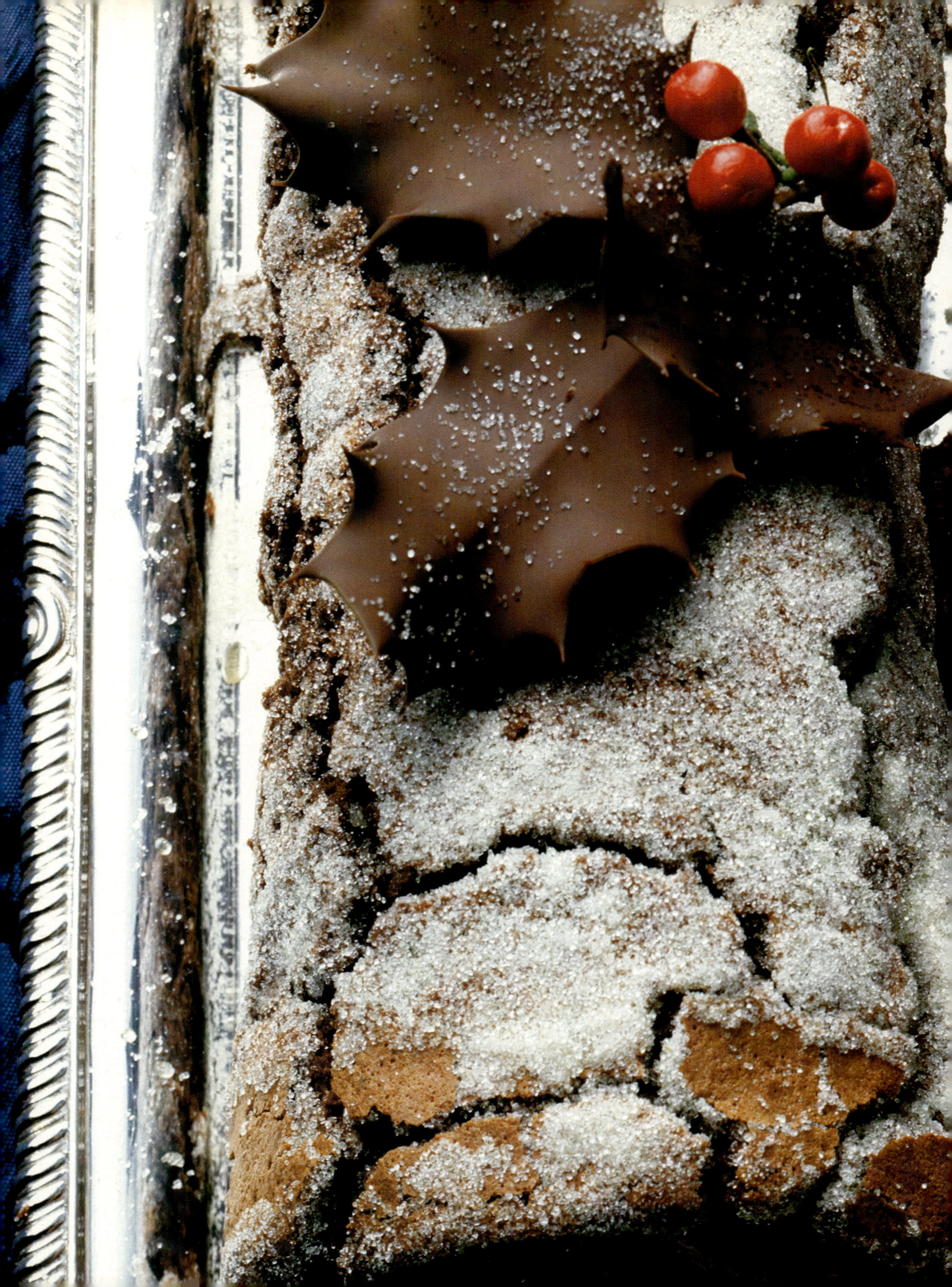

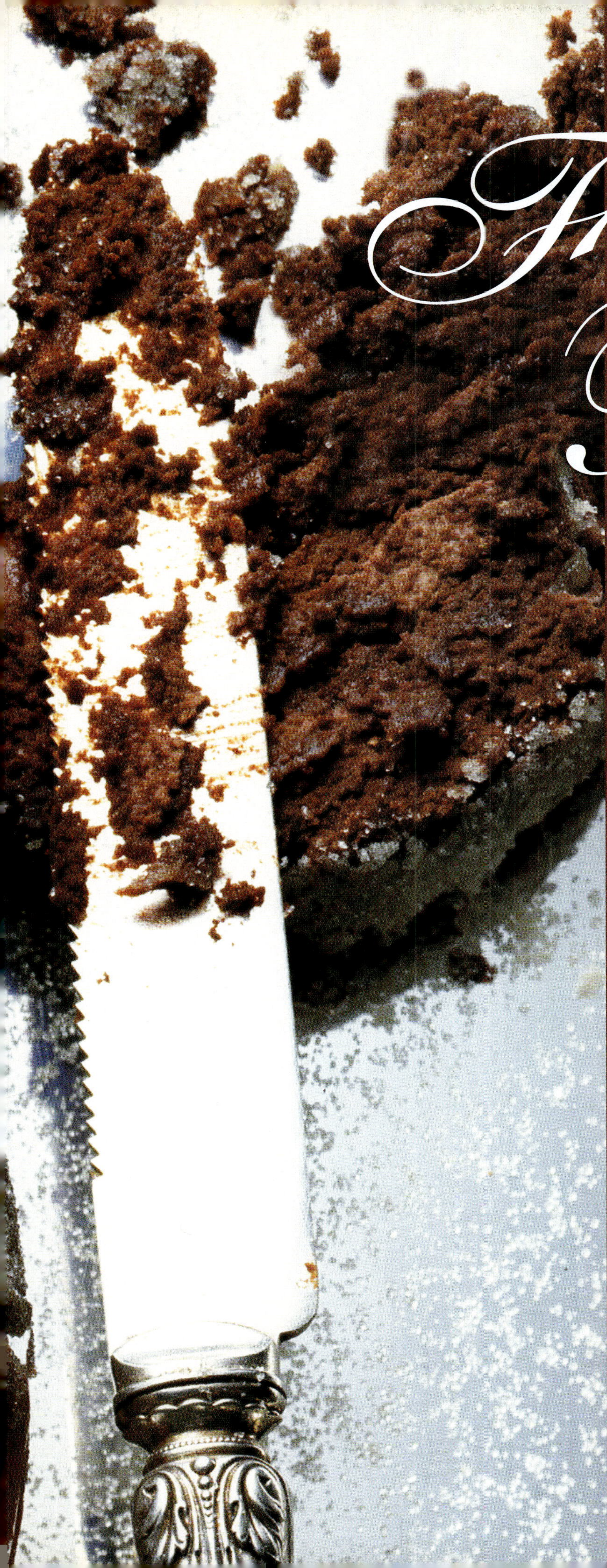

STIR UP A TREAT

Festive Baking

One of the best things at this time of year is the aroma of Christmas baking. Whether you are making a traditional **Christmas cake** or **mince pies**, our variations for these festive favourites will see the plate cleared in a flash. We've also come up with cake decorating tips to make a magnificent centrepiece, including an Antarctic Cake with frolicking penguins that children will love. There are even suggestions for **alternative Christmas cakes** such as Stollen and Kugelhopf. And what could be nicer than giving a friend a **homemade food gift**? From **truffles** and **fudge**, to **pralines** and **biscuits**, there's something here for everyone.

Classic Mince Pies

Hands-on time: for the mincemeat, 20min, plus 24hr soaking; for the pies, 1hr, plus 2½hr chilling
Cooking time: 20–25min
Makes: 2.7kg (6lb) mincemeat – 600g (1lb 6oz) is enough to fill 24 mince pies. This pastry recipe makes 24 mince pies
Vegetarian

FOR THE MINCEMEAT

* **350g (12oz) each sultanas, raisins and currants**
* **150g (5oz) finely chopped candied peel**
* **250g pack shredded vegetable suet**
* **100g pack whole almonds, finely chopped**
* **350g (12oz) demerara sugar**
* **125g (4oz) chopped naturally coloured glacé cherries**
* **2 medium-sized Bramley apples, peeled, cored and grated**
* **4tsp ground mixed spice**
* **Zest and juice of 1 lemon and 1 orange**
* **150ml (¼ pint) brandy**
* **125ml (4fl oz) Drambuie**

FOR THE PUFF PASTRY

* **500g (1lb 2oz) plain flour, plus extra to dust**
* **375g (13oz) chilled, unsalted butter**

* **Milk to brush**
* **Golden icing sugar to sprinkle**

1 To make the mincemeat, combine all the ingredients together in a large mixing bowl. Cover and set aside in a cool place for 24hr, stirring from time to time. Use immediately or spoon into sterilised jars, cover and seal. Store in a cool, dark place for up to three months.

2 To make the puff pastry, sift the flour and 1tsp salt into a mixing bowl. Dice 75g (3oz) of the chilled, unsalted butter, then rub into the flour until it resembles fine breadcrumbs. Add 225–250ml (8–9fl oz) cold water to form a fairly soft, elastic dough. Turn out onto a lightly floured worksurface and knead lightly until just smooth. Wrap in clingfilm and freeze for 1hr (a speedy way to cool down pastry).

3 Put the remaining chilled butter between two pieces of clingfilm and, using a rolling pin, bash it into a 2.5cm (1in) thick oblong. On a lightly floured surface, roll the chilled pastry out to a 45.5x15cm (18x6in) rectangle, with one of the short edges in front of you. Put the butter in the middle of the pastry – both must be cool and just pliable. Fold the bottom third of the pastry up over the butter, then the top third down. Seal the edges by pressing lightly with the rolling pin.

4 Turn the pastry 90° anticlockwise and roll out to the same size as in step 3. Fold and turn as before, then wrap and freeze for 30min. Roll, fold and turn the chilled pastry once more, then roll, fold and turn again. Wrap and freeze for a further 30min. Roll, fold and turn once more, freeze for 30min, then roll and fold one final time. Wrap and chill the pastry in the fridge for up to two days until ready to use. (Don't use ready-made puff pastry as the bases will rise too much. Ready-made shortcrust pastry is the best alternative.)

5 Preheat the oven to 220°C (200°C fan) mark 7. Butter two 12-bun patty tins. On a lightly floured worksurface, roll out half the pastry to 2mm thick. Using a 7.5cm (3in) fluted cutter, stamp out 24 rounds and line the tins. Spoon 1tbsp mincemeat into each. Roll out the rest of the pastry and stamp out 24 rounds with a 5cm (2in) fluted cutter. Put on top of the mincemeat, but don't press down. Brush with milk.

6 Bake for 20–25min until golden, then sprinkle with golden icing sugar. These mince pies taste best on the day they're baked.

To freeze ahead: Freeze the unbaked pies in their tins, covered with clingfilm, for up to one month. **To use:** Cook the mince pies from frozen at 220°C (200°C fan) mark 7 for 25–30min until golden.

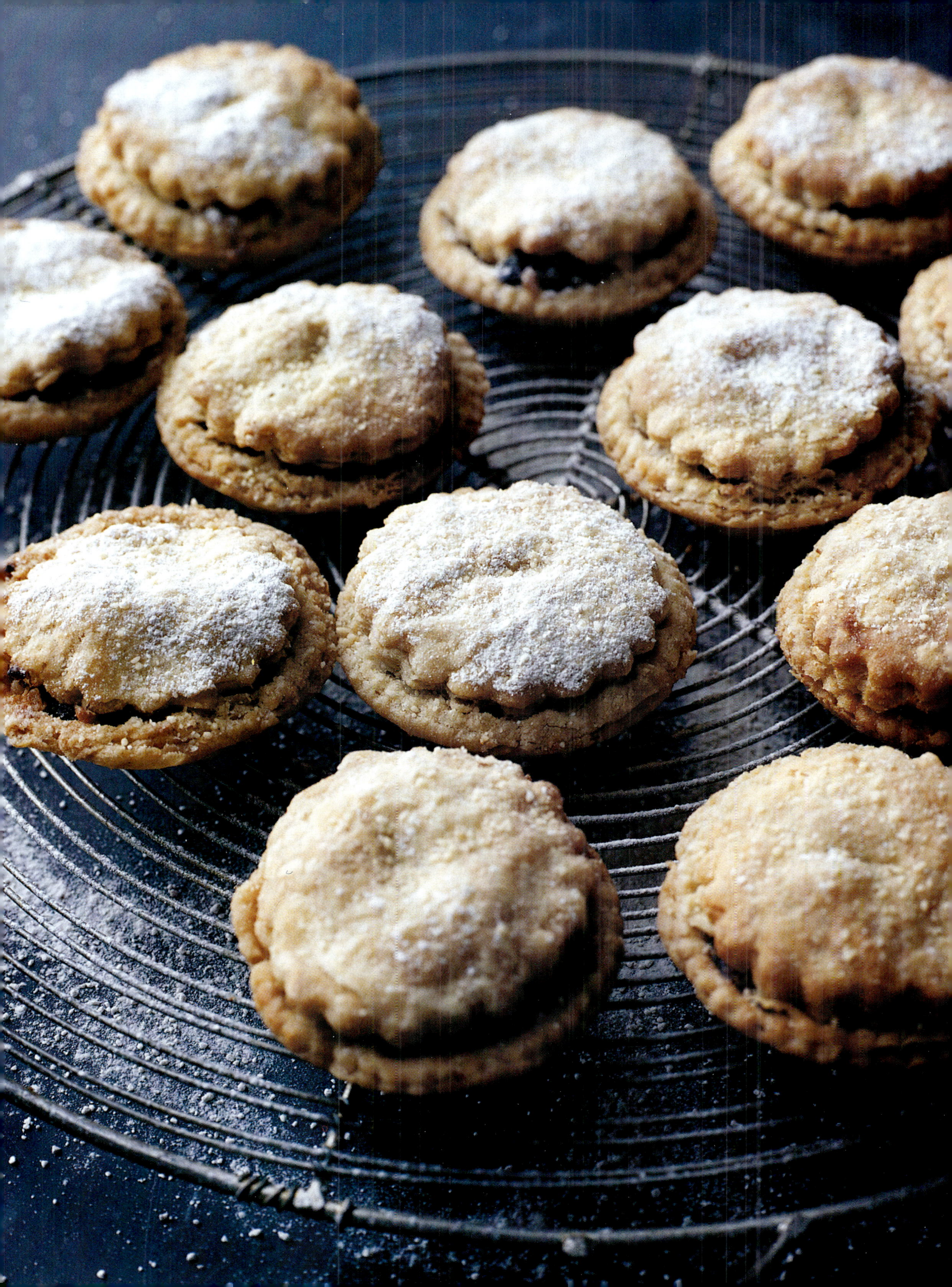

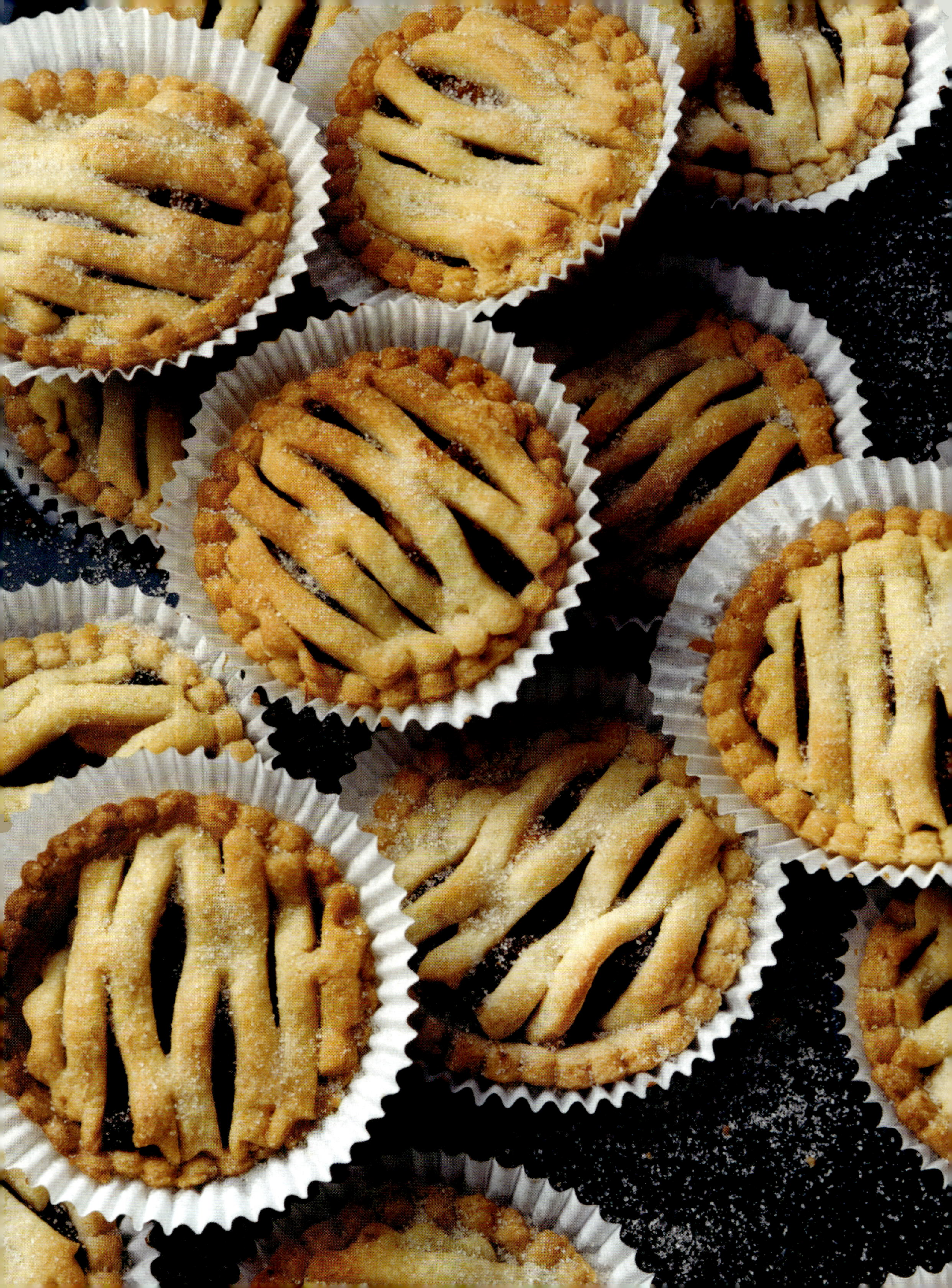

Mince Pies with Orange and Kumquat

Hands-on time: for the mincemeat, 20min, plus 24hr soaking; for the pies, 45min, plus 30min chilling
Cooking time: for the mincemeat, 15min; for the pies, 20–25min
Makes: 2.3kg (5lb) mincemeat – 400g (14oz) is enough to fill 12 mince pies. This pastry recipe makes 12 mince pies
Vegetarian

FOR THE MINCEMEAT

* 225g (8oz) kumquats
* 150ml (¼ pint) Grand Marnier
* 225g (8oz) Bramley apples, cored and chopped
* 350g (12oz) each raisins, sultanas and currants
* 175g (6oz) each light and dark muscovado sugar
* 1tbsp ground mixed spice
* Pinch of ground nutmeg
* Zest and juice of 2 medium oranges

FOR THE PASTRY

* 225g (8oz) plain flour, plus extra to dust
* 2tbsp golden icing sugar, plus extra to sprinkle
* 125g (4oz) unsalted butter, chilled and diced
* A lattice cutter

1 To make the mincemeat, put the kumquats, Grand Marnier and 150ml (¼ pint) water in a pan and bring to the boil. Reduce to a simmer and cook for 15min. Strain, reserving the liquid, and leave to cool. Cut the kumquats in half, discard the pips and chop roughly. Put the kumquats into a mixing bowl with the reserved liquid and the remaining mincemeat ingredients. Stir well. Spoon into sterilised jars, seal and label. Leave for 24hr (it will keep for three months).

2 To make the pastry, put the flour, icing sugar and a pinch of salt into a food processor and whiz for 30sec. Add the butter and whiz until the mixture resembles fine breadcrumbs. Add 1–2tbsp cold water and whiz until the pastry just comes together. Knead on a floured surface, then wrap and chill for 30min.

3 Preheat the oven to 190°C (170°C fan) mark 5. Line a 12-bun patty tin with paper cases. Roll out three-quarters of the pastry on a floured surface. Using a 7.5cm (3in) fluted cutter, stamp out 12 rounds and put in the paper cases. Spoon 1tbsp mincemeat into each and set aside.

4 Add the trimmings to the remaining pastry and roll out into a rectangle. Dust a lattice cutter with flour, then run it over the pastry. Stamp out rounds using a 5cm (2in) plain cutter. Slightly dampen the edges of each pastry case and top with a lattice round. Sprinkle with sugar.

5 Bake for 20–25min or until golden. Cool for 15min, then put on a wire rack. Store in an airtight container for up to two days, warming the pies through for 5min in the oven as you need them.

To freeze ahead: Freeze the unbaked pies in their tins, covered with clingfilm, for up to one month. **To use:** Cook the mince pies from frozen at 190°C (170°C fan) mark 5 for 30–35min until golden.

Cranberry and Apple Mince Pies

Hands-on time: for the mincemeat, 20min, plus 24hr soaking; for the pies, 45min, plus 1hr 10min chilling and 15min cooling
Cooking time: 12–15min
Makes: 2.5kg (5½lb) mincemeat – 400g (14oz) is enough to fill 12 mince pies. This pastry recipe makes 48 mince pies
Vegetarian

For the mincemeat

* 450g (1lb) Bramley apples, cored and chopped
* 225g (8oz) fresh cranberries
* 125g (4oz) candied peel, finely chopped
* 350g (12oz) each raisins, sultanas and currants
* 175g (6oz) each light and dark muscovado sugar
* 1tbsp ground mixed spice
* Pinch of ground nutmeg
* Zest and juice of 2 medium oranges
* 150ml (¼ pint) Calvados

For the almond pastry

* 225g (8oz) plain flour, plus a little extra to dust
* 50g (2oz) ground almonds
* 75g (3oz) golden icing sugar
* 175g (6oz) unsalted butter, chilled and diced
* 2 medium egg yolks

For the shortbread topping

* 75g (3oz) unsalted butter, softened
* 25g (1oz) golden caster sugar, plus extra to sprinkle
* 75g (3oz) plain flour
* 50g (2oz) ground almonds
* A holly cutter

1 To make the mincemeat, combine all the ingredients together in a large mixing bowl. Spoon into five 500ml sterilised jars, seal and label. Leave for at least 24hr (the mincemeat will keep for three months).

2 To make the pastry, put the flour, ground almonds, icing sugar and a large pinch of salt in a food processor and whiz for 30sec. Add the butter and whiz until the mixture resembles fine breadcrumbs. Add the egg yolks and whiz until the mixture just comes together (if it's a little dry, add 1–2tsp cold water). Knead lightly on a floured surface to bring together. Wrap and chill for 1hr.

3 To make the topping, beat the butter and sugar until light and fluffy, then mix in the flour and almonds. Bring together with your hands, then wrap and chill for 15min. Line four 12-bun patty tins with paper cases – if you need to cook the pies in two batches, keep the unused pastry in the fridge.

4 On a floured surface, roll out the pastry to a thickness of 2mm. Stamp out rounds using a 7.5cm (3in) fluted pastry cutter. Put in the paper cases and prick the base with a fork. Chill for 10min. Fill each one with 1tbsp mincemeat. Preheat the oven to 190°C (170°C fan) mark 5.

5 Roll out the shortbread dough pastry to 2mm thick. Using a 4x2.5cm (1½x1in) holly cutter, cut two leaves for each pie. With the back of a knife, mark the leaves with veins and decorate each pie with two cranberries picked out of the remaining mincemeat. Sprinkle with sugar.

6 Bake for 12–15min or until golden. Cool for 15min, then put on a wire rack. Store in an airtight container for up to two days, warming the pies through for 5min in the oven as you need them.

To freeze ahead: Freeze the unbaked pies in their tins, covered with clingfilm, for up to one month. **To use:** Cook the mince pies from frozen at 190°C (170°C fan) mark 5 for 18–20min until golden.

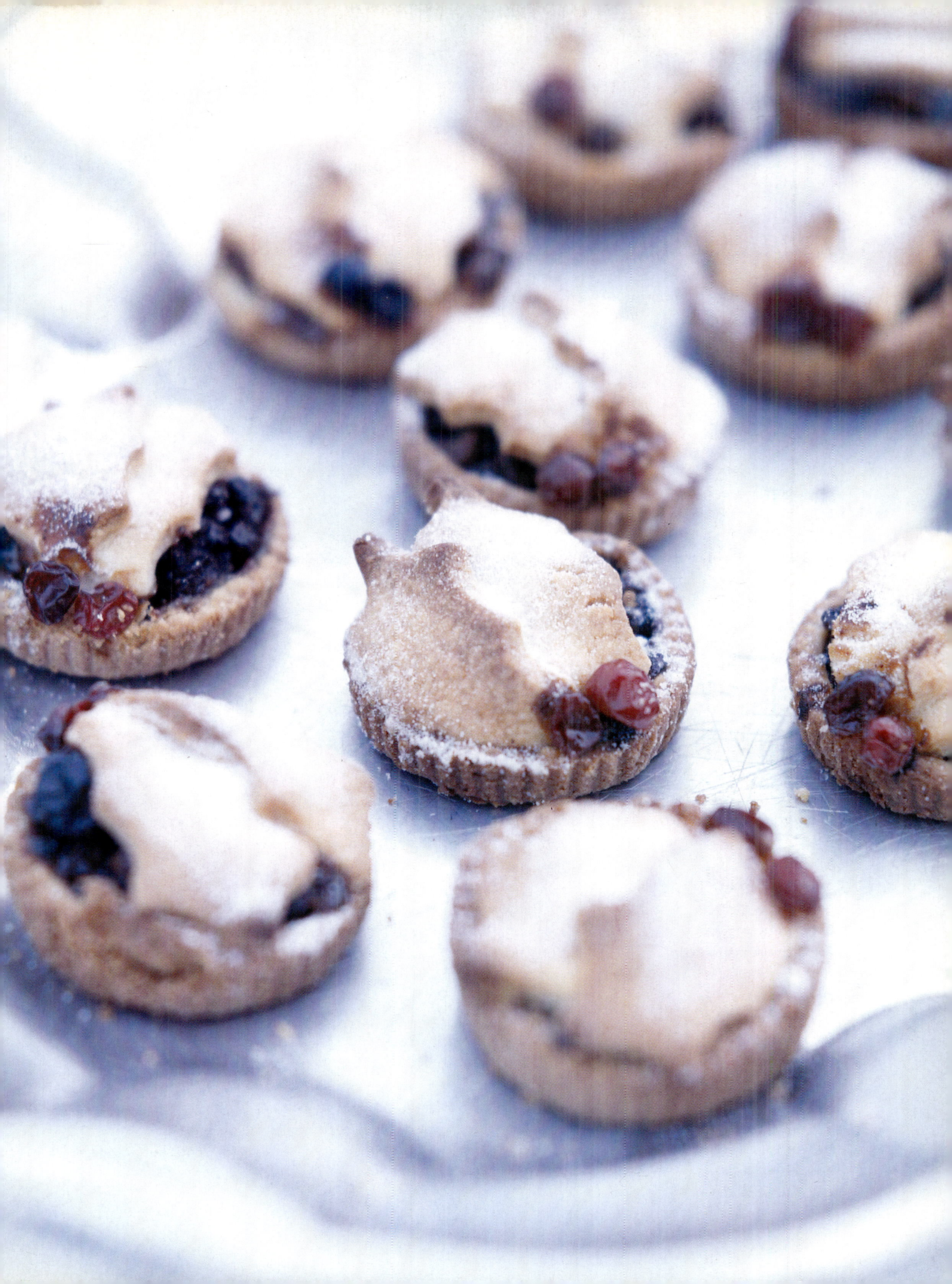

Classic Christmas Cake

Hands-on time: for the cake, 35min, plus 30min cooling; for the almond paste, 30min, plus 1hr chilling and overnight drying; for the royal icing, 25min
Cooking time: 2¾–3hr
Makes: 30–34 slices

Use a 23cm (9in) round cake tin

FOR THE CAKE
* 1½tbsp whole cardamom pods
* 275g (10oz) unsalted butter
* 375g (13oz) light muscovado sugar
* 1.25kg (2¾lb) luxury mixed dried fruit
* Zest and juice of 1½ oranges
* 150ml (¼ pint) sweet sherry or Marsala
* 1tbsp ground allspice
* Butter for greasing
* 125g (4oz) almonds, chopped
* 125g (4oz) ground almonds
* 5 large eggs
* 375g (13oz) plain flour

FOR THE ALMOND PASTE AND GLAZE
* 300g (11oz) ground almonds
* 200g (7oz) golden caster sugar
* 200g (7oz) golden icing sugar, sieved
* Zest of 2 lemons
* 1tsp almond extract
* 2 medium egg whites
* 5tbsp apricot jam
* Cornflour, sieved, to dust

FOR THE ROYAL ICING
* 3 medium egg whites
* 2tbsp lemon juice
* 1tbsp glycerine
* 675g (1lb 7oz) icing sugar, sieved

FOR THE DECORATION
* Fresh or frozen cranberries
* Sprigs of fresh bayleaves
* Icing sugar to dust

1 Crush the cardamom pods using a pestle and mortar to release the seeds. Discard the pods and grind the seeds until they look like coarsely ground black pepper. Alternatively, crush in a bowl using the end of a rolling pin. Put the butter, sugar, dried fruit, orange zest and juice, sherry or Marsala, cardamom seeds and allspice in a large, heavy-based pan and bring slowly to the boil, stirring until the butter has melted. Reduce the heat and simmer for 10min, stirring frequently. Remove from the heat and leave to cool for 30min.

2 Preheat the oven to 150°C (130°C fan) mark 2 and grease and line the cake tin with greaseproof paper.

3 Add the chopped and ground almonds to the pan along with the eggs and stir until combined. Sift the flour into the pan and mix well. Spoon the cake mixture into the prepared tin and level off with a palette knife.

4 Bake on the centre shelf for 2¾–3hr until the cake is dark golden and firm to the touch. The cake is cooked when a fine skewer inserted into the centre comes out clean. Put on a wire rack and leave to cool in the tin. Remove from the tin and peel off the lining paper. Wrap the cake in greaseproof paper, then in foil, and store in an airtight container in a cool, dry place for up to eight weeks.

5 To make the almond paste, mix together the ground almonds, caster sugar and icing sugar in a large bowl. Add the lemon zest, almond extract and egg whites and mix to a firm paste, using your hands if you find it easier. Knead very lightly until smooth, then wrap securely in clingfilm and chill for at least 1hr.

6 If the cake has risen a lot in the middle, use a large knife to level off the surface. Turn it over so the bottom of the cake is now the top and put on a board or serving plate. Heat the apricot jam in a small pan with 1tbsp water until melted, stirring from time to time. Brush over the top and sides of the cake.

7 On a surface heavily dusted with cornflour, roll out the almond paste to a 36cm (14½in) round – 13cm (5½in) larger than the diameter of the cake. Lift the paste over the cake and use your hands to ease it to fit around the sides, trimming off any excess around the base. Cover with greaseproof paper and leave in a cool, dry place overnight for the paste to dry.

Continued over page

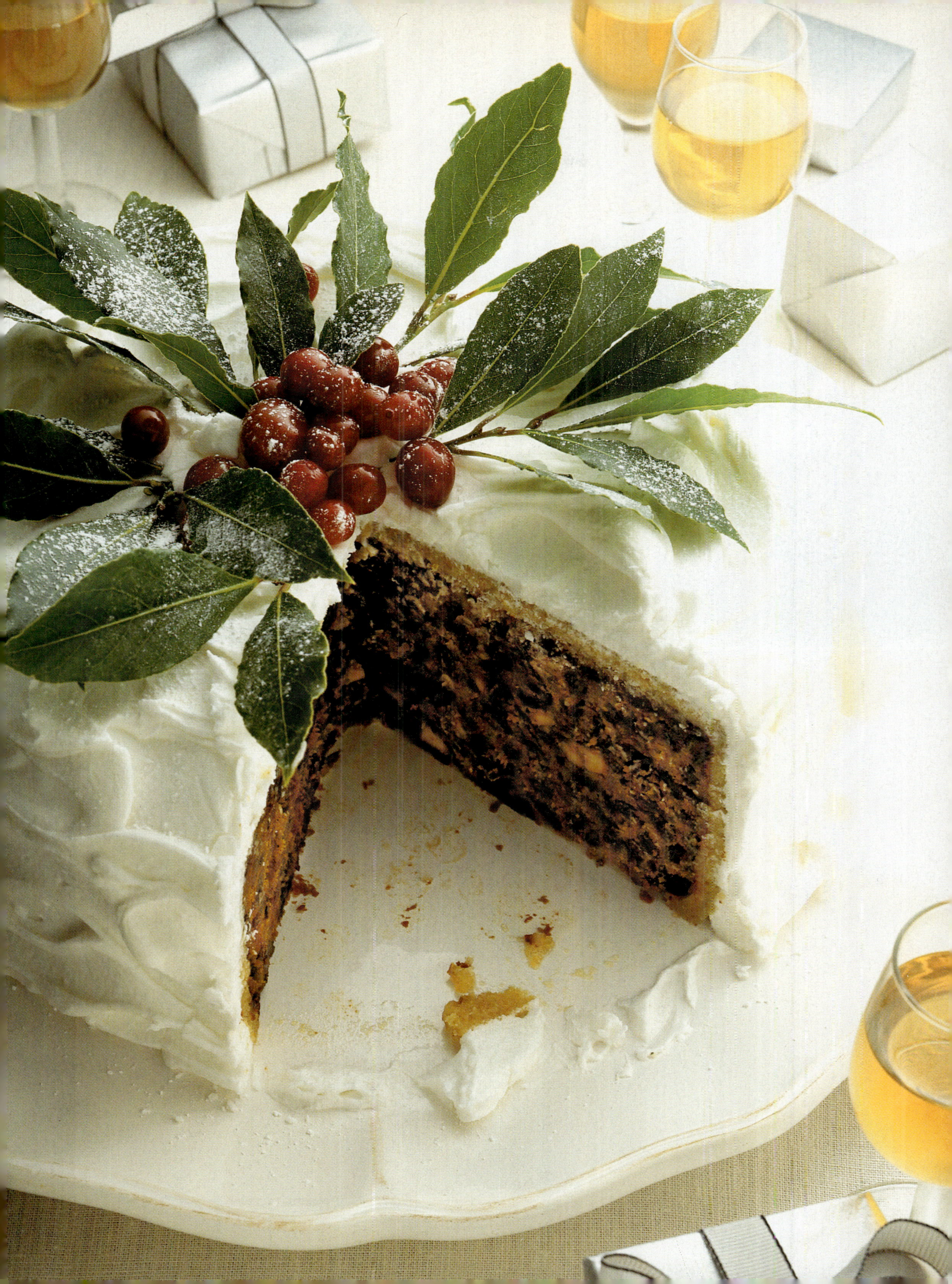

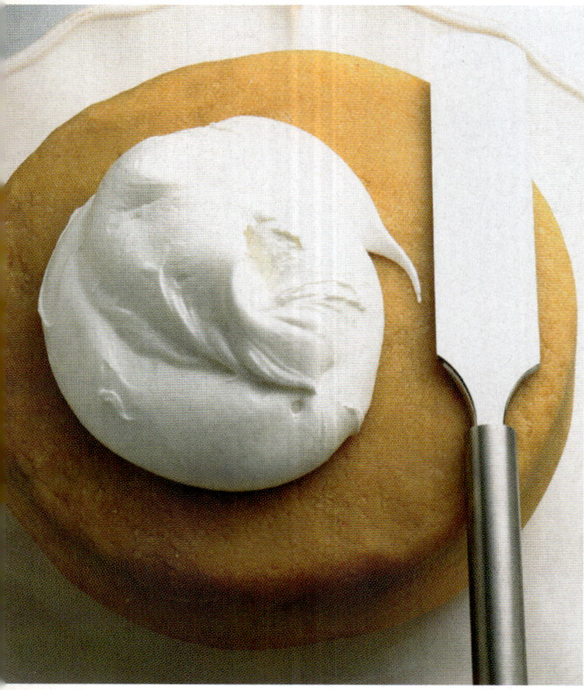

8 To make the icing, put the egg whites in a large, clean bowl and whisk lightly with a freestanding mixer until slightly frothy. Add the lemon juice, glycerine and some of the icing sugar and whisk until smooth. Continue whisking in the icing sugar, a little at a time, until the icing is smooth and softly peaking. To prevent a crust forming, keep the bowl covered with clingfilm until ready to use.

9 When ready to ice the cake, spoon the icing on top and use a palette knife to spread over the top and sides in an even layer, swirling the icing with the knife to give a textured finish.

10 To make the decoration, if using frozen cranberries, thaw and leave on a double sheet of kitchen paper for about 20min to soak up any excess moisture and avoid staining the icing. Wash and dry the bayleaves thoroughly. Snip off leaves in clusters of two or three and arrange on top of the cake with the cranberries. Dust lightly with icing sugar. (For alternative ways to decorate a Christmas cake, see Cake Decorating Ideas.)

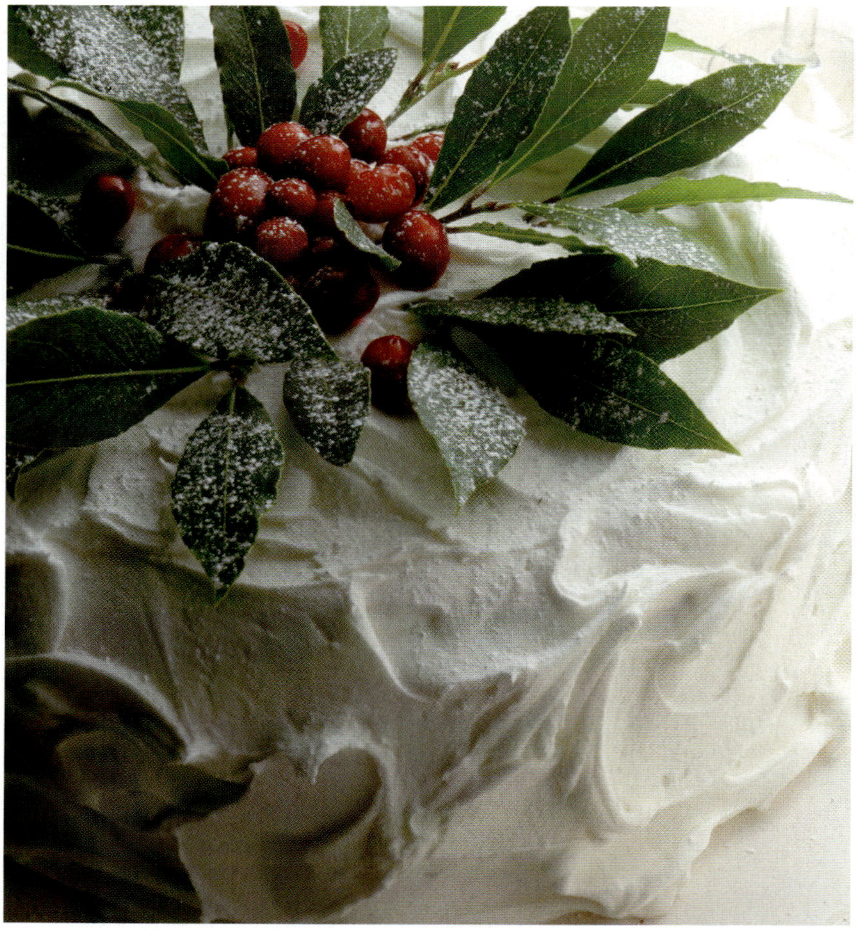

There's nothing more natural.

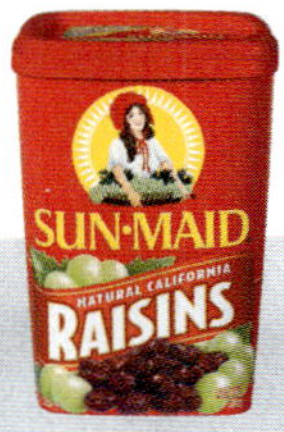

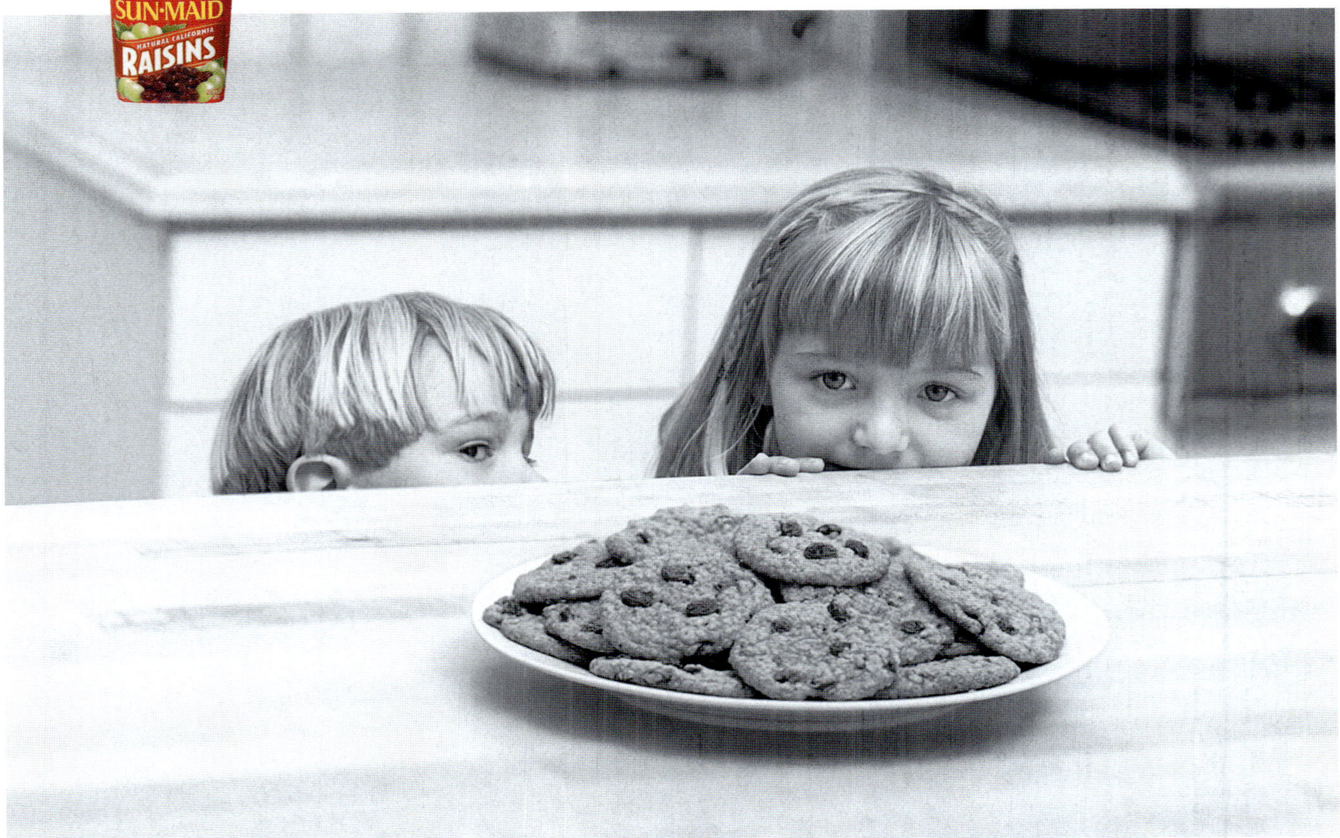

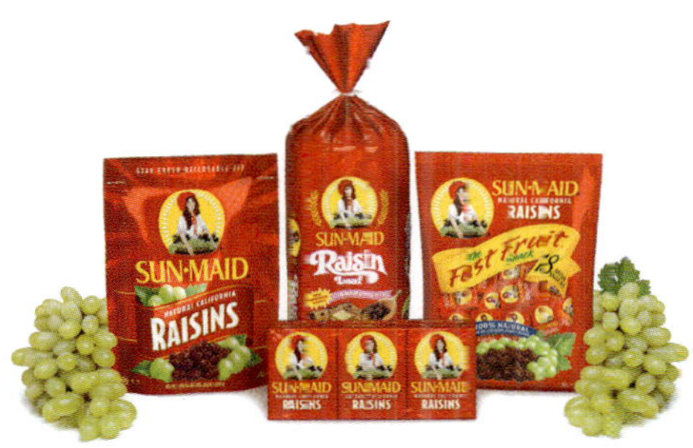

Our best from California.™

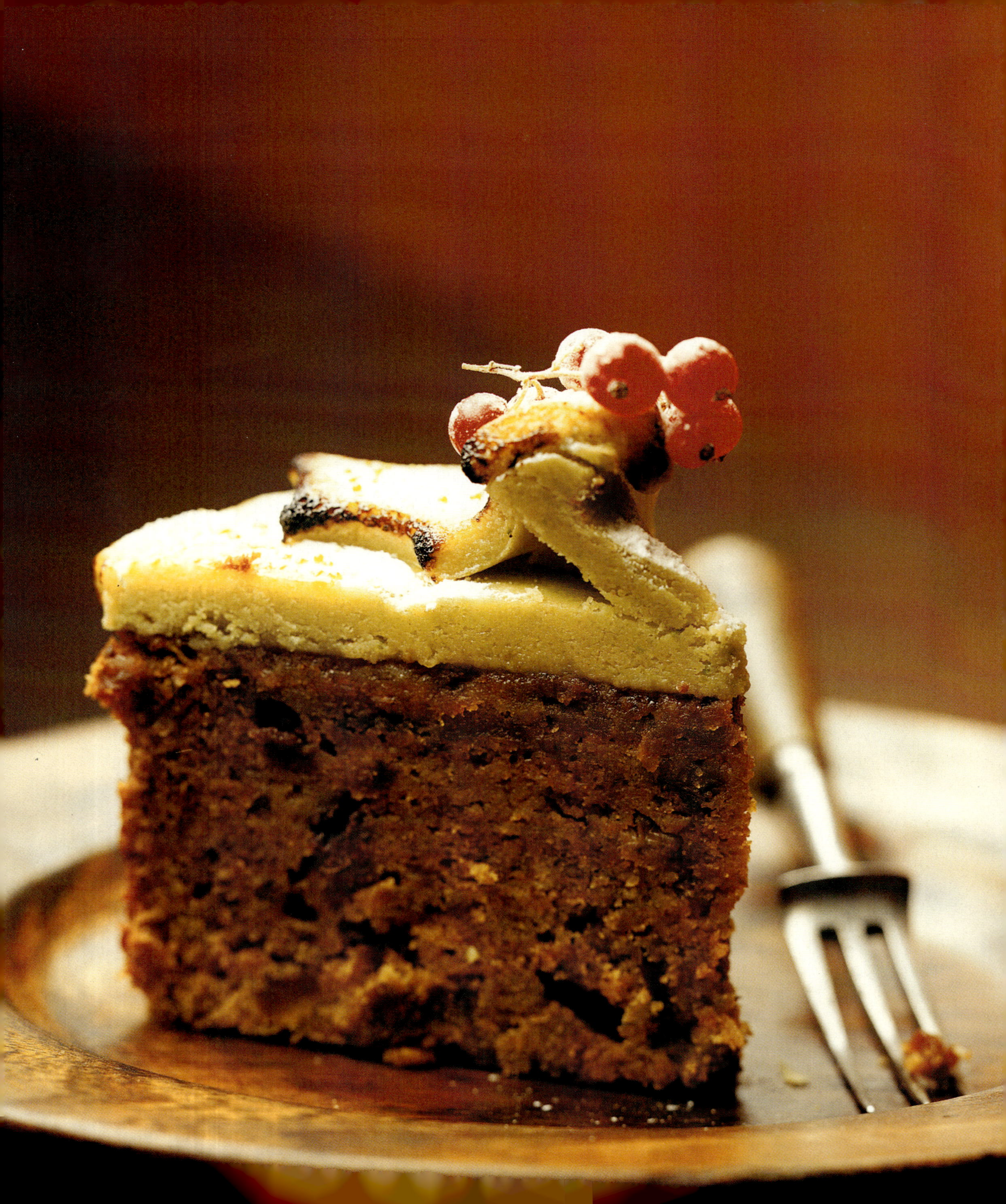

The Booziest Christmas Cake

Hands-on time: for the cake, 45min, plus at least 48hr soaking; for the almond paste, 25min, plus 2–3min grilling time
Cooking time: 3–3¾hr
Makes: 48 slices

Use a deep 25.5cm (10in) round cake tin

For the cake

* 675g (1lb 7oz) mixed dried fruit
* 50g (2oz) stem ginger, chopped
* 200g (7oz) ready-to-eat prunes, chopped
* Zest and juice of 1 large lemon
* 250ml (9fl oz) brandy
* 50ml (2fl oz) ginger wine
* 375g (13oz) butter, softened, plus extra for greasing
* 375g (13oz) dark muscovado sugar
* 5 medium eggs, beaten
* 375g (13oz) self-raising flour
* 1tbsp mixed spice
* 2tsp ground cinnamon
* 2tsp ground ginger
* 100g (3½oz) ground almonds

For the almond paste and glaze

* 175g (6oz) shelled pistachio nuts
* 150g (5oz) ground almonds
* 250g (9oz) golden caster sugar
* 425g (15oz) unrefined golden icing sugar, plus extra to dust
* 2 medium eggs, beaten
* 5tbsp apricot glaze

For the decoration

* Unrefined golden icing sugar to dust
* Sprig of redcurrants or fake berries
* Holly cookie cutters
* 1mx5cm (39x2in) ribbon

1 Put the dried fruit, stem ginger, prunes, lemon zest and juice into a bowl. Pour the brandy and ginger wine over. Cover and soak for at least 48hr.

2 Preheat the oven to 170°C (150°C fan) mark 3. Grease and line the base and sides of the cake tin using a double thickness of baking parchment. Wrap a double thickness of brown paper around the outside and secure tightly with string.

3 Using a small electric whisk or food mixer, beat together the butter and sugar until light and fluffy. Gradually add the eggs, a little at a time, and beat well until smooth (you may need to add a little flour to prevent curdling). Sift the flour, mixed spice, cinnamon and ginger into the cake mixture and carefully fold in, along with the ground almonds, using a large metal spoon.

4 Place half the dried fruit mixture in a processor and whiz to a purée, then fold into the cake mixture with the remaining whole fruit until evenly combined. Spoon the cake mixture into the prepared tin and level off with a palette knife.

5 Bake on the centre shelf for 3–3¾hr, covering with foil after 1½hr. Remove the cake from the oven and test to see if it's done. The cake is cooked when a fine skewer inserted into the centre comes out clean. If it doesn't, return the cake to the oven for a further 15min, then check again. Allow to cool in the tin, then turn out and remove the lining paper. Wrap in greaseproof paper, then in foil, making sure the cake is completely covered, and store in an airtight container in a cool, dry place for up to six weeks.

6 To make the almond paste, whiz the pistachio nuts in a food processor until finely chopped. Add the ground almonds, caster sugar, icing sugar and eggs and whiz together to make a firm paste. Lightly dust a worksurface with icing sugar and knead the pistachio paste until smooth. Set aside one-eighth. Roll out the remainder into a round, 1cm (½in) thick, about the size of the top of the cake. Using the cake tin as a template, cut the almond paste to the right size. Cut a scalloped edge with holly cutters, add the trimmings to the reserved pistachio paste, then knead together and put to one side.

7 Brush the cake with the apricot glaze and lay the almond paste on top, pressing down lightly. Roll out the reserved almond paste to the same thickness as before. Stamp out large holly leaves using cutters and brush one side with a little apricot glaze, then arrange in the centre of the cake. Chill the cake for 1hr, then dust generously with the icing sugar and grill until golden. Leave to cool. Dust the redcurrant sprigs or fake berries with icing sugar and arrange on top of the cake. Tie the ribbon around the cake. (For alternative ways to decorate a Christmas cake, see Cake Decorating Ideas.)

Easy Christmas Cake

Hands-on time: 40min, plus up to 48hr soaking the fruit, six weeks maturing and around 2hr decorating
Cooking time: 2hr
Serves: 12

Use a deep 20.5cm (8in) round cake tin

For the cake

- 75g (3oz) candied peel, finely chopped
- 75g (3oz) glacé cherries, cut in half
- 150g (5oz) seeded raisins
- 150g (5oz) large, seedless raisins
- 200g (7oz) sultanas
- 225g (8oz) currants
- 200ml (7fl oz) brandy, plus 4tbsp for spooning over
- Butter for greasing
- 300g (11oz) plain flour
- 1tsp ground cinnamon
- A little freshly grated nutmeg
- 150g (5oz) softened butter, preferably unsalted
- 150g (5oz) dark muscovado sugar
- 4 large eggs, separated
- 1tsp cocoa powder
- Pinch of bicarbonate of soda

For the decoration

- 6tbsp honey or apricot jam
- Cornflour to dust
- 450g (1lb) white marzipan
- About 900g (2lb) ready-to-roll fondant icing
- Edible silver leaf (from cake decorating shops)
- A length of silver braid

1 Place the candied peel and glacé cherries in a bowl with all the dried fruit and 200ml (7fl oz) brandy. Cover and leave in a cool place for 24–48hr, stirring occasionally.

2 Preheat the oven to 150°C (130°C fan) mark 2. Lightly grease the base of the cake tin, then cover with a disc of greaseproof paper. Halve a double thickness of greaseproof paper 12.5cm (5in) wide and 71.5cm (28in) long. Fold up 2.5cm (1in) along the open edge and cut diagonally at 1cm (½in) intervals. Curl the strip of paper around the inside of the tin, placing the snipped edge on the base. Place a second disc of greaseproof paper in the base of the tin.

3 Sift the flour with the cinnamon, a pinch of salt and a little nutmeg. Using an electric whisk or food mixer, beat the butter until creamy. Add the sugar gradually, beating well between each addition, until light and fluffy. With the whisk or machine at full speed, beat in the egg yolks one at a time. Reduce the speed and add 150g (5½oz) of the flour mixture, the fruit and its soaking liquid, then the remaining flour. In a separate bowl, whisk the egg whites to a foam. Add to the mixture along with the cocoa and bicarbonate of soda, mixing well. Spoon the mixture into the prepared tin and level off with a palette knife.

4 Bake on the centre shelf for 2hr or until a skewer inserted into the centre comes out hot and clean. Allow to cool in the tin for 30min, then transfer to a wire rack. Wrap in greaseproof paper and foil, and store in a cool, dry place for up to six weeks. Wait at least one week before decorating. Every week for the first four weeks, prick the base of the cake and spoon 1tbsp brandy over the top. For the last two weeks, leave to dry.

5 To decorate the cake, warm half the honey or apricot jam and brush a thin layer over the top and sides. On a worksurface dusted with cornflour, roll out the marzipan to a 30.5cm (12in) circle. Position over the top and sides of the cake, press down lightly, then trim any excess. Cover with greaseproof paper and leave in a cool, dry place for two days.

6 Place the cake on a board. Warm the remaining honey or jam and brush over the marzipan. On a worksurface lightly dusted with cornflour, thinly roll out 225g (8oz) fondant icing and cover as with the marzipan. Roll out the remaining fondant icing thinly. Cut a piece of greaseproof paper into a triangle with sides 20.5cm (8in) long and base 4cm (1½in); use this as a template for cutting the icing into about 22 triangles. Re-roll and cut the icing trimmings as needed. Place the icing triangles over the top and sides of the cake, points to the centre, overlapping them and tucking in any excess icing as you go.

7 Roll the final icing trimmings into different-sized balls. Cover some with silver leaf, rolling gently until smooth, then press lightly onto the cake. Decorate the bottom edge of the Christmas cake with a length of silver braid, adding a few of the icing balls to complete. (For alternative ways to decorate a Christmas cake, see Cake Decorating Ideas.)

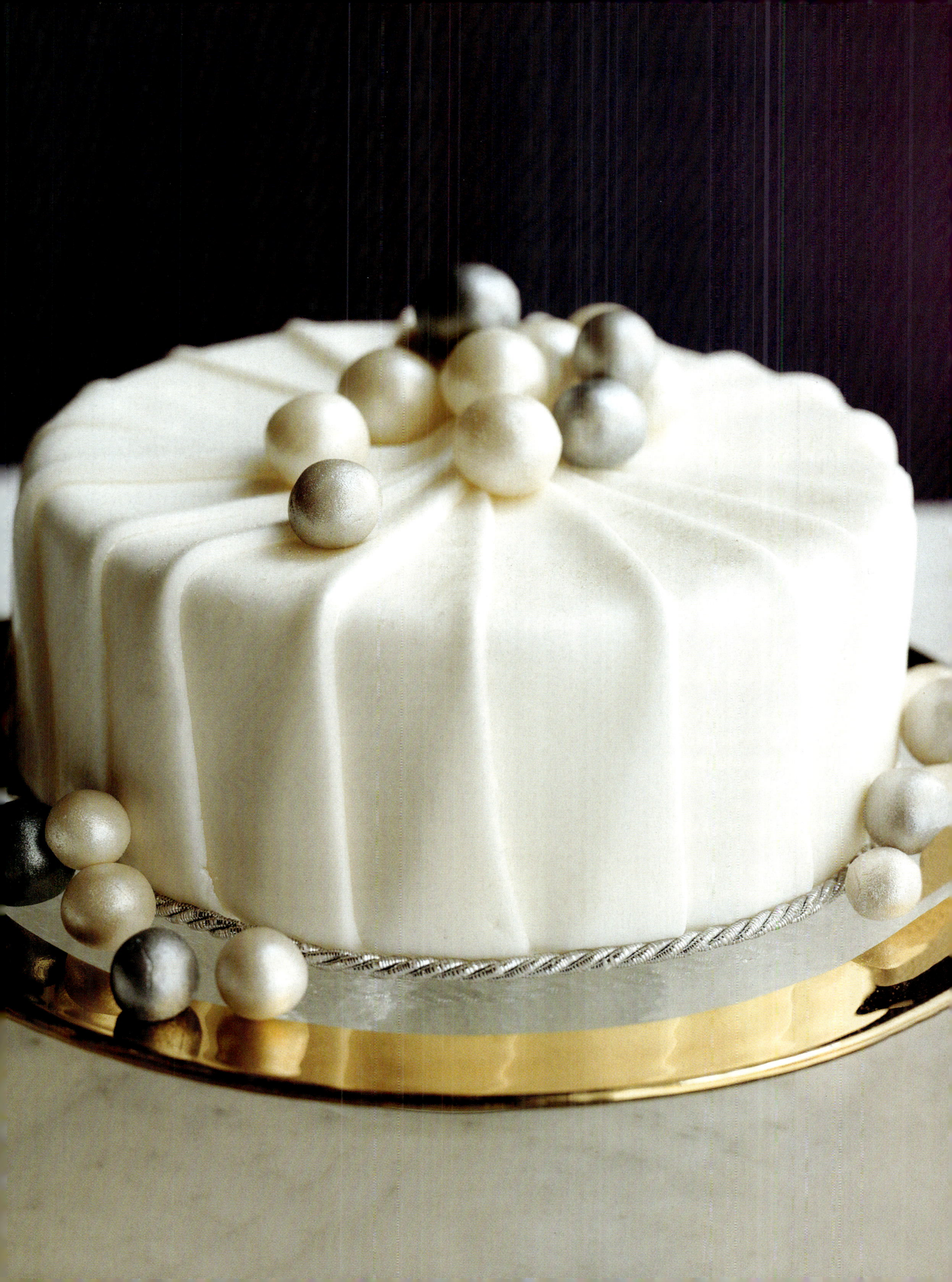

Antarctic Cake

Hands-on time: for the almond paste 25min; for the decoration 35min
Makes: 48 slices

* 25.5cm (10in) round fruit cake (see Christmas Cakes)

For the glaze
* 135ml (9tbsp) honey or apricot jam

For the almond paste
* 450g (1lb) ground almonds
* 225g (8oz) caster sugar
* 225g (8oz) icing sugar, plus extra to dust
* 2 egg whites
* 2tsp lemon juice
* 2tsp sherry
* 3–4 drops of vanilla essence

For the cake
* Ready-made almond paste or 900g (2lb) homemade almond paste (see above)
* Cornflour to dust
* 900g (2lb) ready-to-roll icing

For the decoration
* 1 pack multicoloured icing
* Silver balls
* Blue tissue paper

1 To make the glaze, warm the honey or jam in a pan with 3tbsp water. Strain the mixture through a sieve and brush some of it over a 10in fruit cake.

2 If not using the ready-made almond paste, to make the homemade version, place the ground almonds, caster sugar and icing sugar in a bowl and mix together. In another bowl, whisk the egg whites or a little warm water with the lemon juice, sherry and vanilla essence, then add to the dry mixture. Stir well to mix, pounding gently to release some of the almond oil. Knead with your hands until smooth. This will make 900g (2lb).

3 On a worksurface dusted with icing sugar, roll out half the almond paste to fit the top of the cake. Place it on top of the cake, then smooth over.

4 Cut pieces of string measuring the height and circumference of the cake. Using the string as a guide, roll out the remaining almond paste to a rectangular strip and trim to size. Brush the sides of the cake with the rest of the melted honey or jam. Roll up the almond paste strip, place one end against the side of the cake and unroll to cover it. Use a palette knife to smooth the sides and joins. Flatten the top lightly with a rolling pin. Leave the cake in a cool, dry place for at least three to four days if covering in ready-made paste and five days for homemade paste before icing.

5 Dust a worksurface with cornflour, roll out the ready-to-roll icing and cover the cake with the icing. To make the penguins, take a small piece of black icing and roll into an egg shape. Roll a small piece of white icing into a ball and flatten into an oval. Mould the oval around the front of the penguin's body. Roll a small piece of black icing into a ball and place on top of the body, moulding it to form the head. Make two small holes for the eyes using a cocktail stick. Shape a small piece of red icing into a cone shape and press gently onto the head to form a beak.

6 Using a sharp knife or scalpel, cut each side, about a quarter of the way from the top, and pull each side out to form the penguin's wings. To make the scarf, roll a piece of yellow icing into a long cylinder and snip at the ends. Place around the neck of the penguin. Repeat this process to make six more different-sized penguins.

7 Mould some white icing into iceberg shapes and roll small white balls to create snowballs. Arrange on top of the cake with the penguins. To create the impression of the Antarctic, surround the cake with blue tissue paper and secure with sticky tape. Scatter silver balls on top and dust with icing sugar to give the cake a snowy effect.

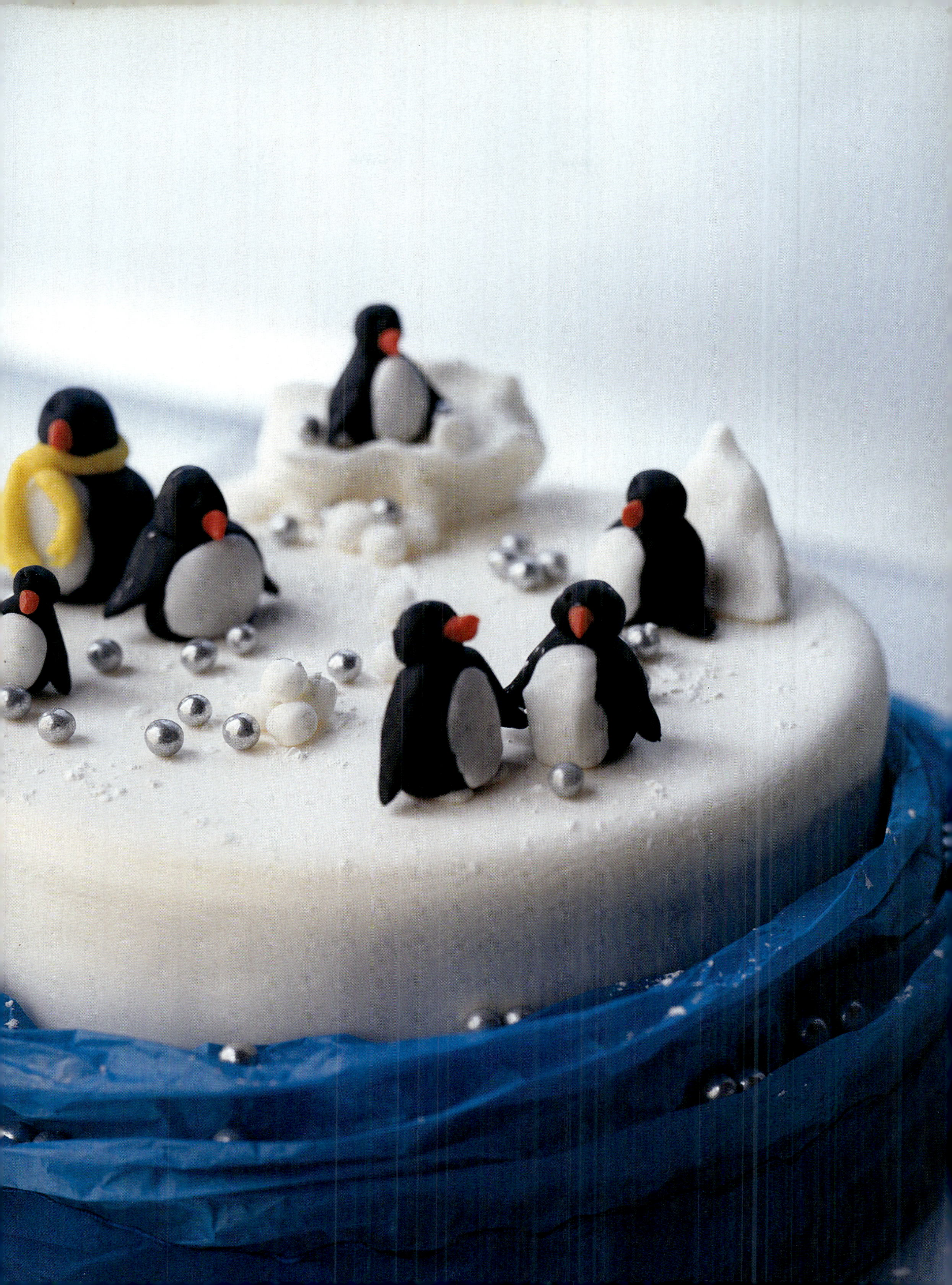

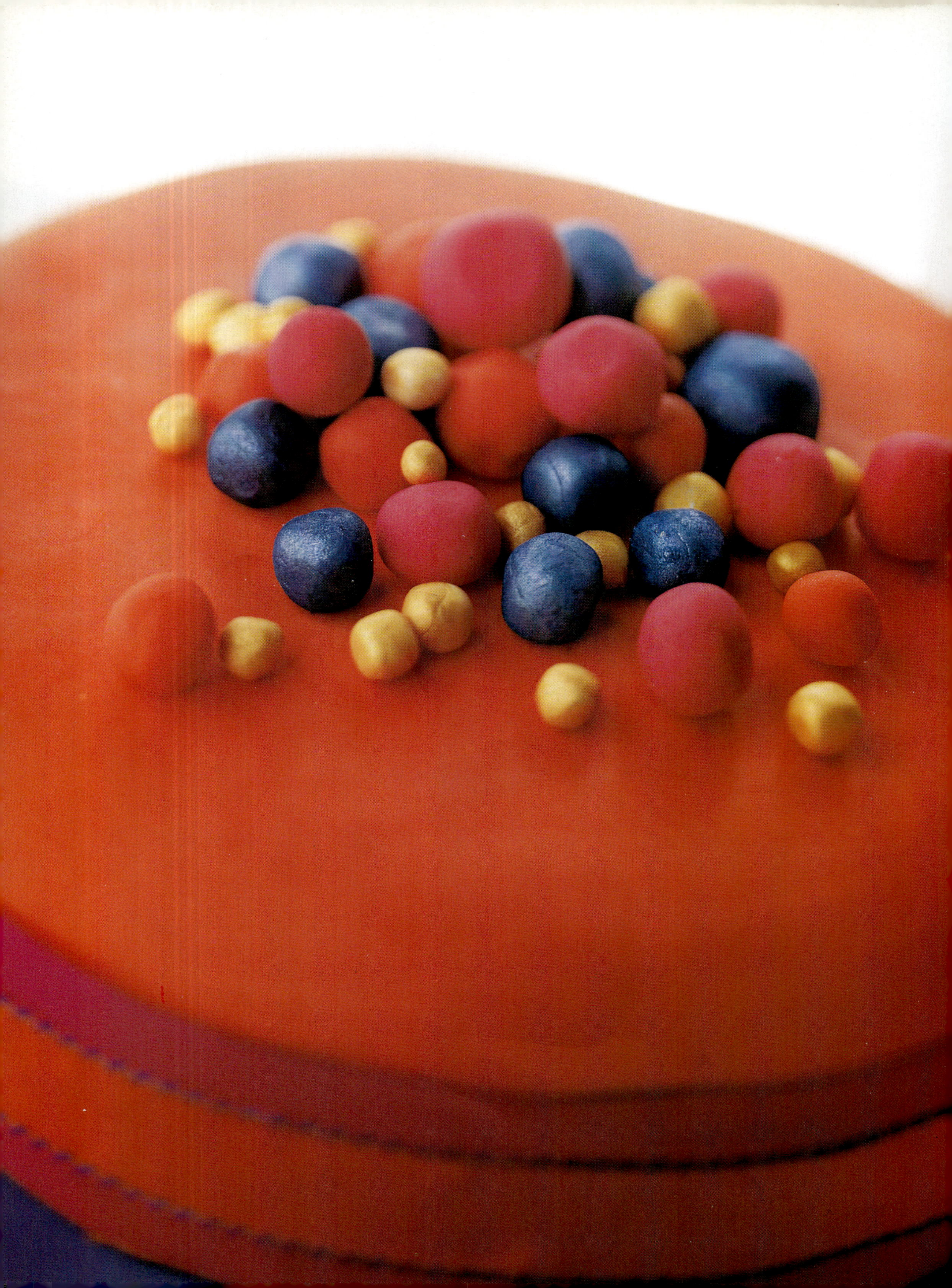

Coloured Snowball Cake

Hands-on time: for the almond paste, 25min, for the decoration 35min
Makes: 48 slices

* 25.5cm (10in) round fruit cake (see Christmas Cakes)

FOR THE GLAZE
* 135ml (9tbsp) honey or apricot jam

FOR THE ALMOND PASTE
* 450g (1lb) ground almonds
* 225g (8oz) caster sugar
* 225g (8oz) icing sugar, plus extra to dust
* 2 egg whites
* 2tsp lemon juice
* 2tsp sherry
* 3–4 drops of vanilla essence

FOR THE CAKE
* Ready-made almond paste or 900g (2lb) homemade almond paste (see above)
* Cornflour to dust
* 900g (2lb) ready-to-roll icing

FOR THE DECORATION
* Orange food paste
* 1kg (2lb 4oz) ready-to-roll white icing
* Midnight blue, light gold and fuchsia pink food colouring
* Pink and orange ribbon

1 To make the glaze, warm the honey or jam in a pan with 3tbsp water. Strain the mixture through a sieve and brush some of it over a 10in fruit cake.

2 If not using ready-made paste, to make the homemade version, place the ground almonds, caster sugar and icing sugar in a bowl and mix together. In another bowl, whisk the egg whites or a little warm water with the lemon juice, sherry and vanilla essence, then add to the dry mixture. Stir well to mix, pounding gently to release some of the almond oil. Knead with your hands until smooth. This will make 900g (2lb).

3 On a worksurface dusted with icing sugar, roll out half the almond paste to fit the top of the cake. Place it on top of the cake, then smooth over.

4 Cut pieces of string measuring the height and circumference of the cake. Using the string as a guide, roll out the remaining almond paste to a rectangular strip and trim to size. Brush the sides of the cake with the rest of the melted honey or jam. Roll up the almond paste strip, place one end against the side of the cake and unroll to cover. Use a palette knife to smooth the sides and joins. Flatten the top lightly with a rolling pin. Leave the cake in a cool, dry place for at least three to four days if covering in ready-made paste and five days for homemade paste before icing.

5 To make the coloured icing, add a little orange food paste to 900 (2lb) white ready-to-roll icing and knead lightly until a uniform colour is achieved. Continue to add extra food paste until the icing is bright orange. Dust a worksurface with cornflour, roll out the coloured icing, then cover the cake with the icing. Reserve any trimmings.

6 To make the coloured snowballs, roll out the icing trimmings into different-sized balls. Take the rest of the ready-to-roll white icing and roll into different-sized balls. Cover some white balls with midnight blue and gold edible food colour and colour the remaining white balls with fuchsia pink food colouring. Allow the balls to dry before arranging them on top of the cake. Wrap some pink and orange ribbon around the outside of the cake.

Chocolate Box Cake

Hands-on time: 25-30min for the decoration
Makes: 30-34 slices

* 23cm (9in) round fruit cake (see Christmas Cakes)

FOR THE GLAZE
* 6 tbsp honey or apricot jam

FOR THE CAKE
* 800g (1¾lb) ready-made white almond paste
* 3tbsp cocoa, sieved
* 2tbsp glucose syrup
* Icing sugar to dust
* 800g (1¾lb) ready-to-roll icing

FOR THE DECORATION
* 18 plain chocolate thins
* Black icing pen
* Sieved cocoa powder to dust
* Truffles, chocolate nuts and gold dragees
* Edible gold balls
* Gold crepe paper, cord and ribbon

1 To make the glaze, warm the honey or jam in a small pan with 2tbsp water. Strain the mixture through a sieve and brush some of it over the 9in fruit cake. Break up the almond paste, then whiz in a food processor with the cocoa and glucose syrup. Turn out and knead on a clean worksurface.

2 On a surface lightly dusted with icing sugar, roll out the almond paste into a circle large enough to cover the top and sides of the cake – about 10cm (4in) bigger than the cake's top. (You can use a piece of string to measure the diameter of the almond paste you need to cover the cake.) Lay the rolled paste over the cake, press gently around the sides, then trim the edges.

3 Warm the remaining glaze and lightly brush it over the paste. Roll the icing until it's about 10cm (4in) bigger than the top of the cake, then lay the icing over the cake. Lightly press down the icing onto the cake and turn the edges using a small sharp knife. (Don't worry if there are any gashes or notches in the icing – they can be smoothed out by buffing. To do this, roll the trimmings into a ball and use this to 'buff' the surface smooth by pressing.)

4 To make the decoration, take 18 plain chocolate thins and stick six together using a black icing pen, overlapping the edges slightly. Lay flat on the greaseproof paper. Repeat with the remaining chocolates to make three strips. Leave in a cool place to harden overnight.

5 Put three strips on top of the cake to form a triangular box, dust all over with the sieved cocoa and fill the box with truffles, chocolate nuts and gold dragees. Scatter edible gold balls over the cake and wrap gold crepe paper around it and secure with pins. Add a gold cord around the base and a gold ribbon around the middle. Keep in a cool place (not a fridge).

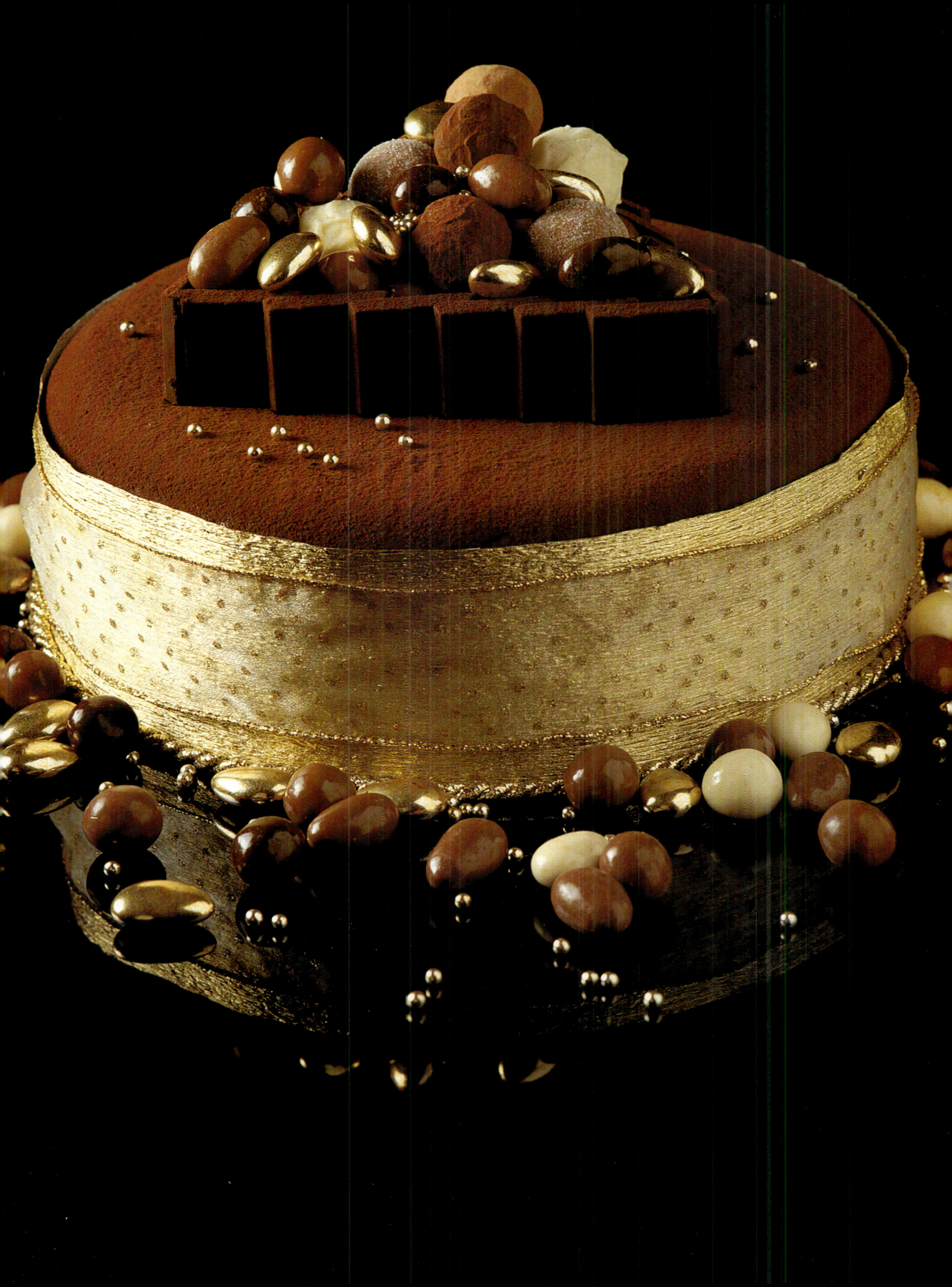

Chocolate and Chestnut Torte

Hands-on time: 1hr, plus 20min chilling, overnight freezing and 1hr freezing
Serves: 8–10

- **200g (7oz) bourbon or chocolate digestive biscuits**
- **50g (2oz) melted butter**
- **225g (8oz) milk chocolate**
- **250g tub mascarpone**
- **75g (3oz) unsweetened chestnut purée**
- **4 large eggs, separated**
- **50g (2oz) golden caster sugar**
- **142ml carton extra-thick double cream**

FOR THE DECORATION

- **175g (6oz) plain chocolate, plus extra for chocolate shavings**
- **White chocolate truffles**
- **Cocoa powder to dust**

1 Whiz the biscuits into fine crumbs in a food processor and mix in the butter. Press the mixture into a 20.5cm (8in) spring-release tin and chill for 20min or until firm.

2 Melt the milk chocolate in a small bowl over a pan of gently simmering water. In a large bowl, beat together the mascarpone cheese and the chestnut purée, then beat in the warm melted chocolate.

3 Using an electric whisk, beat the egg yolks with the caster sugar until pale and thick, then stir into the chestnut mixture using a metal spoon. Fold in the cream.

4 Whip the egg whites until soft peaks form and stir one large spoonful into the chocolate mixture. Fold in the remainder using a large, metal spoon. Pour onto the biscuit base. Wrap in clingfilm and freeze overnight.

5 To decorate the torte, cut two strips of non-stick baking parchment, each 35.5cm (14in) long and 5cm (2in) wide. Melt the plain chocolate in a small bowl over a pan of gently simmering water and spread evenly along the parchment strips.

6 Take the torte out of the freezer, run a palette knife around the outside, then unclip and remove the spring-release tin. Carefully wrap the chocolate-covered strips (with the chocolate side facing inwards) around the torte and return the torte to the freezer for about 1hr.

7 Peel away the parchment strips to leave a thin chocolate 'collar' around the torte, then put in the fridge to thaw overnight. Remove from the fridge, arrange the white chocolate truffles on top around the edge, then dust generously with cocoa powder and grate over some of the extra plain chocolate just before serving.

To freeze: After step 6, over-wrap the frozen torte with clingfilm and put back in the freezer.
To use: Thaw overnight in the fridge and then decorate as above before serving.

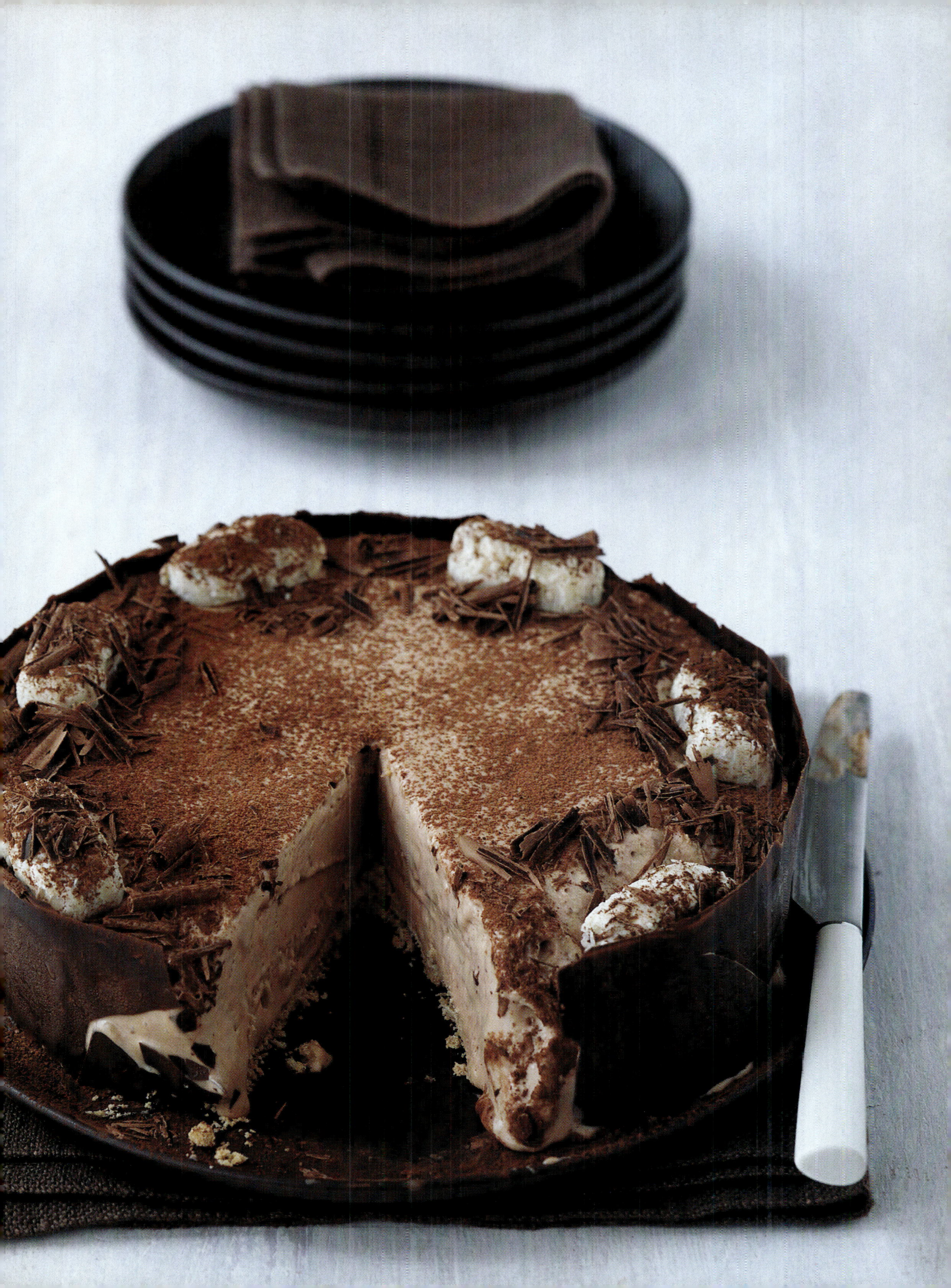

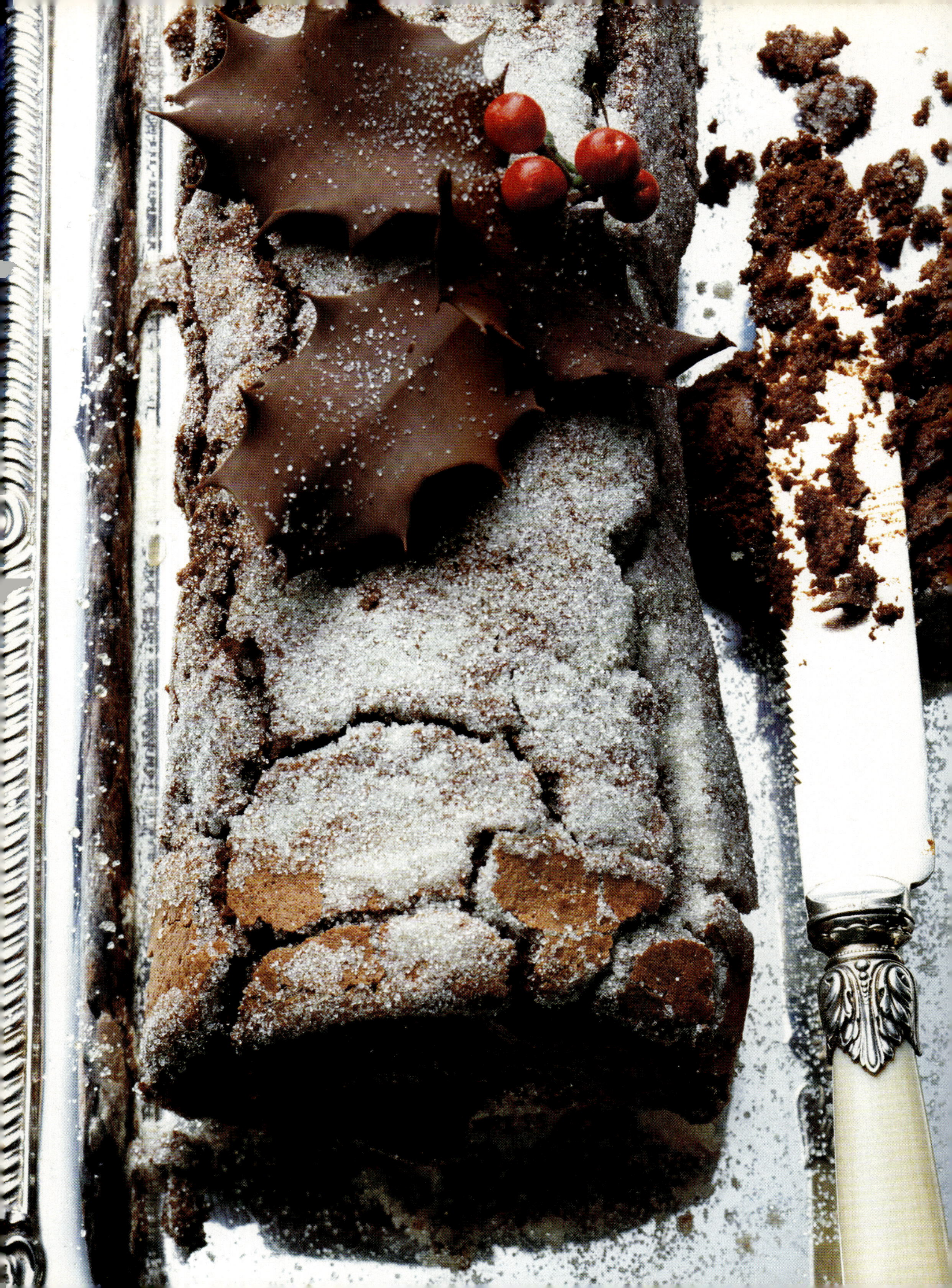

Classic Chocolate Roulade

Hands-on time: 20min, plus 10min cooling and 2hr chilling
Cooking time: 25min
Serves: 8

* Butter for greasing
* 175g (6oz) good quality plain chocolate, with at least 52% cocoa solids
* 6 large eggs, separated
* 175g (6oz) golden caster sugar, plus extra to dust

For the filling

* 250g tub mascarpone
* 2tbsp crème de cacao
* 2tbsp cocoa powder
* 25g (1oz) golden icing sugar

For the decoration

* 75g (3oz) plain chocolate cake covering
* 2–3 holly leaves, washed and patted dry with kitchen paper
* A few fake red berries

1 Grease and baseline a 28x38cm (11x15in) Swiss roll tin with baking parchment. Break up the chocolate and put in a bowl over a pan of simmering water until just melted. Set aside. Preheat the oven to 180°C (160°C fan) mark 4.

2 Put the egg yolks in the bowl of a freestanding mixer with the caster sugar and whisk until pale and thick. Whisk in the melted chocolate until blended.

3 In a clean, grease-free bowl, whisk the egg whites until they form soft peaks. Stir a quarter into the chocolate mixture, then fold in the remainder with a metal spoon. Pour into the prepared tin.

4 Bake the roulade for 25min or until risen – the sponge should spring back slightly when lightly pressed. Cool for 10min, then cover the tin with a clean damp cloth. Once cool, cover with clingfilm and chill for at least 2hr or overnight.

5 To make the filling, put the mascarpone, crème de cacao, cocoa powder and icing sugar into a bowl. Beat until smooth, then set aside.

6 Dust a large sheet of greaseproof paper with plenty of caster sugar and carefully turn out the roulade. Peel away the lining paper, then trim off the short ends. Spread over the mascarpone mixture and roll up tightly from a long side, using the greaseproof paper to help.

7 To decorate the roulade, break up the cake covering and melt as for step 1 – this chocolate has a thinner consistency, so it's better for dipping the leaves. Dip one side of each leaf in the chocolate, then leave to set. Once set, peel off the chocolate leaves and use to decorate the roulade with the berries.

To freeze: Complete the recipe to the end of step 6. Open-freeze until solid, then wrap in clingfilm, put in the freezer and store for up to one month. Make sure you don't put anything on top of the roulade so it doesn't get damaged.
To use: Thaw overnight at room temperature and then complete the recipe.

Traditional Christmas Stollen

Hands-on time: 30min, plus 2hr rising and 1hr proving
Cooking time: 35–45min
Makes: 2 loaves of 12 slices each

- **75g (3oz) fresh yeast, crumbled, or 40g (1½oz) dried yeast**
- **700g (1½lb) plain flour, warmed in the microwave for 2min on defrost**
- **½tsp ground coriander**
- **¼tsp ground nutmeg**
- **100g (3½oz) caster sugar**
- **2 medium eggs, beaten**
- **250g pack butter, softened**
- **300g (11oz) raisins**
- **125g (4oz) currants**
- **150g (5oz) mixed candied peel, finely chopped**
- **4tbsp rum**
- **Zest of 1 large lemon**
- **150g (5oz) blanched almonds, roughly chopped**
- **250g pack white marzipan**
- **250g pack unsalted butter, melted, to brush**
- **50g (2oz) icing sugar to dust**

1 Mix together the yeast and 150ml (¼ pint) warm water. Put the flour and spices into a bowl, make a well, pour in the yeast mixture and sprinkle with a little flour from the sides. Leave for 15min or until the yeast bubbles. Mix the sugar and eggs in a bowl, then pour into the flour. Add the butter.

2 Mix everything together until a rough dough forms. Turn out onto a floured surface and knead for about 5min until smooth. Put into a lightly oiled bowl, cover with clingfilm and a clean tea-towel and leave in a warm place for about 2hr or until doubled in size.

3 Put the raisins, currants and mixed peel in a bowl and add the rum. Cover and set aside. Turn the dough out onto a lightly floured surface and stretch into a rough rectangle measuring about 25.5x35.5cm (10x14in).

4 Tip the fruit into the middle, add the lemon zest, almonds and 1tsp salt, then knead until the fruit and nuts are incorporated. Cut the dough in half. Halve the marzipan and roll each piece into a sausage measuring 25.5cm (10in).

5 Shape the dough into two ovals about 30.5cm (12in) long. Press a rolling pin lengthways down the middle of each to make a trough and put the marzipan into each trough. Fold the dough over the marzipan, put on a baking sheet, then cover with clingfilm and a clean tea-towel. Leave for 1hr.

6 Preheat the oven to 180°C (160°C fan) mark 4 and bake for 35–45min or until the loaves sound hollow when tapped on the base. Cool for 15min, then brush with the melted butter, using it all up – this gives the bread a richer texture and helps keep it fresh for longer. Dust generously with icing sugar just before serving. The Stollen will keep in an airtight container for one to two weeks – be sure to point this out if you are giving the second one as a gift.

To freeze ahead: Complete the recipe except for dusting with the icing sugar. Wrap in clingfilm, put in a freezer bag, secure and freeze.
To use: Thaw at cool room temperature overnight and dust with icing sugar.

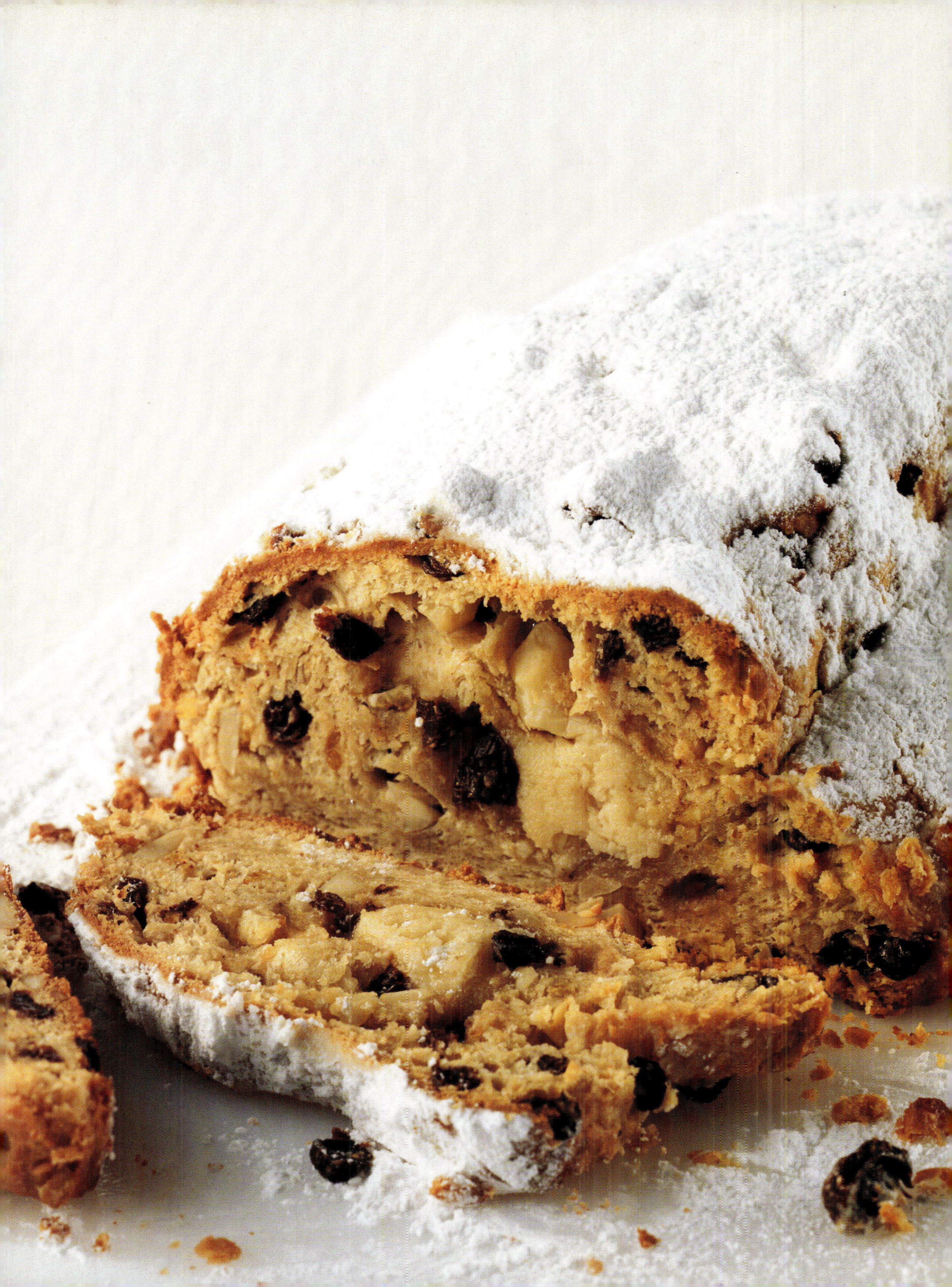

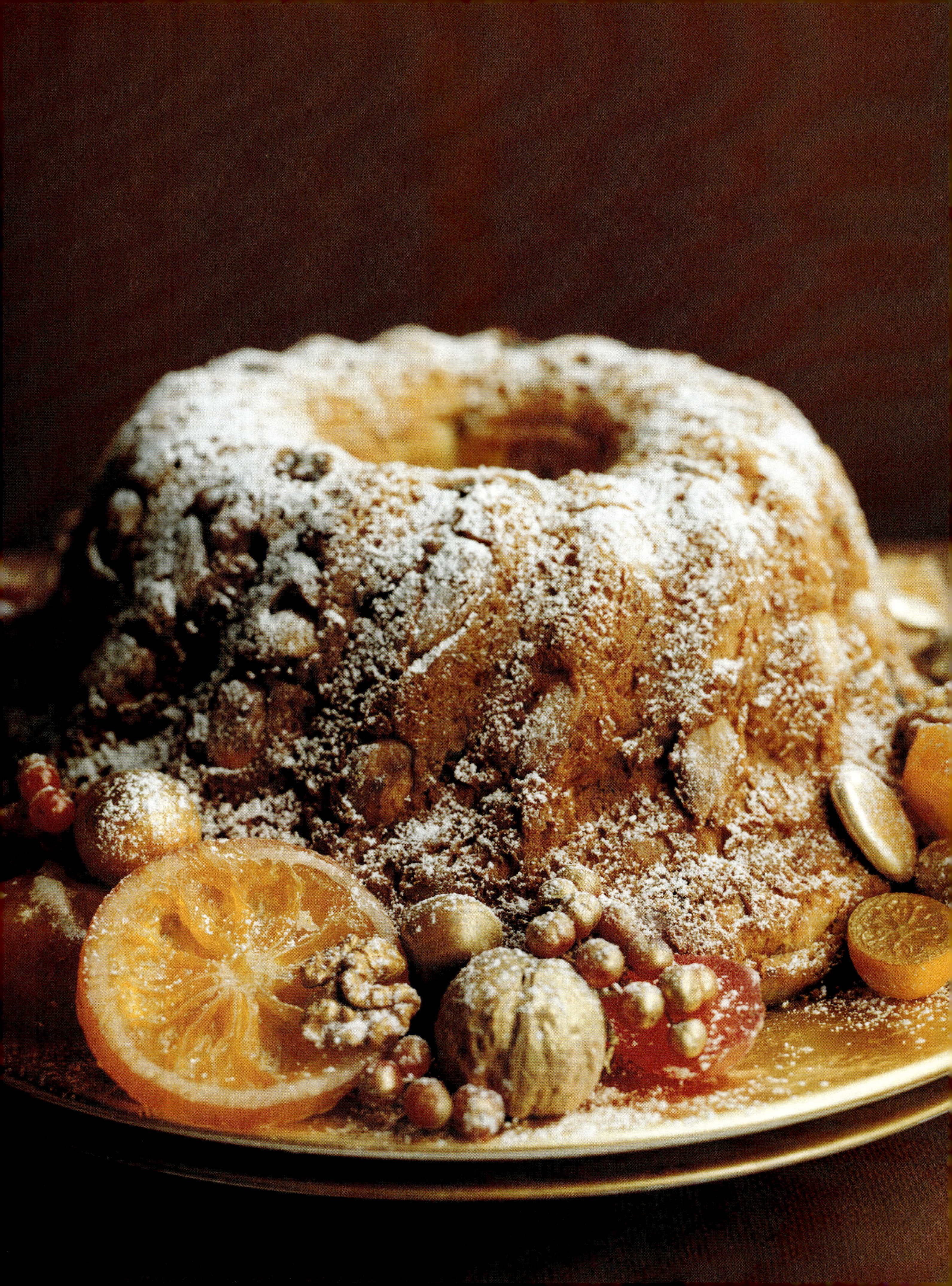

Kugelhopf

Hands-on time: 45min, plus overnight chilling and rising for about 3hr
Cooking time: 50–55min
Serves: 12–14

- 200g (7oz) raisins, preferably black seedless
- 3tbsp light rum
- 2tsp easy-blend yeast
- 300g (11oz) plain white flour
- 4 large eggs
- 100ml (3½fl oz) milk
- 225g (8oz) unsalted butter, softened, plus extra for greasing
- 75g (3oz) caster sugar
- Zest of 1 lemon
- Flour to dust
- 100g (3½oz) split blanched almonds
- Icing sugar to dust
- Whole glacé fruits, nuts and dragées (use gold, silver or a mix of both) to decorate

1 Place the raisins in a small bowl, pour over the rum, cover and leave in a cool place overnight. Place the yeast in a food mixer with the flour. Whisk the eggs and milk together lightly. With the machine running on a slow speed, pour in the egg mixture and mix for about 10min or until the dough is very smooth, shiny and elastic. (If you don't have a beater attachment, use a food processor with a flat plastic blade.)

2 Put the butter in a bowl and beat in the caster sugar, a pinch of salt and lemon zest. With the machine running, add the butter and sugar mixture to the dough, spoonful by spoonful, until evenly incorporated. Turn the mixture into a large, lightly floured bowl, then cover with clingfilm and chill overnight.

3 Lightly toast the almonds. Generously butter a 2 litre (3½ pint) Kugelhopf ring mould. Take a third of the almonds and press onto the sides of the mould. If they won't stay in place, use a little soft butter on each nut to help them stick. Chill. Roughly chop the remaining almonds and mix by hand into the chilled dough, along with the raisins and rum. Carefully place the dough in the prepared mould, then cover and leave for about 3hr in a warm, draught-free place until it feels spongy and has risen to within 2cm (¾in) of the top of the mould.

4 Bake at 200°C (180°C fan) mark 6 on a shelf below the centre of the oven for 10min. Cover with greaseproof paper, turn the oven down to 190°C (170°C fan) mark 5 and bake for 40–45min or until the Kugelhopf sounds hollow when you tap the mould.

5 Allow to cool in the tin for 15min, then turn onto a wire rack to cool completely. Serve dusted with icing sugar and decorated with glacé fruits, nuts and dragées. This cake is made with yeast, so it's best eaten within two days or it will go stale. Wrap and freeze in slices if you have any left over – it's delicious toasted or used for making a special bread and butter pudding.

Gingerbread House

Hands-on time: 4hr, plus 30min chilling and 5hr drying
Cooking time: around 10min
Makes: 4 houses

For the gingerbread

* **350g (12oz) plain white flour, sifted, plus extra to dust**
* **1tsp bicarbonate of soda**
* **2tbsp ground ginger**
* **150g (5oz) butter, plus extra to grease**
* **200g (7oz) light muscovado sugar**
* **2tbsp golden syrup**
* **1 medium egg, beaten**

For the icing and filling

* **1 medium egg white**
* **200g (7oz) icing sugar, sifted, plus extra to dust**
* **75g (3oz) assorted sweets, such as jelly beans, jelly babies, and dolly mixtures**

For the templates (see over)

* **Tracing paper and card – roof pieces 6.5x8cm (2.5x3in); end walls 10x6cm (4x2in); side walls 6x8cm (2x3in)**

For the cake boards

* **4x15cm (6in) cardboard rounds, covered in brown paper**
* **Cellophane and ribbon to wrap**

1 Preheat the oven to 190°C (170°C fan) mark 5. Using the tracing paper, trace the templates pictured overleaf, then cut out of the card.

2 Put the flour, bicarbonate of soda and ginger into a large bowl. Rub in the butter until the mixture resembles fine breadcrumbs, then stir in the sugar.

3 Warm the syrup slightly in a pan, then pour onto the flour mixture, along with the beaten egg, and stir. Bring together with your hands to form a soft dough and knead until smooth. Divide into four pieces, wrap in clingfilm and chill for 15min.

4 On a lightly floured surface, roll out one piece of dough to 3mm (1/8in) thick. Using the templates, cut out two of each, re-rolling the dough as necessary. Put on greased baking sheets and straighten the edges with a palette knife. Do the same with the rest of the dough.

5 Re-roll the trimmings and stamp out four hearts for gift tags. Skewer a hole in the top of each heart, then place on the baking sheets. Chill for 15min.

6 Bake for 8–10min until golden. While the gingerbread is still warm, push a skewer through the holes in the gift tags again. Leave the gingerbread on the trays for 5min, then transfer to a wire rack to cool completely.

7 For the icing, put the egg white into a bowl and gradually beat in the icing sugar until the mixture stands up in peaks. Spoon into a piping bag fitted with a tiny plain nozzle and pipe lines to mark the windows and doors on the side and end walls, and squiggly lines on the roof pieces. Leave to dry for 2hr.

Continued over page

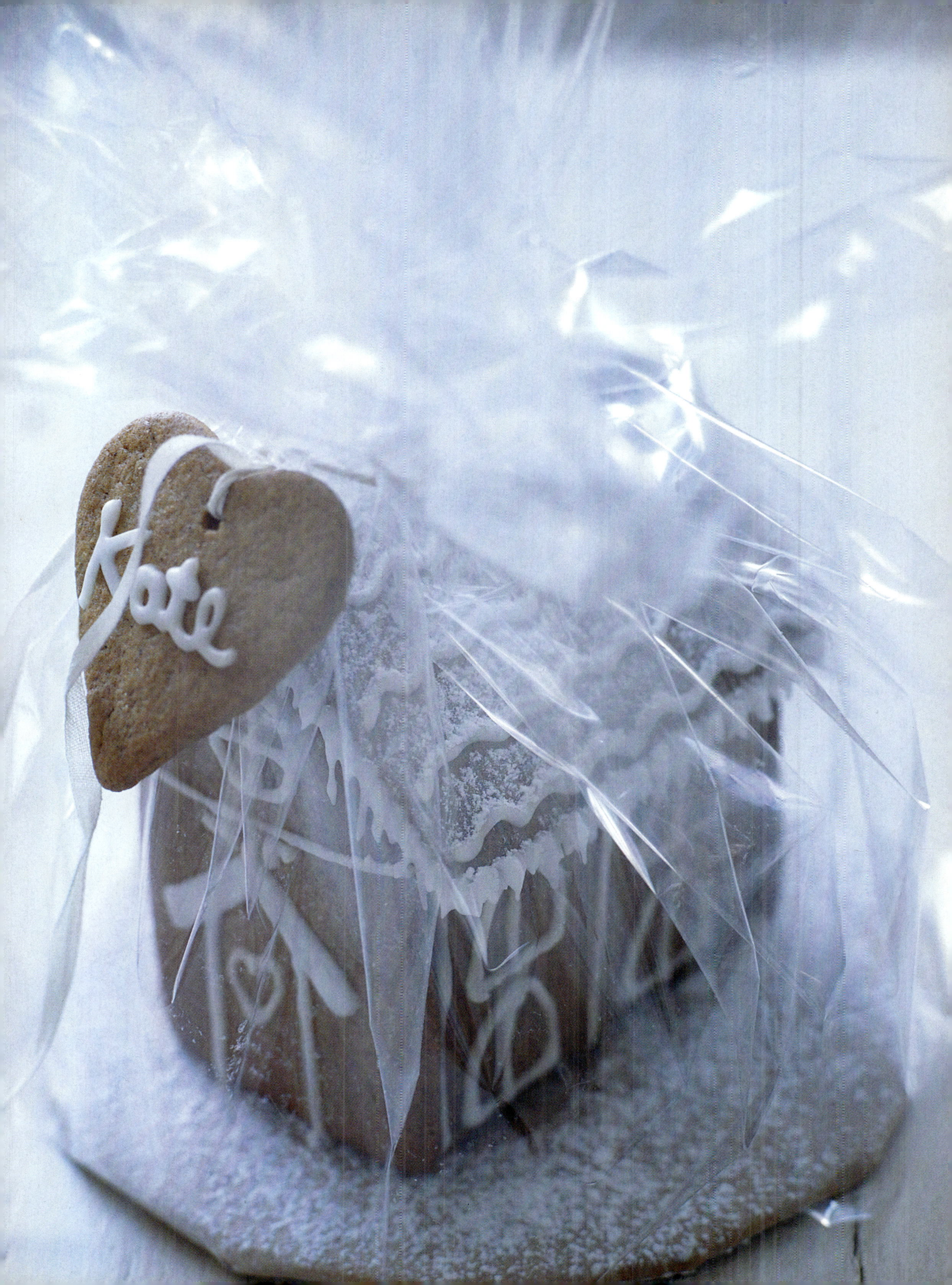
Kate

8 To assemble the houses, pipe a thin line of icing along the short edges of the side walls and stick together with the end walls to form an open-topped box. Leave to dry for 1hr. Put one house on each of the paper-covered cake boards, then fill with sweets. Pipe icing along the top edges of the house and roof pieces. Press the roof pieces gently into position (the roof should overhang slightly) and hold for 1–2min until you feel they're secure, then leave to set for about 2hr. Use the remaining icing to pipe names onto the gift tag hearts. Store in an airtight container until ready to wrap.

9 Lightly dust each house with icing sugar, then put each one in the middle of a piece of cellophane, gather up the corners and tie with ribbon. Thread ribbon through the holes in the gift tags and tie.

To freeze ahead: Complete the recipe up to step 5. Wrap and freeze the gingerbread, on the baking sheets, for up to two months. **To use:** Thaw at cool room temperature for 30min and complete the recipe. Eat within five days.

SIDE WALL

END WALL

ROOF

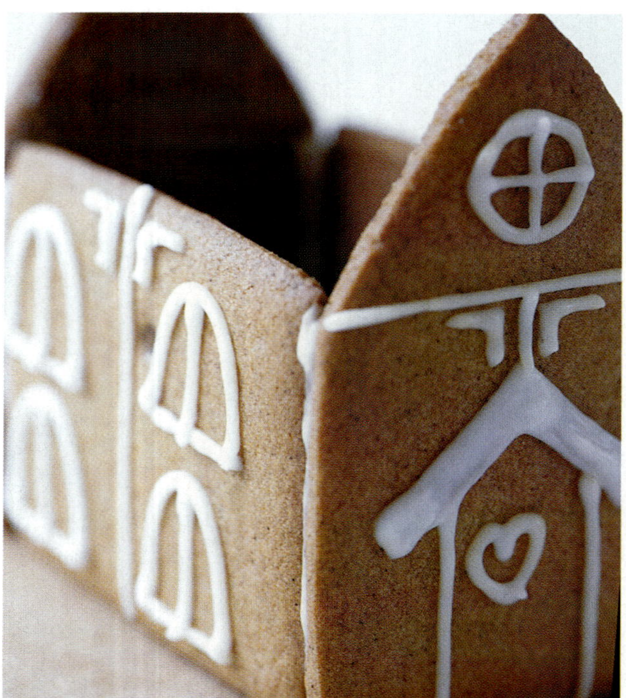

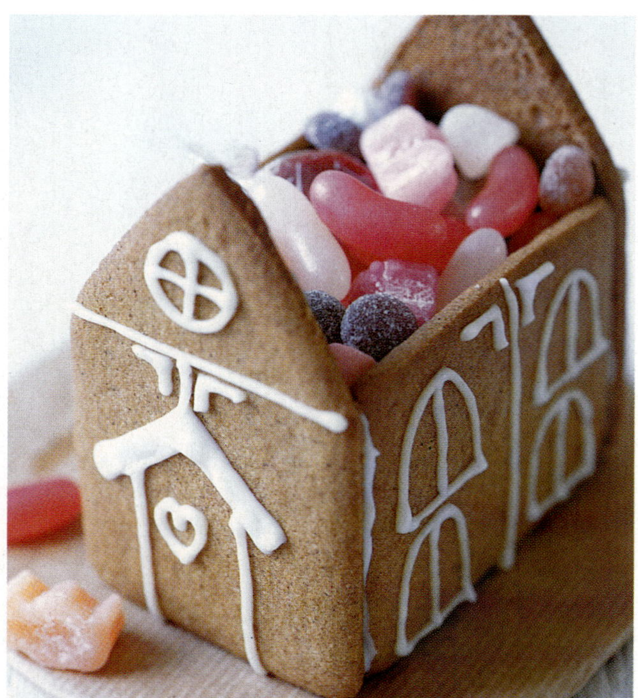

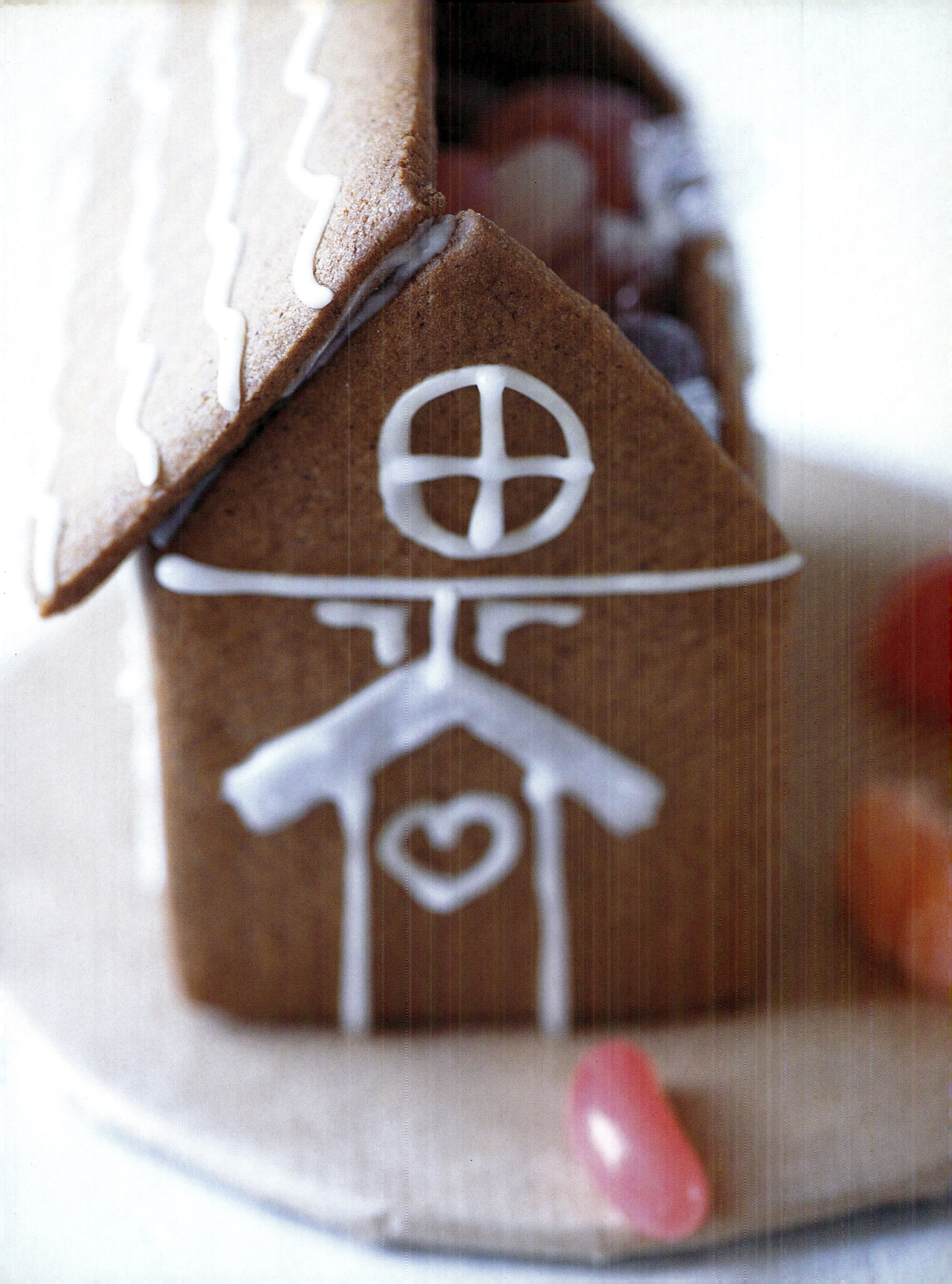

Snowball Truffles

Hands-on time: 20min, plus chilling
Cooking time: 5min
Makes: 25 truffles

- **175g (6oz) plain chocolate (about 50% cocoa solids is best; any higher and the truffles may taste bitter)**
- **150ml (5fl oz) extra-thick double cream**
- **25g (1oz) unsalted butter**
- **2tbsp Baileys Irish Cream, Grand Marnier or brandy**
- **1tbsp crème fraîche**
- **40g (1½oz) icing sugar**
- **Petit four paper cases**

1 Break the chocolate into pieces and put in the bowl of a food processor. Whiz for about 30sec or until the chocolate is very finely chopped.

2 Put the cream, butter and liqueur into a small pan and bring to the boil. Switch on the processor and, with the motor still running, add the hot cream mixture to the chopped chocolate. Blend until evenly mixed.

3 Spoon the chocolate mixture into a bowl and stir in the crème fraîche. Cool, cover with clingfilm and leave in the fridge overnight to thicken.

4 Arrange the petit four cases on a tray. Sieve the icing sugar onto a baking sheet lined with foil or greaseproof paper. Drop teaspoonfuls of the chocolate mixture onto the icing sugar and roll to cover. Use two forks to lift them and drop them carefully into the paper cases – to get the pretty pink lining, turn the cases inside out.

5 To gift wrap, pack each truffle in its paper case into a decorative box. Tie a pretty ribbon around the lid and cover the box. Label with storage instructions and an eat-by date. The truffles can be kept in the fridge in an airtight container for up to one week.

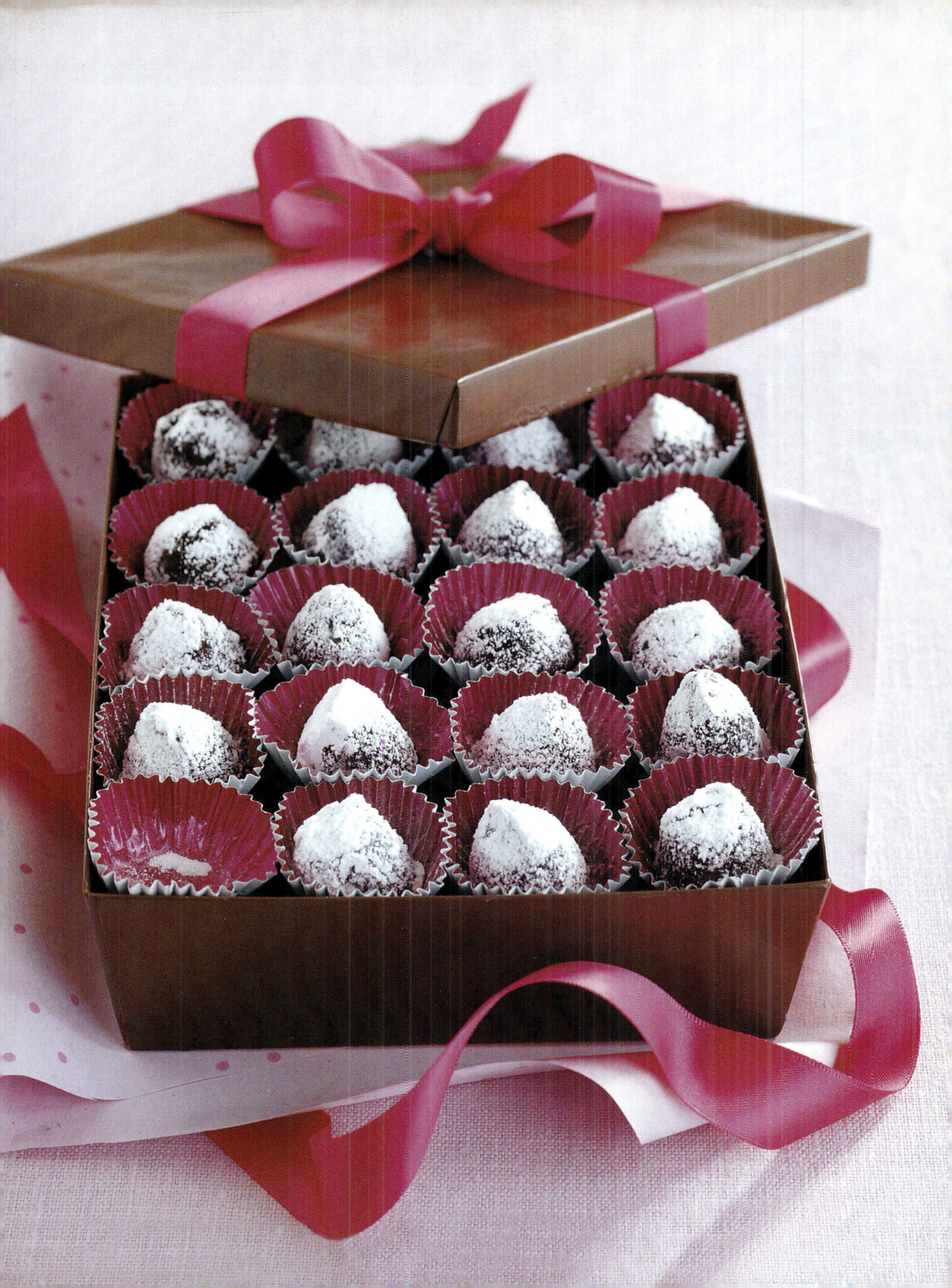

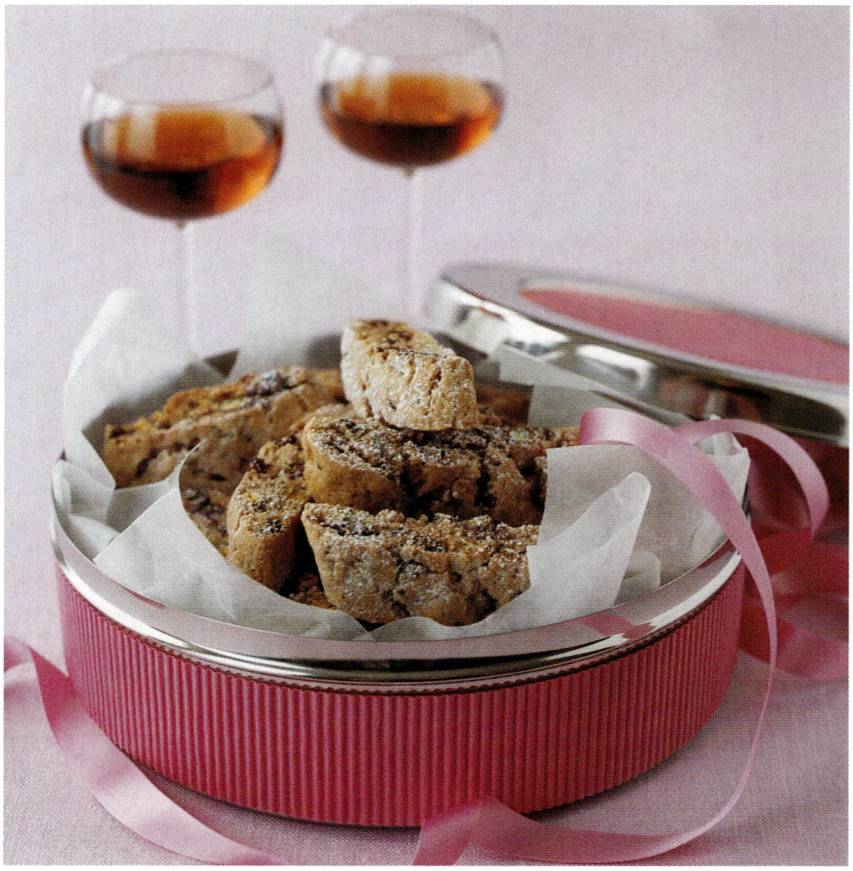

Chocolate and Pistachio Biscotti

Hands-on time: 15min
Cooking time: 1hr 10min
Makes: 30 biscuits, enough to fill two medium-sized biscuit tins

- **300g (11oz) plain flour**
- **75g (3oz) cocoa powder**
- **1tsp baking powder**
- **150g (5oz) plain chocolate chips**
- **150g (5oz) shelled pistachio nuts**
- **75g (3oz) unsalted butter, softened**
- **225g (8oz) granulated sugar**
- **2 large eggs, beaten**
- **1tbsp icing sugar**

1 Preheat the oven to 180°C (160°C fan) mark 4. Line a large baking sheet with non-stick baking parchment.

2 Mix together the flour, cocoa powder, baking powder, chocolate chips, pistachio nuts and 1tsp salt.

3 Using an electric whisk, beat together the softened butter and sugar until light and fluffy. Gradually whisk in the beaten eggs.

4 Stir the dry ingredients into the mixture until it forms a stiff dough. With floured hands, shape the dough into two slightly flattened logs, each about 30.5x5cm (12x2in). Sprinkle with icing sugar.

5 Bake the logs for 40–45min or until they are slightly firm to the touch. Cool on the baking sheet for 10min, then cut diagonally into 2cm (¾in) thick slices. Arrange them, cut side down, on the baking sheet and bake again for 15min or until crisp. Cool on a wire rack.

6 To gift wrap, line a pretty airtight tin with some greaseproof paper and put the biscotti inside. Decorate the outside with coloured paper, then tie with a ribbon and label with an eat-by date. The biscotti can be kept in an airtight container for up to one week, or in the freezer for up to one month.

Shortbread Biscuits

Hands-on time: 15min, plus 30min chilling
Cooking time: 15min
Makes: 12 biscuits

- 175g (6oz) unsalted butter, softened, plus extra for greasing
- 75g (3oz) golden caster sugar
- 200g (7oz) plain flour, sieved
- 50g (2oz) cornflour
- White caster sugar to sprinkle

1 Cut the softened butter into pieces and whiz in a food processor with the sugar for 1min until pale and fluffy. Add the flours and whiz until the mixture just comes together. Wrap and chill for 30min. Heat the oven to 190°C (170°C fan) mark 5.

2 On a lightly floured surface, roll out the dough until it's 1cm (½in) thick. Cut 12 x 7cm (2¾in) rounds with a fluted cutter and put onto a greased baking sheet. Gently press a 4cm (1½in) plain cutter into the centre of each and prick with a fork.

3 Bake for 15min or until pale golden. Sprinkle with the caster sugar and cool on a wire rack.

4 To gift wrap, line two oval wooden boxes with greaseproof paper and put six biscuits in each. Tie with ribbon and label with an eat-by date. The shortbread can be kept in an airtight container for up to five days.

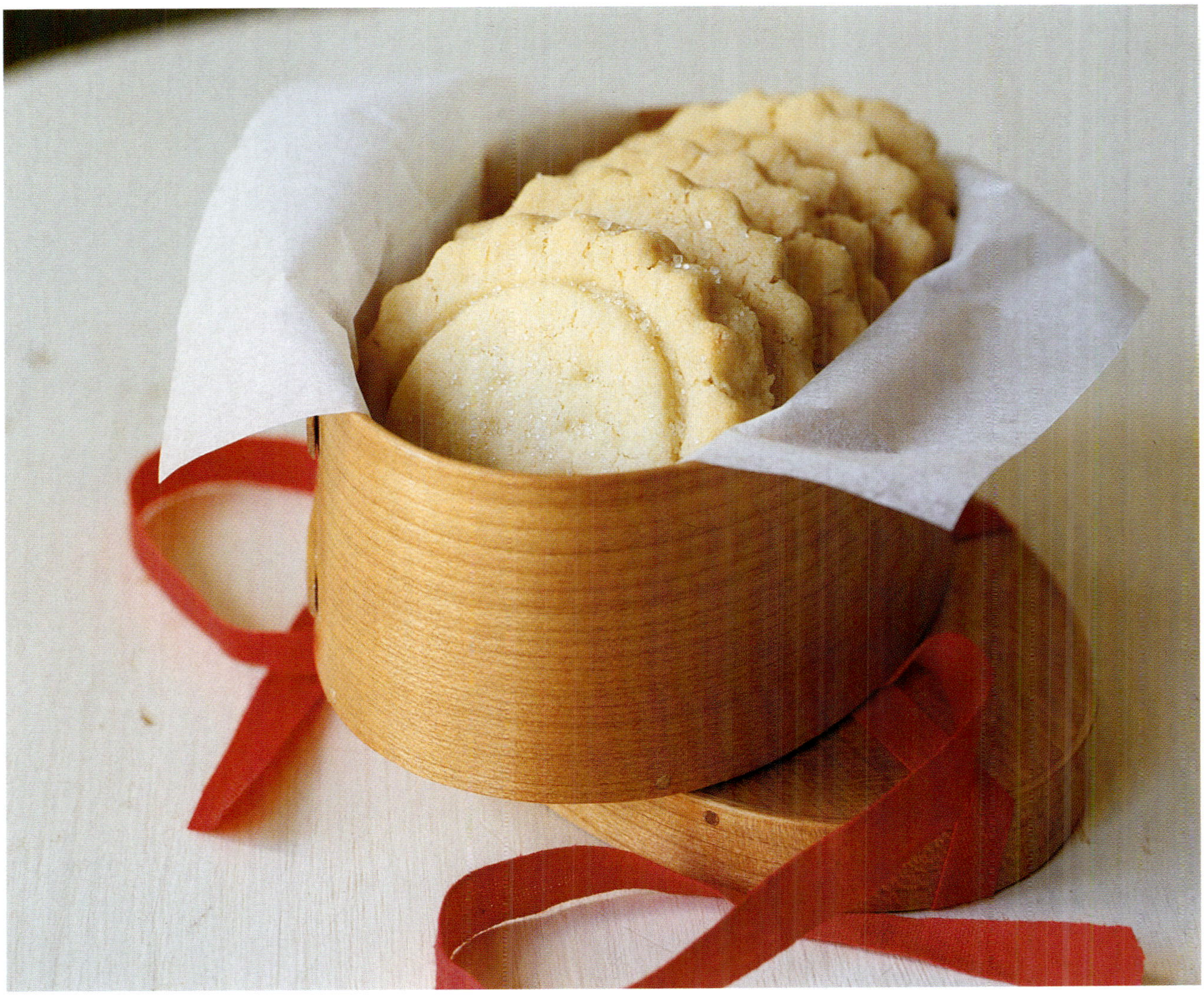

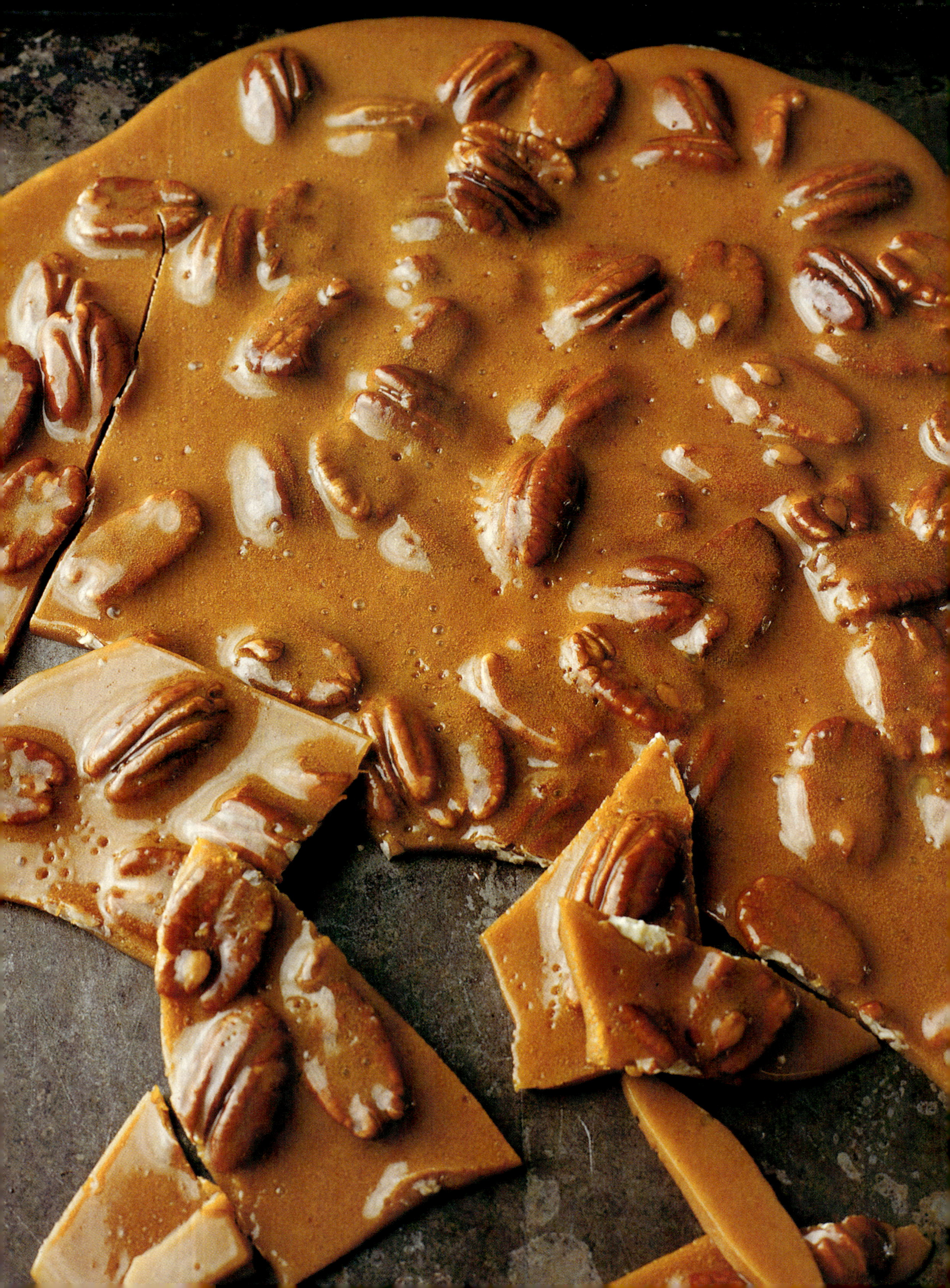

Pecan Pralines

Hands-on time: 10min
Cooking time: 15min
Makes: 4 gift packs

* 200g (7oz) granulated sugar
* 125ml (4fl oz) golden syrup
* 150g (5oz) pecan halves
* ½tsp vanilla extract
* 50g (2oz) unsalted butter, plus extra for greasing
* ¾tsp bicarbonate of soda
* A sugar thermometer

1 Lightly grease a large baking sheet. Put the granulated sugar and golden syrup into a large, heavy-based pan and heat gently, stirring constantly until the sugar dissolves in the syrup.

2 Once dissolved, increase the heat so the mixture boils and reaches a temperature of 110°C on the sugar thermometer.

3 Add the pecan halves to the pan and continue to cook, stirring to coat all the nuts with the syrup, until the mixture reaches 150°C.

4 Remove the pan from the heat and stir in the vanilla extract, butter, bicarbonate of soda and a pinch of salt until everything is thoroughly combined. Tip the mixture onto the prepared baking sheet spreading it thinly. Set aside until completely cooled and hardened, then break into pieces.

5 To gift-wrap, divide the praline into four piles and put each on a piece of cellophane measuring 20.5x20.5cm (8x8in). Gather up the corners and tie with a pretty ribbon to secure, attaching a label with an eat-by date. The pralines can be stored in an airtight container, layered between baking parchment, for up to 10 days.

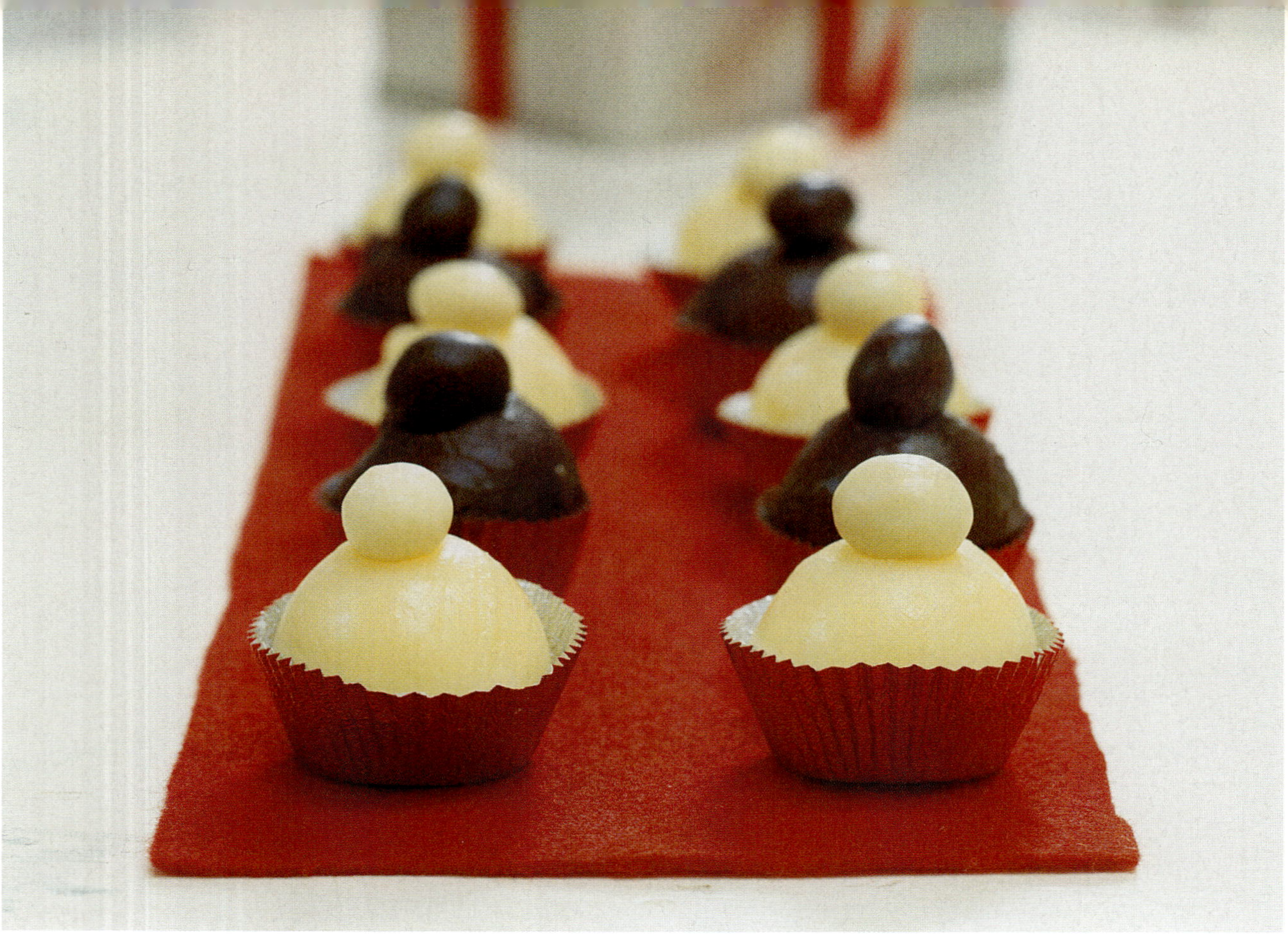

Mocha Truffles

Hands-on time: 50min, plus 2½hr cooling
Cooking time: 2min
Makes: 12 dark and 12 white truffles

- 200g (7oz) plain chocolate, at least 50% cocoa solids
- 142ml carton thick double cream
- 25g (1oz) unsalted butter
- 1tbsp Tia Maria
- 1tbsp Baileys Irish Cream
- 24 chocolate-coated coffee beans

FOR THE COATING

- 200g (7oz) plain chocolate
- 200g (7oz) white chocolate cake covering
- Petit four paper cases

1 Put the chocolate for the truffles into a bowl and set over a pan of barely simmering water to melt. Meanwhile, put the cream into a separate pan and bring just to the boil, then remove from the heat.

2 Remove the melted chocolate from the heat and beat in the butter until smooth. Add the cream and beat again until smooth. Divide the truffle mixture between two bowls. Add the Tia Maria to one bowl and the Baileys to the other, and stir. Transfer to separate shallow containers and chill for at least 2hr until firm.

3 Taking one batch of the mixture, scoop out spoonfuls with two spoons, then quickly roll into 12 balls between your hands. Put onto a baking tray, press a coffee bean into the top of each and return to the fridge until firm. Repeat with the remaining mixture.

4 In two separate bowls, melt the plain chocolate and the white chocolate cake covering as before. Put aside until just cool. Dip the Tia Maria truffles into the plain chocolate and the Baileys truffles into the white chocolate. Leave to set.

5 To gift wrap, put each truffle in a paper case and pack into decorative boxes. Tie with a pretty ribbon and label with storage instructions and an eat-by date. The truffles can be kept in the fridge in an airtight container for up to two weeks.

Tiffin

Hands-on time: 40min, plus cooling and overnight chilling
Makes: 8 pieces

* 50g (2oz) raisins
* 75g (3oz) dates, chopped
* 4tbsp brandy
* 200g bar plain chocolate
* 150g (5oz) butter
* 3tbsp golden syrup
* 250g (9oz) digestive biscuits, roughly crushed
* Zest of ½ large orange

FOR THE TOPPING

* 150g (5oz) dark chocolate, at least 70% cocoa solids

1 Grease and baseline a 20.5cm (8in) round tin with a depth of 4cm (½in).

2 Put the raisins, chopped dates and brandy in a bowl and leave to soak for 30min.

3 Melt the dark chocolate, 125g (4oz) butter and golden syrup in a pan over a gentle heat.

4 Add the biscuits, orange zest, raisins, dates and any remaining brandy. Mix well, pour into the tin, cool and chill for 1hr.

5 To make the topping, melt the dark chocolate in a pan with the remaining butter. Pour over the biscuit layer. Chill overnight.

6 To gift wrap, cut into wedges and pack into decorative boxes. The cake can be kept in the fridge in an airtight container for five days.

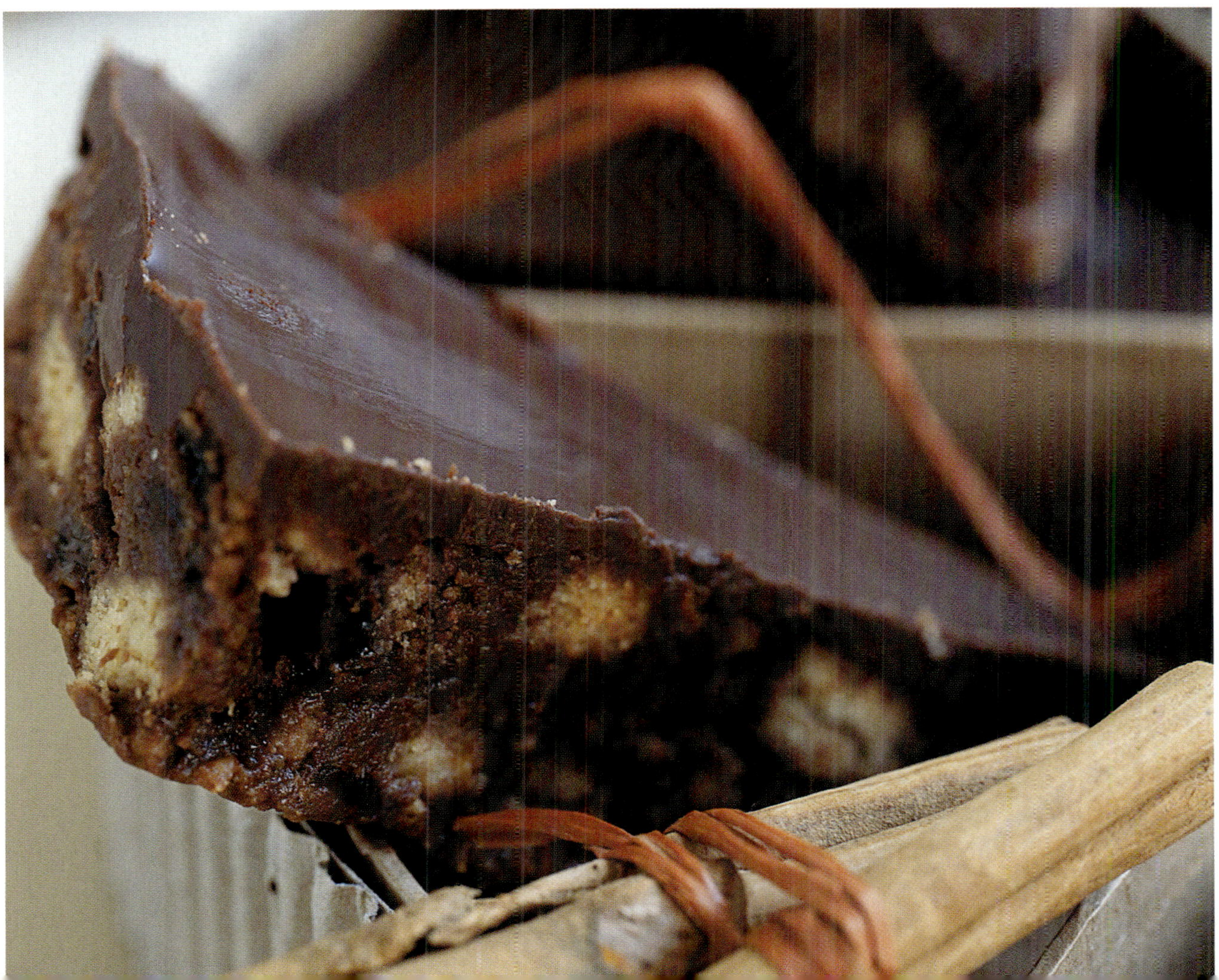

Cookies and Cream Fudge

Hands-on time: 10min, plus overnight chilling
Cooking time: 15min
Makes: 36 pieces

- A little sunflower oil for greasing
- 125g (4oz) unsalted butter
- 200ml (7fl oz) evaporated milk
- 450g (1lb) golden caster sugar
- 1tsp vanilla extract
- 75g (3oz) plain chocolate, chopped
- 25g (1oz) hazelnuts, toasted and roughly chopped
- 6 Oreo cookies or bourbon biscuits, roughly chopped

1 Lightly grease a 450g (1lb) loaf tin with a little sunflower oil. Put the butter, evaporated milk, caster sugar, vanilla extract and 50ml (2fl oz) water in a large solid-based pan, set over a low heat and stir constantly until the butter has melted and the sugar has dissolved.

2 Increase the heat to a gentle boil and continue to cook until the fudge forms a soft ball when half a teaspoonful is dropped into a cup of cold water – this will take about 10min – stirring all the time.

3 Remove the pan from the heat and, working quickly, divide the fudge mixture between two bowls. Add the chocolate to one of the bowls and allow it to melt into the fudge. Stir the mixture gently until smooth.

4 Pour half the chocolate fudge into the tin and smooth the surface, then scatter over half the hazelnuts and half the biscuits. Pour the vanilla fudge into the tin on top of the nuts and biscuits, then top with the remaining nuts and biscuits. Finish with a final layer of the chocolate fudge. Set aside to cool.

5 Cover with clingfilm and leave in the fridge overnight to set firm. Once set, remove the fudge from the loaf tin and cut into slices, then chop up each slice to make 36 pieces in total.

6 To gift wrap, place small piles of the fudge in clear cellophane and tie with a pretty ribbon, then attach a label to each parcel with an eat-by date and a note to store the fudge in the fridge. The fudge must be eaten within two weeks of being made.

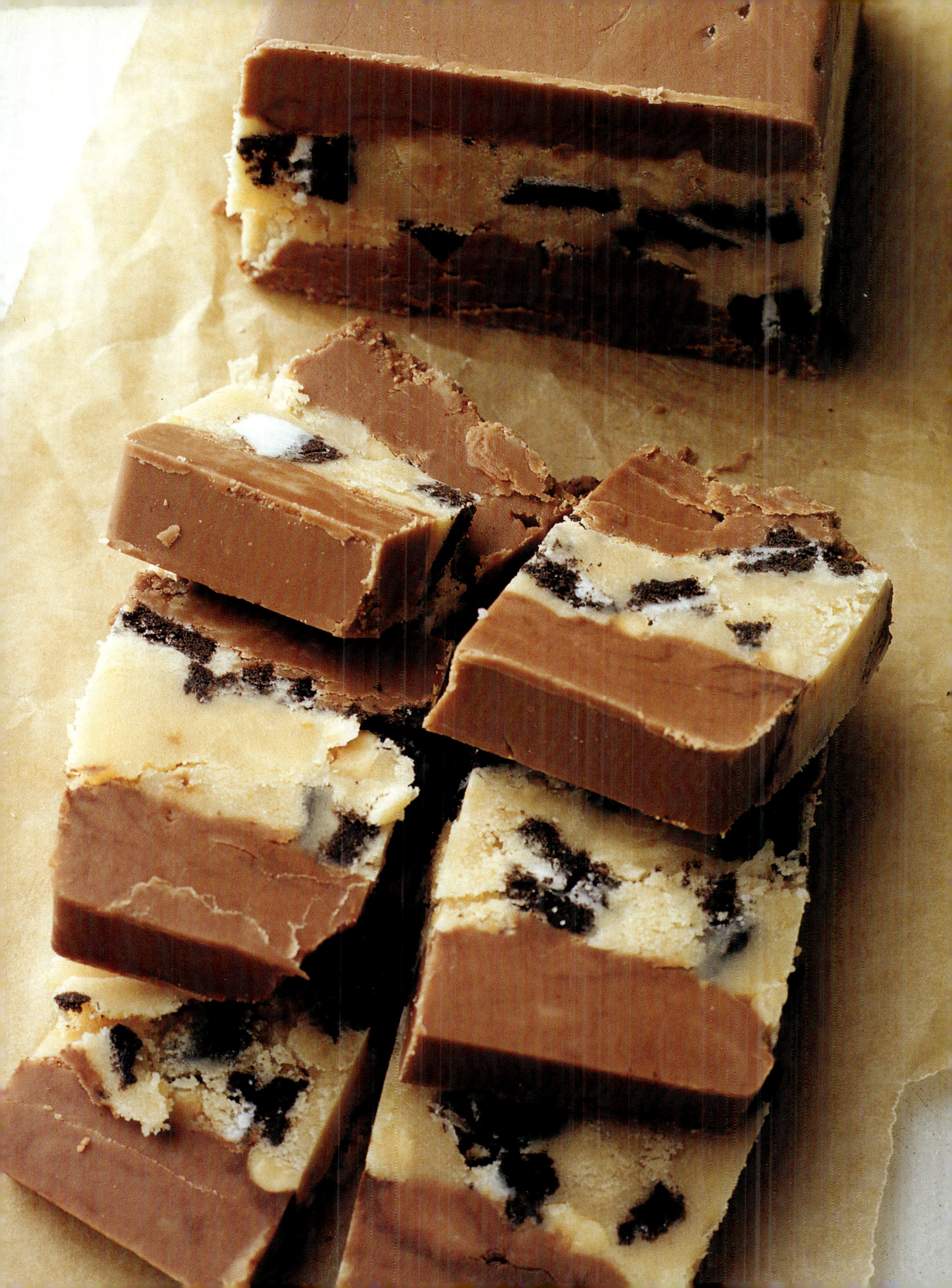

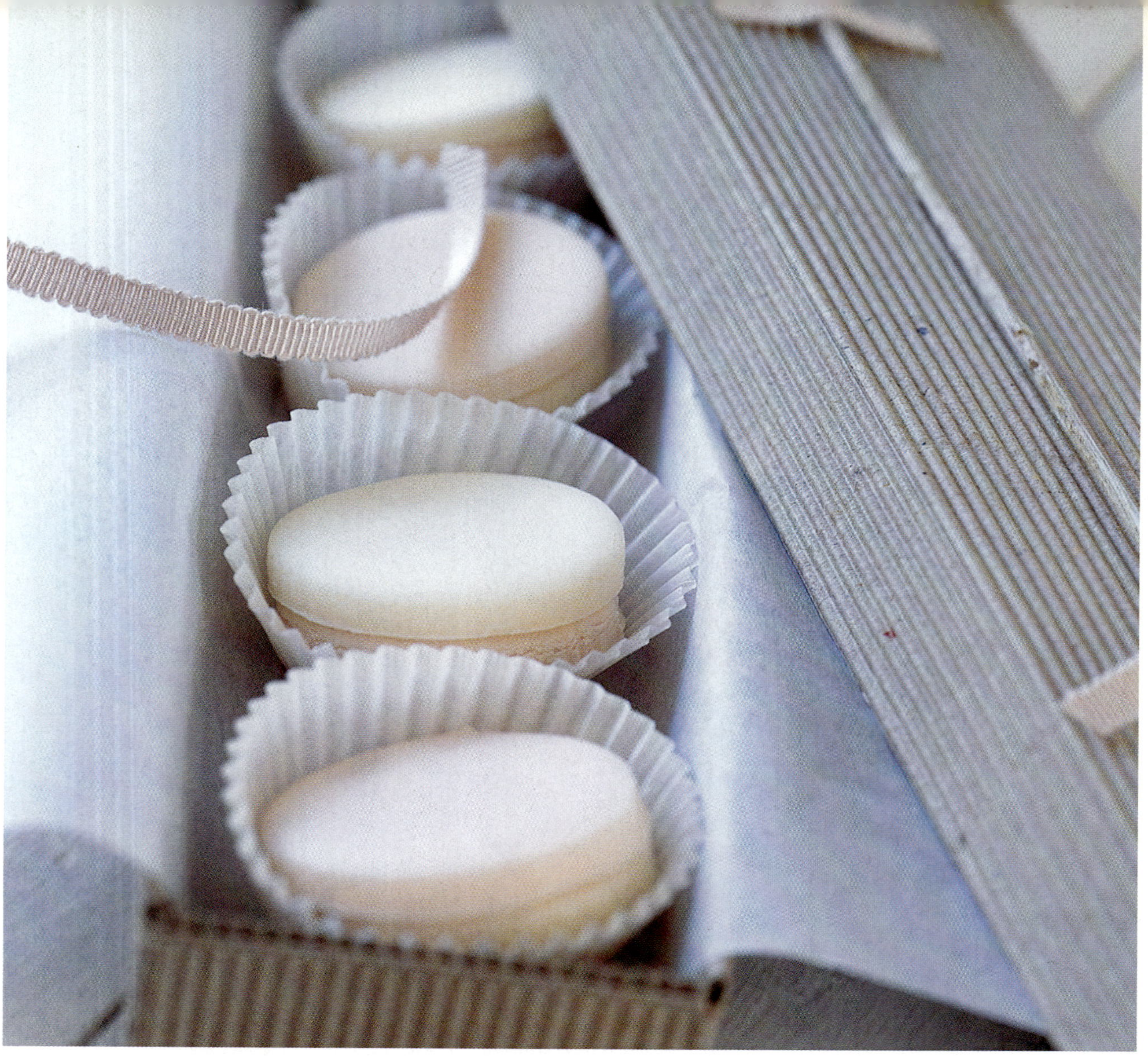

Peppermint Creams

Hands-on time: 45min
Makes: 50 mints

* **450g (1lb) icing sugar, sieved, plus extra to dust**
* **½tsp cream of tartar**
* **4–5tbsp evaporated milk**
* **2tsp peppermint essence**
* **Red food colouring (optional)**

1 Put the sugar and cream of tartar into a bowl. Add the milk and peppermint and stir together. Use your hands to bring together into a ball. Knead on a surface dusted with icing sugar to make a smooth fondant. If making both white and pink mints, cut in half; wrap one piece in clingfilm.

2 Dust the surface with more icing sugar. Roll out the unwrapped half of the icing to about 5mm (¼in) thick. Stamp out 4cm (1½in) rounds. Put on a tray lined with parchment. Dry out overnight.

3 Meanwhile, dip a skewer into the food colouring, press onto the other half of icing and knead until pink. Stamp out 4cm (1½in) rounds, then dry on a lined tray, as above. (Alternatively, use all the icing for white peppermints.)

4 To gift wrap, put a couple of mints each in the paper cases (you could mix and match the white and the pink if wished), pack in decorative boxes and tie with a pretty ribbon. Store the mints in airtight containers until ready to use. The mints will keep for up to three weeks.

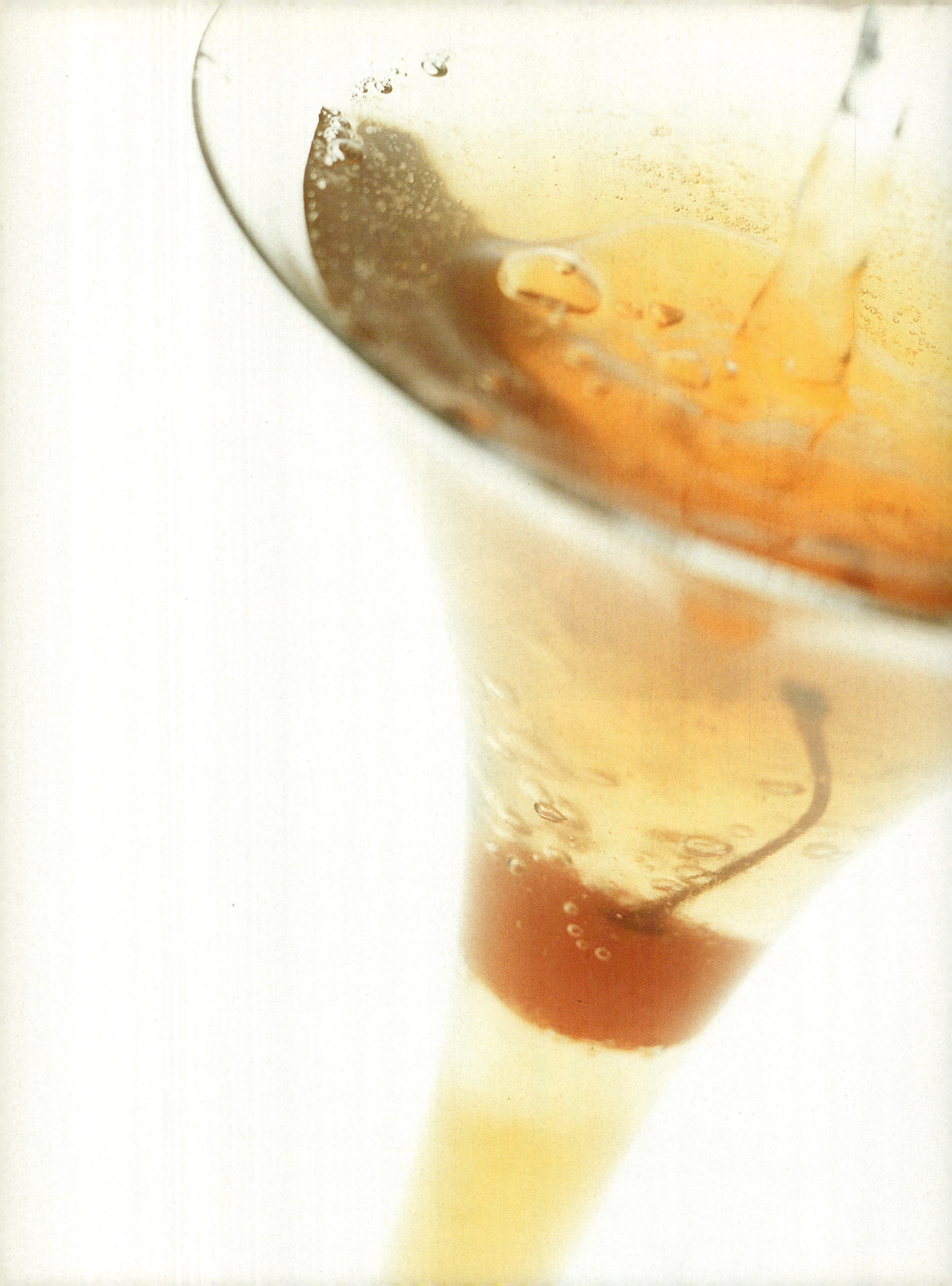

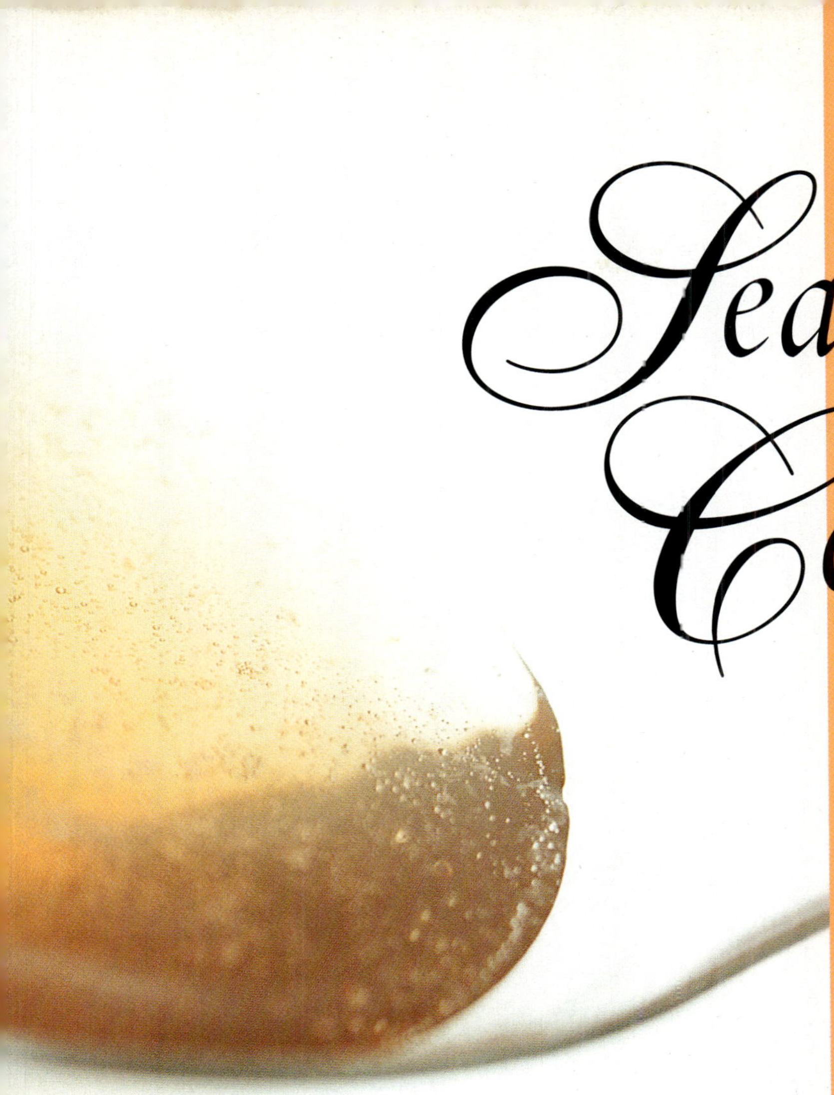

ENTERTAINING IN STYLE

Seasonal Celebrations

Let the festivities begin. And whether you're throwing a big party or just having the neighbours round for a drink, you'll need to serve something more exciting than cheese straws to complement a glass of fizz. **Homemade canapés** taste so much better than shop-bought ones – and our **party snacks** can be made in no time, use only a few ingredients and taste great. As for the **drinks**, we've chosen cocktails to serve individuals, mulled wine for a crowd, and a couple of non-alcoholic drinks for drivers. And if you're the one making the cocktails, it would be good to have a few helpers so you don't get stuck behind the bar all night.

Smoked Salmon Croustades

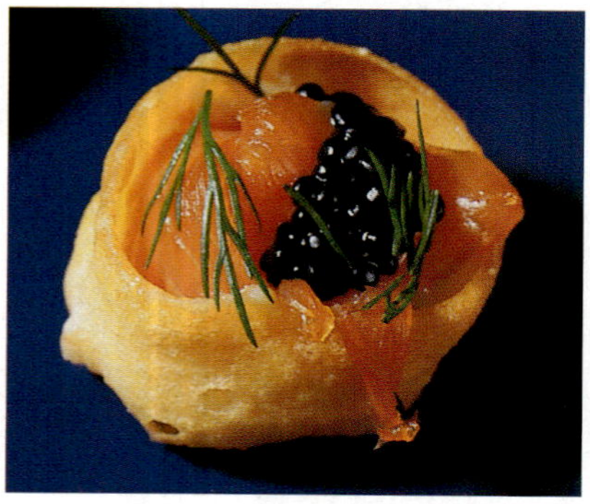

Hands-on time: 15min
Makes: 24

* 100g (3½oz) crème fraîche
* 1tbsp freshly chopped dill, plus dill sprigs to garnish
* 24 mini croustades
* 100g (3½oz) smoked salmon, cut into small squares
* 55g jar Avruga (black herring roe)

1 Put the crème fraîche and chopped dill into a bowl and mix together. Season with a pinch of salt. Spoon a little of the mixture into each croustade and top with a square of smoked salmon.

2 Dab a little Avruga on top and garnish with dill sprigs. Serve within 1hr (or the croustades will soften).

Mozzarella Nibbles

Hands-on time: 15min
Makes: 30

* 85g pack Parma ham
* 2 x 125g tubs mini mozzarella balls, drained
* 397g jar pitted black and green olives, drained and halved
* 125g (4oz) each roast artichokes and peppers, cut into small bits
* A bunch of basil leaves

1 Wrap a little Parma ham around each mozzarella ball. Push a halved olive onto a cocktail stick, add a piece each of artichoke and pepper, a basil leaf, then the Parma and mozzarella ball. Repeat to make 30 nibbles. Serve immediately or cover and chill for up to 1hr.

Tangy Chicken Bites

Hands-on time: 10min
Makes: 48

* 2 x 50g packs mini croustades
* Around 275g (10oz) fruity chutney
* 2 roast chicken breasts, skinned and torn into small pieces
* 250g tub crème fraîche
* Thyme sprigs to garnish

1 Spread out the croustades on a board. Spoon around ½tsp chutney into each one. Top with a few pieces of chicken, a small blob of crème fraîche and a sprig of thyme. Serve immediately.

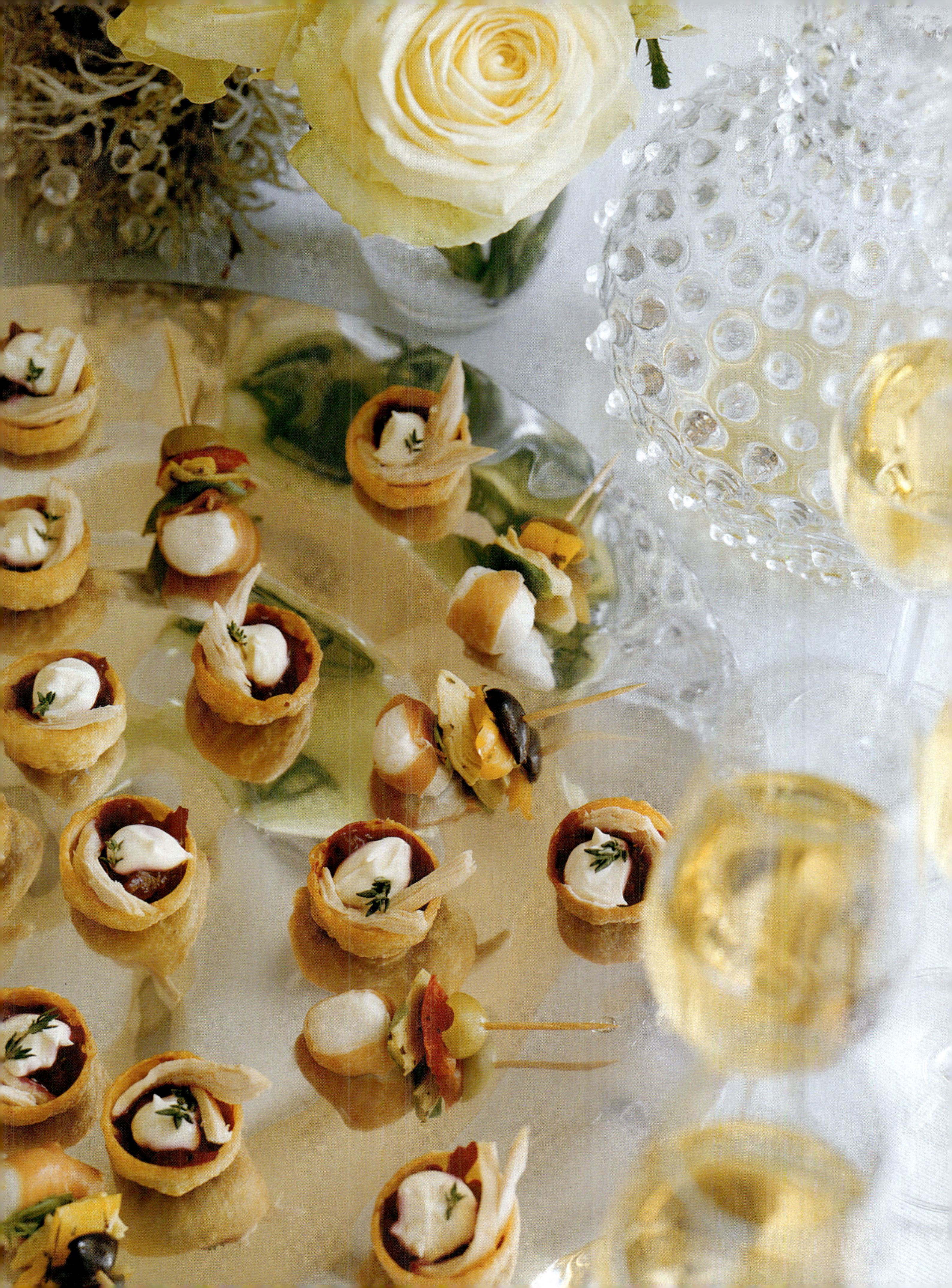

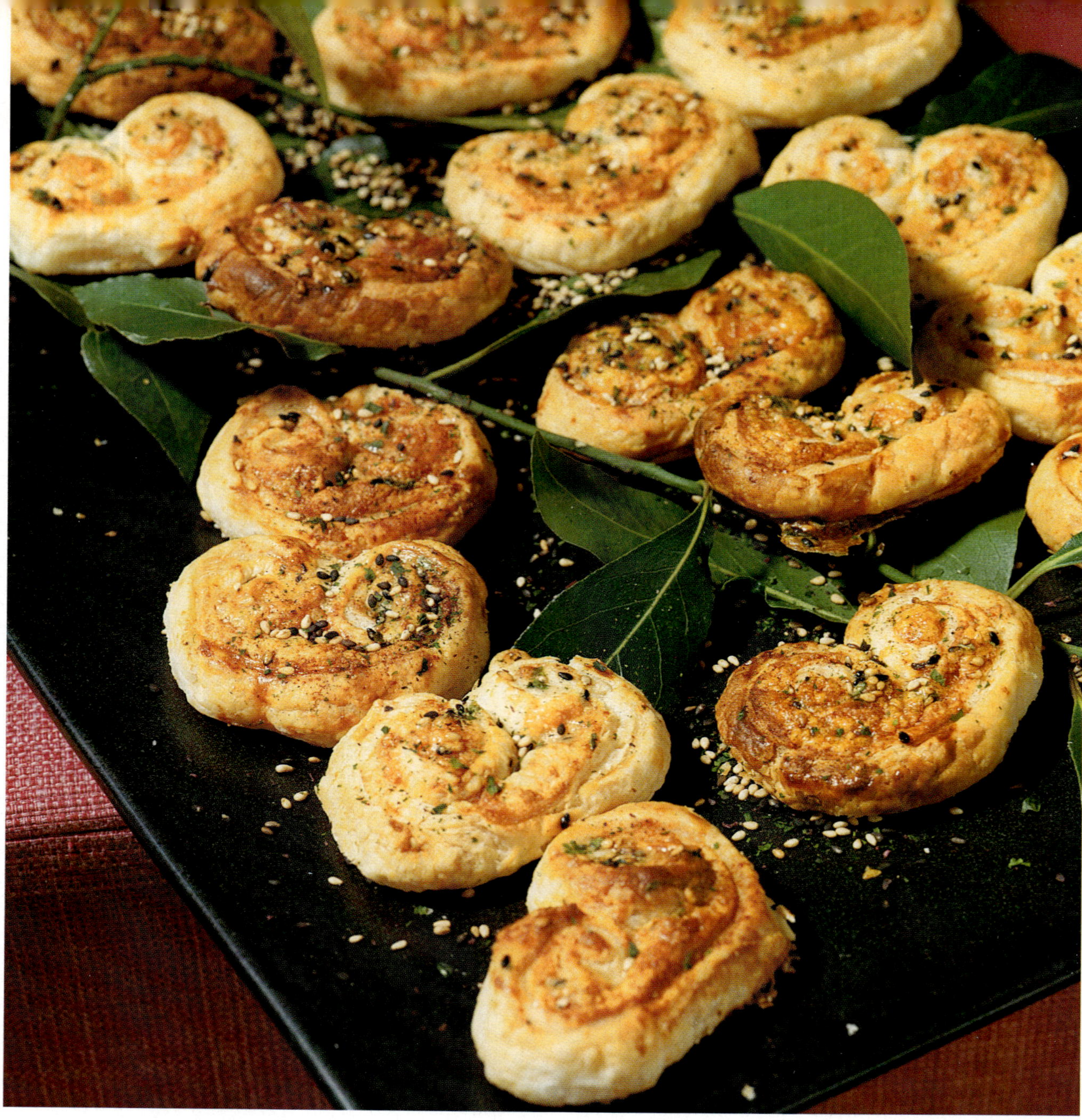

Spiced Puff Pastry Hearts

Hands-on time: 15min, plus 20min chilling
Cooking time: 20min
Makes: 36

- **Flour to dust**
- **500g pack puff pastry**
- **1 medium egg, beaten**
- **2tbsp sesame seeds or Sanchi Furikake Japanese Seasoning**

1 Dust a clean worksurface and rolling pin with a little flour and roll out the puff pastry along the narrow width until it measures 68.5x16cm (27x6½in). Roll up each long side tightly until the two sides meet in the middle.

2 Cut the pastry into 1–2cm (½–¾in) slices, making 36. Lay each slice on its side, then gently roll out flat to make a heart shape. Put on a baking sheet (you'll need three sheets in total) and chill for 20min. Preheat the oven to 200°C (180°C fan) mark 6.

3 Take the baking sheets out of the fridge. Brush each pastry heart with a little beaten egg, then sprinkle over a little of the sesame seeds or Japanese seasoning. Bake for 20min until puffed and golden. Use a palette knife to lift the pastry off the baking sheets and cool on a wire rack.

New Potatoes with Herby Cheese

Hands-on time: 10min, plus 5–10min cooling
Cooking time: 35min
Makes: 24

* 750g bag baby new potatoes
* Olive oil
* 80g portion soft herb cheese
* 1tbsp finely chopped chives to garnish

1 Preheat the oven to 200°C (180°C fan) mark 6. Put the potatoes in a pan of cold, salted water, cover and bring to the boil. Cook for 10min until tender. Drain well.

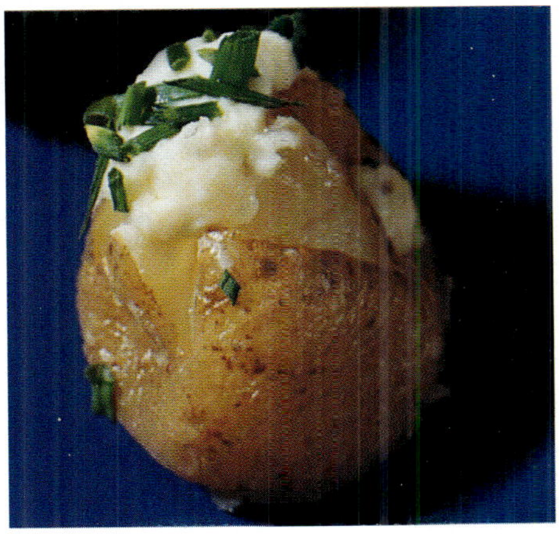

2 Tip the potatoes into a roasting tin, add a little olive oil and season. Toss well. Roast for 25min, then cool for 5–10min.

3 Cut a cross in the top of each potato. Squeeze them a little and spoon a little soft herb cheese into each one. Sprinkle with chives. Serve warm or at room temperature.

Goat's Cheese, Pimiento and Mint Wraps

Hands-on time: 10min, plus 15min chilling
Makes: 40

* 2 x 150g tubs soft goat's cheese, chilled
* 4tbsp fresh chopped mint
* 400g can pimientos, drained
* 4 large flour tortillas
* Mint sprigs to garnish

1 Beat together the goat's cheese and chopped mint, then season and chill. Sandwich the drained pimientos between sheets of kitchen paper. Press down lightly with your hands until they're completely dry, then cut the pimientos into rough pieces.

2 Spread each tortilla with a quarter of the goat's cheese mixture and scatter the chopped pimientos on top. Starting from the nearest end, begin to roll up as tightly as possible.

3 Wrap the filled tortillas in clingfilm and chill for about 15min. (They can be kept in the fridge for up to 2hrs before serving.)

4 To serve, remove the clingfilm and slice each roll into 10 pieces. Garnish with the mint sprigs.

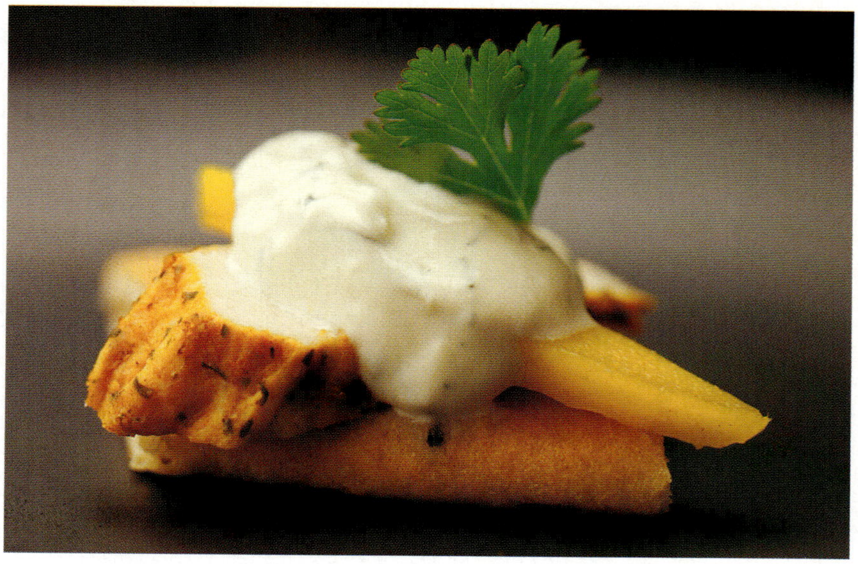

Tandoori Chicken with Mango on Naan

Hands-on time: 20min
Cooking time: 2min
Makes: 30–36

- 300g pack ready-to-eat tandoori chicken breasts
- 1 large ripe mango, thinly sliced
- Juice of 1 lemon
- 300g pack naan bread
- 2tbsp olive oil
- 2tbsp sea salt
- 200g tub tzatziki
- Coriander leaves to garnish

1 Cut each chicken breast into thin, diagonal slices. Toss the mango in the lemon juice and season. Cover with clingfilm.

2 Preheat the oven to 200°C (180°C fan) mark 6. Prick the naan bread with a knife, drizzle with olive oil and sprinkle with sea salt. Warm in the oven according to the instructions on the pack.

3 Cut the warmed naan into 30–36 bite-size pieces and top each one with a slice of chicken and mango. Spoon over a little tzatziki and garnish with a coriander leaf. (As these don't take long to assemble, you can prepare them up to 1hr ahead and top with the tzatziki just before serving.)

Roquefort and Cranberry Chipolatas

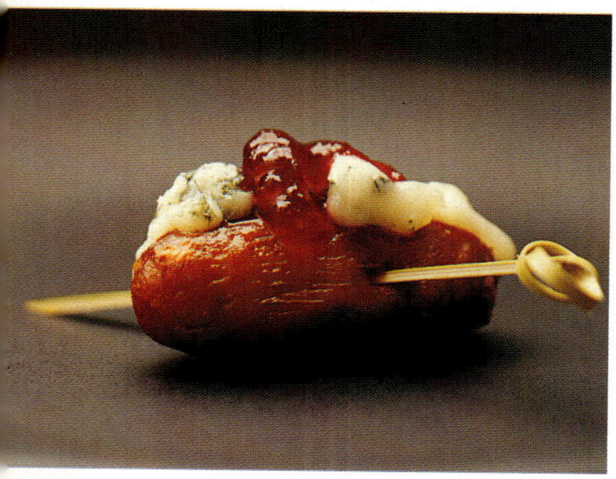

Hands-on time: 15min
Cooking time: 2min
Makes: 40

- 400g pack ready-to-eat cocktail sausages
- 75g (3oz) Roquefort, sliced
- 3tbsp cranberry sauce

1 Preheat the grill. Cut the sausages lengthways to make a slit, then stuff each one with a small slice of Roquefort and put on a baking sheet.

2 Cook the cheese-filled sausages under the preheated grill for about 2min or until the cheese starts to melt. Skewer each sausage onto a cocktail stick and top with a little cranberry sauce to serve. (The sausages can be prepared up to 2hrs ahead and grilled just before serving.)

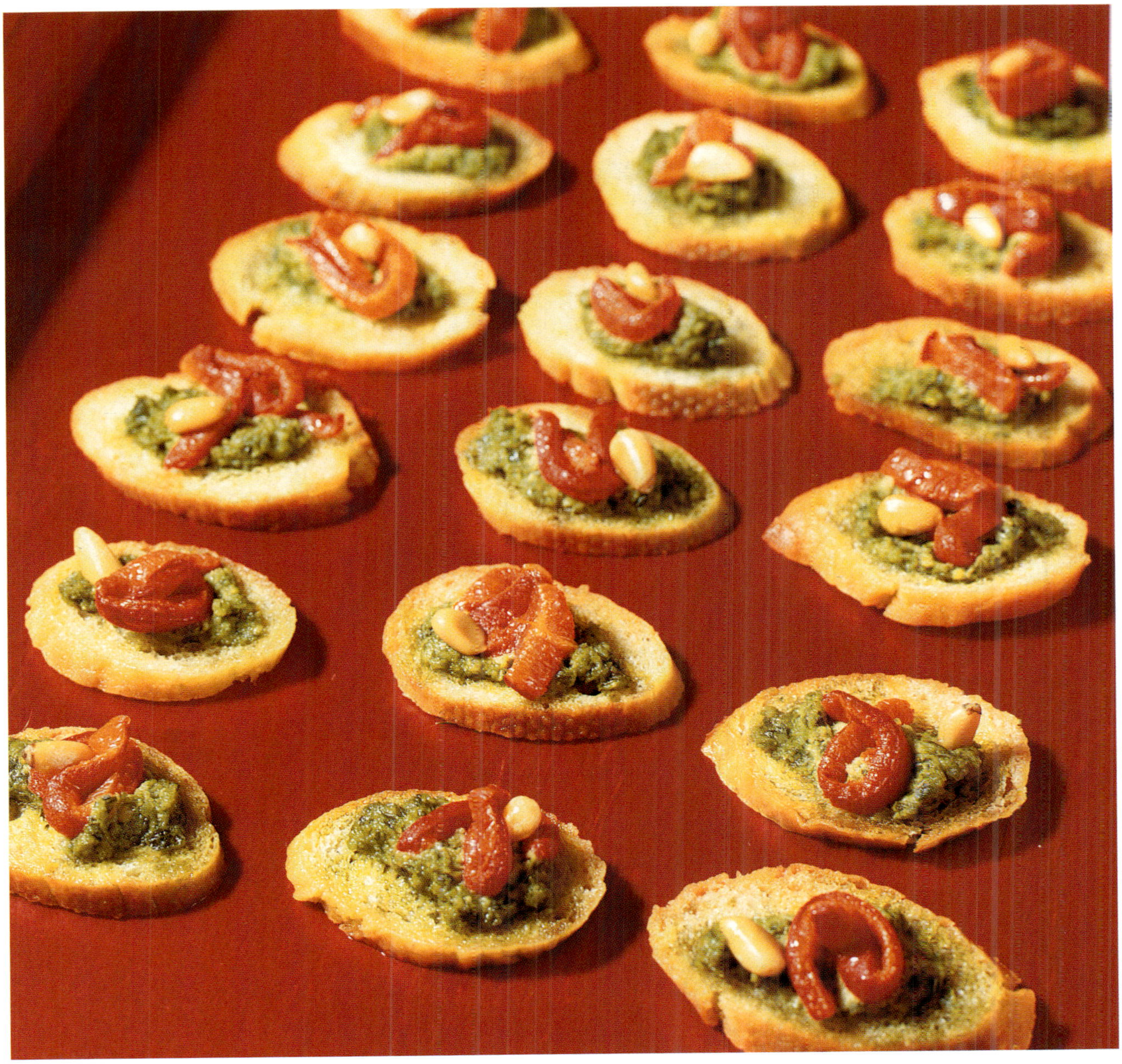

Red Pepper Pesto Croutons

Hands-on time: 20min, plus a little cooling
Cooking time: 15–20min
Makes: 24

- 1 thin French stick, sliced into 24 rounds
- Olive oil to brush
- 190g jar ready-made fresh pesto
- 4 pepper pieces (from a jar of marinated peppers), each sliced into 6 strips
- 24 pine nuts to garnish

1 Preheat the oven to 200°C (180°C fan) mark 6. Brush both sides of the bread with olive oil, then put on a baking sheet and bake for 15–20min.

2 Spread some of the pesto on each croûton and top with a pepper strip and a pine nut. Serve immediately.

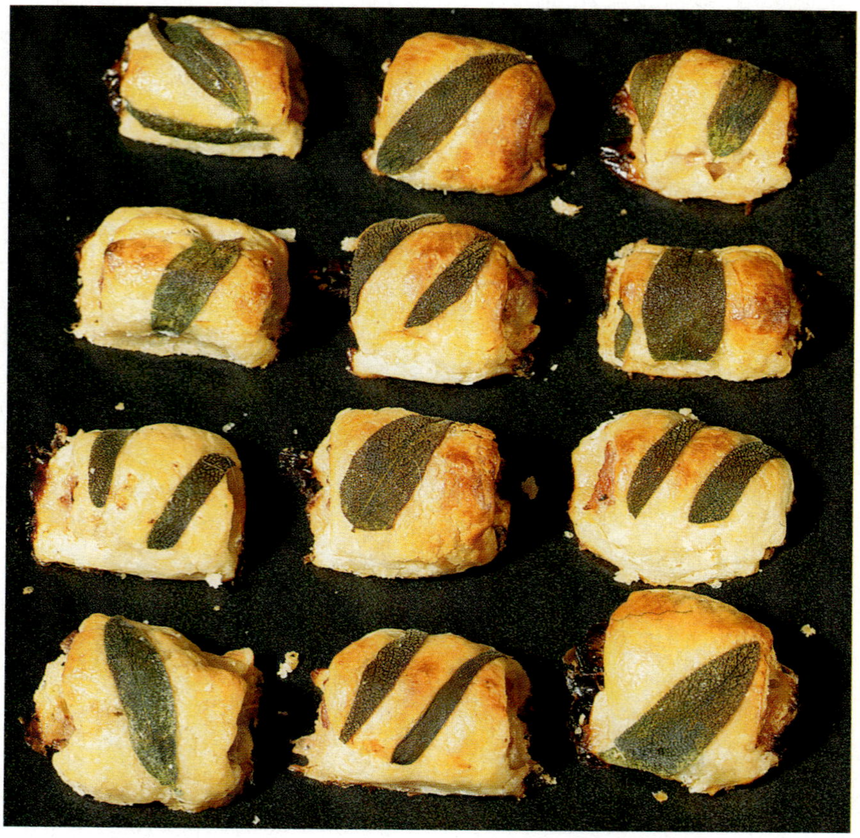

Sausage and Sage Rolls

Hands-on time: 20min, plus 15min chilling
Cooking time: 25min
Makes: 24

* 6 good quality pork sausages
* Flour to dust
* 375g pack ready-rolled shortcrust pastry
* 1 medium egg, beaten
* 36-48 sage leaves to garnish

1 Slit the sausage skins and remove the meat. Put it into a bowl and mix it well, using your hands.

2 Dust a clean worksurface with a little flour and open out the pastry. Roll slightly until it's about 1cm (½in) bigger. Cut in half lengthways to make two long strips. Position one strip so that the longest edge is nearest to you.

3 Dust your hands with flour. Take half the sausagemeat, roll into a long sausage, then lay down the middle of one pastry strip. Season the egg with a pinch of salt and brush along the long edge of the pastry furthest away from you. Take the near edge and roll over the sausagemeat to give a neat roll. Trim the long and short edges with a sharp knife, then cut the roll into 5cm (2in) pieces. Repeat with the rest of the pastry and sausagemeat.

4 Brush each roll with the beaten egg, put one or two sage leaves on top, then brush again. Put on a baking sheet and chill for 15min. Preheat the oven to 200°C (180°C fan) mark 6. Bake the sausage rolls for 25min or until they are crispy and golden.

Melon, Parma Ham and Cheese

Hands-on time: 20min
Makes: 30

* ½ ripe Charantais melon, peeled and deseeded
* 70g pack Parma ham
* 30 small basil leaves
* 75g (3oz) Manchego cheese, from the supermarket deli counter (if unavailable, try Pecorino or mozzarella)

1 Cut the melon into 30 bite-size pieces. Cut the ham into slices and wrap around the melon.

2 Thread the wrapped melon pieces on to cocktail sticks, followed by a basil leaf and a small chunk of cheese. (These can be made up to 1hr before serving.)

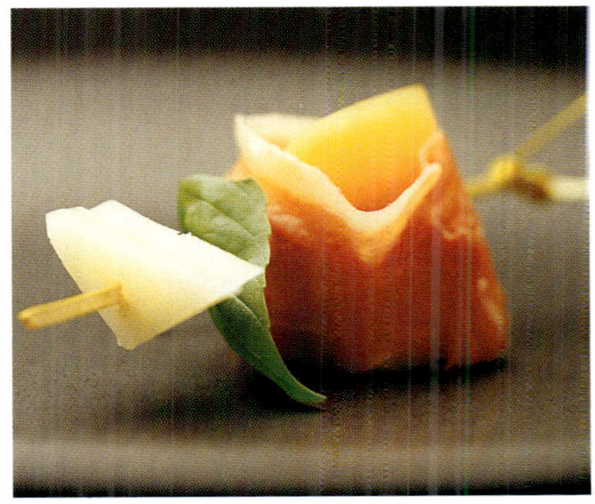

Gravadlax on Rye Bread

Hands-on time: 15min
Makes: 32

* 4 slices rye bread
* 2 x 140g packs gravadlax with mustard and dill sauce (minimum 4 large slices)
* 1 lemon
* Dill sprigs to garnish

1 Spread the rye bread with the mustard and dill sauce from the gravadlax (you may not need it all). Cut each slice of bread lengthways into four strips, then widthways in half to make eight pieces.

2 Cut the gravadlax into strips and crumple a strip over each piece of rye bread. Cover with clingfilm. (These can be prepared up to 1hr ahead.)

3 Just before serving, squeeze over a little lemon juice, season with black pepper and garnish with a dill sprig.

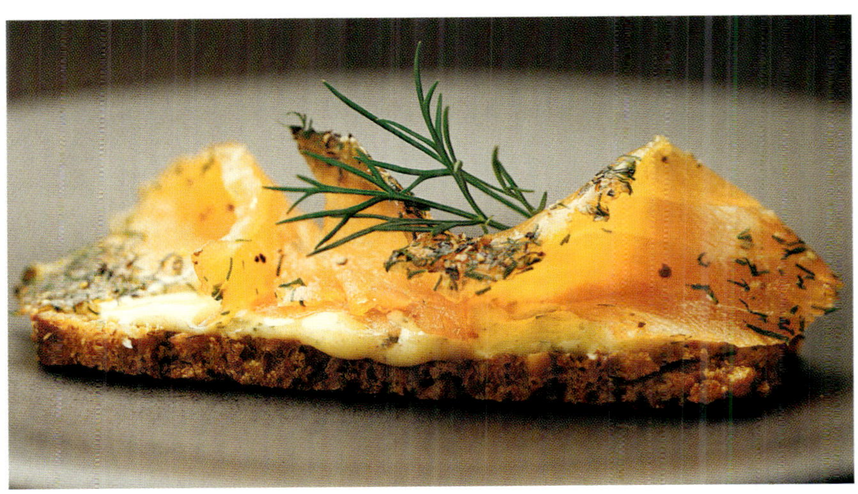

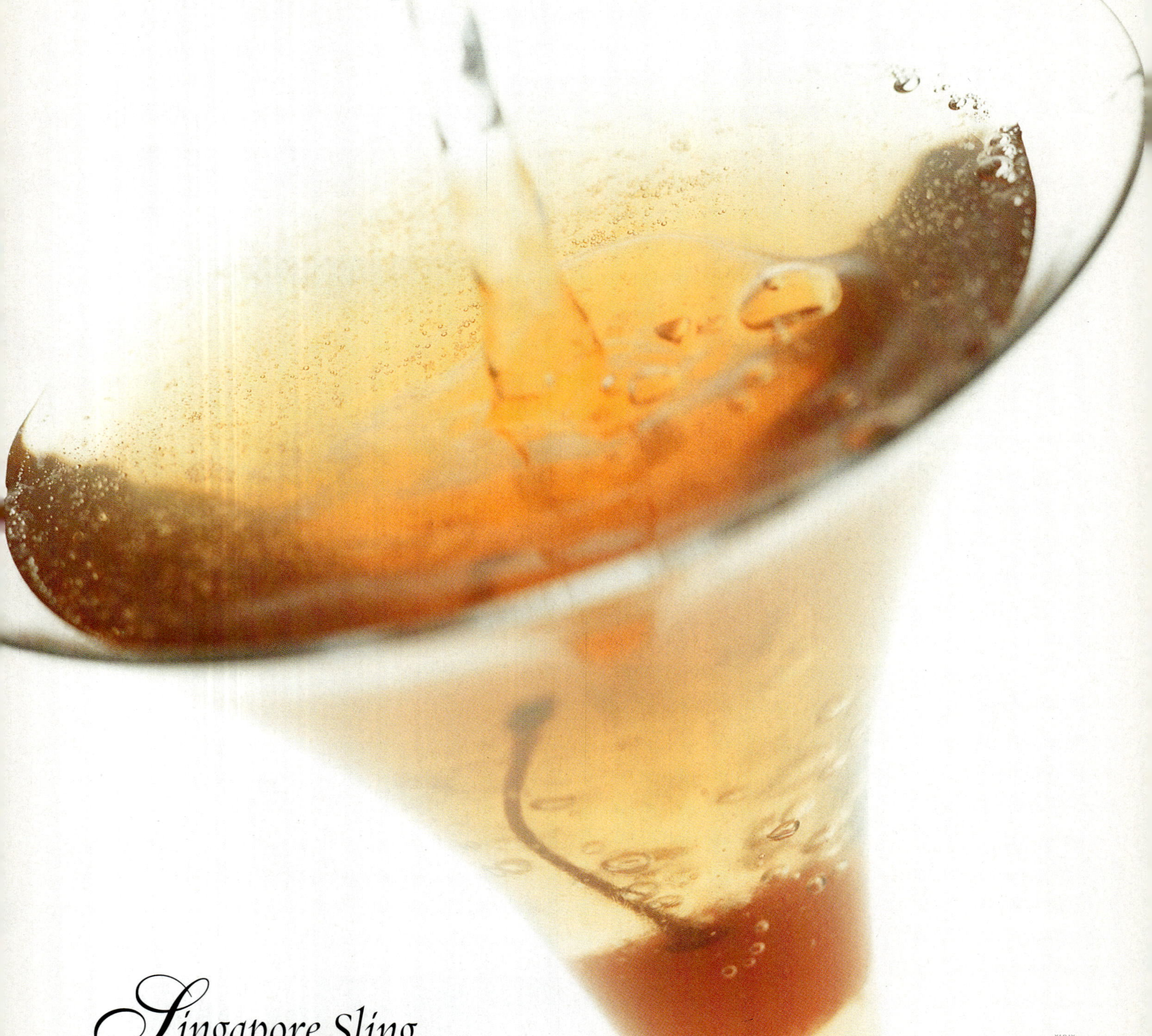

Singapore Sling

Serves: 1

- 1 measure (25ml) gin
- 2 measures (50ml) cherry brandy
- Juice of ½ lime
- 1–2 drops of Angostura bitters (optional)
- 1 cocktail cherry (optional)
- 150ml (¼ pint) soda water

1 Mix the gin, cherry brandy and lime juice, plus the Angostura bitters, if using – this will give the drink an extra kick. Pour into a trumpet-shaped glass.

2 Add the cocktail cherry, if you like, and plenty of ice cubes and then top up with the fizzy soda water. Serve immediately.

Mulled Wine

Serves: 6

- 2 medium oranges, cut into 12 wedges
- 12 cloves
- 75cl bottle red wine
- 2 measures (50ml) brandy or Cointreau
- 1 cinnamon stick, broken, plus 6 whole cinnamon sticks
- ½tsp mixed spice
- 2tbsp golden granulated sugar

1 Spike each of the orange wedges with 1 clove. Put six wedges with the red wine, brandy or Cointreau, cinnamon stick, mixed spice and sugar into a stainless steel pan. Warm gently over a low heat. Turn off the heat and let the flavours infuse for 10min.

2 Ladle the wine into glasses, leaving out the orange wedges and straining out the cinnamon bark.

3 Take the 6 remaining orange wedges, make a cut between the pith and the flesh and hook onto the side of the glasses. Add the fresh cinnamon sticks to serve.

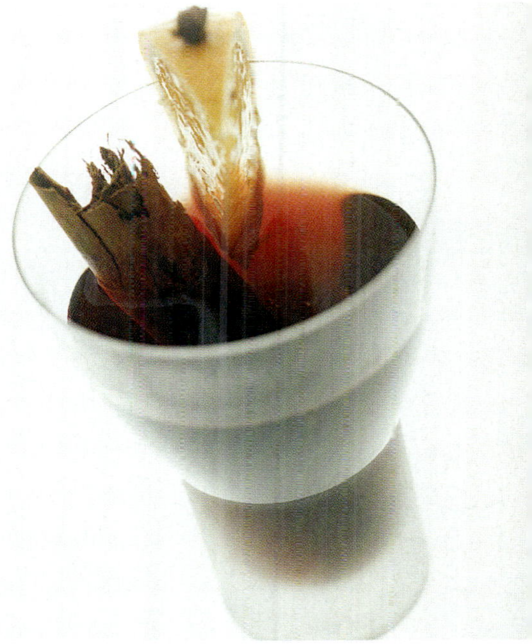

Bloody Mary

Serves: 1

- 2tsp Worcestershire sauce
- 1 dash Tabasco
- 1 measure (25ml) vodka, chilled
- 150ml (5fl oz) tomato juice
- Lemon juice to taste
- Celery salt to taste
- 1 celery stick, with leaves left on, to serve

1 Pour the Worcestershire sauce, Tabasco, vodka and tomato juice into a long glass and stir.

2 Add ice and the lemon juice and celery salt to taste. Serve with the celery stick.

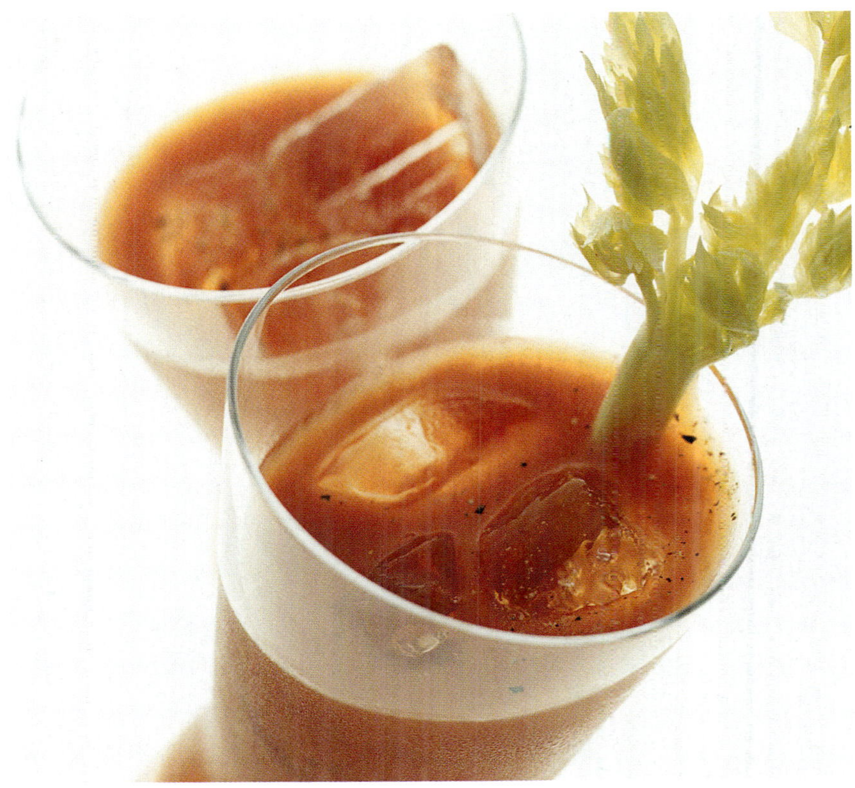

Champagne Cocktail

Serves: 8

* 125ml (4fl oz) Grand Marnier
* 75ml (3fl oz) grenadine
* 1 large orange, cut into 8 wedges
* 8 sugar cubes or sugar sticks
* 75cl bottle chilled champagne, cava or sparkling wine

1 Measure out the Grand Marnier and grenadine and divide among eight champagne glasses.

2 Add an orange wedge and a sugar cube or stick to each glass.

3 Top up the glasses with the champagne, cava or sparkling wine and serve immediately.

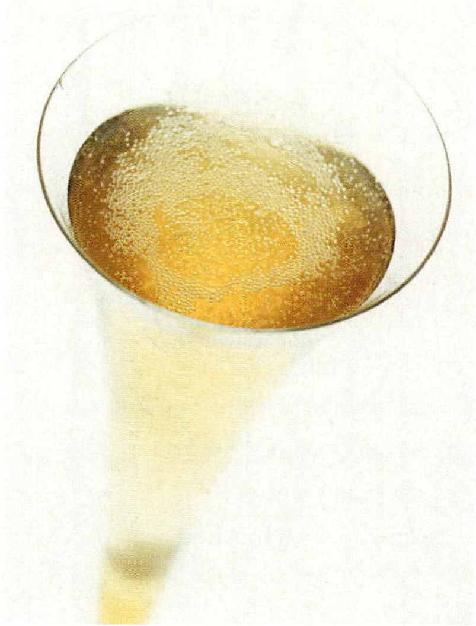

Elderflower Sparkle

Serves: 20, with enough for top-ups

* 37.5cl bottle elderflower cordial
* 6–7x75cl bottles sparkling wine

1 Chill the elderflower cordial and sparkling wine well. Half an hour before serving, pour a splash of cordial into each champagne flute.

2 When ready to serve, fill each glass with sparkling wine. This is an elegant but simple aperitif, so for best results use a good-quality sparkling wine.

Rum Punch

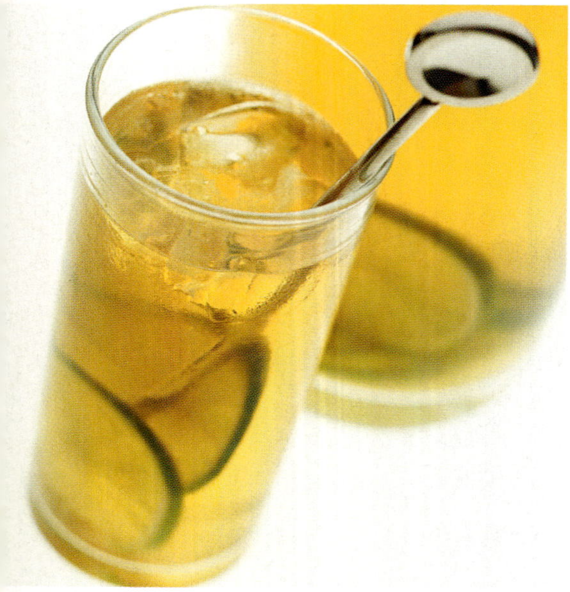

Serves: 1

* Juice of 1 lime
* 2tsp golden caster sugar
* 2 measures (50ml) dark rum
* 1 dash Angostura bitters
* Soda or mineral water to taste
* Lime slices to serve

1 Mix the lime juice and sugar in a tall glass. Add the dark rum, Angostura bitters and ice.

2 Top up with the soda or mineral water and then serve with slices of lime.

Cranberry Crush

Serves: 14

* 75cl bottle sparkling wine, such as cava, chilled
* 300ml (½ pint) Calvados
* 1 litre (1¾ pint) cranberry juice, chilled
* 450ml (¾ pint) sparkling water, chilled
* 1 small orange, washed and thinly sliced into rounds

1 Pour the sparkling wine, Calvados and cranberry juice into a large glass bowl.

2 Just before serving, stir in the sparkling water and add the orange slices and 10–12 ice cubes.

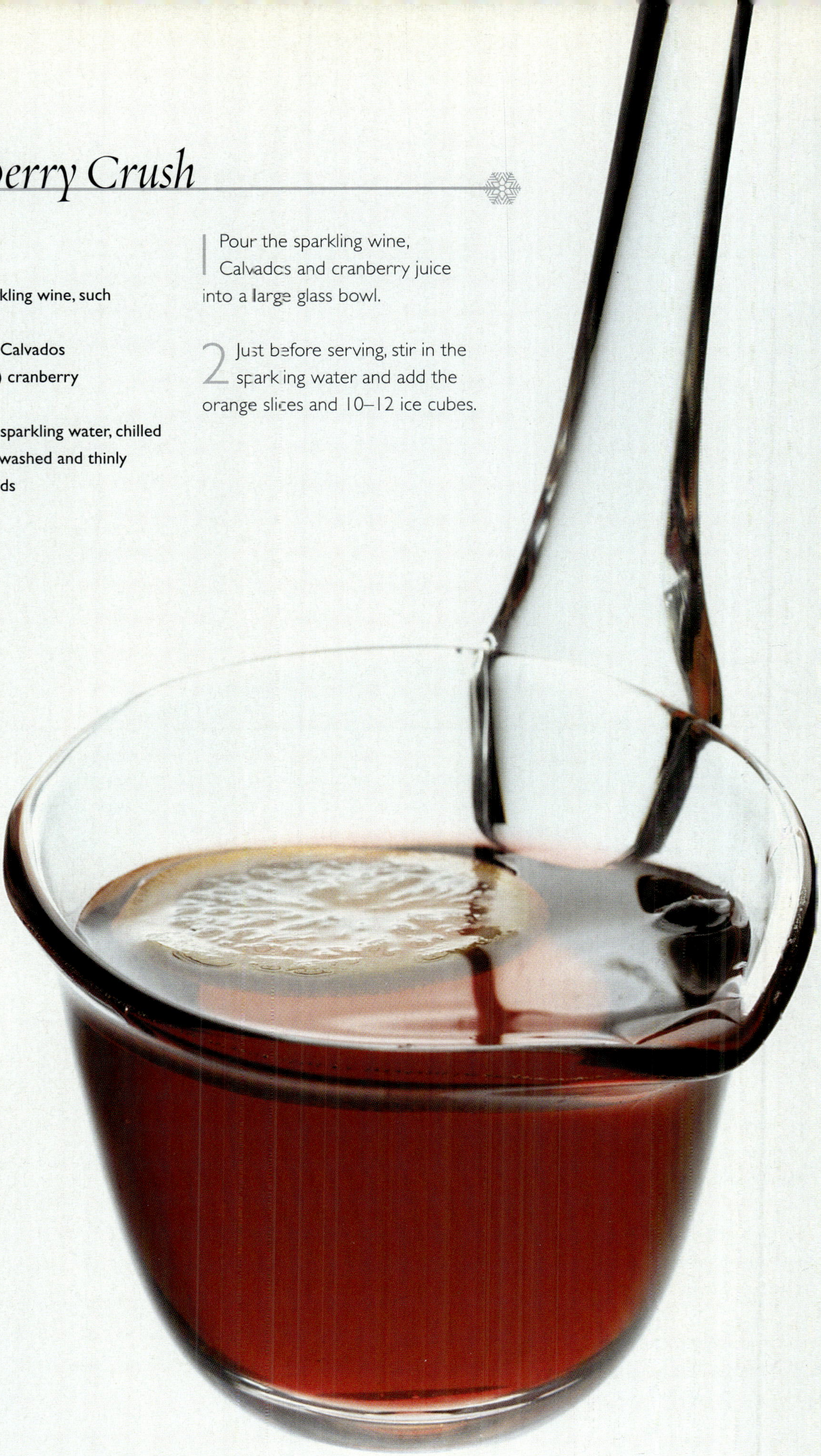

Cranberry Cooler

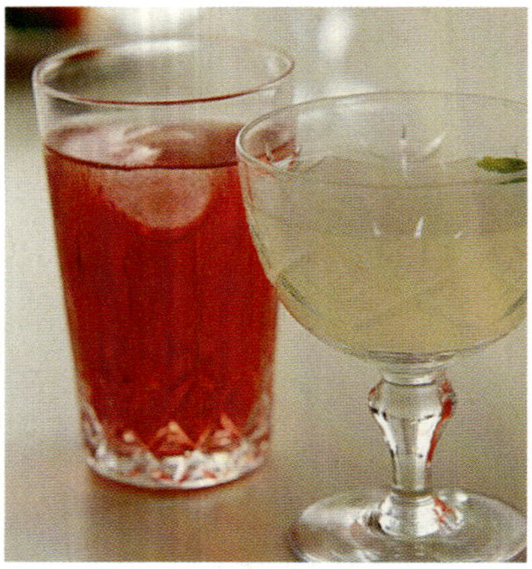

Serves: 1
Non alcoholic

- 75ml (3fl oz) cranberry juice
- Lemonade or sparkling water to taste
- 1 slice of lemon to serve

1 Pour the cranberry juice into a tall glass, half-filled with ice.

2 Top up with lemonade. If you would like your drink to be less sweet, double the amount of juice and top up with sparkling water.

3 Mix together and serve with a slice of lemon.

Fruity Punch

Serves: 8
Non alcoholic

- 1 litre (1¾ pints) apple juice
- 1 litre (1¾ pints) ginger ale
- 2 apples, sliced and cut into stars

1 Put the apple juice, ginger ale and apple shapes into a large bowl and mix together to make a refreshing, non-alcoholic punch.

2 Pour into a large jug and serve. With its fun star shapes cut from unpeeled apples, this drink will go down well with children.

Brandy Cocktail

Serves: 1

- 1 measure (25ml) brandy
- ½ measure (12.5ml) Cointreau
- 1 dash Angostura bitters

1 Put the brandy, Cointreau and Angostura bitters in a brandy glass with 4–5 cubes of ice.

2 Swirl around to chill, then lift out the ice with a slotted spoon and discard. Drink immediately.

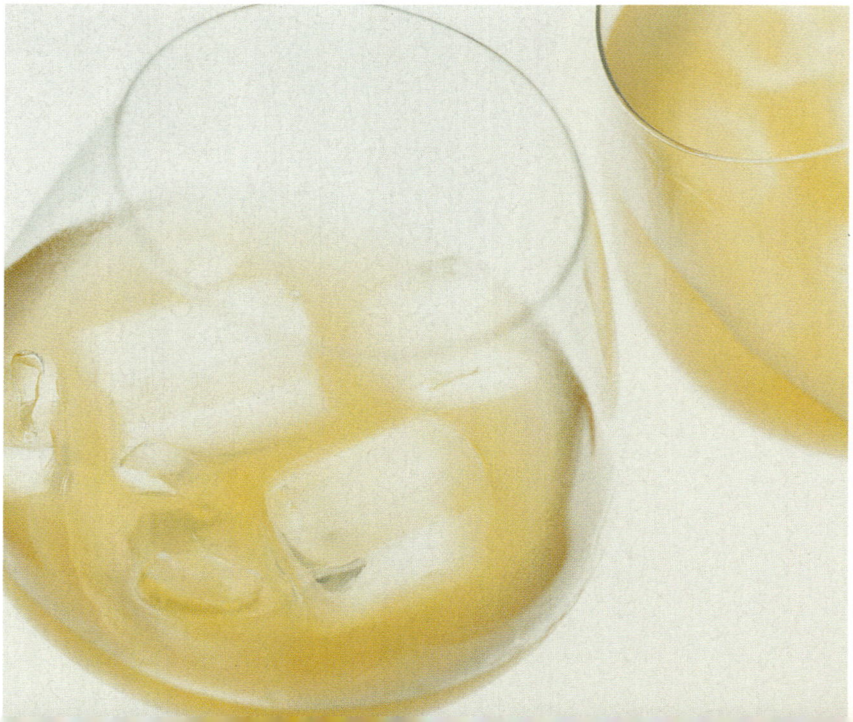

Special Christmas Eve Supper

SERVES 6

Parsnip Soup with Parmesan Crisps

* * * * *

Guinea Fowl with Prunes, Apples and Bacon

* * * * *

Ginger Parfait

Traditional Christmas Lunch

SERVES 8–10

Smoked Salmon and Boursin Terrine

* * * * *

Lemon and Herb-roasted Turkey
Spiced Cranberry and Orange Relish
Luxury Bread Sauce
Turkey Gravy
Pork, Spinach and Apple Stuffing
Roast Potatoes with Rosemary and Garlic
Lemon and Orange Carrots
Roast Parsnips with Honey Glaze
Herby Buttered Brussels Sprouts

* * * * *

The Ultimate Christmas Pudding
Brandy Butter

Classic Christmas Lunch

SERVES 8–10

Twice-baked Cauliflower Cheese Souffles

* * * * *

Goose with Roasted Apples and Onions
Cranberry Sauce
Luxury Bread Sauce
Orange, Sage and Thyme Stuffing
Mustard Roast Potatoes and Parsnips
Lemon and Orange Carrots
Herby Buttered Brussels Sprouts

* * * * *

Boozy Christmas Pudding
Fresh Vanilla Custard

Vegetarian Christmas Lunch

SERVES 8–10

Leek, Mushroom and Artichoke Croûte

* * * * *

White Nut Roast
Cranberry, Orange and Port Sauce
Roast Parsnips with Honey Glaze
Caramelised Carrots
Creamy Brussels Sprouts
Spicy Red Cabbage

* * * * *

Chocolate and Chestnut Torte

Relaxed Boxing Day Lunch

SERVES 8

Ginger and Honey-glazed Ham
Red Cabbage and Beetroot Salad
Roasted Sweet Potatoes with Sage

* * * * *

White Chocolate and Red Fruit Trifle

Festive Afternoon Tea

SERVES 12 OR MORE

Gravadlax on Rye Bread

* * * * *

Traditional Christmas Stollen
Classic Mince Pies
Easy Christmas Cake
Shortbread Biscuits

* * * * *

Serve with Earl Grey Tea

Easy Lunch

SERVES 6

Cheese and Chive Tart
Serve with a tossed green salad

* * * * *

Spiced Pears in Mulled Wine Syrup

Party for Friends

SERVES 12 OR MORE

Smoked Salmon Croustades
Tandoori Chicken and Mango on Naan
Spiced Puff Pastry Hearts
New Potatoes with Herby Cheese
Melon, Parma Ham and Cheese

Simple Family Supper

SERVES 4

Salmon and Fennel Rosti

* * * * *

Mango Ice Cream Terrine

Vegetarian Supper for Friends

SERVES 6

Mushroom Baskets

Roasted Vegetable Moussaka
Serve with a tossed green salad and crusty bread

* * * * *

Chocolate and Cherry Gateau

Supper with Leftovers

SERVES 6

Turkey, Pepper and Haricot Casserole
Serve with garlic bread and tossed green salad

* * * * *

Christmas Pudding Parfait

Fish Supper

SERVES 6

Roquefort Leek and Walnut Tarts

* * * * *

Provençale Fish Stew

* * * * *

Jewelled Cheesecake

Turkey Planner

TO PREPARE YOUR TURKEY TO PERFECTION, FOLLOW OUR SEVEN EASY TIPS FOR A STRESS-FREE CHRISTMAS LUNCH

Thawing Leave a frozen turkey in its bag and thaw at a cool room temperature, not in the fridge. Remove any giblets as soon as they are loose. Once there are no ice crystals in the body cavity and the legs are flexible, cover and store in the fridge. Cook within 24hr.

Stuffing Remove the wishbone before stuffing the turkey to make it easier to carve. Loosely stuff the neck end only. Allow about 225g (8oz) stuffing for each 2.3kg (5lb) dressed weight of bird and stuff just before cooking. Sew up the neck skin and secure with skewers or cocktail sticks, or sew with a trussing needle threaded with fine string.

Cooking instructions Weigh the bird after stuffing. Calculate the complete cooking time to be ready 30min before carving – this allows time for the meat to firm up, making carving easier. Spread with butter and season. Wrap loosely in a 'tent' of foil, then cook in a preheated oven at 190°C (170°C fan) mark 5. Remove the foil about 1hr before the end of its cooking time to brown. Baste regularly.

Ready to eat? To tell if the turkey is cooked, pierce the thickest part of the leg with a skewer. The juices that run out should be golden and clear with no traces of pink; if they're not, return the bird to the oven.

Finishing touches A little garnish will help to make the cooked turkey a stunning centrepiece. Put the bird onto a platter, then gather a bunch of fresh parsley and rosemary sprigs and tuck the stalks into the cavity of the bird.

Carving First remove the legs. Using a carving fork and sharp knife, push the fork into the breast to steady the turkey. Cut downwards between the thigh and breast, then use the flat of the knife to push the thigh out and cut through the hip joint, removing the leg. Repeat on the other side. To carve the breast, use the fork to secure the turkey. Slice the meat, starting at the neck cavity carving it into long thin slices. To remove the wing, secure the bird with the fork and cut through the corner of the breast until you feel the wing joint. Cut through it and serve a wing with a slice of breast.

Storing Don't forget the leftover turkey when lunch is finished – never leave it standing in a warm room. Cool it quickly in a cold place, then cover and chill.

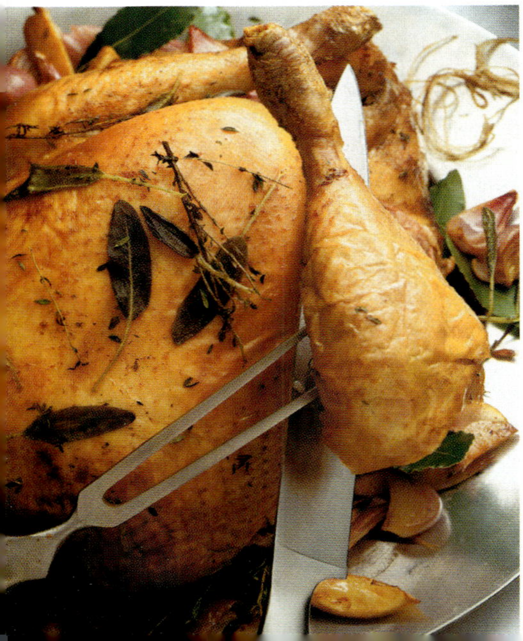

TURKEY ROASTING TIMES

Calculated for an oven temperature of 190°C (170°C fan) mark 5

Oven-ready weight (at room temp)	Approximate no. of servings	Approximate thawing time	Cooking time foil-wrapped
550g-1.4kg (1¼-3lb)	2-4	4-10hr	1-1½hr
1.4-2.3kg (3-5lb)	4-6	10-15hr	1½-2hr
2.3-3.6kg (5-8lb)	6-10	15-18hr	2-3hr
3.6-5kg (8-11lb)	10-15	18-20hr	3-3¼hr
5-6.8kg (11-15lb)	15-20	20-24hr	3¼-4hr
6.8-9kg (15-20lb)	20-30	24-30hr	4-5½hr

Index

Good Housekeeping Institute
TRIED · TESTED · TRUSTED